W9-CGQ-332

Ferguson's Surgery of the Ambulatory Patient

Ferguson's Surgery of the Ambulatory Patient

Fifth Edition

edited by

MARK W. WOLCOTT, M.D., F.A.C.S.

*Professor of Surgery and
Associate Dean for Veterans' Affairs
University of Utah College of Medicine
Chief of Staff, Veterans Administration
Hospital, Salt Lake City, Utah*

With 14 Collaborators

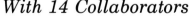

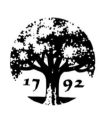

J. B. LIPPINCOTT COMPANY
Philadelphia and Toronto

FIFTH EDITION

Copyright © 1974 by J. B. Lippincott Company
Copyright © 1966, 1957 by J. B. Lippincott Company
Copyright 1947, 1942 by J. B. Lippincott Company

ISBN   0-397-50333-4

Library of Congress Catalog Card Number 74-1439

Library of Congress Cataloging in Publication Data

Ferguson, Lewis Kraeer
  Ferguson's Surgery of the ambulatory patient.

  Includes bibliographies.
  1. Surgery, Minor. I. Wolcott, Mark W., ed.
II. Title. III. Title: Surgery of the ambulatory
patient. [1. Ambulatory Care—Surgery, Minor.
DNLM: WO192 F352s 1974]
RD111.F4   1974   617'.024   74-1439
ISBN   0-397-50333-4

Printed in the United States of America
4

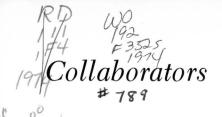

Collaborators

Douglas S. Dahl, M.D.

Associate Professor of Surgery-Urology, Division of Urologic Surgery, University of Utah College of Medicine, Salt Lake City, Utah

Andrew A. Gage, M.D., F.A.C.S.

Chief of Surgery, Veterans Administration Hospital, Buffalo, New York; Professor of Surgery, School of Medicine, State University of New York at Buffalo

John R. Groh, M.D.

Associate in Department of Surgery, Graduate School of Medicine, University of Pennsylvania, Philadelphia; Surgeon, Good Samaritan Hospital, Lebanon, Pa.

John B. Herrmann, M.D., F.A.C.S.

Professor of Surgery, University of Massachusetts Medical School; Chief of Surgery, Worchester City Hospital, Worchester, Mass.

J. Gary Maxwell, M.D.

Associate Professor of Surgery, University of Utah, College of Medicine, Salt Lake City, Utah

Richard G. Middleton, M.D.

Associate Professor of Surgery-Urology and Head, Division Urologic Surgery, University of Utah College of Medicine, Salt Lake City, Utah

Hugo V. Rizzoli, M.D.

Professor and Chairman, Department of Neurological Surgery, The George Washington University Medical Center, Washington, D. C.

Andrew C. Ruoff III, M.D.

Associate Professor of Surgery-Orthopedics, University of Utah College of Medicine; Chief of Orthopaedic Surgery, Veterans Administration Hospital, Salt Lake City, Utah

Edwin Rushia, M.D.

Professor of Anesthesiology, University of Virginia School of Medicine, Charlottesville, Virginia

Luis F. Sala, M.D., F.A.C.S.

Chairman, Department of Surgery, Damas Hospital, Ponce, Puerto Rico
Professor ad Honorem, Department of Surgery, University of Puerto Rico School of Medicine

William A. Shaver, M.D.

Associate, Department of Surgery, Graduate School of Medicine, University of Pennsylvania, Philadelphia; Surgeon, Good Samaritan Hospital, Lebanon, Pa.

Clifford C. Snyder, M.D., F.A.C.S.

Chief of Surgery, Veterans Administration Hospital; Professor and Chairman, Division of Plastic Surgery, University of Utah College of Medicine, Salt Lake City, Utah

Morton A. Stenchever, M.D.

Professor of Surgery, Obetetrics, and Gynecology; Head, Division of Obstetrics and Gynecology, University of Utah College of Medicine, Salt Lake City, Utah

David K. Wagner, M.D.

Associate Professor of Medicine, Medical College of Pennsylvania, Philadelphia, Pa.

Mark W. Wolcott, M.D., F.A.C.S.

Professor of Surgery and Associate Dean for Veterans' Affairs, University of Utah College of Medicine; Chief of Staff, Veterans Administration Hospital, Salt Lake City, Utah

Preface To Fifth Edition

The fifth edition of what has become a classic in the field of ambulatory surgery is an encyclopedia of minor surgical procedures, most of which can be done in an outpatient setting, either in the private office or clinic or in the new ambulatory surgical units being built as free-standing units or in hospitals. Since the fourth edition, the crisis of health care delivery has begun to engulf us. The increased use of outpatient surgery is part of the solution to this problem. Plans in operation of ambulatory surgical unit clinics in several settings–hospitals, offices, private or community clinics–are present in a new chapter developed by Dr. David K. Wagner, which deals also with the overall problem of health care delivery.

All of the chapters have been updated to incorporate the changes that have occurred over the last few years. "Anesthesia for Ambulatory Surgery" was done by Dr. Edwin Rushia. Dr. John Herrmann wrote chapters on "Open Wounds" and "Management of Infections." Dr. Clifford C. Snyder totally revised the chapter on "Snakebites and Insect Bites" as well as the chapter on "Scalp and Face." Dr. Andrew Gage has contributed a chapter on "Cryosurgery." Dr. Luis F. Sala has revised the chapter on "The Abdomen," and Drs. William Shaver and John Groh have rewritten the chapter on "Perianal Region and Anal Canal." Dr. Hugo Rizolli has rewritten the chapter on the "Back." Drs. Richard Middleton and Douglas Dahl revised the chapter on "Genitourinary System." Dr. Morton Stenchever has contributed a new chapter on gynecology. Dr. Andrew C. Ruoff revised all the material on fractures. A new chapter, "Shunts and Fistulas for Hemodialysis," has been added. Although many chapters have been revised, the text still reflects the ever-relevant surgical acumen of L. Kraeer Ferguson.

It is the hope of the authors that the book will be of great relevance at this time as the Profession attacks the huge problem of taking better care of greater numbers of people with a disproportionately small increase in its own numbers.

Mark W. Wolcott

Contents

1

Health Care Delivery Today and Tomorrow in Surgery

Mark W. Wolcott, M.D.

The surgery of ambulatory patients is a subject that has been much neglected in present-day medicine. Surgeons who have large hospital practices often, as a matter of convenience and because of a lack of alternative mechanisms, admit to the hospital patients requiring minor surgical procedures. The result of all of these forces has been to crowd hospitals and, more significantly, to start an escalation of costs that has nearly priced the average citizen out of the health care market. A procedure done on an ambulatory patient is only one-third as costly as one done on an inpatient.

The patients with minor lesions tend to be lost in the surgeon's more intense interest in gallbladder disease, carcinoma of the bowel, vascular and cardiac lesions, and other more impressive and dramatic fields of major surgery.

The training programs of many young surgeons have tended to emphasize the unusual, the bizarre, and major surgery. Good surgical technique, learned in whatever environment, is applicable to all surgery; however, lack of familiarity with many, many procedures that can and should be done for a patient who can then go home, leads to unwillingness, or even inability, to perform such procedures.

The general practitioners and the young surgeons who see many of the surgical conditons for which ambulatory care should be given are frequently ill-prepared to deal with them because of lack of experience, equipment, or assistance. This book has been written particularly to aid this group. No procedure is described which has not actually been carried out in ambulatory patients and which cannot easily and safely be performed when adequate equipment and assistance are available.

The development of ambulatory surgical units in the hospital, often next to the operating room or the emergency room of the hospital, has further broadened the number and the complexity of surgical procedures that can quite safely be performed on the ambulatory patient.

SOME GENERAL CONSIDERATIONS

It is probable that more poor surgery is performed on minor lesions of the hand than is performed, for instance, on major brain lesions. The highly trained specialist working almost exclusively in one region becomes expert in his field. In contrast with this intensive specialization, the lesions falling within the field of ambulatory surgery tend to be varied and

1

to be distributed over all parts of the body. Ambulatory surgery, therefore, never can be restricted regionally, nor can it be considered the exclusive field of any specialist. On the contrary, it is an integral part of the work of the general surgeon.

With all signs pointing toward more and more emphasis on ambulatory care as well as on preventive medicine, the need for improvement in the teaching, learning, and care of minor surgical lesions is of great importance.

ADVANTAGES AND DISADVANTAGES

Methods of treatment which permit the patient to be ambulatory have many advantages. Usually, the patient is able to pursue his regular occupation with little or no disability. This, combined with the fact that he can stay in his own home, means a considerable saving of money and much less inconvenience. The patient's morale is markedly improved, and the need to move and ambulate for himself restores his self-confidence as well as improving his physiology.

From the point of view of the surgeon, there are also many advantages. Fewer complications develop after operations on ambulatory patients than develop after the same operations performed on hospitalized patients. For instance, in a large experience with anal operations in ambulatory patients, retention of urine has never been encountered as a complication, although this is well known and a frequent and troublesome complaint in hospital patients. In the second place, the end results are satisfactory, comparing favorably with those obtained in similar lesions treated in hospital patients. In most hospitals, the problem of noscomial infections is significant, and these can be shown to relate to the length of stay in a hospital environment in which an incidence of 10 to 30 percent of hospital-acquired infections is not unusual.

The rising costs of hospital care are now being recognized as an increasing burden on the various types of health insurance agencies. Employers who buy health insurance for their employees are beginning to question the necessity for the hospitalization of patients who have lesions that can be treated on an ambulatory basis. Pressure is being brought to bear by labor-management councils, state departments of health, insurance commissions, commercial health insurance companies, and Blue Cross/Blue Shield, as well as by the Federal Government, to stop the unnecessary admissions to the hospital. All recognize that one way to conserve the public's health-care dollar is to reserve the use of hospital beds for patients who need inpatient care. Studies, examinations, and therapy which can be performed in an office, an outpatient department, or even a hospital's operating room, but which permit the patient to be ambulatory and to return home the same day, are of value to reduce overutilization of costly hospital beds.

Surgery in the ambulatory patient is not always advisable, even though possible. The patient should not be permitted to go home after an operation without a friend or a relative to accompany him. Sometimes home care is required following operations. In the case of the patient who should be confined to his room for a day or two but would have to go out for his meals, it is perhaps wiser to take advantage of the facilities of a hospital. Several recent developments may extend the benefits of ambulatory surgery to some of the people now excluded because of these problems. The first of these is the development of "In-Out" ambulatory surgical facilities in some hospitals. Here a patient may remain for several hours until he has recovered completely and is able to go home alone, or until a friend or relative can conveniently come and get him. The second is the concept of a motel-type facility attached to a hospital, where a patient who is ambulatory after a minor, or even a major, procedure can stay for short to longer periods of time. The cost is half, or less than half, that of a hospital bed.

Ambulatory surgery requires that the physician be available for call should a problem arise after his patient returns home. Emergency care is necessary only infrequently, but safety demands that it be available.

SELECTION OF PATIENTS AND PRECAUTIONS

In the selection of patients for ambulatory care there should be no question as to the advisability or the possibility of completing the therapy decided upon. Major surgery requiring a close watch over the postoperative course should not be attempted. When the diagnosis is in doubt or the extent of the lesion is not definitely known, the operation should not be performed on an ambulatory patient.

Constant care must be exercised in doubtful cases. Smallness is not always synonymous with unimportance, and the surgeon must be constantly on his guard. Moreover, the general practitioner who will usually recognize acute appendicitis and will send his patient to the hospital for immediate surgical attention will frequently fail to recognize or to evaluate the danger of a small malignant growth or of a boil on the upper lip.

Even though the lesions are insignificant, operations upon patients with blood dyscrasias, such as hemophilia or leukemia, are performed best in the hospital because of the danger of post-operative bleeding. In diabetics, even minor operations should be performed in the hospital because of the danger of metabolic complications. Emotionally disturbed individuals usually are not good candidates for ambulatory surgery.

Today, with more hospitals developing ambulatory facilities within the hospital itself, the protection of the patient against any untoward or unexpected development has been further increased, since all the services of a hospital are immediately available should a complication arise.

Ambulatory surgery should be safe surgery!

2

The Surgical Ambulatory Care Unit

D. K. Wagner, M.D.

During the decade of 1960 to 1970, inpatient per diem costs increased an average of 279 percent in the United States. Speculation as to the future varies from a moderately conservative social security administration estimate of a rise of 70 percent by 1975, to the estimate of other government officials who state that, by 1980, costs will average $1,000 a day at major urban hospitals, $600 in medium-sized communities, and $400 in rural areas. During the same decade, construction for new hospital bed space rose to an average per-bed cost of approximately $100,000 in 1970. Concurrently, sophisticated advances in surgical technology relating to the areas or organ transplantation and corrective cardiac surgery have increased the need for available intensive and maximal care beds. This combination of elevated per diem rates, increasing construction costs, and demands for in-service beds has precipitated the need for fiscal economies in the delivery of medical services where such can be accomplished without the compromising of patient care. For many communities, this will mean the establishment of an ambulatory surgical unit.

SURGICAL PROCEDURES AMENABLE TO AN AMBULATORY CARE UNIT

Forty years ago, an inguinal hernia in a child was considered an occasion for a major surgical undertaking. Twenty-five years ago, this procedure required an average of five days' hospitalization. In 1973, in a properly functioning ambulatory surgery unit, this same procedure can be carried out on an ambulatory basis in the vast majority of cases, and with a diminished incidence of postoperative complications as compared with those of the hospitalized child. This transition has resulted not so much from an improvement in surgical technique as from the development of efficient ancillary support services and from an improved understanding of the disease process. The pediatric inguinal hernioplasty typifies an ever-increasing list of surgical procedures that can be done safely on an ambulatory basis.

Almost any operative procedure that does not involve major invasion of the abdominal or thoracic cavity may be considered for outpatient surgery. The limitations are primarily imposed by post-operative management. Any procedure, therefore, that occasionally produces postoperative bleeding is generally contraindicated. In this category, one must include tonsillectomies. In addition to the surgical procedure, there are situations in which the physical status of the patient limits the feasibility of ambulatory surgery. The patient with diabetes or severe heart disease is a candidate only under unusual circumstances. Finally, the outpatient route is also contraindicated for patients who are psychologically unprepared or who find the concept emotionally threatening. In general, an operating time of 90 minutes or less should be required of the surgeon, and an anesthetic recovery time of less than 4 hours anticipated.

A list of the 20 most commonly performed in-the-hospital surgical procedures is shown in Table 2-1. These 20 procedures comprise approximately 2/3 of all in-the-hospital surgery. Of these 20 procedures, 2/3 are candidates for ambulatory consideration. An examination of these conditions, listed in Table 2-2 for one institution in the year 1971, reveals that between 52 and 73 per-cent of all inpatient procedures potentially could have been carried out on an ambulatory basis.

The realignment of these surgical activities has financial implications for the health care system. A cost comparison between a hospital and an ambulatory unit is shown in Table 2-3. These figures can be expected to vary from location to location, but usually when the procedure is done on an ambulatory basis, the cost is reduced to between 1/3 and 1/2 of the inpatient expense.

THE PLANNING PROCESS

The development of a successful ambulatory surgical unit entails a planning process which incorporates input from those component groups of people who will subsequently be influenced by its function. There are three general areas to be represented: the provider segment, as

Table 2-1. Most Frequent In-Hospital Procedures

Rank	Procedure(s)	Percent of all Inpatient Hospital Surgery
1.	Tonsillectomy-adenoidectomy	14.4
2.	Dilatation and curettage*	7.2
3.	Hernioplasty*	5.1
4.	Cystoscopy*	4.7
5.	Hysterectomy	4.6
6.	Excision of tumors— not elsewhere classified*	3.8
7.	Appendectomy	3.0
8.	Hemorrhoidectomy*	3.0
9.	Cholecystectomy	2.7
10.	Excision of breast cyst*	2.4
11.	Sigmoidoscopy*	1.7
12.	Repair of varicose veins*	1.7
13.	Colpoplasty	1.5
14.	Cataract removal	1.3
15.	Bronchoscopy*	1.2
16.	Prostatectomy	1.2
17.	Salpingo-oophorectomy	1.1
18.	Submucous resection*	1.1
19.	Reduction of fracture of radius, ulna*	1.0
20.	Strabismus correction*	1.0

*Can be done on an ambulatory patient.

Table 2-2. Potential Ambulatory Surgical Procedures*†

General surgery	643	1217	52%
Gynecologic	1209	1969	60%
Urologic	306	416	73%
Orthopedic	128	233	54%

*Medical College of Pennsylvania—1971
†By analyzing the annual surgical load, the potential and the size of the ambulatory surgical unit are determined.

exemplified by physicians, nurses, and hospital administrative personnel; the patients or recipient consumers; and the management, or board of trustees, for the involved institution. This planning group for each institution and its medical community must decide the following:

1. Is it desirable to develop an ambulatory surgery unit?
2. Is it feasible?
3. How should it be organized?

Table 2-3. Average Inpatient Hospital Charges Compared with Hospital Outpatient and Ambulatory Surgical Unit (Surgicenter) Fees

Procedure	Hospital Inpatient	Hospital Outpatient	Surgicenter (Path. Fee Inc.)	Savings Per Case
Dilatation and	$265.00	——	$105.00	$160.00
curettage	——	$148.90	105.00	43.90
Excision of skin	253.00	——	85.00	168.00
lesions	——	141.00	85.00	56.00
Bilateral myringo-	228.33	——	95.00	133.33
tomy, with tubes	——	134.31	95.00	39.31
Bilateral inguinal	245.00	——	150.00	95.00
herniorrhaphy				
Vasectomy	——	100.00	85.00	15.00
Excision of ganglion	265.00	——	105.00	160.00
Cystoscopy	295.00	——	125.00	170.00
	——	175.00	125.00	50.00
Excision of foreign	210.00	——	125.00	85.00
body	——	165.00	125.00	40.00
Adenoidectomy and	236.75	——	95.00	141.75
myringotomy				
Tonsillectomy and	210.00	——	125.00	85.00
adenoidectomy				

4. Where will it be; e.g., will it share existing facilities or construct a new area?

5. How will it be financed?

In addition, the planning group will need to consider the following:

1. Who will be in charge?

2. How will professional standards be established?

3. What procedures are allowable, and by whom?

4. What are the technical constraints; i.e., type and length of anesthesia, required laboratory data, and mechanisms for data base acquisition, storage, and retrieval?

To further focus on these questions, it is useful to plan in depth for the work force, the finances, and, finally, the facility itself.

Planning the Work Force

The work force consists of business, technical, and professional categories.

The business work force includes reception, interview, clerical, and unskilled technical activities. The tendency is always to plan too conservatively in this area. The success of the unit will inevitably depend on its ability to function efficiently, pleasantly, and effectively for both patient and physician. Concern for the ancillary comforts of the patient and his family are of paramount importance, and the business work force provides this image. Anything that makes the patient's visit unsafe, prolonged, uncomfortable, unpleasant, or inconvenient should be eliminated at the earliest possible moment. The development of a business work force that facilitates an efficient and pleasant operation is consequently essential. It is better that a receptionist be intelligent than that she be beautiful; an interviewer, perceptive to human signals rather than rigidly occupied with boring detail; a financial secretary, skilled in human relations as well as in daily bookkeeping.

Following the reception, a brief interview of all patients takes place. Since a patient will previously have had a professionally obtained history and physical examination, a repeat at this point is unnecessary. It is, however, essential that a check-list of conditions which might have recently arisen be established.

The recovery room attendant is the prime component of the skilled technical work force. This person has an extended role of a recovery room nurse, which includes both preinduction and postinduction monitoring and observation of the patient. This individual acts as a second barrier, screening the patient before he receives an anesthetic, and represents a higher degree of technical competence than does the initial screening interviewer. He should be capable not only of taking vital signs but also of auscultation of the heart. Upon termination of the operative procedure, this individual carries out the usual recovery room functions. The presence of higher levels of consciousness in postanesthetic patients will be part of this individual's concern. In addition, the presence of an anxious parent will require sensitivity to concerns not normally encountered in the recovery room. Consequently, the ability to deal with these anxieties is an added requirement for this member of the work force.

Physicians active in an ambulatory surgical unit must have certain flexibilities which are not universally called for in the inpatient setting. For instance, the anesthesiologist should be ready to complete the screening process of any patient in question; or the surgeon may need to vary his usual approach to hemorrhoids, breast masses, or varicose veins. Many surgical training programs do not emphasize ambulatory techniques, and it may be necessary for the trained surgeon to consider new procedures which his residency years did not make available.

A projected case load of 10 per day requires a work force of about 6 persons, exclusive of physicians and housekeeping personnel. This increases to approximately 9 full-time equivalents if the case load doubles. For the unit anticipating less than 10 cases per day, part-time equivalents are proportionately planned.

FINANCIAL PLANNING

It is important to establish the ambulatory surgery unit as a cost center with separate accounting for services provided. A tentative cost analysis for each of the anticipated common procedures should be carried out. With these available, contact is made with public and private carriers. Third-party insurers have been traditionally geared toward inpatient payment, and to alter this habit may take prolonged negotiation. Consequently, it is wise to begin this dialogue early in the planning process. The experience of areas with active units would indicate that virtually all public and private insurers will eventually realign their reimbursement to ambulatory coverage when the potential savings are indicated. Professional physicians' services, responsibilities, and fees are generally not diminished when surgery is conducted in an ambulatory setting.

PLANNING THE FACILITY

The facility may be built as a freestanding enterprise, such as the "Surgicenter" (Fig. 2-1), or it may be developed by making minor alterations and using the facilities common to most hospitals (Fig. 2-2). Most evidence would indicate that a unit which can utilize existing facilities is most economical to develop and operate. This is particularly true where institutional planners foresaw a shift toward ambulatory activities and real and/or potential square footage was appropriately allocated. The facility has four component parts. These are the reception, interview, procedure, and recovery areas.

In the reception area, a well-appointed, comfortable, homey atmosphere is desirable. A personal telephone where waiting parents or friends may make contact with home or work activities is necessary. In addition, the presence of a television set, educational material, coffee, and snack foods add to the chaperone's comfort. A

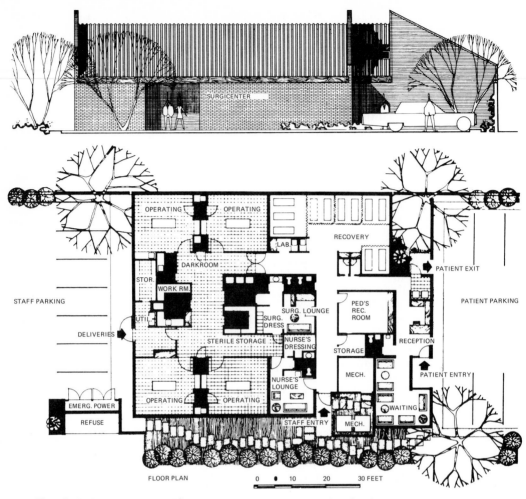

Fig. 2–1. Surgicenter in Phoenix, Arizona—an example of a freestanding ambulatory surgery unit.

private area for interview is not only conducive to accurate information retrieval but also simulates the intimacy of the private office setting. A small room, which may double as a dressing facility, serves this purpose well. A locker is necessary for personal belongings. A toilet facility is necessary, but need not be complex. Unless the volume anticipated is high, separate facilities for the sexes are usually not indicated. The location of the reception and interview sections should provide easy access to procedure and recovery areas. It is particularly comforting to children to sense that their parents are not far removed. It is even more desirable that the reception and interview areas have easy access to laboratory and x-ray testing, for it appears that, in most institutions, these areas often provide a maze from which patients have difficulty escaping. The limited amount of laboratory information necessary for the majority of ambulatory surgical procedures may call for consideration of a small facility in the immediate reception area. There are no national criteria for laboratory requirements necessary for ambulatory surgery. Consequently, each local facility must establish its own standard with respect to

FLOOR PLAN OF IN AND OUT SURGERY

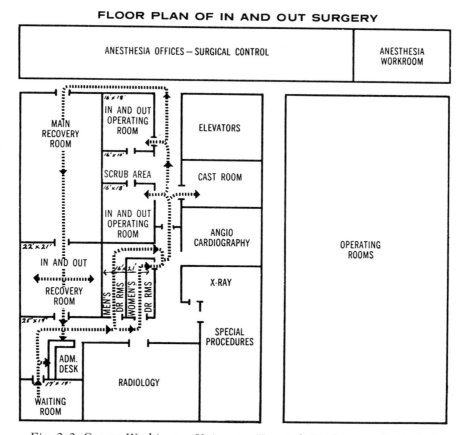

Fig. 2–2. George Washington University Hospital, Washington, D. C. Ambulatory surgery unit—an example of an in-hospital facility. (Levy, M. L., and Coakley, C. S.: Southern Med. J., *61*:995, 1968)

laboratory testing. For those institutions which require a hemoglobin, a hematocrit, and a urinalysis within 48 hours of giving a general anesthetic, the ability to obtain these tests in the reception area is desirable.

Since the ambulatory surgery unit will engage in manipulations categorized as major surgery, the procedure area must conform to the operating room standards of the Joint Hospital Association and to those established by federal regulation to qualify for Hill-Burton construction support. Traffic flow in and out of the operative area must be controlled as in all operating rooms and must be restricted to individuals in the proper attire. In constructing a new operative area, it may be possible to reduce costs by the elimination of conductive flooring.

The recovery area must be designed to accommodate patients who will remain until they are essentially fully recovered from effects of anesthesia. It should be large enough to allow some screening and separation of patients. If possible, the recovery area of the ambulatory unit should be separate from the general recovery room of the major operating suite. The pediatric portion must be large enough to allow a comfortable chair for an accompanying parent. A stretcher bed that resembles the type commonly found in intensive care units should be used for transport and recovery. This includes a sponge pad, 6 inches thick and 30 inches wide, and provides for the patient's comfort when he is awake, yet allows access to the patient during the recovery phase. Narrow, thinly padded stretchers are to be condemned for the adult patient. Cribs provide excellent recovery vehicles for infants, allowing access, comfort, and protection during the recovery phase. The recovery room must have access to basic liquids, which are made available to patients before their return to the reception-discharge area. Standard resuscitative recovery room equipment is necessary.

THE MODEL UNIT

The model ambulatory surgical unit becomes a reorganization of ongoing health services within a community. It calls for broad-based planning of the work force, the finances, and the facilities. It may be a newly constructed unit or one developed from existing facilities. It has an excellent potential for growth. It thrives on proper organization and serves to exemplify the physician's interest in improved surgical care and fiscal responsibility for health costs.

BIBLIOGRAPHY

Alexander, E. L., Burley, W., Ellison, D., and Valleri, R.: Care of the Patient in Surgery, Including Techniques. St. Louis, C. V. Mosby, 1967.

Avnet, H. H.: Physician Service Patterns and Illness Rates. New York, Group Health Insurance, 1967.

Calnan, J., and Martin, P.: Development and practice of an autonomous minor surgery unit in a general hospital. Brit. Med. J., 4:92, 1971.

Crouch, B. L., Ford, J. L., and Reed, W. A.: The surgical center: concept, care, cost in freestanding facility. Hosp. Top., Dec., 1971.

Eastman, P. F., and Applebaum, I. A.: Critical evaluation of internal hemorrhoidal ligation as an outpatient procedure. Am. J. Proctol., 20:109, 1969.

Levy, M. L., and Coakley, C. S.: Survey of "in and out surgery"—first year. Southern Med. J., 61:995, 1968.

McGibony, J. R.: Principles of Hospital Administration. New York, G. P. Putnam's Sons, 1969.

Nabatoff, H. A.: Three thousand stripping operations for varicose veins on a semi-ambulatory basis. Surg., Gynec. Obstet., 130:497, 1970.

Roemer, M. I., and DuBois, D. M.: Medical costs in relation to the organization of ambulatory care. New Eng. J. Med., 280:988, 1969.

Rudd, W. W. H.: Hemorrhoidectomy in the office: method and precautions. Dis. Colon Rectum, 13:438, 1970.

Rupnik, E. J., Williams, E. L., and Johnson, W. C.: Breast biopsy, an outpatient procedure using local anesthesia. Milit. Med., 133:743, 1968.

Somers, A. R.: Health Care in Transition; Directions for the Future. Chicago, Hospital Research and Educational Trust, 1971.

Williams, J. A.: Outpatient operations — 1. the surgeon's view. Brit. Med. J., 1:174, 1969.

3

Anesthesia for Ambulatory Surgery

Edwin L. Rushia, M.D.

INTRODUCTION

The convenience and favorable economics of performing surgery on an ambulatory basis are very appealing. This arrangement should not be utilized without recognizing the presence of surgical and anesthetic risks. Thus, certain prerequisites for surgery and anesthesia must be observed if uniformly satisfactory results are to be obtained and tragedy averted. The history and physical examination, preoperative and postoperative instructions, written permission for operation, and close observation during and after the procedure are all important. If the patient is considered a poor surgical or anesthetic risk, admission to the hospital, where more sophisticated medical and surgical evaluation and equipment are available, should be seriously considered.

The history and physical examination are mandatory. It should be remembered that we are especially interested in knowing about the patient's past responses to the administration of various drugs, and how he reacted to local or general anesthesia. Physical examination should include an assessment of his apparent attitude—is he calm or nervous, cooperative or suspicious, happy or depressed? Our assessments should make considerable difference as to whether we operate on this patient as an outpatient at all, and certainly as to whether we select local or general anesthesia as the method of obtunding pain.

The securing of informed consent for surgery and anesthesia is becoming increasingly important regardless of the magnitude of the procedure contemplated. Time spent in giving a lucid explanation of the procedure as well as in listening to the patient's questions and expression of feelings about the anesthesia and surgery is important if the patient is to give an informed consent.

Instructions given the patient before his arrival for the performance of surgery are very important and should be in writing. No set of instructions can be completely routine; each must be tailored to suit the individual circumstances and the individual patient. The patient should arrive approximately an hour before surgery to permit adequate premedication and the regaining of composure, which is frequently lost in the scramble to meet the appointment. Regardless of the anesthetic procedure planned, it is well to ask the patient to neither eat nor drink after midnight, the night before surgery. A simple local anesthetic procedure can change rapidly into a respiratory crisis should consciousness and protective reflexes be lost due to an untoward response to drugs administered. When general anesthesia is contemplated, an empty stomach is, of course, mandatory if one is to avert the aspiration of vomitus. The patient or his parents should be evaluated regarding their capabilities or willingness to carry out directions. Many tragedies have resulted from the provision of food preoperatively to a child by a well-intentioned parent or other relative.

Continual observation by trained attendants from the time the patient reaches the office or clinic until an appropriate time after anesthesia and surgery is important. The patient should be able to perform appropriate tests of coordination and to demonstrate his ability to exercise judgement and follow instructions before acute vigilance is terminated. During operation the surgeon's attention should be upon the operative procedure and not the general response of the patient to anesthetic drugs. Many untoward drug reactions can be detected and reversed effectively if there is careful observation of the blood pressure, pulse, and respiration. The appearance of flushing or blanching of the skin or of perspiration are clues to future trouble. Irrational speech and abnormal thought content are clues to central nervous system problems and can be detected only if verbal contact is maintained between the patient and the nurse or other trained office personnel.

After surgery, no patient should be discharged except in the company of an observant adult chaperone who can take appropriate action should the patient become nauseated, unstable, or sleepy. Transportation, too, should be the responsibility of a person other than the patient. He cannot be expected to be immediately capable of driving or performing other skilled tasks. It is best that he not return to his job the day of surgery if he can possibly avoid doing so.

After careful consideration has been given to the evaluation of the ambulatory patient, the anesthesiologist can decide whether local or general anesthesia should be used, as well as what type of premedication is needed. The preanesthetic medication must be appropriate if the patient is to be without anxiety or side effects of the anesthetic drugs. The duration of action of the premedication and that of the anesthetic selected are of critical importance. The patient must be able to leave the surgical area walking without assistance and feeling safe to go home with only a relative to accompany him.

PREMEDICATION

Preanesthetic medication, appropriate in both type and amount, must be given if a technically satisfactory operative result and a satisfied and psychologically unshaken patient are the ultimate goals of the effort. Often this "premedication" will consist only or predominantly of assurance before and during the surgical procedure, but therapy in this very important part of the procedure must be individualized.

Our concerns about premedicants center about type of drug, dosage, and route of administration, and all of these factors are closely interrelated.

Time and Route of Administration

This is quite a critical factor when considering the outpatient for anesthesia. In spite of our best planning for the patient to arrive 1 to 1½ hours prior to surgery, we are often confronted with the necessity of inducing anesthesia 30 minutes after his arrival, and of selecting a drug and a route of administration which will produce the desired effect in this time. The rate of absorption of an orally or rectally administered drug varies, and, unless 1 to 2 hours is available preoperatively, these routes are of doubtful value in premedication for our purposes. Parenteral drug administration appears to be the best from the standpoint of time. The fastest route, and one too often neglected, is the intravenous route. Most narcotics when given intravenously reach their peak of action in approximately 5 minutes and, if given slowly and in moderate doses, they cause no significant circulatory or respiratory depression. Next in speed of action and onset time is the intramuscular administration route. Anticholinergic drugs, most narcotics, and a variety of tranquilizing drugs adapt well to outpatient circumstances when given intramuscularly. Most of these agents have an appreciable effect in 30 to 45 minutes when given intramuscularly. The recently introduced fentanyl (Sublimaze) has an intramuscular onset time of about 10 minutes and thus competes, timewise, very nicely with intravenously administered drugs.

DURATION OF EFFECT

Most ambulatory patients, even those requiring for their surgery 30 to 60 minutes of general anesthesia, should be in condition to be discharged within an hour of the completion of surgery. The anesthetics themselves are usually excreted or detoxified within this time. Care, then, must be taken in choosing premedicants if one is to avoid somnolence, dizziness, or other instability protracted beyond the hour after the completion of surgery.

DRUGS AND DOSAGES

Good premedication should effectively dispell fear and anxiety and produce an attitude of drowsiness and unconcern without clinically significant depression of the circulation or respiration. In addition, when general anesthesia is to be used, premedication should include an anticholinergic drug to inhibit pharyngeal secretions and to control the effects of vagal stimulation. The amount of premedicants used varies with age and weight, and with patient management. A few minutes spent in reassurance of the patient and explanation of the contemplated anesthetic and surgical procedures will go far toward elimination, or at least reduction, of the need for sedative drugs before surgery. Furthermore, the tactful removal of well-intentioned but nervous relatives from the preoperative scene and the provision of a quiet and dimly lit patients' waiting room will do wonders for permitting sedative drugs to perform their pharmacologically intended task optimally.

Barbiturates

The barbiturates have little or no analgesic value, and this lack of capacity to raise the pain threshold makes them distinctly inferior to narcotic preparations when pain is being experienced preoperatively or is anticipated, as is the case with most any surgical procedure. Even when given intravenously or intramuscularly, the short-acting barbiturates, of which pentobarbital (Nembutal) and secobarbital (Seconal) are the best known examples, are a bit too long-acting for our purposes in ambulatory procedures; this, coupled with their rather minimally suitable pharmacological properties, makes the value of their use in this setting decidedly limited. The conception, commonly held previously, that barbiturates are of help in lowering the dangers of reactions from local anesthetic drugs appears to be without merit, and thus this can no longer be given as a valid reason for their use.

Narcotics

These compounds undoubtedly offer the best solution for preoperative medication, and when the shorter-acting members of the group are chosen, one can be reasonably certain of accomplishing adequate analgesia and permitting rapid recovery and ambulation. The narcotics do an effective job of raising the pain threshold and lowering metabolic function, thus decreasing the amount of general anesthetic needed and rendering the patient unmindful of minor but otherwise bothersome stimuli during conduction (local or regional) anesthesia. Of the many opiates and opioid compounds available to us, probably the best for our purposes, because of their short duration of action, are meperidine (Demerol), alphaprodine (Nisentil), and fentanyl (Sublimaze).

Meperidine (Demerol). Meperidine has long had a place in the analgesic drug realm. It is significantly shorter-acting than morphine, and its use carries a lower incidence of nausea. It has little tendency to depress the circulation and even when given intravenously, slowly and in conservative doses, does not greatly depress respiration. Meperidine should be used with great care in infants under two years of age, and frequent observations should be made of the adequacy of respiration. In these infants, effective analgesia and sedation are obtained with 0.7 to 1.0 mg. per kg. of meperidine. Three concentrations are available; 50, 75, and 100 mg. per ml.; and of these, the 50 mg. per ml. is by far the most common.

Alphaprodine (Nisentil). This drug has been about for some time but has probably not received the popularity it deserves. Its onset of action is a bit more rapid, and its duration of effect is decidedly less, than that of meperidine. Mild cardiovascular depression occasionally is seen following its administration. As with meperidine, alphaprodine can be given intravenously to shorten the onset time; or it can be given intramuscularly or subcutaneously if this factor is not a pressing problem. One mg. per 5 pounds of body weight is a good dosage guide. It is assumed that one will infrequently, if ever, use this or other narcotics on infants of under 20 pounds in weight. When alphaprodine is given intravenously to adults, it is well to give an initial 20 mg. and to augment this dose very slowly, observing the patient closely not only for the amount of sedation produced but also for the occurrence of undue respiratory or circulatory depression.

Fentanyl (Sublimaze). This is an exceedingly potent piperidine compound supplied in a concentration of 0.05 mg. per ml. Circulatory depression attending its use is exceedingly uncommon, but one must be very attentive to the possibility of the development of respiratory depression, or of muscular rigidity in which the muscles of respiration take part, rendering voluntary or artificial ventilation difficult. Fortunately, this latter complica-tion does not occur often, except as an accompaniment of intravenous fentanyl administration, and it can be effectively controlled by the use of ventilatory assis-tance plus the use of narcotic antagonists and/or muscle relaxants in appropriate dosage. Naloxone (Narcan) is a relatively new and promising narcotic antagonist that can be given in 1 ml. (0.4 mg.) doses with great effect. The amount of fentanyl to be given is 0.01 mg. (0.2ml.) per 20 pounds of body weight. The usual adult dose recommended is 0.05 mg. to 0.1 mg. The analgesia produced is rapid, satisfac-tory, and evanescent, making this a good premedicant to consider for the ambu-latory patient.

Tranquilizing Drugs

Many partisans have arisen crying the virtues or the pitfalls of a group of drugs varied in chemical structure but related in their capacity to reduce anxiety. Most of these compounds diminish the tendency to nausea and provide mild sedation but offer very little in the way of pain relief. Their effect when used concurrently with narcotics is additive at the very least, and thus considerable caution is in order when such combinations are employed. Of the phenothiazine drugs available, promethazine (Phenergan) is probably the most useful for our purposes. Its greatest usefulness is realized when it is used in combination with meperidine in a 1 (Phenergan) to 2 (meperidine) relation-ship, and by the intravenous route, for making a patient sleepy and carefree dur-ing conduction anesthesia. It is best to dilute the combination by giving it slowly into a freely flowing infusion line. Phenergan is somewhat irritating to the tissues and can produce phlebitis if given in concentrated form. For the average-sized adult, 25 mg. is usually an adequate dose. Diazepam (valium) is frequently used for the same purpose. Doses of 5 to 10 mg. in the adult are effective, and, as with the phenothiazines, vascular irrita-tion and pain must be prevented by slow administration, preferably via a rapidly running infusion. A combination of droperidol (Inapsine) and fentanyl has been popularized as a producer of a state of neuroleptanalgesia. Whatever be the virtues of the compound, the duration of action of droperidol appears to be a bit too long for its routine use in ambulatory surgery. Its fine qualities as an antiemetic may compensate for this drawback, however. The dose is 2.5 to 5.0 mg., and it can be given intravenously as well as by other routes.

Anticholinergic Drugs

The most common compounds in clinical use are, of course, atropine and scopolamine, and they are used in like amounts for the chief purposes of (1) inhibition of saliva formation, which produces an unobstructed dry airway in the patient receiving general anesthesia; and (2) the obtunding of the cardiac portion of the vagi and, thus, protection of the patient from the side effects of vagal hyperactivity, such as bradycardia, seen with increasing frequency in this era of light anesthesia. There is no clear-cut and final indication of the superiority of one drug over the other. For our purposes, the additional advantage of scopolamine in providing a degree of amnesia and drowsiness is outweighed by its tendency to produce excitement and even hallucinations. Thus, in the outpatient, atropine is to be considered as our drug of choice for the production of anticholinergic effects. The use of any drug of this type before the use of condution anesthesia should be avoided, since dryness of the mouth is a disagreeable sensation and accomplishes little in reversing the possible respiratory depression from depressant drugs. If one has an unexpected need for general anesthesia, intravenous atropine administration is recommended, and the effect of the atropine is quickly available. For use in premedication, atropine is commonly prepared in concentrations of 0.4 mg. or 0.5 mg. per ml, and it can be given subcutaneously, intramuscularly, or intravenously, depending on the speed of action desired. The dosage range is not great, 0.1 mg. not being considered excessive in the infant and 0.4 mg. being quite adequate in all but the largest adults.

CONDUCTION ANESTHESIA

This increasingly used term embraces any anesthesia obtained by the blocking of impulse conduction through nerve fibers and employing, almost exclusively, local anesthetic drugs. In surgery for ambulatory patients, relief of pain is obtained most frequently through the use of one of the many available local anesthetic drugs in some local or regional technique.

Conduction anesthesia of the head, the neck, or the trunk for the ambulatory patient can usually best be managed by local infiltration or field block. This includes anesthesia for simple herniorrhaphies performed on an ambulatory basis. The alternatives for this operation (epidural or subarachnoid block) are considered ill advised due to the occasionally prolonged obtundation of kinesthetic sense after either and cephalalgia following the latter. Caudal anesthesia can be used for certain anorectal procedures in ambulatory patients, but here, too, anesthesia of the legs is frequently inadvertently obtained, so that rapid ambulation is unsafe.

The use of vasoconstrictors, chiefly epinephrine (adrenalin), was introduced for the combined purpose of slowing systemic absorption of local anesthetic drugs (and thus lowering toxicity) and of prolonging the local activity of these agents, thereby permitting the performance of longer procedures in a "drier" field than was previously possible. If epinephrine is used in the proper concentrations, and if one respects its propensities for the production of tachycardia, tachyarrhythmias, dangerous tissue ischemia in critical areas, anxiety, syncope, and a variety of adverse psychic responses, it is a very excellent and helpful drug. Little or no advantage is to be gained by the use of greater than 1:200,000 adrenalin concentration in the anesthetic solution, and much is to be lost in terms of adverse reactions. Certainly no more than 1 ml. of the usual 0.1 percent (1:1000) solution should be used. Assuming the use of a 1:200,000 epinephrine concentration, this is adequate for 200 ml. of anesthetic solution, a volume rarely required to produce anesthesia for ambulatory surgical procedures. A "rule of thumb," that 15 drops, or minims, of a solution equals 1 ml., has long been drawn upon for the adding of epinephrine to local anesthetic solutions when solutions to which epinephrine has not already been added by the manufacturer are used. Drops vary greatly in size, depending both on the physical characteristics of the substance being added and on the size of the orifice at which the drop is formed. Thus, dilutions are much more accurately effected by using a syringe graduated in fractions of a milliliter, and by using 0.1 ml. of the 1:1000 epinephrine concentration per 20 ml. of anesthetic solution. Adverse reactions to epinephrine, which occasionally arise even following the use of proper concentrations and doses of epinephrine, can be distinguished from local anesthetic drug reactions by the presence of tachycardia, often above the rate of 120 beats per minute. This rarely if ever is seen when the reaction results from toxicity of any local anesthetic except cocaine. This tachycardia and the accompanying symptoms are evanescent and of no great moment unless the overdose is considerable and extreme hypertension or ventricular fibrillation results.

Enhancement of the diffusive properties of local anesthetics has in the past been effected by the addition of hyaluronidase to the local anesthetic-epinephrine combination in the ratio of 1 turbidity unit per ml. of anesthetic. This practice has been found to be decreasingly necessary with the advent of the recently introduced, highly diffusible compounds such as lidocaine, mepivacaine, prilocaine, and chloroprocaine.

LOCAL ANESTHETIC DRUGS

Cocaine. Because of its toxicity, cocaine is now used only for topical anesthesia. The concentration used depends on the mucosa being anesthetized. One to 5 percent is used for corneal anesthesia; 10 to 20 percent is commonly used in the nose and throat. Concentrations of 10 percent and over have decided vasoconstricting properties; these help to provide a bloodless field and to decrease the absorption of toxic amounts of the drug.

There is great individual variation in toxicity. Severe toxic reactions occur at the level of 1 g. Reactions have been reported after doses as low as 20 mg.

Procaine (Novocaine). Procaine is used extensively for all types of conduction anesthesia. The optimum concentration varies from 0.5 percent for local block to 2.0 percent for the blocking of large nerve trunks.

Toxic responses vary not only with the dose but also with the rate of absorption into the blood stream, which in turn is dependent on the vascularity of the area injected and the presence or absence of vasoconstrictor substances in the anesthetic solutions.

Although a great range of maximum safe doses is given by various authors, we feel that a maximum of 500 mg. within a one-hour period provides a good rule of thumb. One can feel relatively safe in using 100 ml. of an 0.5 percent concentration of procaine (100 x 5 mg./ml. = 500 mg.) for local infiltration. This volume should certainly be adequate for infiltration anesthesia for most ambulatory surgical procedures. This assumes, of course, the absence of intravascular injection and recognizes the increased safety provided by the use of a 1:200,000 concentration of epinephrine for inhibition of absorption.

Following the above tenets, one sets a maximum dose of 50 ml. of a 1 percent procaine solution, and 25 ml. of a 2 percent solution. Note should be made in passing that in the performance of spinal anesthesia, a total dose of 200 mg. should not be exceeded.

Rarely are true allergic reactions to procaine and chemically related compounds seen. These range in severity from a few skin wheals to the potentially lethal subglottic edema requiring tracheostomy and, often, resuscitative measures.

Tetracaine (Pontocaine). Tetracaine is

a very potent drug and a toxic one; it is stated to be ten times as potent but also ten times as toxic as procaine. Although its definitely longer duration of action as compared with procaine recommends it in a few procedures, it has been largely relegated to use as a spinal anesthetic drug (10 to 20 mg. dose), where it still enjoys great popularity, and to topical anesthesia (0.5 percent concentration in the eye and 2.0 percent in the nose and throat).

Lidocaine (Xylocaine). Lidocaine has been used in all types of conduction anesthesia. Its very great current popularity is attributable to its low toxicity, rapid diffusibility, topical activity, and chemical stability. Although a concentration of 4 percent is required for the production of dependable anesthesia, concentrations of 0.5, 1.0, 1.5, and 2.0 percent are used, much as procaine is used, for anesthetizing progressively larger nerves and nerve groups. Also, as with procaine, a total dose of 500 mg. should not be exceeded if toxic reactions are to be averted.

Mepivacaine (Carbocaine). This compound is similar to lidocaine in structure, and it has similar toxicity and potency. It is mentioned because a bit faster onset time and slightly longer duration of action. Unlike lidocaine, mepivacaine is not available in solutions to which epinephrine has been added.

Toxic Reactions to Local Anesthetic Drugs and Their Treatment

The vast majority of untoward reactions to local anesthetic drugs result not from any idiosyncrasy but from the presence in the blood stream of excessively great amounts of unmetabolized drug, whether this be the result of intravascular drug injection, rapid absorption from a vascular area, or the use of excessive amounts of drug.

Untoward reactions are divided into central nervous system and cardiovascular effects. *Central nervous system phenomena* range from slight giddiness requiring no treatment to the startling and much feared generalized convulsions, sometimes with respiratory failure. To differentiate it from another type of reaction, of psychogenic origin, seen frequently in outpatients is difficult. Pain and fear in these frequent anxious, unprepared, and unpremedicated persons can lead to vasomotor disturbances which may progress to a lowering of the blood pressure (particularly if the patient is in a sitting position), syncope, and even convulsions. Fortunately the treatment is similar to that of toxic reactions, and the outcome can be expected to be a happy one if the treatment outlined for toxic reactions is immediately instituted.

Toxic central nervous system reactions have been explained in two ways. Steinhaus (1957) found that the cerebral cortex and other higher centers are stimulated by local anesthetics, as opposed to the depression manifest in the pons and medulla. More recently, Frank and Sanders (1963) have postulated that the hyperkinesis seen during toxic reactions may represent ultimately a depression of neurons that connect higher and lower centers, resulting in the release of the latter from higher control.

Whatever be the source of the convulsions and the gradations thereof, oxygen demand increases markedly, and this demand must be met by the immediate administration of oxygen by face mask at the first suggestion that something is amiss. At this time also preparation should be made for starting an infusion, not only for the enhancement of blood volume, but especially to provide an avenue for the rapid intravenous administration of drugs should they prove to be needed (Table 3-1).

If convulsions do occur, immediate steps must be taken to control them while the excess of the drug is being detoxified by the usual metabolic processes. The time-honored method of treating convulsions from this source is the use of a barbiturate. Although premedication with barbiturates for this type of anesthesia is of little or no prophylactic value, the intravenous administration of short-acting or, better still, ultra-short-acting

Table 3-1. Contents of Resuscitation Tray

Drug	Proprietary Name	Preparation	Average Dose
Sympathetic and Sympathomimetic Drugs			
Epinephrine	Adrenalin	1 mg./ml.	0.2–1 mg.*
Norepinephrine	Levophed	2 mg./ml.	Diluted*
Phenylephrine	Neosynephrine	10 mg./ml.	2–10 mg.
Ephedrine	Ephedrine	25 mg./ml.	25–50 mg.
Isoproterenol	Isuprel	0.2 mg./ml.	0.02–0.2 mg.*
Belladonna Drugs			
Atropine	Atropine	0.4 mg./ml.	0.4 mg.
Scopolamine	Scopolamine	0.4 mg./ml.	0.4 mg.
Barbiturates			
Pentobarbital	Nembutal	50 mg./ml.	50–100 mg.
Secobarbital	Seconal	50 mg./ml.	50–100 mg.
Cardiac Drugs			
Procaine amide	Pronestyl	100 mg./ml.	50–100 mg.*
Deslanoside	Cedilanid	0.2 mg./ml.	0.4–1.6 mg.
Digoxin	Lanoxin	0.25 mg./ml.	0.5–1 mg.
Antihistaminic Drugs			
Diphenhydramine	Benadryl	10 mg./ml.	10–50 mg.
Tripelennamine	Pyribenzamine	25 mg./ml.	25 mg.
Narcotic Drugs			
Morphine	Morphine	10 mg./ml.	5–10 mg.
Codeine	Codeine	30 mg./ml.	30–60 mg.
Meperidine	Demerol	50 mg./ml.	50–100 mg.
Narcotic Antagonists			
Levallorphan	Lorfan	1 mg./ml.	0.5–1 mg.
Adrenal Cortical Hormone			
Hydrocortisone	Solu-Cortef	100 mg./1.8 ml.	100 mg.
Insulin			
Insulin	Regular Insulin	40 U/ml.	10–50 U

*Give slowly and with great caution

barbiturates, such as thiopental (Pentothal) and like drugs, is valuable. The barbiturate should be given intravenously for immediate action, and the dose should be the minimum amount needed to control the convulsion if too profound a psychic, cardiovascular, and respiratory depression is to be avoided. Long-acting barbiturates should be avoided because they cause prolongation of the central nervous system depression.

A promising newcomer in the controlling of convulsions due to local anesthetics is diazepam (Valium). Given intravenously, in doses of 5 to 35 mg., this drug is very effective, and it is much less likely to produce respiratory and vasomotor depression than are the barbiturates.

The intense convulsive muscular contractions can, of course, be obliterated by peripheral neuromuscular blockade, and this form of therapy, using succinylcholine in doses of 50 to 100 mg. given intravenously (or intramuscularly if no vein is available), has much merit, particularly if large amounts of barbiturates are found to be required for convulsion control. Two precautions should be mentioned: (1) this treatment can be used on conscious patients only, because of the psychic effect of the widespread paralysis on the conscious person;

and (2) the materials and skill for providing respiratory support for the paralyzed patient must be at hand.

Toxic cardiovascular reactions are attributable chiefly to the depression of intracardiac impulse conduction and myocardial contractility, with resulting hypotension and even cardiac arrest. Symptoms and signs range from those of mild cerebral hypoxia through complete unconsciousness and, ultimately, to cardiac standstill. Treatment consists of placing the patient in the supine, moderately head-down position, and of supplying the sluggish circulation with a high oxygen concentration (100 percent oxygen furnished the lungs via suitable apparatus using artificial ventilation if the patient's own respiratory effort is inadequate). Naturally, a patent airway is necessary for adequate ventilation, and if the patient is unconscious, an oropharyngeal airway device or even a carefully inserted endotracheal tube may be required. Hypotension can best be corrected by the intravenous use of vasopressors. A great number of these are available to us, and two dangers accompany their use; too little effect and too great effect; the latter sometimes produces an uncontrolled and potentially dangerous hypertension. Mild hypotension is often very satisfactorily managed by the intravenous administration of 12 to 25 mg. of ephedrine (assuming the patient to be an adult of around 70 kg. in weight). Persistent and profound hypotension is better managed by using phenylephrine (Neo-Synephrine) in an infusion, 10 mg. of the drug being added to 500 ml. of any common infusion solution. Its action is evanescent and overdosage is easily corrected. This dilute "drip" technique provides for individualization of the administration of the drug, the need for which is difficult to predict from moment to moment and from patient to patient.

Allergic reactions can frequently be prevented by obtaining a history that includes past responses to local anesthetics. It must be remembered that far more persons receive local anesthesia in connection with dental procedures than for any other reason, and that the sitting position, anxiety, and response to the use of high epinephrine concentration in the anesthetic all may provide statements of "I can't take local anesthesia." True hypersensivity manifests itself in the development of urticaria or swelling of the mucosa of the nose, the pharynx or the larynx. It can best be treated by the immediate administration of 0.1 to 0.5 ml. of 1:1000 epinephrine subcutaneously if this has not already been used with the anesthetic itself. Corticosteroids such as dexamethasone (Decadron), given intravenously in a dosage of 4 to 20 mg., or hydrocortisone, 100 to 500 mg., are often of great benefit. It is very important that one be aware of the possibility of the airway's being closed off by edema, making immediate endotracheal intubation and/or tracheostomy mandatory.

PRINCIPLES OF CONDUCTION ANESTHESIA

1. Preoperative anxiety should be guarded against by proper explanation and premedication (see section on premedication) if psychic reactions are to be kept at a minimum.

2. The circulation should be monitored at least by determination of blood pressure at regular, frequent intervals, particularly early in the procedure.

3. Whenever the demands of the operative procedure permit, the patient should be placed in the supine position for anesthesia and surgery.

4. Minimum amounts of the lowest effective drug concentration should be used.

5. Except in the case of anesthesia on fingers, toes, and any other "end circulation" areas, epinephrine, in a concentration of 1:200,000, should be used in the anesthetic not only to prolong its effect and minimize bleeding but also to delay drug absorption into the bloodstream.

6. Oxygen, airway devices, intravenous fluids, vasopressors, and barbiturates should be readily at hand for the treatment of drug reactions.

7. Whenever local infiltration can be

effectively utilized, it is unwise to subject the patient to regional block, which carries an increased possibility of nerve damage.

8. In preparing the skin for conduction anesthesia the minimum amount of antiseptic which will adequately cover the skin of the exposed area is adequate. Too generous application of antiseptic materials results in running of the antiseptic all over the area, an unnecessary and esthetically unappealing situation.

9. When a skin wheal is produced in preparation for deeper placement of the needle, the patient should be alerted as to what is about to happen, and the needle should be inserted intracutaneously with steady pressure (no jabbing!) and slow injection made as the needle is being inserted. During the formation of the wheal, anesthesia is only partial, and the practice of injecting as much anesthetic material as possible is to be discouraged. Overdistension of the tissue is painful, and only a minute wheal is required.

10. When the touching of bone is necessary as part of the block procedure, this should be accomplished gently. Touching of the periosteum by the probing needle is painful.

11. Incision and drainage of small abscesses always presents a problem. Use of the frequently recommended ethyl chloride spray usually provides little more than a hard, difficult-to-incise surface, and there will be pain over the whole area due to the pressure required for incision. In spite of the acidity of the tissues and the resulting difficulty in obtaining anesthesia in this area by the use of local anesthetic drugs, it should be stated that one can usually obtain anesthesia for incising these lesions, and without spreading the infection, by careful injection of a minute quantity of dilute anesthetic solution. The injection should be made with a short 25-gauge needle at the point of the summit of the abscess.

EQUIPMENT FOR CONDUCTION ANESTHESIA

The equipment necessary for local anesthesia need not be elaborate, but it must be kept in good condition at all times. Luer-Lok glass syringes of 5 ml. and 10 ml. capacity, with metal tips, are the most satisfactory. Metal rings for the fingers, which permit a firmer grip and better control of the syringe, are preferred (Fig. 3-1). Needles must be carefully selected. A 25-gauge, $^3/_4$-inch needle with a sharp, beveled point is used for the initial skin wheal, or endermic infiltration. A selection of 22-gauge needles, of 2, 3, and 4 inches, should be available for deep infiltration and nerve blocks.

TECHNIQUES OF CONDUCTION ANESTHESIA

Local Infiltration

Local anesthesia is produced most commonly by direct infiltration of the tissues with the anesthetic solution. Thus, suitable anesthesia may be obtained for superficial tumors, cysts, thrombosed external hemorrhoids, and a number of other superficial lesions. Acute fractures may be reduced easily after the direct infiltration of the hematoma about the fracture site with the anesthetic solution. Superficial infections, contrary to general opinion, may be opened under local anesthesia by infiltration of the skin along the line of the proposed incision without fear of spreading the infection.

Procaine hydrochloride, 0.5 percent, is used for local infiltration for removing superficial lesions, suturing small wounds, skin grafting, and incising superficial abscesses. An initial skin wheal is first made, using the small 25-gauge hypodermic needle. The point of the needle is inserted, with the bevel down, directly into the skin. In places where the skin is loose, it should be held under tension during this injection. The anesthetic solution is injected as the needle is inserted into the skin. Thus a cutaneous wheal, which should be about 1 cm. in diameter, is produced with little or no pain to the patient. Then a longer needle is attached to the syringe, inserted through the anesthetized skin at the site of the wheal, and a subcuntaneous linear

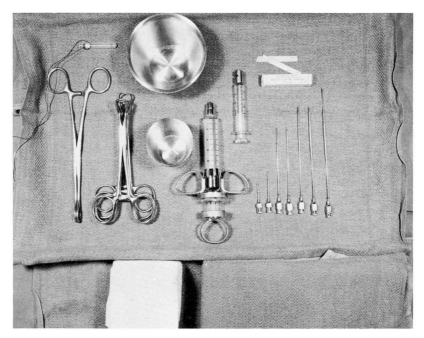

Fig. 3–1. Equipment for local anesthesia tray. One 10-ml. Luer-Lok syringe. One 2-ml. Luer-Lok syringe. Needles: 1 3/4-inch, 24- or 25-gauge; 1 2-inch, 22-gauge; 2 31/2- or 4-inch, 22-gauge; 2 5-inch, 20-gauge. One 1-ml. ampule of epinephrine, 1:1000 dilution. Two metal solution containers (200 ml.) for antiseptic solution, one (250 ml.) for local anesthetic solution. One sponge-holding forceps. Four towel clamps. Two dozen sponges, 2 × 2 or 3 × 3 inches. Five towels for draping operative field. One Diack indicator.

or elliptical line of infiltration is produced; or the intradermal infiltration may be continued from the original wheal. When the infiltration is to be continued subcutaneously, it may be necessary to make more than one cutaneous wheal; or, better still, the longer needle may be inserted into the cutaneous layer from beneath, at the end of the subcutaneous infiltration, a wheal produced, and the subcutaneous infiltration continued further by reinserting the needle through this wheal.

Infiltration of the skin along the line of proposed incision of a superficial abscess will not spread the infection if adequate drainage is obtained, and the abscess may be opened with no discomfort to the patient if pain produced by pressure is prevented. Incision and drainage of superficial abscesses may be easily performed.

After the skin has been anesthetized, it is grasped with a towel clip, or between two towel clips, and is lifted up while the incision is made. Thus, deep pressure over the inflamed area is avoided, and painless incision can be performed, since the skin has been anesthetized. No epinephrine is used in the anesthetic solution.

Anesthesia for the reduction of acute fractures of any of the bones of the extremities may be obtained readily by the direct infiltration of a local anesthetic solution at the fracture site. The longer, 2-inch or 3-inch needle is introduced through one or more skin wheals toward the fracture line, avoiding the larger vessels and the nerves. After contacting the bone, the needle may be partially withdrawn and reinserted until aspiration of bloody fluid indicates that the hematoma

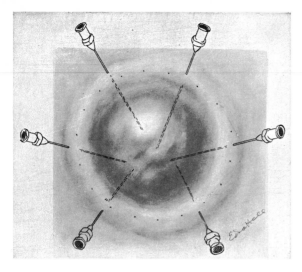

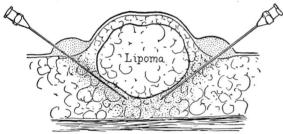

Fig. 3–2. Field block. By inserting the long needle through the initial skin wheal a complete wall of the anesthetic solution is infiltrated round the operative field. In this way all sensory impulses from the operative site are blocked without actual infiltration in the field or distortion of tissues.

about the fracture has been reached. Occasionally, one may be able to feel the needle slip between the bone fragments at the line of fracture. The fact that bloody fluid may be aspirated at several levels indicates that the hematoma has been pierced, rather than that an accidental venipuncture has been performed. The blood aspirated from a hematoma of several hours' duration may also be identified by its dark appearance.

Procaine hydrochloride, in 1 or 2 percent solution, preferably with epinephrine, is used for the infiltration about a fracture. Not more than 30 ml. of the 2 percent solution, or more than 60 ml. of the 1 percent solution, should be used routinely, and the injection always should be performed slowly and cautiously in order to avoid systemic reactions. Full anesthesia is not obtained until at least 15 minutes after the injection.

The best results with infiltration anesthesia for the reduction of fractures are obtained with early, acute fractures. After from 48 to 72 hours, the hematoma about the fracture site becomes organized, making it more difficult to obtain satisfactory infiltration. However, this anesthesia may be used with almost any fracture of less than 48 hours' duration and is the most efficient anesthesia in such cases. Reduction may be performed safely under fluoroscopic guidance, and the full cooperation of the patient maintained throughout the procedure; this greatly facilitates the reduction and the subsequent application of splints or plaster casts for immobilization. It is a distinct advantage in the reduction of fractures in a dark fluoroscopic room and at times when an anesthetist is not available. It is the anesthesia of choice for the reduction of fractures in ambulatory patients.

Field Block

Diffuse infiltration of an anesthetic solution through all tissues containing sensory nerves leading from the field of

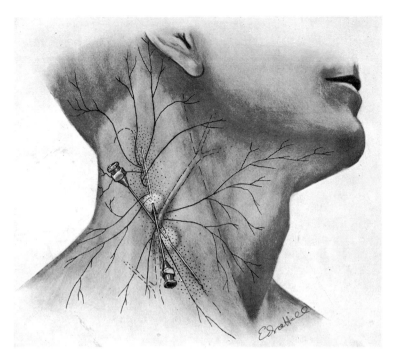

Fig. 3–3. Superficial cervical block. The superficial branches of the cervical plexus may be blocked as they cross over the posterior border of the sternocleidomastoid muscle. The long needle is inserted through an initial skin wheal, and the injection is made deep to the external jugular vein but directly overlying and along the posterior edge of the muscle.

proposed operative intervention effectively blocks sensory impulses in these nerves and their branches. Anesthesia of the operative field is thus produced without direct infiltration at the operative site. This is known as fieldblock anesthesia, and it is a procedure intermediate between purely local infiltration and nerve block. A wider zone of anesthesia, which usually lasts longer, may be obtained with smaller quantities of anesthetic solution than would be required for local infiltration of the entire operative field. In addition, it requires less technical skill than does nerve block and therefore may be used to advantage when the operative site is supplied by a number of small sensory nerves.

Fieldblock anesthesia may be preferred to direct local infiltration for the removal of sebaceous cysts, lipomas, benign tumors, and other superficial lesions of the body surface, as the tissues at the site of operation are not distorted by infiltration with the anesthetic solution. The anesthetic solution is injected into the skin and the subcutaneous tissues through an initial skin wheal to form an elliptical or diamond-shaped zone of infiltration around the operative field. Procaine hydrochloride, 0.75 or 1.0 percent, should be used for this type of anesthesia (Fig.3–2).

The Scalp. Anesthesia of the scalp may be obtained by a zone of infiltration encircling the lesion, since all the sensory nerves pass upward in the subcutaneous tissues. Thus any portion of the scalp may be anesthetized conveniently by a field block with 0.5 to 1.0 percent procaine hydrochloride.

The Neck. The majority of operations

about the neck on ambulatory patients may be accomplished by the use of local infiltration anesthesia. Deep cervical block, which may be used for more extensive operations, is not indicated, although superficial cervical block, a form of field block anesthesia, may be useful occasionally in conjunction with local infiltration. The superficial branches of the cervical plexus may be blocked as they cross over the posterior border of the sternocleidomastoid muscle. Twenty to 30 ml. of 0.5 percent procaine are injected on the posterior border of this muscle where the superficial jugular vein crosses it (Fig. 3-3).

The Thoracic Wall. Any desired area of the thorax may be blocked by simple infiltration of all its layers with a 0.5 percent solution of procaine. Wider areas of anesthesia may be produced by intercoastal nerve block. Wheals are raised in the midaxillary line along the inferior borders of the desired ribs. A 5–cm. needle is introduced through the wheal until the rib is contacted. It is then withdrawn slightly and reintroduced, passing beneath the lower border of the rib in a cephalad direction. It is advanced 0.5 cm. beyond the rib border. After aspiration, 4 ml. of 1 percent procaine are injected at this site (Fig. 3-4). To complete the block, it may be necessary to infiltrate the skin and subcutaneous tissues with 0.5 percent procaine.

The Abdominal Wall. Rarely will it be necessary to provide extensive abdominal wall anesthesia for the ambulatory patient. Infiltration of the layers of the abdominal wall with procaine will produce satisfactory anesthesia. Abdominal field block for operations of greater magnitude may be produced by the injection of the thoracic nerves as they traverse the abdominal wall. With the patient lying in the supine position, skin wheals are raised over the xyphoid process, at the point along the 10th costal cartilage where the lateral border of the rectus abdominis muscle crosses it (on the side of the abdomen to be anesthetized), and along the lateral border of the rectus abdominis muscle a few centimeters

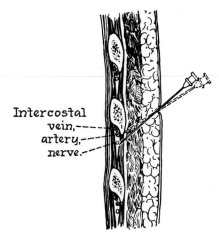

Fig. 3–4. Intercostal nerve block. The dotted figure shows the position of the needle as it is introduced through a cutaneous wheal until the rib is contacted. The needle then is withdrawn slightly and reintroduced so that it passes just beneath the lower border of the rib. At this point the anesthetic solution is injected.

above and below the umbilicus. An 8-cm. needle is passed through these wheals to join them together in straight lines by subcutaneous injections of 0.5 percent procaine. The needle is again passed through each wheal toward the fascia of the rectus muscle. Procaine is injected as the needle pierces the superficial fascia and then passes through the fascia of the rectus muscle. Injection of several milliliters is made into the muscle. The position of the needle is then changed in fanlike manner, and repeated injections are made into the muscle.

The Penis. Block anesthesia for circumcision or other operations on the penis may be obtained by a subcutaneous injection encircling the base of the penis, supplemented by the injection of 1 to 2 cc. of 1 percent procaine beneath the fascia (Buck's) on each side. Procaine solution of 1 or 2 percent should be used (Fig. 3-5).

For circumcision, a simple form of infiltration anesthesia is practiced more commonly. The foreskin is reflected, and,

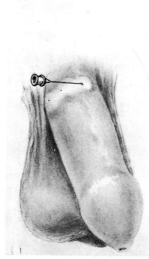

Nn. dorsalis penis

Section near base
of penis.

Fig. 3–5. Block anesthesia of the penis. The nerves of the penis may be blocked by a subcutaneous injection encircling the base of the penis. The cross section shows the dorsal nerves of the penis beneath Buck's fascia, which must also be blocked by the injection beneath the fascia of 1 or 2 cc. of the anesthetic solution.

with 1 percent procaine solution, a circle of infiltration anesthesia is deposited under the skin, close to the base of the glans. Special care must be taken to infiltrate the frenulum, in which there is a rich plexus of sensory nerves. After this infiltration has been completed, the foreskin is replaced over the glans, and a second circle of infiltration is made in the skin at the same level, at the base of the glans. This dual infiltration is not time consuming and gives excellent anesthesia (Fig. 3-6). In cases in which the foreskin cannot be retracted easily, the superficial skin anesthesia is induced first, and then the anesthetic is carried deeper into the foreskin near the base of the glans. A line of infiltration is injected downward to the edge of the foreskin. With this anesthesia, it is possible to incise the edge of the foreskin sufficiently to permit retraction and the completion of the anesthesia.

The Anus and the Rectum. The sensory nerves which go to the anal canal and the anal orifice may easily be blocked as they traverse the fatty tissues of the ischiorectal fossa. These nerves arise from the perineal nerve as it passes in Alcock's canal along the ramus of the pubis. They traverse the ischiorectal fossa, from behind, forward and medially, to reach the anal canal. In addition, there are a few small so-called coccygeal nerves which

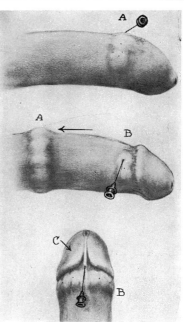

Fig. 3–6. Technique of local infiltration anesthesia for circumcision. The foreskin is reflected over the glans and a circle of the anesthetic solution is infiltrated subcutaneously at the level of the base of the glans at (A). The foreskin is retracted and a circle of the anesthetic solution is deposited under the skin close to the edge of the glans at (B). Special care must be taken to infiltrate the frenulum and its sensory nerve (C).

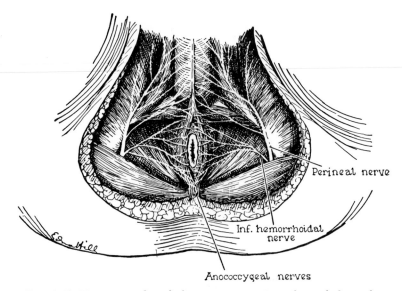

Perineal nerve

Inf. hemorrhoidal
nerve

Anococcygeal nerves

Fig. 3–7. Nerve supply of the perineum. Branches of the inferior hemorrhoidal and perineal nerves cross forward and medially from the lateral wall of the ischiorectal fossa. In addition, a few sensory fibers pass directly forward from the region of the coccyx. To block the nerves of this region, therefore, it is important that most of the anesthetic solution be deposited round the posterior half of the circumference of the anal canal. (Ferguson, L. K.: Surg. Clin. N. Am., *19*:1513, 1939).

pass directly forward from the region of the coccyx to the anal canal. Therefore, it is possible to block completely all the nerves which reach the anal canal by introducing a wall of anesthetic solution outside it, in the ischiorectal fossa (Fig. 3-7).

This is accomplished best with two injections. The first is the infiltration of an anesthetic, usually 1 percent procaine solution containing epinephrine, into the skin of the perianal region. This may be done without fear of subsequent infection if the area has been cleaned with soap and water, followed by the application on one of the commonly used antiseptic solutions. The local infiltration is begun at the midline posteriorly and is carried laterally on each side to anesthetize completely the skin surrounding the anal orifice.

After skin infiltration, a deeper injection must be made to block the nerves as they traverse the ischiorectal fossa. Since these nerves pass, from behind, forward and medially, it is most important that the

anesthetic solution be introduced around the posterior half of the circumference of the anal canal. With the index finger of the left hand introduced through the anal orifice (Fig. 3-8); the injection is begun just to the lateral side of the midline. The patient should be warned of some slight feeling of discomfort as the needle is introduced deeply into the ischiorectal fossa. Failure to give this warning may cause the patient undue apprehension; and if he moves, considerable difficulty may ensue, even the puncturing of the anal canal or the rectum with the needle. The needle is carried in a fanlike direction around the anal canal, forward and backward. The injection is made at a distance of about ³⁄₄ inch to 1 inch away from the canal, the nerves being blocked as they approach the canal itself. It should be carried throughout the entire length of the anal canal, about 20 ml. of 1 percent procaine being used on each side. Occasionally, it is necessary to make an anterior injection.

In making these injections into the is-

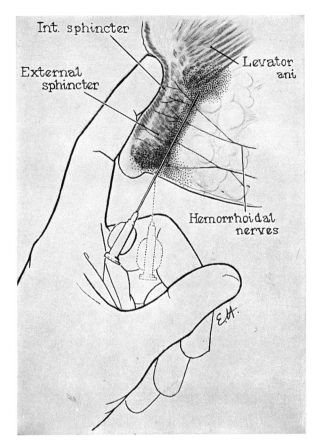

Fig. 3–8. Technique for block of the nerves to the anal region. Following local infiltration of the skin of the perianal region, a deeper injection is made to block the sensory nerves as they cross the ischiorectal fossa. With the index finger of the left hand in the anal canal as a guide, the long needle is inserted into the midline posteriorly, and the injection is carried out in a fanlike direction on either side of the anal canal and about 1 inch from it. (Ferguson, L. K.: Surg. Clin. N. Am., *19*:1513, 1939).

chiorectal fossa for block of the nerves to the anal canal, it is important that only a small amount of the solution be deposited in one place. The needle must be kept moving practically all the time, and the injection must be made continuously. If too much solution is deposited at any one place, a painful slough may result.

Local infiltration produces almost immediate anesthesia and causes relatively slight distortion. The addition of epinephrine, 3 drops of a 1:1000 solution to 30 ml. of the anesthetic solution, not only prolongs the anesthetic effect but also markedly reduces the amount of bleeding. This type of anesthesia is especially valuable for anal-fissure operations, hemorrhoidectomy, and the removal of anal polyps and anal crypts. It may be contraindicated in infected areas, such as abscesses and complicated fistulas. The incidence of postoperative urinary retention following anal operations is less after local infiltration and block anesthesia than after any of the other types of anesthesia used for anal operations.

Nerve Block

Sensory anesthesia may be produced by the injection of an anesthetic solution into or immediately around the nerve or a plexus of nerves. The production of long-lasting anesthesia of a rather large area with a minimum amount of drug is the chief advantage of nerve block anesthesia. Its only disadvantage is that a fair degree of technical skill and experience is required to master the various nerve block procedures. With increasing experience, however, one will find a few of the various types of nerve block very useful and suitable for operations on ambulatory patients.

Digital Nerve Block. The dorsal and the volar digital nerves may be blocked

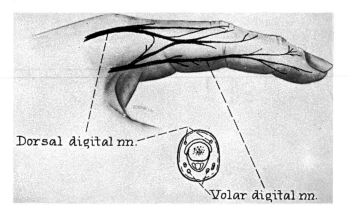

Dorsal digital nn.

Volar digital nn.

Fig. 3–9. Digital nerve block. Operations on the fingers and the toes may be performed by blocking the digital nerves. The needle is inserted through intradermal wheals at the base of the digit, and the anesthetic solution is deposited in the region of the dorsal and the volar digital nerves shown in the figure.

within the soft tissues at the base of the fingers or of the toes for operations on the digits. Intradermal wheals are raised on each side at the base of the digits, and the needle is introduced into the deeper tissues through these wheals. The anesthetic solution is deposited close to the bone, near the anterior and the posterior digital nerves (Fig. 3-9). From 3 to 5 ml. of 1 percent procaine will produce adequate anesthesia. It must be remembered that, with a digital block or any other type of conduction anesthesia, one must wait a short time for the full anesthetic effect. Usually, from 5 to 10 minutes must elapse from the time of injection for complete anesthesia of the digit. A tourniquet (rubber band) may be applied at the base of the digit to control bleeding. Epinephrine is usually omitted.

Brachial Plexus Block. Other than digital blocks, which are very useful and technically simple in operating on the fingers, most conduction anesthesia for operations on the arm and hand is effectively performed by the use of the block of the brachial plexus at one of these sites:

1. Axillary approach. This block has gained much popularity over the past ten years, and for a good reason. The plexus at the level of injection is quite superficial and quite easily identifiable by its close association to the brachial artery. If care is taken not to injure the plexus or to inject the anesthetic intravascularly, the complication rate is low. Because of its technical simplicity, the procedure can be used in children, where it is an excellent

aid to the correction of fractures and other acute lesions of the lower arm and hand. An important consideration in the selection of the axillary approach for outpatients is that there is no danger of invasion of the pleura, with resulting pneumothorax, as is true of the supraclavicular type of block. Of course, one cannot expect to obtain anesthesia of the shoulder cap (supraclavicular nerve, C_3 and C_4) or of the small segment of the inner upper arm supplied by the intercostobrachial nerve (T_2). The lack of anesthesia in the latter occasionally may result in some tourniquet pain when this equipment is used during surgery for provision of a bloodless field. This block is particularly well described and illustrated in Eriksson's excellent book, Illustrated Handbook in Local Anesthesia.

2. Supraclavicular approach. This time-honored technique is mentioned only to be condemned for use in outpatients because of the rather high incidence of pneumothorax resulting from invasion of the dome of the pleura, which lies in close relation to the site of approach to the plexus.

3. Scalene approach. The fascial sheath which surrounds the brachial plexus as it descends into the arm arises from the anterior and posterior tubercles of the transverse processes of C_3, C_4, C_5, and C_6, along with the origins of the anterior and the smallest scalene muscles. The plexus thus can be blocked very proximally with little danger to the pleura or to the neck structures by placing anesthetic solution

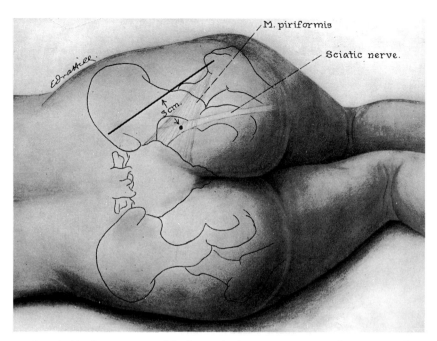

Fig. 3–10. Sciatic nerve block. With the patient in Sims's position, the side to be injected uppermost, an imaginary line is drawn between the posterior superior iliac spine and the superior border of the greater trochanter. This line is bisected by a perpendicular line drawn upon its midpoint. Three cm. down on this perpendicular line an intradermal wheal is raised. Through this wheal a long needle is inserted at right angles to the skin to deposit the anesthetic solution for the block.

within the sheath between these muscles near the base of the neck. By injection of rather large volumes of solution, the anesthesia can be extended over sufficiently high segments to include anesthesia of the shoulder as well as of the arm. An excellent description of the block is given by Winnie and Collins (see Bibliography).

Sciatic and Femoral-Sciatic Blocks. The sciatic nerve may be blocked easily near its exit from the sciatic foramen. The resulting anesthesia may be used for the reduction of fractures about the ankle or for operations on the posterior aspect of the thigh. However, sciatic block is chiefly employed for the diagnostic and the therapeutic management of sciatic neuralgia.

A satisfactory approach to the sciatic nerve is obtained with the patient in Sims's position (Fig. 3-10). An imaginary line is drawn between the posterior superior iliac spine and the superior border of the greater trochanter. This line is bisected, and an intradermal wheal is raised 3 cm. beneath its midportion. An 8- to 10-cm. needle is introduced through this wheal and inserted at right angles to the skin for a distance of 6 to 8 cm., depending on the habitus of the patient. The point of the needle should strike bone at this depth. If no paresthesias are obtained, the needle should be withdrawn and reinserted. It is usually quite easy to elicit paresthesias, as the sciatic nerve is large at this point. Fifteen ml. of 2 percent procaine are injected.

Much more satisfactory, however, when local or field block will not suffice, is the combined femoral-sciatic block described very adequately in most any treatise on the subject. Both nerves are extremely easy to locate and can be blocked with ease for operations below the knee. The knee itself can be manipulated with the use of this procedure, but open operation is not possible because of the contribution to the innervation of the knee by the obturator and lateral femoral cutaneous nerves.

Intravenous Regional Anesthesia

Intravenous regional anesthesia, applied much more often to the arm than to the leg, was introduced by Bier in 1908 but enjoyed only limited use until about 1965. It has since been employed increasingly in the field of orthopedics, both in surgery of acute trauma and in correction of more chronic or congenital defects of the hand and forearm.

Any of the commonly used local anesthetics (without a vasoconstrictor) may be employed in dilute, usually 0.5 percent, concentration. With a needle or an intravenous catheter inserted into the vein as near the lesion as possible, as much blood is drained from the arm as possible, either by elevation of the arm for several minutes or by application of an Esmarch bandage; and then a dependable tourniquet, usually placed about the upper arm, is inflated to a pressure that is 50 to 150 mm. Hg above the patient's systolic pressure. When this has been accomplished, anesthetic solution is injected into the indwelling needle or catheter in the dosage of 2 to 3 mg. per kg. of body weight, the volume ultimately depending on the volume of the limb.

The onset of anesthesia and of muscular relaxation is fairly rapid (5 to 15 minutes), and the duration of anesthesia is limited by the safe occlusion time for the extremity, which is certainly not over 90 minutes. Care should be taken to have the muscle under the tourniquet relaxed during inflation of the tourniquet, and to defer deflation of the tourniquet until a minimum of 15 minutes has passed after injection of the anesthetic. Care must be taken to deflate the tourniquet slowly, having in mind the entry of the anesthetic

solution into the general circulation. With these two provisions, untoward drug reactions are relatively rare. When the tourniquet is released after the use of lidocaine, there is a fainting or dizzy sensation, which lasts for only a few seconds. The problem of pain due to pressure from the tourniquet can be solved by using two tourniquets or a double tourniquet unit, now commercially available, with preliminary inflation of the proximal cuff followed by inflation of the distal cuff over the anesthetized area once the block has been established. In spite of the excellent anesthesia produced, some surgeons do not prefer this form of conduction anesthesia because of a certain amount of wetness of the tissues.

GENERAL ANESTHESIA

Although the majority of ambulatory surgery is and should be accomplished with the aid of conduction anesthesia, there are valid indications for the employment of general anesthesia in this situation.

1. Age. Although simple procedures can often be performed even on small children without general anesthesia, depending on the stability of the child and the presence or absence of friendship for, and confidence in, the surgeon and/or anesthetist, general anesthesia is sometimes necessary. Children are notorious for the frequency with which they somehow contrive to eat just before arriving at surgery, however; therefore, regional anesthesia, when it can be used without psychic trauma to the child, has a distinct advantage over general anesthesia, because with the latter there may be aspiration of vomitus.

2. Temperament of the patient. Aversion to "knowing anything about it" is quite common in patients coming to surgery, and frequently no amount of reasoning or premedication can change this attitude. It is a mistake to force conduction anesthesia upon these persons when general anesthesia can safely be employed.

These are the chief reasons for resorting to general anesthesia, and one need only add, as indications for general anesthesia occasional instances in which attempts at conduction anesthesia are unsuccessful or in which a history of untoward drug reactions makes it potentially dangerous.

Once one assures himself of the immediate availability of equipment for treating any complication of general anesthesia likely to arise, he can proceed with the selection of the proper drugs to be used and the proper technique for their use. Fortunately, the equipment and the drugs necessary for safe anesthesia and for treating complications are similar (see Table 3-1). The presence of devices of proper sizes to produce and maintain a patent airway and of their companion pieces, is mandatory; this will assure complete control of respiration by any of a variety of ventilating devices, ranging from those for mouth-to-mouth ventilation, through simple bag-and-mask combinations, and on to sophisticated anesthesia machines. Added to these, of course, should be a source of oxygen for the provision of this gas in higher concentration than is found in room air, and a readily available and efficient suction apparatus for the removal of pharyngeal secretions and vomitus, should they unexpectedly appear.

Competence and good judgement in the use of these airway devices are necessary, and they can be learned most effectively by experience gained from others performing anesthetic procedures. Maintenance of the patient's normal cardiovascular function during anesthesia demands the careful and frequent recording of pulse and blood pressure and that drugs for the support of the circulation be readily at hand. The conscientious use of simple monitoring devices will go far toward early detection and treatment of cardiovascular problems before they become serious and will minimize the need for more sophisticated equipment. An intravenous infusion need not be provided for all patients having minor surgery, but the provision of this access to the circulation for immediate use should disaster strike, whether during general or regional anesthesia, is a great source of comfort. There is no frustration greater than that caused by the frequently unsuccessful attempts to perform a venipuncture for the administration of corrective drugs in the middle of a convulsive seizure or cardiovascular collapse.

GENERAL ANESTHETIC DRUGS

The possession by the anesthetist of a fair degree of expertise in the use of equipment and drugs is a basic necessity. The use of any anesthetic drug without the user's being familiar with its virtues and drawbacks alike is foolhardy, and the safest drug in the world can thereby be made a lethal one.

From the long list of general anesthetics available at present, some drugs can be selected, on the basis of duration of action, to meet the time demands of ambulatory surgery.

Gases

Nitrous Oxide. Nitrous oxide is being used in greater quantity than ever before. It is rather sweet smelling, is easily synthesized from ammonium nitrate, and has the distinct advantage of being nonflammable. Its oil/water solubility coefficient is 3.2, and its blood/gas solubility coefficient is 0.47, characteristics which promote its rather rapid uptake and pharmacologic effect. It enters into no chemical combination in the body and thus is eliminated rapidly when administration is concluded. Its effect on any and all organ ·systems is minimal, and we have here a very excellent drug, the value of which is limited only by the fact it is a rather weak anesthetic and is not capable of producing anesthesia in most persons without exclusion of the amount of oxygen necessary for a normal metabolic function. The happy alternative to yielding to this unphysiologic circumstance is to provide the oxygen concentration necessary for the patient and to compensate for the deficiency in potency by the addition of other anesthetics, sedatives, and hypnotic drugs. Currently most popular in use for this purpose are halothane and other volatile fluorinated hydrocarbons; narcotics, such as morphine, meperidine, fentanyl, and other drugs otherwise more commonly thought of as pain relievers; and ultrashort-acting barbiturates. Many methods for the use of nitrous oxide have been described. For our purposes, the safest and most practical technique is to supply the gas along with adequate oxygen through an anesthesia machine, using a high-flow, semiclosed system and venting excess gas through an escape valve on the machine. In an effort to wash nitrogen out of the patient's tissues and lungs, providing for a more nearly nitrogen-free atmosphere of respired gases, administration is commonly begun and continued for 5 to 10 minutes with flows of nitrous oxide and oxygen of 7 and 3 liters per minute respectively. After this period, the nitrogen can be considered to be nearly "washed out" and the more economical flows of nitrous oxide, 3.5 liters per minute, and oxygen, 1.5 liters per minute, can be started, adjusting the flow of oxygen upward in response to the development of any evidence of hypoxia, and adding more adjuvant drug in response to the appearance of light anesthesia. Certainly the oxygen flow should not be reduced, nor the nitrous oxide increased, in response to the need for increasing anesthetic depth.

Ethylene. This drug is a gas with a potency 10 to 15 percent greater than that of nitroux oxide, and it is administered by the same technique. Ethylene has fallen into disfavor in recent years because of the rather marked explosion hazard associated with its use and because it is only slightly more potent than nitroux oxide.

Cyclopropane "won its spurs" in the period between 1930 and 1940 as a very potent agent permitting rapid induction into, and emergence from, the anesthetic state. Its potency allowed for the provision of high oxygen concentrations during anesthesia; thus it was recommended for patients with any degree of cardiovascular impairment tending to compromise tissue oxygenation. Unfortunately, cyclopropane possesses several undesirable

properties, and its use brings with it the necessity to circumvent them. It is a rather marked respiratory depressant, and some respiratory assistance is necessary during its use if hypoxemia and hypercarbia, with its attendant arrhythmia production, are to be avoided. Ventricular arrhythmia is also a danger when the use of adrenalin is required during surgery. Probably the greatest reason for the fading popularity of cyclopropane, however, is its flammability over a wide concentration range. It is used in a closed anesthetic system in a concentration of 10 to 25 percent, and is given either intermittently or by continuous flow, with careful respiratory support and monitoring of the circulation.

Volatile Anesthetics

Diethyl ether is a very pungentsmelling, flammable, potent anesthetic, capable of providing profound anesthesia and muscular relaxation when concentrations of below 4 percent are inspired. It can be administered by a great variety of techniques and equipment. Lack of acceptance by the patient, and flammability, in the era of less nauseating and nonflammable drugs, have led to its decline as a popular anesthetic drug. In addition, its rather slow uptake and its excretion characteristics make it a very poor choice for anesthesia for ambulatory patients.

Halothane. Next to nitrous oxide, halothane is undoubtedly the most frequently administered inhalation anesthetic in use today, chiefly because of a rather benign odor, nonflammability, and excellent potency and rapidity of anesthesia induction and emergence. The incidence of postoperative nausea and vomiting is very low. It is commonly administered along with nitrous oxide-oxygen mixtures through a "copper kettle" or Vernitrol vaporizer, or through a vaporizer specifically made and calibrated for its use. Open drop administration is rather easily managed, but this technique is seldom employed because of the excessive cost involved and the risk of overdose due to the high vapor pressure of this agent.

The concentrations required for attaining surgical anesthesia in the premedicated patient vary from 0.5 to 1.5 percent. Halothane is a respiratory depressant, commonly compromising tidal volume with no decrease in respiratory rate. Circulation is also frequently depressed, and this results from a decrease in both peripheral vascular resistance and cardiac output. The fact that both of these changes appear to be dose-related cautions us to use the lowest effective concentration of the drug possible. Its great capacity to cause uterine dilatation qualifies halothane for use in situations in which the uterus must be rapidly dilated, but appears to contraindicate its use otherwise in a patient with a gravid uterus because of the attendant increased bleeding.

For several years, a dispute has waxed and waned over the effect of halothane on the liver and its implication in cases of acute liver necrosis. The dispute remains unsettled, but these facts and bits of advice appear to be valid. The incidence is extremely rare, and the pathologic findings compatible with this diagnosis occur much more frequently in adults than in children. When possible, it is probably best to administer halothane to a patient no oftener than every four weeks, at least for the first three or four administrations. A history of previous liver damage from whatever cause contraindicates the use of halothane. The occurrence of unexplained postadministration fever and leukocytosis with eosinophilia contraindicates subsequent use of the drug.

Intravenous Agents

Barbiturates. Enjoying great and deserved popularity, not only as adjuvants to nitrous oxide but also for the induction of hypnosis before any type of general anesthesia, are the ultrashort-acting barbiturates. The best-known members of this group are the sodium salts of thiopental (Pentothal), thiamylal (Surital), and methohexital (Brevital). With minor differences, the three are quite similar, and our discussion will be related to thiopental as representative of the group.

In common with all barbiturates, thiopental is a compound of malonic acid and urea. Its alkaline salt is very water soluble, and it is commercially prepared as a crystalline product for dilution by sterile saline, distilled water, or 5 percent dextrose solution. A 2.5 percent solution is considered the safe maximum in this country because of the great danger that more concentrated solutions will produce tissue irritation and necrosis when extravasation inadvertently occurs. Once in solution, thiopental maintains its potency well for about 48 hours at room temperature, or approximately a week when refrigerated. Reviewing the drug pharmacologically, we find that, following a single injection, it rapidly finds its way into the central nervous system, only later to be concentrated in various nonfatty tissues of the body, and, finally, in the poorly perfused fatty tissues. Less than 1 percent of the thiopental injected is excreted unchanged through the urinary tract; the remainder is broken down in the liver at the rate of approximately 20 percent per hour. The clinical uses for thiopental in ambulatory surgery are as great as they are in any other facet of anesthesia, owing to the speed and simplicity of intravenous induction of the anesthetic state and rapid emergence therefrom when the total dosage (and thus tissue saturation) is kept to a minimum. Ordinarily, when anesthetizing a premedicated, 70-kg. patient, 250 mg. of the drug should be adequate for the induction of the hypnotic state. The maximum dose is 2 g., and, in combination with 70 percent nitrous oxide, 1 g. is sufficient for most ambulatory surgical procedures.

Ketamine. A newcomer to the field of intravenous agents is a cyclohexanone compound known variously as Ketamine, Ketalar, and Ketaject. It is designated a "dissociative anesthetic" because of its apparent capacity for selective interruption of certain central nerve pathways concerned with pain perception and reaction while leaving other pathways intact. Pharyngeal and laryngeal reflexes remain normal, and therefore there is no need of artificial devices for the preservation of a patent airway; this accounts for much of the appeal of the drug. Muscular tone remains unchanged, or somewhat increased, and a rise in blood pressure is frequently seen, making the use of this drug in severe hypertensive patients impractical. Although Ketamine can be used for induction or in combination with other anesthetics, it is commonly used independently for minor procedures in children. The age exclusion is relative and is based on the frequent occurrence in adults of disturbing dreams. These are said to be minimized considerably by the use of Valium or droperidol and, more particularly, by guarding the awakening patient from verbal and tactile stimuli. Although Ketamine can be administered intramuscularly as well as intravenously, the latter route is much preferred because of the sometimes alarmingly long wake-up time seen after intramuscular administration. This is particularly true when the length of the surgical procedure necessitates a repeat dose. The dose is calculated on a weight basis, 1 to 2 mg. per pound being given intravenously, and 5 to 7 mg. per pound intramuscularly. Anesthesia induction (intravenous) occurs within 1 minute, and the anesthesia lasts approximately 10 minutes. The need for drug supplementation is manifested by the onset of purposeful muscular movements, and approximately one half of the induction dose is usually required. Although Ketamine is a very interesting and potentially useful compound, its future for adult application, and that of similar drugs sure to follow, will hinge upon the absence of (or ability to cope with) the all-too-frequent psychic phenomena accompanying emergence.

BIBLIOGRAPHY

Physiology

de Jong, R. H.: Physiology and Pharmacology of Local Anesthesia. Springfield, Ill., Charles C. Thomas, 1970.

Guyton, A. C.: Textbook of Medical Physiology. ed. . Philadelphia, W. B. Saunders, 1966.

Pharmacology

American Medical Association. Council on Drugs: AMA Drug Evaluations. ed. 1. Chicago, 1971.

Goodman, L. S., and Gilman, A.: The Pharmacological Basis of Therapeutics. ed. 3. New York, Macmillan, 1965.

Conduction Anesthesia

Eriksson, E.: Illustrated Handbook in Local Anesthesia. Chicago, Year Book Medical Publishers, 1969.

Labat, G.: Regional Anesthesia, Its Technic and Clinical Application. Philadelphia, W. B. Saunders, 1922.

Moore, D. C.: Regional Block. ed. 3. Springfield, Ill., Charles C. Thomas, 1961.

Winnie, A. P., and Collins, V. J.: The subclavian perivascular technique of brachial plexus anesthesia. Anesthesiology, *25*:353, 1964.

General Anesthesia

Corssen, G.: Dissociative anesthesia with Ketamine hydrochloride. Proc. Inst. Med. Chicago, *27*:341, 1969.

Smith, R. M.: Anesthesia for Infants and Children. ed. 3. St. Louis, C. V. Mosby, 1968.

Wylie, W. D., and Churchill-Davidson, H. C.: A Practice of Anesthesia. ed. 3. London, Lloyd-Luke, 1972.

Toxic Reactions to Local Anesthetic Drugs

Frank, G. B., and Sanders, H. D.: A proposed common mechanism of action for general and local anesthetics in the central nervous system. Brit. J. Pharmac. Chemother., *21*:1, 1963.

4
Dressings and Bandages

Mark W. Wolcott, M.D.

The requirements of dressings and bandages for ambulatory patients are somewhat more exacting than are those for patients in hospitals or at home in bed. In addition to fulfilling the requirements of any dressing, which are to absorb secretion, protect the part, serve as wet compresses, or exert pressure, the dressings must be comfortable and not burdensome or inconvenient. Also, they must stay absolutely in place until time for the next dressing, and they should permit the patient as far as possible to resume or continue his normal activities with the least inconvenience.

DRESSINGS

The original dressing applied at the time of operation should provide sufficient absorbent material to take care of the wound secretions for at least 24 to 48 hours, and it should be applied well enough to remain in place for that period of time. It should provide sufficient pressure to aid in producing hemostasis. Experience in the care of operative wounds in ambulatory patients permits the surgeon to gauge very well the amount of absorbent dressing necessary for a given wound. When packing has been inserted into an infected wound following incision, a gauze dressing or the commercial type of gauze dressing containing a film of cotton should be applied over the wound. Pressure is obtained by placing one or two strips of adhesive across the dressing and onto the skin and applying a firm bandage. In the application of a simple dry dressing, as in the application of all dressings to ambulatory patients, it should be remembered that the dressing need be no larger than the wound to be covered. It is, therefore, quite permissible, and even to be recommended, that the sterile gauze be cut with sterile scissors to fit the wound rather than that a large dressing be applied to a small wound. The gauze may be held in place by either adhesive or bandage, depending on the situation of the wound.

RE-DRESSINGS

The time for re-dressing depends upon the type of wound, or more exactly, upon the amount of secretion from it.

Dressing Clean Wounds. In the case of clean wounds, unless pain, swelling, or other evidence of infection appears, re-dressing is not necessary until it is time to remove the sutures. Every patient with a clean wound, therefore, is instructed to return in 3 days or sooner if the lesion does not become increasingly more comfortable. At the third-day visit, the dressing is inspected; if it is not soiled and if there is no discomfort in the region of the wound, the patient is asked to return on the fifth to the seventh day for removal of the sutures. When there is some soiling of the superficial parts of the dressing, the gauze on top may be changed, care being taken not to disturb the layers underneath, where there is usually a brownish hard stain of dried blood which acts as an excellent splint for the wound.

When the patient complains of some discomfort in the area of the wound and, on inspection of the bandage, some edema of the tissues is noted, the dressing is removed and the wound is inspected. This state of affairs is usually found in cases in which there has been considerable dissection in the subcutaneous fatty tissues and a low-grade localized cellulitis has resulted. In such cases it is rarely necessary to open the wound, although removal of one or two sutures to relieve tension may be helpful. Experience has shown that this type of wound reaction will subside in 24 to 48 hours if 70 percent alcohol is applied to the dressing, and the patient is instructed to apply this three or four times a day. Simple cleansing with soap and water is often desirable. No ointments are to be used because they tend to macerate the tissues.

At the patient's second visit, on the fifth to the seventh day after operation, the sutures are removed. In cases in which the integrity of the wound may be affected by movement of the part, splints are included as a part of the dressing for a week or so after removal of the sutures. In other cases, adhesive strips may be applied across the wound at right angles to its long axis. These provide continued support to the wound edges and may be left in place for a week or 10 days if desired. They are especially valuable for wounds of the shoulder and back, where the skin is quite thick and motion tends to pull the wound edges apart.

Dressing Infected Wounds. The patient with an infected lesion should be asked to return for dressing on the second day after operation. As a rule, it is unwise to change the dressing on the day follow-

ing operation, as to do so usually sets up renewed bleeding, and the secretions are usually not excessive enough to demand a change of the dressing.

On the second day after operation, the superficial dressings are removed and the wound is inspected with the packing or the drain still in place. The surgeon then decides as to the type of dressing to be applied, and this must be done before the instruments and the dressing tray have become soiled. He should be provided with sufficient cotton balls soaked in hydrogen peroxide to wash away the dried secretions on the edge of the wound and to use as sponges in removing purulent secretions from the wound itself. A few alcohol sponges are useful for a final cleaning of the skin around the wound. If packing is to be replaced, sterile instruments should be reserved for removing packing from its sterile container and for cutting it without contaminating the remainder. Unless the packing in the wound seems to be acting as a plug and preventing drainage of the wound secretions, it is usually wise to leave it in place or to remove it only in part at this dressing because, at this time, a sufficient amount of inflammatory induration has not developed in the walls of the wound to keep its lips from falling together. It should be mentioned in passing that, when gauze packing is adherent to the edges of the wound, considerable pain is produced by pulling it away at this second-day dressing, whereas it usually is easily removed without pain at later renewals of the dressing

After this initial dressing, the interval between future dressings depends to a great extent upon the amount of secretion. If it is profuse, daily dressings are necessary, whereas, if the breakdown of sloughing tissue is slow, dressings may be maintained for 2 or 3 days. Usually, at the second dressing all packing is removed from the wound, and by this time, if an adequate incision has been made, an opening of sufficient size remains. Unless the infected area is deep, there is no necessity for reinserting packing or other drainage material. The inflammatory induration in the walls of the wound will not permit its closure until all the purulent material has been discharged. When the wound is exposed, an effort should be made to remove all the liquid necrotic material and as much of the loosened necrotic tissue as possible.

Two methods are of particular value for the removal of liquid material. The easier and less painful method is the irrigation of the wound with warm sterile saline solution. The glass syringes with rubber bulbs or the disposable sterile plastic bulb syringes have been found to be most useful; either type can be handled with one hand, and the force of the stream can be regulated so that the solution may be forced with good pressure into the deeper recesses of the wound cavity. This method of cleaning the wound is of particular value when the wound is deep and when there is considerable sloughing fascia and connective tissue. Hanging a bottle of sterile saline and connecting an intravenous tube to it provides copious gentle irrigation. Large bottles of solutions for irrigation are now available commercially; these contain up to 2 liters apiece. In surface infections, the liquid secretion and the slough may be removed by mopping the wound surface gently with a cotton sponge moistened with saline or hydrogen peroxide. Once the wound and the surrounding tissues have been cleaned of purulent material, areas of sloughing tissue that has not yet liquefied may be seen. Often these areas may be loosened gently by applying slight tension with forceps; or they may be cut away carefully with scissors from the surviving tissue adjacent to them. If the sloughs are not loose, it is better to leave them alone until the next dressing rather than to run the risk of causing the patient pain and of setting up bleeding.

When the wound and the surrounding tissues have been cleared of purulent secretions, it is often well to bathe the skin around the wound with 70 percent alcohol on a cotton sponge. This may prevent the infection of the hair follicles in the adjacent skin and the furunculosis which not infrequently occur. When the

secretion is profuse, an excoriation of the surrounding skin may develop. This is treated by applying a small amount of zinc oxide ointment after the skin has been thoroughly cleaned with 70 percent alcohol.

Dressings are continued daily or every other day as long as there is much drainage from the wound. Moistening the dressings prevents crusting and permits the escape of the wound secretions. It should be borne in mind, however, that the best results are obtained and maceration of the skin is avoided by permitting the dressing to dry at frequent intervals, so that after the fourth or fifth day the dressings need be moistened only once or twice a day.

As soon as all the slough has disappeared and the wound has become covered with a base of granulation tissue, an effort may be made to hasten the closure of the wound by pulling its lips together with adhesive straps. Generally, this is necessary only in cases in which there has been considerable skin slough, as, for instance, following incision and drainage of a carbuncle. In a few such cases, epithelization may be hastened by the application of pinch skin grafts. These can be taken under local anesthesia in the office and placed on the granulating bed.

HOT WET DRESSINGS

In the treatment of inflammatory lesions, hot moist dressings are applied both before and after incision. The requirements of a wet dressing are that it can be kept warm for a considerable period and that it be one from which drying may take place. In addition, because the patient is ambulatory, some provision must be made to protect his clothing with waxed paper, Saran Wrap, or cellophane, which are most useful. Special attention must be paid to the security of the dressing. In almost all hot moist dressings of the extremities, a splint or some other form of immobilization is employed to keep the part at rest. The inflammatory lesion is overlaid with several gauze compresses. These are applied dry and are so

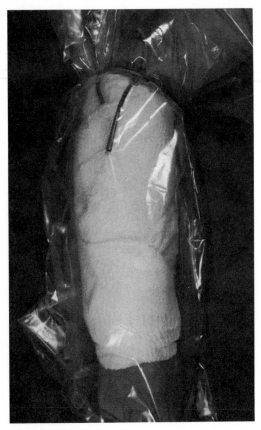

Fig. 4–1. Hot wet dressing technique for extremities.

placed and built up over the wound as to provide a large dressing of gauze, fully ¹/₂ inch thick at its center, which spreads for a considerable distance on all sides of the infected wound. In order to keep the moisture and heat from escaping, a protection of 1 or 2 layers of crumpled waxed paper, cellophane, or Saran Wrap is then applied over the compress. A disposable plastic trash-can liner makes an excellent outer cover (Fig. 4-1). In some cases a plastic tube or a rubber catheter, through which solutions may be added, is placed between the gauze layers and is brought out to the surface above the protective covering. The whole is then securely wrapped with a gauze bandage. Finally, the securing strips of adhesive are applied in circles, so that the end of each strip lies on adhesive. When the dressing is applied

to the hand or the forearm, a sling is provided. The patient is then instructed to moisten the gauze compress with a designated solution. This is best done with a small rubber ear syringe, the nozzle of which is inserted at one end of the bandage while the part is so held that the solution will moisten the gauze compress by gravity and by capillary attraction. When a plastic tube is used, the solution may be introduced through it. This directs the solution onto the gauze compresses, and, as a rule, a smaller amount of solution may be used because there is no doubt about its getting to the right place. Dressings do not need to be moistened oftener than 3 or 4 times a day.

When hot wet dressings are to be applied to large areas, as, for instance, in the treatment of a lymphangitis of the arm, and when there is no open wound, it is often possible to use nonsterile materials, such as absorbent cotton or surgical lint. These two materials make excellent large absorbent applications. The arm is flexed at a right angle, and the entire arm, from hand to shoulder, is covered with the cotton or lint and then with crumpled waxed paper or with Saran Wrap, which in turn is held in place by bandages. In such cases, openings may be left in the waxed paper and marked on the surface of the bandage; through these the patient later may moisten the dressing at intervals.

DRESSINGS FOR INDIVIDUAL PARTS

Finger and Toe. For dressings of the fingertip, as, for instance, following an incision and drainage of an infection of the distal closed space, the 3-inch gauze compress is cut as shown in Figure 4-2. The loose ends are then folded over the fingertip, and the dressing is completed with circular turns of a bandage about the gauze and recurrent turns over the tip of the finger; the latter are finally held in place by additional circular turns. The bandage is then anchored with a longitudinal adhesive strip held in place by circular anchoring strips. In many cases it

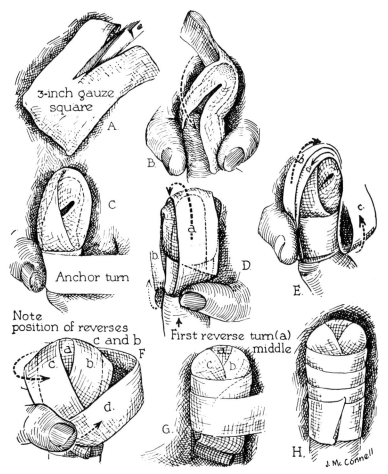

Fig. 4–2. Dressing for the finger.

is advisable to apply a hairpin or opened-paper-clip splint as extra protection. (Fig. 4-3).

In the case of lesions at the base of the finger, as, for instance, a furuncle of the proximal phalanx, there is frequently a considerable amount of associated cellulitis and edema over the dorsum of the hand. In these cases, it is well to apply a splint that includes the adjacent finger. The splint which has been found to be most useful is the swab-stick-adhesive splint (Fig. 4-4). This is applied with 2 or 3 circular turns of adhesive which include the sterile gauze over the lesion. More gauze is then applied as indicated, and the whole is held in place by a 1-inch bandage wrapped about the palm and the proximal fingers. Circular turns of 1/2-inch adhesive anchor the dressing.

Dressings for the toe are applied in the same manner as that described for the finger.

The Hand. Dressings for the palm and the dorsum of the hand are best applied with 2-inch bandage and must be anchored by figure-of-eight turns around the hand and the wrist (Fig. 4-5). The new but somewhat expensive, loose-weave bandages are extremely useful for bandaging irregularly shaped regions of the body. When a splint is used with this dressing, it should be long enough to include the entire length of the fingers

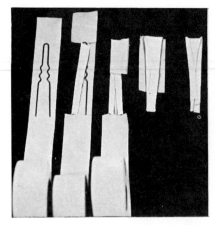 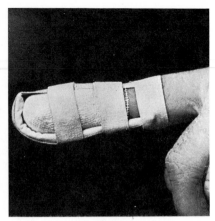

Fig. 4–3. (*Left*) Hairpin splint. This splint is easily available and useful in immobilizing fingers. It is small, compact, and molds readily to the part. (*Right*) Hairpin splint applied to the finger. The splint is molded to fit over the finger dressing, covering the palmar surface of the finger and the fingertip. It is held in place with a longitudinal strip of adhesive, which begins and ends on the skin and is anchored by 3 circular turns of adhesive applied in such a way that the ends lie on adhesive. In this way, the dressing may be soaked without fear of its coming loose. (Ferguson, L. K.: Penn. Med. J., *40*:909, 1937).

and to extend upward beyond the mid-forearm. Padding should be provided in the palm to allow the fingers to lie comfortably in partial flexion.

The Forearm. Dressings for the forearm are held in place with 2-inch gauze bandage applied in spiral and spiral-reverse turns. The bandage should be anchored by diagonal strips of ½-inch adhesive applied to the skin above and below the bandage; these in turn are fixed by circular turns of ½-inch adhesive (Fig. 4-6).

The Elbow. For dressings at the elbow, large gauze compresses are used, usually 4 x 8 inches in size. With the elbow flexed at a right angle, these are anchored by a circular turn or two of 2-inch bandage on the forearm side. The bandage is then applied in figure-of-eight turns, one loop above and one below the elbow, until the area is covered. Longitudinal anchoring strips of ½-inch adhesive are applied to the skin above and below the bandage, and circular fixation turns are used to hold these in place (Fig. 4-7).

The Upper Arm. Dressings here are applied in the same way as they are to the

forearm, except that in this area reverse turns are less often necessary.

The Axilla. Dressings are most often applied to this area for superficial infections or abscesses. After a sufficient amount of gauze has been used to cover the wound, one large piece of gauze should be spread out to cover the entire underlying dressing and to extend for a distance of about 3 or 4 inches downward along the lateral chest wall and for the same distance along the inner side of the upper arm. A strip of 1-inch adhesive is then placed across the middle of the gauze in the uppermost part of the axilla; the adhesive should be long enough so that the cut ends reach over the top of the shoulder (Fig. 4-8). The arm is then placed down against the side of the chest wall, and the adhesive is attached to the skin in front and back, one end overlying the other over the acromion. The arm then is raised, and a second strip of adhesive is applied over the gauze and fixed front and back over the chest wall. A third strip is applied in the same manner over the gauze and around the upper arm.

The Shoulder. A spica bandage is used

A   B   C

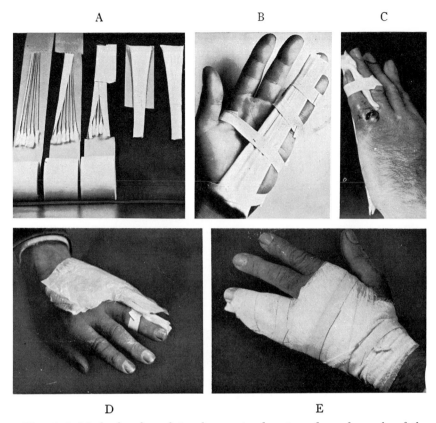

D   E

Fig. 4–4. Methods of applying hot moist dressings for a furuncle of the dorsal surface of the proximal phalanx. The swab-stick splint (*A*) is made and is applied to the hand with adhesive (*B*). The fingers are separated with gauze (*C*); sterile gauze dressings are applied and overlaid with waxed paper (*D*), and the entire dressing then is enclosed in gauze bandage held in place with adhesive circles (*E*). (Ferguson, L. K.: Penn. Med. J., *40*:909, 1937)

occasionally for the application of dressings to the top of the shoulder and the upper chest. It is applied in what amount to figure-of-eight turns, beginning in the axilla of the normal side and coming up across the anterior portion of the chest and the shoulder and around the arm from behind forward. Sometimes a circular turn is made around the arm in the first lap of bandage and then the roll is carried across the back to its original starting place in the sound axilla. These turns are repeated, crossing each other higher and higher on the shoulder, each succeeding turn overlapping about one half of the previous one, until sufficient turns have been applied to cover the de-

sired area. A 3-inch gauze bandage or Kerlix gauze is best for this purpose. The spica is fixed with 1-inch adhesive strips (Fig. 4-9).

The Neck. Dressings are most often applied to this area for furuncles or carbuncles at the back of the neck or for abscesses of the cervical glands in the anterior neck. After the application of a sufficient number of gauze compresses, the dressing is held in place by circular turns of 2-inch gauze bandage; Kerlix gauze is extremely helpful. This dressing cannot be applied well with the patient lying down. Therefore, when it is to be applied immediately after operation, it is best to hold the dressing in place until the

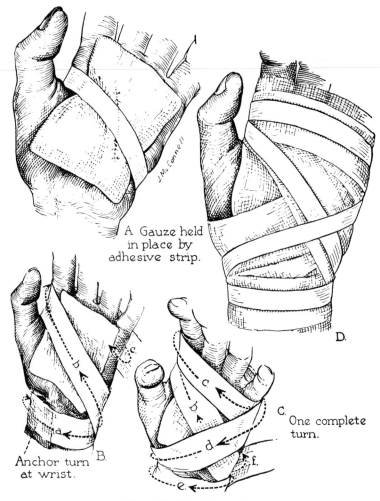

A. Gauze held in place by adhesive strip.

B. Anchor turn at wrist.

C. One complete turn.

D.

Fig. 4–5. Hand dressing.

patient has recovered sufficiently from the anesthetic and can sit up. The dressing is usually wider at the site of the lesion than it is at other portions of the circumference of the neck, and the bandage should be so applied at this area as to cover completely and to hold in the top and the bottom of the gauze compresses. The bandage is anchored in place by ½-inch adhesive strips. Experience has shown that it is more secure if the adhesive strips are applied first at the site of the lesion, at the top and the bottom of the bandage, and in such a manner as to form an ellipse; the ends are then covered by a circular strip

of adhesive applied over the middle of the bandage. (Fig. 4-10). After such a dressing has been applied, it should be inspected carefully to make sure that it is not tight enough to cause compression of the veins of the neck, with resulting venostasis of the face and the head. Occasionally it is necessary to snip the bandage a little in several places to relieve this compression.

The Lower Face and the Jaw. As a rule, ordinary dressings of the face and the jaw may be applied with gauze and adhesive, or a spray adhesive may be applied. In some instances, however, and especially

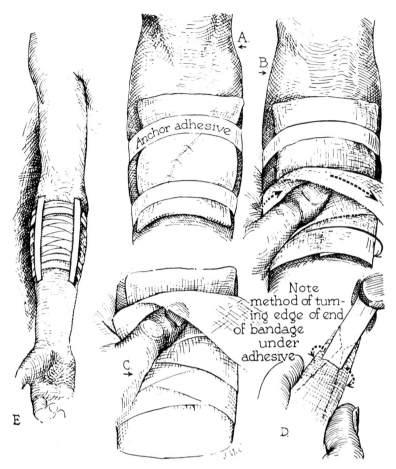

Fig. 4–6. Forearm bandage dressing.

following trauma or operation, a dressing must be held in place with bandage for compression or for the application of hot wet dressings. In these cases, the use of loose-knit roller dressing is ideal (Fig. 4-11).

The Back of the Neck and the Head. Dressings of the back of the neck and the lower scalp are held in place best by figure-of-eight turns around the head and the neck. The bandage is started at the back of the neck, carried forward around the head and above the ears to its starting place, thence around the neck and back again to its beginning. Several such turns are applied to cover the compress. The bandage is strengthened by a figure-of-eight turn of ½-inch adhesive applied over it (Fig. 4-12).

The Scalp. Most traumatic or operative wounds of the scalp may be treated by the application of a spray adhesive dressing. When the ooze has been controlled by digital or palmar pressure, the wound is sprayed with the adhesive. A small amount of fluff cotton is then applied over the wound while the adhesive is still moist, and the cotton is moistened with additional spray. This dries rapidly, and, as a rule, no further dressing need be applied. Occasionally, there is a slight ooze, which may be absorbed by the application of a small amount of gauze over the wound for a short time.

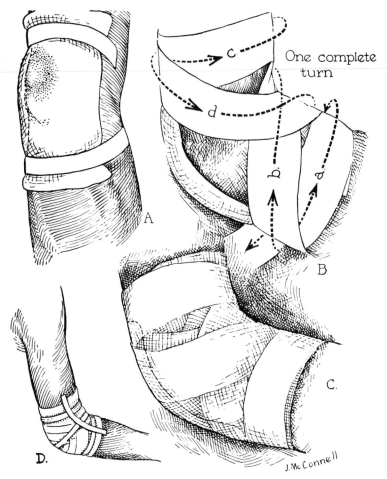

Fig. 4–7. Method of applying a dressing and bandage at the elbow.

When there is considerable secretion from an infected wound, or hemorrhage demanding pressure, a skullcap dressing is most satisfactory. Gauze compresses are placed over the lesions, and the entire skull is then covered by two of the 4 x 8 gauze compresses, which have been unfolded so as to make a double layer of gauze about 8 x 8 inches. These pieces of gauze are held tightly over the scalp by an assistant while the surgeon applies 2 or 3 circular turns of 3-inch or 4-inch loose-weave gauze bandage snugly around the scalp below the occiput and well down over the forehead (Fig. 4-13). When the gauze has thus been anchored, it is pulled down snugly in all directions, so as to provide pressure over the gauze compress and the lesion. The edges of the gauze are then turned upward and are included in additional circles of bandage, some turns of which extend well down behind the occiput and high on the forehead, while others extend low on the forehead and high on the occiput. Half-inch strips of adhesive are then applied over the gauze across the head from before backward and from side to side. Finally, two anchoring circles of ½-inch adhesive are applied, the first extending well down

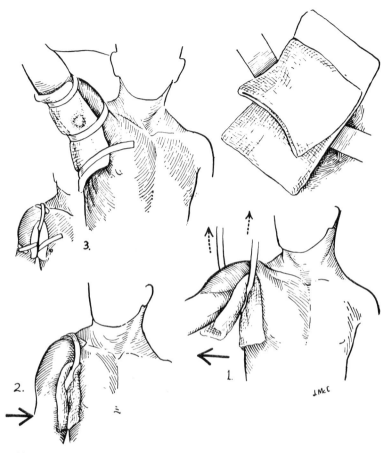

Fig. 4–8. Method of applying a dressing to the axilla, using adhesive.

behind the occiput and high over the forehead and the second passing across the forehead at the lowermost part of the bandage and high up on the occiput. This dressing will be found to give excellent compression and will remain securely in place for 5 or 6 days if necessary.

The Breast. These dressings are most often applied for inflammatory lesions, either before or after incision. Gauze compresses are placed over the lesion and are held in place with transverse circles of 3-inch loose-weave gauze bandage. The transverse turns of the bandage are so placed that they lie above and below the breast. As a rule, those turns lying above the involved breast are pulled downward so that they lie below the opposite breast, and those which are applied below the involved breast cross the chest in an upward direction to lie above the normal breast. In effect, the bandage is therefore a cross bandage of the breast. Circular strips of adhesive and, occasionally, longitudinal ones are also applied (Fig. 4-14). This bandage must be applied with the patient in the sitting or standing position.

The Groin. A spica bandage of the groin is usually applied to provide pressure or to hold compresses in place. Here the loose-weave roller gauze such as Kerlix or Kling, is a great help. It is begun with a circular turn around the upper

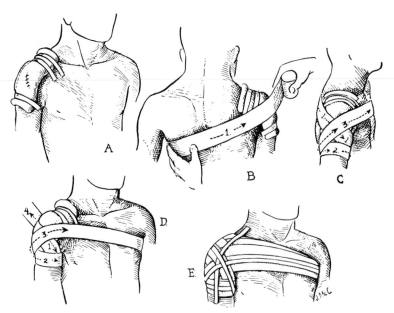

Fig. 4–9. Application of a dressing to the shoulder, showing the use of the spica bandage of the shoulder.

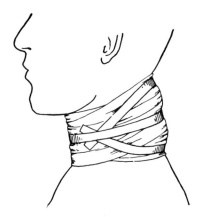

Fig. 4–10. Neck dressing. Note method of applying adhesive strips.

thigh and is best applied with the patient standing and holding the legs spread slightly apart. After the first circular, or anchoring, turn, the bandage is carried upward across the groin and the lower abdomen. A circular turn is then made round the low back and downward across the groin to the thigh. This constitutes one turn of the bandage; several such turns are applied, and the bandage is anchored with a similar turn of $\frac{1}{2}$-inch or 1-inch adhesive (Fig. 4-15).

If elastic adhesive is used, a groin dressing is more easily applied as follows: after the compress has been fixed with 1 or 2 strips of adhesive, the elastic adhesive is started below and lateral to the anterior spine of the iliac crest and is carried down parallel to and below Poupart's ligament and around the thigh to finish on the original turn. The ends of the bandage are fixed with strips of 1-inch adhesive to prevent rolling (Fig. 4-16).

The Thigh and the Leg. When dressings are to be applied to these conical parts, it is usually wise to fix the compresses in place with 1 or 2 transverse strips of 1-inch adhesive. Then the bandage is applied in spiral and then spiral-reverse turns until the compress is covered sufficiently. Two longitudinal strips of adhesive fix the bandage to the skin above and below, and the whole is

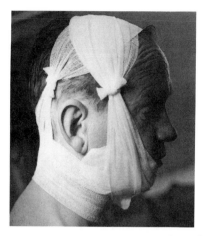

Fig. 4–11. Barton type bandage for lesions of the jaw. Note method of tightening bandage with ties of gauze.

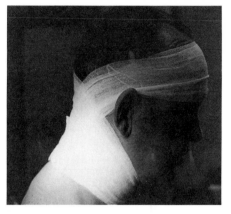

Fig. 4–12. A figure-of-eight bandage for neck and back of the head and forehead.

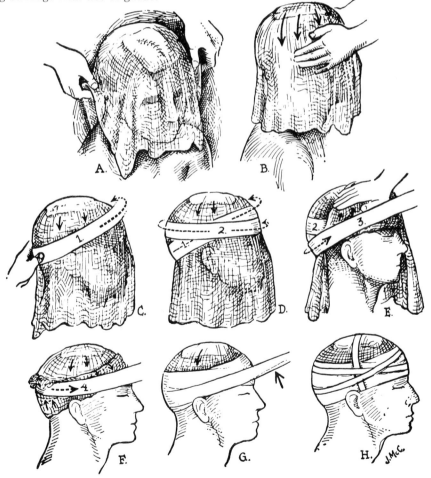

Fig. 4–13. Steps in the preparation of a Frazier head dressing for lesions of the scalp.

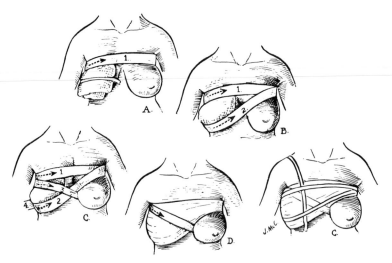

Fig. 4–14. Method of applying a bandage to the breast.

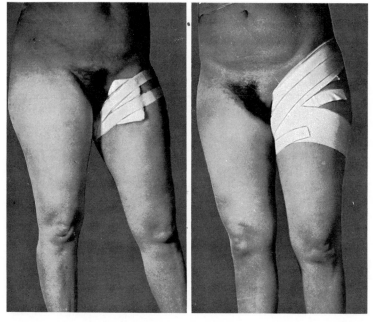

Fig. 4–16. Method of applying a dressing to the groin using elastic adhesive. This gives firm compression and does not necessitate a bandage round the abdomen; therefore, it is more convenient and is especially serviceable following ligations of varicose saphenous veins.

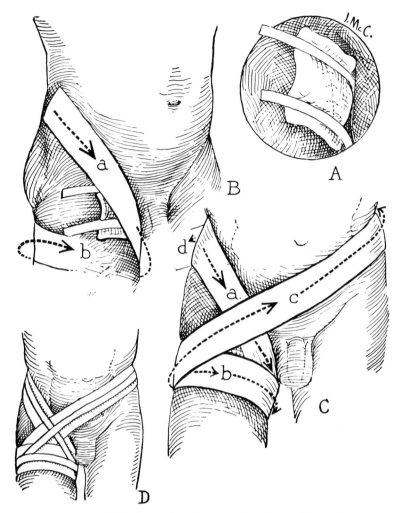

Fig. 4–15. Method of applying a dressing to the groin.

held in place by 2 or 3 fixation circles of 1/2-inch or 1-inch adhesive. When the lesion is anterior, in placing the adhesive circles on a conical part, the adhesive should be stretched and applied to the back of the part first. The cut ends are then brought round the part; to lie flat they must ascend slightly. Dressings are applied to the opposite side of the part, in a similar manner. Three-inch bandage is best for the thigh, and 2-inch is best for the leg.

The Ankle and the Foot. Bandages for the ankle and the foot are most conveniently applied in figure-of-eight turns around the foot and the ankle. Two-inch bandage is usually used, with fixation by 1/2-inch adhesive (Figs. 4-17 and 4-18).

The Perineum. It is difficult to hold perineal dressings in place with adhesive. The best is composed of one sterile gauze pad over the wound, held in place by the ordinary sanitary pad (Kotex). The elastic sanitary belt is easily available to secure

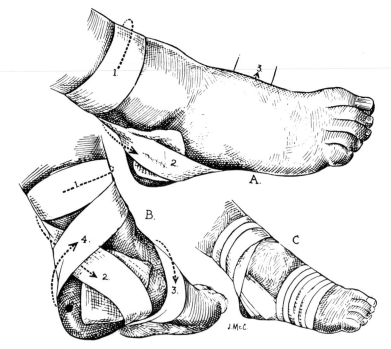

Fig. 4–17. Method of applying a dressing to the heel.

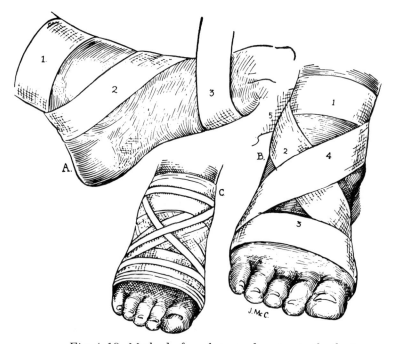

Fig. 4–18. Method of applying a dressing to the foot.

Fig. 4–19. Fuller Shield. A protective pouch designed to hold anal, perianal, and sacral dressings in place without binding and without adhesive. It may be used in male or female patients. (Fuller Pharmaceutical Co.)

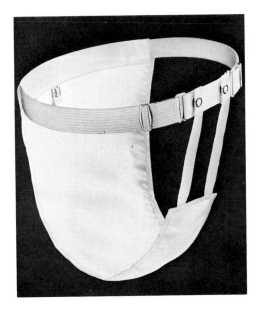

the sanitary pad. The sanitary belt that may be applied with a snap is the most convenient type.

There is also available a protective dressing designed especially to hold anal, perianal, and sacral dressings in place without the use of adhesive tape. It is rubberized to prevent soiling and is held in place by an adhesive adjustable waistband (Fig. 4-19).

5

Open Wounds

John B. Herrmann, M.D.

Accidental wounds are one of the most common surgical conditions treated on an ambulatory basis by physicians. Sound surgical judgment and careful attention to proper wound management will result in success in the vast majority of cases, and needless and expensive hospitalization will be avoided. Certain injuries and certain patients, however, require hospital care, and misguided attempts at ambulatory management may result in serious complications. In general, injuries which involve vital structures, such as nerves, tendons, or major vessels, or in which there is penetration of one of the body cavities require hospital care. Evidence or suspicion of such involvement may be apparent on initial examination or may not be apparent until later. In either case, ambulatory management should be abandoned and hospitalization arranged. Patients with complicating diseases, such as diabetes, blood dyscrasias, bleeding disorders, and other major systemic diseases, are generally more safely treated in a hospital. Hospital management of such injuries and patients is beyond the scope of this chapter, but the basic principles of wound care as described here for the ambulatory patient apply equally to the hospitalized patient.

PRINCIPLES OF WOUND CARE

The healing mechanism has a high biologic priority and is almost impossible to stop once it has been initiated by an injury. Thus, the role of the surgeon in wound management is not to effect healing, but to provide an environment in which optimum healing can occur. The primary objective in management is to restore tissue continuity in the least possible time with a minimum of deformity and loss of function.

LOCAL AND SYSTEMIC FACTORS THAT AFFECT THE REPAIR MECHANISMS

The repair mechanism is complex and involves many diverse factors. It is apparent, therefore, that alterations in one or more of these factors may significantly change the rate of healing. Accelerated healing produced by varying some of these factors remains a laboratory phenomenon for the present. On the other hand, a multitude of local and systemic factors which significantly impair clinical healing have been recognized.

The primary local factors which may result in delayed healing are infection and the presence of foreign bodies, devitalized tissue, or dead space in the wound. Every accidental wound contains some bacteria which may result in an infection which will delay healing. Even surgical wounds produced in a "sterile" operating room contain some bacteria that are brought in from the skin during the incision or that settle in the wound from the surrounding air. Whether or not the surgical or accidental wound becomes infected depends upon the number and virulence of the organisms, as well as upon the local condition of the wound and various systemic factors of host resistance. Wound infection remains the single most important factor in delayed healing; therefore the role of the surgeon in the management of traumatic wounds must be strongly directed toward the prevention of infection. Attention must be directed toward removing contaminating organisms from the wound by careful irrigation and cleansing, and toward avoiding inoculation of the wound with virulent organisms by adhering to the principles of strict aseptic technique. Careful attention must be given to the local and systemic factors which predispose to infection and delayed wound repair. Removal of foreign bodies, débridement of devitalized tissue, control of hemorrhage, and careful approximation of tissues to avoid dead space are cardinal principles of local wound management.

The recognition and proper management of regional or systemic conditions may be crucial in the proper overall management of the wound. Deficient regional blood supply, poor tissue perfusion, hypovitaminosis C or A, protein deficiency, severe anemia, uremia, coagulation defects, and the administration of cortisone or immunosuppressive drugs are but a few of the many factors which may adversely affect wound repair and resistance to infection.

METHODS OF WOUND MANAGEMENT

In the management of a traumatic open wound, the surgeon has a number of options available regarding the treatment of the wound. These include *primary closure, delayed primary closure, open treatment,* and *secondary closure.*

The decisions as to which technique should be used in a specific case, and whether or not ancillary measures should be employed, must be based on a thorough knowledge of the repair mechanism. A careful history should be taken, with particular attention to the time of the injury and the causative agent. Close inquiry should be made into those systemic factors which may influence healing. A careful inspection of the wound itself is absolutely necessary. The most important factor in making this decision is the physician's estimate of the risk of infection—a judgment made on the basis of the above information. Repeated reevaluation during the course of healing may dictate a change in method.

Primary Closure. In this technique, the tissues of the wound are carefully approximated after thorough cleansing and débridement of foreign material and devitalized tissue. Most surgical incisions are managed in this fashion, and the technique can be applied to many accidental wounds which are clean and in which the risk of infection is considered small. A variation of this technique is the immediate application of a skin graft to an avulsion injury. Primary healing produces minimal scarring and deformity and the least functional impairment. Because of the dangers of infection in a closed space, primary closure should not be performed when infection is considered to be more than a minimal risk. In the management of accidental wounds, a drain should not be placed in the subcutaneous tissue to allow accumulated blood and serum to escape following primary closure. Careful attention to hemostasis should make its use unnecessary, and the placement of a drain to provide a route for escape of pus should infection occur later indicates poor judgment in the choice of wound management technique. Paradoxically, such a drain may allow bacteria to enter and infect a wound. If the risk of infection is considered high enough to suggest the use of a drain, primary closure should not have been the technique employed.

Delayed Primary Closure. This modification of the primary closure technique is applicable to many dirty wounds. It may be used with excellent results when the degree of contamination or the delay between injury and treatment is such that the risk of infection appears high. It is the standard method adopted by the military for most battlefield injuries. In this technique, the wound is debrided and irrigated as in the primary repair technique, but instead of being closed immediately, the wound is carefully packed open, and a sterile dressing is applied. The wound is inspected daily, using strict sterile precautions. If by the third or fourth day there is no evidence of infection, and the entire wound appears healthy without any necrosis or debris, closure is accomplished. Since closure is accomplished prior to the proliferative phase of healing, no delay in healing is measurable, and repair progresses in the same fashion and with the same benefits as outlined above. If, however, infection or necrotic debris is evident on inspection, the technique of delayed primary closure should be abandoned, and open treatment, as described below, should be employed.

Open Treatment. Open treatment is the method of choice in infected or grossly contaminated wounds and in wounds in which devitalized tissue is known or suspected to be present. It should also be used in wounds which have been closed primarily, but which have later become infected. The technique employed is essentially that of open wound management, and the mechanism of healing is by wound contraction, granulation tissue formation, and epithelialization. Although ultimate results in terms of function and deformity may be quite good,

considerable delay in healing and excess scar tissue formation can be anticipated with this method of wound management.

Secondary Closure. Healing by third intention refers to the mechanism of healing which occurs when an open granulating wound is converted to a closed wound by excision and suture or by skin grafting (secondary closure of the wound). Delayed primary closure is technically a variant of healing by third intention, although if accomplished within the first 4 or 5 days the results are almost indistinguishable from primary healing. If closure is delayed beyond the first week, the walls of the wound become covered with granulation tissue, and the resulting scar is thicker than that formed by a wound closed primarily.

THERAPEUTIC CLASSIFICATION OF OPEN WOUNDS

From the point of view of management, open wounds can be classified as *superficial* or *deep, simple* or *complex*, and *clean* or *dirty*. For therapeutic purposes, this is a far more useful classification than is a descriptive one.

Superficial Wounds are those which involve skin, subcutaneous tissue, fascia, and/or muscle, but do not involve vital deep structures, such as nerve, tendon, blood vessel, bone, or viscera.

Deep Wounds are injuries which involve the deep structures mentioned above or which cause sufficient concern on the part of the physician that deep structures may be involved, even though definite proof of such involvement may not be apparent on physical examination. In the initial evaluation of a wound, a careful assessment of pulses, sensation, and motor function is essential, and a thorough knowledge of anatomy is important. If deep involvement is discovered or strongly suspected, the patient should be hospitalized for further evaluation and treatment and should not be managed on an ambulatory basis. The management of such injuries is beyond the scope of this chapter.

Simple Wounds are those in which there is interruption of tissue continuity but no significant tissue loss or implantation of foreign debris. Cuts, puncture wounds, lacerations, and low velocity penetrating injuries are wounds of this type.

Complex Wounds are those in which there is loss or damage of tissue or which contain foreign debris. Lacerations, avulsions, crush injuries, high velocity injuries, and burns are wounds of this type.

Clean Wounds are those which contain minimal bacterial contamination and which can be expected to heal after primary closure. Considerable judgment on the part of the physician must be employed in classifying a wound as clean. In addition to careful inspection of the wound, factors such as time elapsed since injury, location of the wound, causative agent, local blood supply, and general health of the patient must be considered when making a decision.

Dirty Wounds are those which, in the judgment of the physician, are likely to become infected if closed primarily. The same factors listed above are considered in making this evaluation. It is beyond the scope of this chapter to describe in detail the multiple factors which enter into the decision whether to classify a wound as clean or dirty. Almost all of the factors are relative, and proper evaluation of them is based upon experience, attention to details, and a thorough knowledge of wound healing and infection. At best, however, there is always an element of risk because all of the facts are not usually available. In general, a delay of more than a few hours between injury and treatment predisposes to bacterial multiplication and infection; a contaminated instrument of injury predisposes to infection; impaired local circulation and systemic conditions, such as diabetes, uremia, malnutrition, steroid therapy, etc., predispose to infection.

---

*Reprinted with permission from Bull. Am. Coll. Surgeons, 57:32, DEC. 1972.

GENERAL APPROACH TO THE TRAUMATIC WOUND

The following general steps should be observed in the management of any traumatic wound:

Initial Classification. The initial steps in the management of the wounded patient include a pertinent history and physical examination. The circumstances of the injury, the injuring agent, the time of injury, and any first-aid treatment given should be carefully noted. Associated symptoms and other pertinent medical data, such as tetanus immunization, allergies to drugs, and other medical diseases, should be recorded. A careful examination of motor and sensory function and arterial pulses distal to the wound should be made. Examination of the wound itself should be carried out under sterile precautions; and, after initial inspection, the wound should be covered with a sterile gauze bandage. Based upon this examination, a tentative classification of the wound (superficial vs. deep, simple vs. complex, and clean vs. dirty) can be made. Wounds suspected or proven to be other than superficial should be managed in a hospital without further delay. Classification at this point must be considered tentative because additional factors may become apparent during the course of surgical exploration.

Tetanus Prophylaxis. This is an extremely important and necessary step. The status of the patient's immunity to tetanus should be established, and appropriate procedures to prevent this dread complication instituted according to the procedures outlined by the American College of Surgeons' Committee on Trauma.

A Guide to Prophylaxis Against Tetanus in Wound Management*

GENERAL PRINCIPLES

1. The attending physician must determine for each patient with a wound, individually, what is required for adequate prophylaxis against tetanus.

2. Regardless of the active immunization status of the patient, meticulous surgical care, including removal of all devitalized tissue and foreign bodies, should be provided immediately for all wounds. Such care is essential as part of the prophylaxis against tetanus.

3. Each patient with a wound should receive adsorbed tetanus toxoid† intramuscularly at the time of injury, either as an initial immunizing dose, or as a booster for previous immunization, unless he has received a booster or has completed his initial immunization series within the past 5 years. As the antigen concentration varies in different products, specific information on the volume of a single dose is provided on the label of the package.

4. Whether or not to provide passive immunization with tetanus immune globulin (human) must be decided individually for each patient. The characteristics of the wound, conditions under which it was incurred, its treatment, its age, and the previous active immunization status of the patient must be considered.

5. To every wounded patient give a written record of the immunization provided, instructing him to carry the record at all times and, if indicated, to complete active immunization. For precise tetanus prophylaxis, an accurate and immediately available history regarding previous active immunization against tetanus is required.

6. Basic immunization with adsorbed tetanus toxoid requires three injections. A booster of adsorbed tetanus toxoid is indicated 10‡ years after the third injection or 10‡ years after an intervening wound booster. All individuals, including pregnant women, should have basic immunization and indicated booster injections.

SPECIFIC MEASURES FOR PATIENTS WITH WOUNDS

For Previously Immunized Individuals

A. When the patient has been actively immunized within the past 10‡ years:

1. To the great majority give 0.5 cc. of adsorbed tetanus toxoid† as a booster unless it is certain that the patient has received a booster within the previous 5 years.

2. To those with severe, neglected, or old (more than 24 hours) tetanus-prone wounds, give 0.5 cc. of adsorbed tetanus toxoid† unless it is certain that the patient has received a booster within the previous year.

B. When the patient has been actively immunized more than 10‡ years previously:

1. To the great majority, give 0.5 cc. of adsorbed tetanus toxoid.†

2. To those with severe, neglected, or old (more than 24 hours) tetanus-prone wounds:

    a) Give 0.5 cc. of adsorbed tetanus toxoid,†#

    b) Give 250 units§ of tetanus immune globulin (human),#

    c) Consider providing oxytetracycline or penicillin.

For Individuals NOT Previously Immunized

A. With clean minor wounds in which tetanus is most unlikely, give 0.5 cc. of adsorbed tetanus toxoid† (initial immunizing dose).

---

†The Public Health Service Advisory Committee on Immunization Practices in 1972 recommended DTP (diphtheria and tetanus toxoids combined with pertussis vaccine) for basic immunization in infants and children from two months through the sixth year of age and Td (combined tetanus and diphtheria toxoids: adult type) for basic immunization of those over six years of age. For the latter group, Td toxoid was recommended for routine or wound boosters; but, if there is any reason to suspect hypersensitivity to the diphtheria component, tetanus toxoid (T) should be substituted for Td. (Morbidity and Mortality Weekly Report. Vol. 21, No. 25, National Communicable Disease Center).

---

‡Some authorities advise 6 rather than 10 years, particularly for patients with severe, neglected, or old (more than 24 hours) tetanus-prone wounds.

#Use different syringes, needles, and sites of injection.

---

§In severe, neglected, or old (more than 24 hours) tetanus-prone wounds, 500 units of tetanus immune globulin (human) are advisable.

B. With all other wounds:
1. Give 0.5 cc. of adsorbed tetanus toxoid† (initial immunizing dose),#
2. Give 250 units§ of tetanus immune globulin (human),#
3. Consider providing oxytetracycline or penicillin.

Precautions regarding passive immunization with tetanus antitoxin (equine):

If the patient is not sensitive to tetanus antitoxin (equine), and if the decision is made to administer it for passive immunization, give at least 3,000 units.

Do not administer tetanus antitoxin (equine) except when tetanus immune globulin (human) is not available within 24 hours, and only if the possibility of tetanus outweighs the danger of reaction to heterologous tetanus antitoxin.

Before using tetanus antitoxin (equine), question the patient for a history of allergy and test for sensitivity. If the patient is sensitive to tetanus antitoxin (equine), do not use it, as the danger of anaphylaxis probably outweighs the danger of tetanus; rely on penicillin or oxytetracycline. Do not attempt desensitization, as it is not worthwhile.

NOTE: With different preparations of toxoid, the volume of a single booster dose should be modified as stated on the package label.

Local Preparation. The area surrounding the wound should be cleansed and possibly shaved. Any of the mild antiseptic soaps and skin prep solutions are satisfactory for this purpose. Harsh germicides and solutions containing alcohol should be avoided because of irritation and possible tissue damage. Routine shaving is a ritual which has limited merit under most circumstances and need not be religiously adhered to except to facilitate care of the wound in hirsute areas. The eyebrow should never be shaved because of the possible failure of proper regrowth.

Anesthesia. Adequate anesthesia can be obtained by infiltration of procaine, lidocaine, or another suitable anesthetic into the wound margins. The same agents can be used to obtain a field block of the area or a regional nerve block. Regional blocks are of considerable value in the management of traumatic wounds, particularly of the upper extremity and face, because the danger of spreading contamination from the wound to surrounding tissue is eliminated. Experience and skill in their use, however, is required, and sufficient time must be allowed for the block to become fully effective. General sedation and administration of analgesics may be indicated in certain patients, but general anesthesia is seldom necessary. When it is, it should be administered in a hospital under the supervision of a competent professional.

Initial Cleansing of the Wound. After achieving adequate anesthesia, the wound should be thoroughly cleansed and irrigated to remove loose foreign material, blood clots, and bacteria. Foreign bodies in a wound hinder the normal process of wound repair. These may be driven into the wound at the time of injury, as, for instance, splinters, dust, grease, or soil; or they may result from the injury, that is, clots of blood. The early removal of these foreign materials permits wound repair to take place normally without interference.

Removal of contaminating bacteria and foreign bodies is best accomplished by mechanical means. Thorough irrigation with an irrigating syringe or irrigating set and the use of sterile gauze sponges to gently cleanse the tissues are helpful.

Antiseptics are not used in the effort to remove contaminating bacteria from a wound. Any antiseptic capable of killing organisms also kills tissue, a factor which should not be added when tissues are already devitalized. The highly colored antiseptics are especially bad because they mask the color and the condition of the tissues.

Hemostasis. Cleaning and irrigating the wound will often result in bleeding which was formerly controlled by blood clot. Major bleeding points should be controlled by individually ligating vessels, using fine hemostats and fine absorbable sutures. A mass of ligatures should

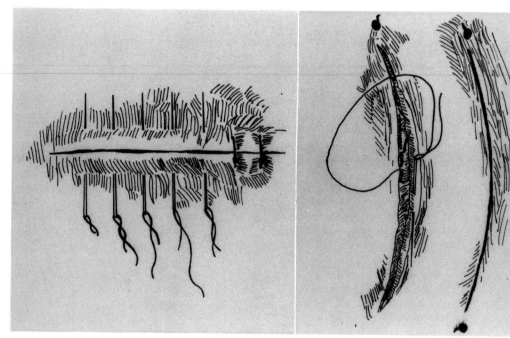

Fig. 5–1. Closure of a simple clean wound with interrupted sutures of fine silk or synthetic material. (Multiple needles are for purpose of emphasis on spacing.)

Fig. 5–2. Closure of a simple wound by a subcuticular stitch. (Note small lead shot used at each end rather than tying the suture.)

be avoided. The temporary control of bleeding necessary to locate the specific injured vessel can usually be obtained in an extremity by compression of proximal blood supply by an assistant. Tourniquets are rarely necessary and should be used with caution. Minor bleeding and oozing can be controlled by pressure and should not require multiple ligatures. It must be remembered that all suture material, absorbable and nonabsorbable, left in a wound acts as a foreign body and may promote infection and delay healing.

Débridement. At this point a careful search should be made for any foreign bodies and dead or devitalized tissue. All such materials should be removed as thoroughly and completely as possible. Jagged skin edges can be excised, but extensive débridement of skin is not normally indicated. Subcutaneous tissue,

fascia, and muscle, however, should be more widely debrided if there is a question of damage or devitalization. In certain unusual or extensive wounds, complete débridement of questionable tissue would result in severe deformity or functional disability. Sound judgment would dictate a more conservative approach relying on natural body defenses and repeated surgical débridement to minimize tissue loss.

Final Irrigation. The wound should be thoroughly irrigated with large amounts of sterile saline. This procedure is effective in reducing the numbers of contaminating bacteria present in the wound. It is also effective in removing debris too minute to be removed effectively by other means.

Final Classification. The initial classification of the wound should be confirmed or revised at this time. Further wound management will depend on an accurate classification at this stage.

MANAGEMENT OF SPECIFIC WOUNDS

After the initial steps in wound management listed above have been accomplished, a decision must be made as to whether or not immediate wound closure should be attempted. An accurate classification of the wound is helpful in reaching this decision.

Simple Clean Wounds. Primary closure is the obvious treatment of choice. This is accomplished by careful approximation of tissue layers, including skin, by fine interrupted sutures (Fig. 5-1). Nonabsorbable sutures of silk, cotton, or Dacron may be used because the risk of infection is minimal. Many surgeons prefer absorbable materials in deep layers because of occasional extrusion of nonabsorbable sutures after healing has occurred. The recently introduced polyglycolic acid absorbable suture is ideal for this purpose because it does not evoke the inflammatory reaction associated with the resorption of catgut. Skin sutures are removed anywhere from two days to two weeks later, depending on the location and the condition of the wound. Early removal (2 to 5 days) from the face and neck, is recommended, and, from the lower extremity and back, delayed removal (10 to 14 days). In other areas, sutures may be removed in about a week, but the final decision must be made after careful inspection of the individual wound. In many cases, skin sutures are neither necessary nor desirable, since a certain amount of extra scarring is always associated with their use. Alternatives include approximation of skin edges with a subcuticular running suture (Fig. 5-2), the use of sterile adhesive strips (Fig. 5-3), or the suturing together of adhesive strips which have been applied to the lips of the wound (Fig. 5-4). These last two methods cannot be used when there is any tension on the wound, and the wound must be protected from strain and motion during the healing phase. Tincture of benzoin applied to the skin is helpful in preventing premature separation of the tape. In many simple cuts, the use of these techniques can effect closure without the necessity of using local anesthesia. This avoids the "needles" and

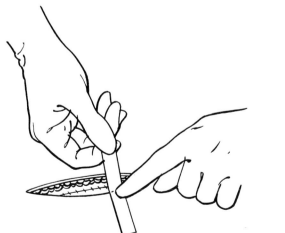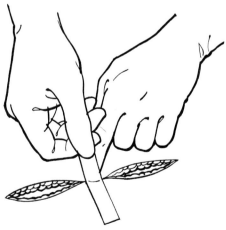

Fig. 5–3. Method of applying Steri-strip adhesive for wound closure. The strip is applied first on the skin on one side of the wound (*left*) and the edges of the wound approximated as the strip is carried across the wound and fixed to the skin of the opposite side. As many strips are used as is necessary to close the wound. (Minnesota Mining & Manufacturing Co.)

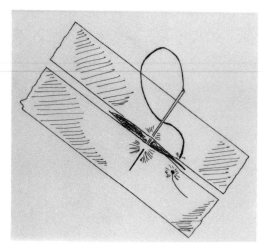

Fig. 5–4. In small wounds approximation of the edges can be secured by first placing two strips of tape along the edge of the wound and then sewing the tape together. A painless method.

"stitches" which are so frightening to children. Care must be taken, however, not to neglect the basic essentials of care, such as hemostasis and thorough cleansing of the wound.

Simple stab wounds can be closed by primary suture provided that hemostasis is not a problem and that injury to deep vital structures has been ruled out. A soft rubber catheter attached to an irrigating syringe is helpful in irrigating the wound.

Complex Clean Wounds. Primary closure is the treatment of choice if tissue loss has not been too great and tissue layers can be approximated without tension. Care must be taken to avoid dead space, which may be more of a problem in complex than in simple wounds. Primary split-thickness skin grafts should be used if skin closure cannot be obtained. These can be obtained freehand, using a sterile disposable razor or prep blade or one of the new battery-operated dermatomes with disposable heads (Davol). Pedicle grafts and other plastic procedures are usually best deferred until after initial healing has occurred.

Simple Dirty Wounds. Primary closure should be avoided in these wounds because of the increased risk of infection.

Delayed primary closure is the method of choice. After thorough cleansing, débridement, and irrigation, a culture is taken, and the wound is left open and is covered with a layer of sterile fine mesh gauze. A bulky occlusive dressing is applied and is changed daily, with thorough inspection of the wound using strict aseptic technique. If no evidence of infection is present by the third or fourth day, the wound is closed in the same fashion as described for the simple clean wound. If evidence of infection is found, the wound should be cultured and treated as an open infected wound. Secondary closure can often be accomplished after the infection has been cleared by treatment with wet dressings and systemic antibiotics selected on the basis of the initial and subsequent cultures. Some evidence exists that local antibiotics and antiseptics are of help in clearing the infection and aid the healing process by lowering bacterial concentrations on the surface of the wound. The local use of antibiotics that are normally used systemically should be avoided because of possible sensitivity reactions and emergence of resistant strains of bacteria. Mild hypochlorite solution (Dakin's solution) is probably as effective and certainly far less expensive than other agents.

Complex Dirty Wounds. A wide variety of wounds, from abrasions containing ground-in foreign material to gunshot injuries, fall into this category. Some of the injuries tax the surgeon's skill and experience to the ultimate. Careful attention to the basic elements of initial wound management is important, but judgement may dictate modifications necessary for ultimate functional restoration. Extensive injuries with incompletely defined areas of devitalization may well indicate staged conservative débridement in an effort to conserve tissue and protect vital structures beneath. Multiple wounds from shotgun pellets are best treated conservatively, removing only those pellets which are superficial and easy to reach. Likewise, low velocity bullet injuries are treated without undue efforts to remove the bullet unless it is near the surface or in the vicinity of a vital structure. High velocity bullet injuries and close range shotgun blasts require extensive débridement because of the blast injury to surrounding tissue as it absorbs the kinetic energy of the missiles. One of the most difficult problems encountered in débridement is the determination of viability of muscle. Contractibility when pinched with forceps and bleeding when cut are the two most important signs indicating viability.

ADJUNCTIVE MEASURES IN WOUND MANAGEMENT

Dressings, Bandages, and Splints. Sound wound management in the ambulatory patient includes the proper use of dressings, bandages, and splints. A simple dry dressing of sterile gauze held in place by adhesive tape is suitable for most simple wounds treated by primary closure. The primary purpose of such a dressing is protection of the wound, and therefore it must be securely fastened so that it will not become displaced before the next visit to the doctor. In addition, it will absorb any oozing from the wound and will serve to splint the area to some degree. A nonadherent layer of Telfa gauze, Adaptic gauze, or Vaseline gauze should be used next to the wound in cases of abrasions and fresh skin grafts. A bulky dressing should then be applied to absorb exudate. Fine mesh gauze is used next to exposed tissue in preparation for delayed primary closure, with an overlying protective and absorptive bulky dressing.

Wet dressings are used primarily in the management of open wounds, particularly if inflammation is present. In order to be maximally effective, they must be changed at least four times per day. Most patients and their families can be instructed to use the proper aseptic technique necessary for ambulatory management. Sterile saline (2 teaspoonfuls of table salt in 1 quart of water boiled for 15 minutes) is the simplest and safest solution. Dakin's solution is useful when débridement of patchy areas of necrotic tissue is necessary, but the solution

should be diluted and the skin edges protected with Vaseline gauze if any irritation occurs. For maximum débridement effect, dressings should be applied wet and removed without remoistening. If débridement is not necessary, remoistening prior to a dressing change will usually prevent additional trauma to the wound and unnecessary discomfort to the patient.

Bandages of gauze, cloth, or elastic material may be used for additional fixation of dressings, partial immobilization, or compression. Splints of plaster, wood, metal, or other rigid material may be used for further immobilization. This is particularly indicated when a wound is located in close proximity to a joint and would be subject to excessive motion. Slings and crutches are valuable protective devices for wounds of the upper and lower extremities, respectively.

Heat. The use of heat is a valuable adjunctive measure in the management of inflammation. A well-insulated and well-padded electric heating pad is excellent for this purpose. The local application of heat increases local blood flow, local metabolic activity, and phagocytosis. This aids the body defense mechanisms and repair process. Caution must be observed to avoid excessive heat, particularly in the aged and the very young. Application of heat is contraindicated in areas of circulatory impairment.

Elevation. Elevation of an injured part, usually an extremity, is effective in limiting the edema associated with trauma or inflammation. This results in improved circulation and aids healing. It is of particular importance in injuries involving the lower extremity and can be accomplished by recumbency and support of the extremity above heart level by the use of pillows. This is probably of minor importance in trivial injuries, but increases in value with the extent of the injury.

Antibiotics. The routine use of prophylactic antibiotics in patients with clean wounds is to be condemned. Their use in situations where body defense mechanisms are impaired, however, is certainly justified. Prophylactic antibiotic treatment of dirty wounds is still controversial, but clinical experience and experimental evidence tend to support their use in many injuries of this type. Antibiotics do not, however, substitute for strict adherence to proper wound care. An infected wound with surrounding cellulitis is a clear indication for systemic antibiotic therapy. Cultures should always be taken prior to institution of antibiotic treatment. Broad-spectrum drugs should be used at least until culture results are obtained.

Enzyme Treatment. There is no good evidence that the oral or intramuscular administration of various enzymes has any beneficial effect upon wound healing. Their use cannot be recommended on the basis of present evidence.

The topical use of proteolytic enzymes to aid in the débridement of necrotic debris in open wounds is also controversial. It is the author's personal experience that careful surgical débridement and proper dressing techniques are at least as effective in aiding natural mechanisms, and that enzyme therapy neither offers additional benefit nor substitutes for good surgical management.

BIBLIOGRAPHY

Bernard, C. W., Herrmann, J. B., Woodward, S. C., and Pulaski, E. J.: Healing of incisions closed with surgical adhesive tape, Am. J. Surg., *107*:591, 1964.

Crile, G., Jr.,: Treatment of wounds. Cleveland Clin. Quart., *12*:48, 1945.

Dunphy, J. E. (Ed.): Wound Healing. New York, Medcom Inc., 1971.

Dunphy, J. E., and Van Winkle, W., Jr. (Eds.): Repair and Regeneration. New York, McGraw-Hill, 1968.

Fritz, M., and Tanner, E. K.: The Novocain pack; a contribution to the therapy of fresh accidental wounds. New York J. Med., *35*:1217, 1935.

Gosis, M.: Painless rendering closure of superficial wounds. Am. J. Surg., *44*:400, 1939.

Lawrence, R. R.: Infection and healing in superficial wounds. Calif. Med., *100*:100, 328, 1964.

Mason, M. L.: The surgical principles involved in the treatment of open injuries. West J. Surg., *45*:239, 1937.

Moorhead, J. J.: The general management of injuries. Surg., Gynec. Obstet., *64*:397, 1937.

Peacock, E. E., and Van Winkle, W., Jr.: Surgery and Biology of Wound Repair. Philadelphia, W. B. Saunders, 1970.

Reid, M. R.: The study of wound healing. Ann. Surg., *105*:982, 1937.

Reid, M. R., and Carter, B. N.: The treatment of fresh traumatic wounds. Ann. Surg., *114*:4, 1941.

6
Management of Infections

John B. Herrmann, M.D.

Infections encountered in the ambulatory surgical patient are generally of one or two types: (1) those resulting from accidental or surgical wounds, or (2) infections of nontraumatic origin for which surgical therapy must be considered. Most infections of both types are superficial, involving skin or mucous membranes and subjacent tissues.

The function of the surgeon in the treatment of an inflammation due to infection is to favor or help the processes which the body has already initiated. In the early, or invasive, stage, treatment consists of the application of heat to enhance the active hyperemia, elevation of the part to reduce the swelling, and application of splints and dressings to provide physiologic rest and to protect the area from trauma. Specific antibiotic therapy is used to augment the body defense mechanisms. To these measures are added incision and drainage when fluctuation and pus are present. In addition to these principles of local care, some consideration must be given to relief of the patient's pain and discomfort.

Depending upon the type and extent of the infection, systemic symptoms of varying degree arise as a result of infection: malaise, anorexia, fever. These all subside promptly with control of the infection.

THE LOCAL CARE OF INFECTION

Although the same principles apply in all cases, the local treatment of an infection must vary with the type and situation of the infection. The treatment of a "closed" infection, such as a boil or cellulitis, differs from that of an "open" infection, such as an infected wound.

Application of Heat. Heat in any form, when applied locally to an area of the body surface, causes an increased rate of blood flow due to vasodilatation. This results in a rise in capillary pressure associated with an increased rate of transfer of fluid from the blood to the tissues, accelerated metabolic activity, and an increase in phagocytosis. The greatest rise in temperature occurs at the point of contact, where the energy exchange is greatest. After a sufficiently long period of contact with the heat locally, deeper structures, as a result of conduction, also show a temperature rise. Excessive local temperature is prevented by the distribution of heat throughout the body by increased blood flow.

Prior to the availability and the use of specific chemotherapeutic agents for the treatment of infections, the use of either dry or moist heat was routine adjunctive treatment in the therapeutic regimen. Its use afforded relief of pain and spasm and favored drainage. Since antibiotics are now employed regularly in the management of infections, the application of heat, particularly in the form of hot soaks or hypertonic solutions, has largely given way to dry treatment. Although the "hot soaks" almost universally applied by the laity certainly do no harm and in many cases are beneficial, the principal indication for moist heat at the present is the open infection, in which moist heat helps to loosen crusts and tissue debris and so favors drainage. A physiologic or a slightly hypertonic solution of sodium chloride (2 teaspoonfuls salt to 1 quart of water) or of magnesium sulfate (from 4 to 5 heaping tablespoonfuls to 1 quart of water) is used.

Warm solutions applied to an open wound must be sterile. In ambulatory patients, the chosen solution is sterilized by boiling for 10 minutes. The sterility is maintained by applying the solution with a previously boiled glass syringe with a rubber bulb or a rubber ear syringe. The temperature of the solution should not exceed 110° F.; i.e., it should be cooled until it can be tolerated comfortably by the skin on the inner side of the elbow. The solution may then be applied to the entire dressing with a syringe, or the dressing may contain several small rubber tubes, through which the warm solution may be introduced. Moisture and heat, if continued for more than 24 hours, predispose to increased swelling, the narrowing of drainage exits by sodden tissues, and satellite infection and superinfection.

The electric pad, if well protected from wetting by waxed paper, oiled silk, or a rubberized cover, is probably the most effective method of applying heat for long periods of time. Care must be taken that the pad does not become wet, since a short circuit and burning may occur. Rubber cases are available for some pads, and there are others made with the heating unit enclosed in rubber.

There are other precautions which must be considered in the use of heat. Extreme care must be exercised to avoid producing a troublesome burn, particularly in very young children, in old people, in patients who are debilitated, and in those who are suffering from chronic disease, such as arteriosclerosis or other forms of impaired peripheral circulation.

Elevation. Elevation as a therapeutic measure may be carried out readily when the infection is in one of the extremities; it is less easy when the infection is in other parts of the body. For elevation to be effective, the infected area should be above the level of the heart, so that a patient with an inflammation of the extremity should lie down. However, a marked degree of swelling may be prevented, and venous and lymphatic drainage aided, by making sure that the part is not dependent; thus, to sit with a leg on a chair or to carry an arm or a hand in a sling is better than to put the leg on the floor or to permit the hand to hang at the side. As a rule, because of the marked relief of pain, patients are quite willing to undergo the restraint that elevation may place upon their activities.

Immobilization. For the lesions which are treated in ambulatory patients, physiologic rest demands, in most cases, some degree of immobilization of the part. The extremities are best immobilized by the use of splints or bandages, slings, and adhesive strappings. The methods of effecting immobilization will be discussed in the chapters on regional surgery. However, some mention must be made here of the protection of inflammatory lesions from external trauma. The most common type of trauma is the pinching and squeezing of local infections by the patient or by the energetic physician. There is no better way of breaking down the protective wall of induration and of producing an extension of the inflammatory process, and it is mentioned only to be condemned. Other forms of trauma, such as bumping or striking an area of infection, have the same result; hence the necessity for protection of the area with dressings and splints.

Timed Surgical Intervention. The nature of the lesion and the character of its response to treatment determine the need for surgical intervention. The extraordinary efficacy of antibiotic therapy in such hemolytic streptococcal lesions as cellulitis and lymphadenitis is evidenced by rapid control and resolution of the infection. Surgical intervention is necessary only in the case treated late in which localized abscess and/or gangrene has occurred. As a general rule, drainage is required in most fluctuant staphylococcal lesions, in order to limit further breakdown of the affected tissues, to reduce tension in the area of inflammation, to relieve pain, to provide ingress of bloodborne antibiotics and phagocytes, and to allow wound healing. The removal of sutures and the reopening of infected incisional wounds and the removal of foreign bodies, infected necrotic tissue, and sequestra are important for the same reasons. Although effective chemotherapy has resulted in a marked reduction in the number of cases requiring extensive drainage for resolution, incision and drainage are still indicated when (1) the infection has localized and fluctuation is evident, (2) there is no likelihood of spontaneous rupture with adequate drainage, and (3) there is no danger of extension of infection as a result of surgical trauma.

Technique of Incision and Drainage. Although specific details may vary somewhat depending on the nature and location of the infection, certain general principles of surgical incision and drainage should be followed. Strict aseptic technique should be used to prevent spread of the patient's infection to others, and to prevent new and possibly more virulent organisms from spreading to the patient. This includes a careful skin prep, sterile drapes and instruments, gloves, mask, etc. Local infiltration with procaine or lidocaine is satisfactory, but care must be taken not to spread infection to surrounding tissue. Local intradermal infiltration in the proposed line of incision is safe in this regard. Regional nerve blocks are ideal and are applicable in many circumstances.

The surgical incision should be precise and only as long as necessary to provide adequate drainage. The contents of the abscess cavity should be evacuated and a specimen taken for culture and determination of antibiotic sensitivity. The cavity should be carefully explored to detect and open any undrained pockets of pus. Continued drainage may be provided by a rubber Penrose drain or gauze strip. Packing of an abscess cavity serves no useful purpose and prevents collapse and healing of the lesion. Drains should be used until the cavity has disappeared and drainage has virtually ceased. However, they may be shortened or changed every two to three days if necessary.

The Treatment of an Open Infection

The treatment of an infected wound due to trauma or of an area of infection after an incision for drainage differs somewhat from the programs outlined above. There is now an open wound to be treated rather than an infection below the surface of the skin; consideration must therefore be given to prevention of secondary infections and to the treatment of a wound which must heal by granulation.

In the treatment of an open infection, the danger of introducing secondary infection can be reduced to a minimum by the application of strict asepsis in the care and the dressing of the wound. An all-instrument technique should be employed. In any open infection, the first requisite is macroscopic cleanliness. The wound itself should be cleaned mechanically of liquid pus and necrotic tissue. The surrounding area should be kept free of pus and crusts and should be protected from excoriation due to irritating discharges.

The surface of the wound is covered lightly with fine dry mesh gauze, over which compression dressings are applied. An absorbent dressing permits early and rapid removal of the liquefied wound secretions and thus promotes a continued flow of serum, lymph, and leukocytes into the wound. It should be bulky enough to avoid soaking through. The use of constrictive circular bandages should be avoided. Elastic cotton bandages are useful, but care must be exercised in applying them, for they, too, may cause constriction if they are too tight. Dressings are changed only as necessary, since too frequent changing enhances the possibilities of contamination and increases exudations. Since bacteria from the external environment readily penetrate moist gauze, open wounds should have waterproofed external dressings if practicable.

The beneficial effects of heat, moist dressings, elevation, and immobilization upon healing have been discussed in previous paragraphs.

The role of topical antiseptics, antibiotics and other chemotherapeutic agents in the management of open infected wounds is still highly controversial. If our theoretical conception of nature's method of handling infections be true, the so-called biologic antisepsis, then there is no place for antiseptics and topical antibiotics in the treatment of infected wounds unless it can be shown that they enhance the action of the natural processes. It is clear that antiseptics are ineffective against organisms residing beneath the surface of a wound. Furthermore, the destructive action of most antiseptics is exerted against all cells with which they come in contact, be they tissue cells or bacteria. The result is a lowering of local tissue vitality and a retardation of healing. There is therefore no rational basis for the use of these agents in the treatment of open infected wounds.

In recent years, however, topical chemotherapeutic agents have been developed which have a definite antibacterial effect without appreciable toxicity for tissues. Aqueous silver nitrate (0.5%) and Sulfamylon are two such agents which have revolutionized the treatment of burns. The effectiveness of these agents in the management of open infected wounds other than burns has not been established. Nitrofurazone (Furacin) has also been used for topical application to infected wounds, but hypersensitivity and superinfection with resistant organisms have been problems. Povidone-iodine (Betadine) and other organic iodine prep-

arations have also been used for this purpose.

Numerous topical antibiotic preparations have also been developed. Because of the risk of sensitization, it has generally been considered unwise to use for topical application antibiotics which are normally employed systemically. Most topical preparations therefore contain antibiotics which are rarely used systemically. These include neomycin, bacitracin and polymyxin. Even when used in combination these agents are not effective against all bacteria. Because of this, topical antibiotics have been generally ineffective in the treatment of burns. Consequent to their use, overgrowth of resistant organisms may occur. Local hypersensitivity has also been observed.

It appears, therefore, that, despite wide usage, there is little rationale for the use of topical antibiotics and antiseptics. Personal experience indicates that these often expensive preparations offer little advantage over simple moist saline dressings. There is, however, some experimental and clinical evidence that high concentrations of surface bacteria impede wound healing and that reduction of surface population with appropriate antibacterial agents results in improved healing. Thus, the topic is still controversial. At the present stage of our knowledge it appears rational to avoid using these topical agents (except in burns) unless their use is clearly indicated by evidence of delayed healing. Cultures for both bacteria and fungi taken at this time may provide help in selecting appropriate agents. Intensive topical treatment may also be indicated in the preparation of a granulating surface for skin grafting. Marked surface contamination, particularly with hemolytic streptococcus and Pseudomonas, appears to be detrimental to successful grafting.

The chronically infected indolent skin ulcer remains a therapeutic problem in many instances despite correction of underlying conditions, such as postphlebitic stasis, and intensive topical therapy. The recent use of fresh and cryogenically preserved allografts of split thickness skin as biologic dressings has shown considerable promise in this area, as well as in the treatment of burns.

SYSTEMIC TREATMENT OF INFECTION

Although antibiotic therapy has revolutionized the treatment of infections, due consideration must also be given to various supportive measures designed to maximize host resistance. Antibiotic therapy is, in reality, no more than an adjunctive measure employed to regulate the balance between parasite and host, and represents only a part of the total care picture of bacterial disease. Both antibiotic therapy and general support of host resistance must be equally considered.

Antibiotic Therapy

There are two basic requirements for effective antibiotic therapy of an infection:

1. The antibiotic must be capable of inhibiting the growth of the agent or agents causing the infection. This requires an identification of the infecting bacteria and a selection of an antibiotic effective against that organism.

2. A therapeutically effective concentration of the antibiotic must reach the infected tissues for a period of time long enough to permit the antimicrobial activity of the compound to be effective. This requires a knowledge of that dosage of the antibiotic (by mouth or by injection) which gives antimicrobial concentration in the blood, and it requires a blood supply capable of delivering the antibiotic in the blood to the infected tissues. The reader should remember that because necrotic tissue and pus have no blood supply there is still the necessity for incision and drainage in the cases of abscess formation.

In the majority of cases of well-localized staphylococcal infections requiring incision and drainage, antibiotic therapy is unnecessary. Natural defense mechanisms are more than adequate to effect a cure once drainage has been established. Cultures should be obtained at the time of drainage so that in the occasional case which does not rapidly respond an appropriate drug can be used.

The general incidations for systemic antibiotic therapy are lesions associated with (1) a wide area of cellulitis, (2) lymphangitis and lymphadenitis, (3) systemic symptoms, such as fever, chills, or malaise; or (4) depressed host resistance due to other illnesses. In addition, multiple simultaneous lesions and lesions of the face and neck and hands should be treated with systemic antibiotics.

Selection of Antibiotic Therapy

In most cases of infection seen in an office or an outpatient clinic the physician is called upon, at first, to make an empirical selection of an antibiotic without laboratory identification of the bacteria or without specificity tests. As a general rule he should be able to distinguish the type of inflammation produced by streptococci (spreading cellulitis, lymphangitis, lymphadenitis) from that produced by staphylococci (boils, carbuncles, paronychiae). This should give the physician sufficient information to make a primary selection of an antibiotic, because most infective inflammations seen in ambulatory patients are produced by one of these two organisms. If the infection responds to the drug selected, culture and specificity tests are not needed. It is known, however, that many species of staphylococci have developed resistance to some antibiotics, especially to penicillin. In such cases culture and specificity tests are important, and laboratory help is necessary to obtain the information required for antibiotic selection.

The empirical choice of antibiotic therapy for staphylococcal infections depends on whether the patient developed the infection in the hospital or outside the hospital, and, to a certain degree, on whether he did or did not receive antibiotic therapy within the period of, say, 3 months prior to onset of the present illness. In the nonhospitalized patient who has not received penicillin before, or in recent months, the chances are excellent that the staphylococci causing the infection are susceptible to penicillin. In the occasional patient of this type whose lesion does not respond to penicillin, and in the patient who is sensitive to penicillin, erythromycin or one of the tetracyclines is usually effective. For infections acquired in the hospital, culture and sensitivity tests become more important because of the varying pattern of resistance found in these infections. Penicillinase-resistant penicillins, the cephalosporins, and lincomycin are frequently effective alternative drugs.

The prophylactic use of antibiotics in the management of traumatic wounds appears logical if the antibiotic is administered in the early, pre-invasive phase, before bacteria, although present, have become established in the wound. Despite ample experimental evidence to support this concept, there is no clinical evidence that antibiotic prophylaxis has any influence on the course of soft tissue wounds that have been adequately and promptly débrided and cleansed. Routine prophylaxis is therefore no longer employed in the treatment of simple soft tissue injuries. Prophylactic antibacterial therapy is reserved for extensive musculoskeletal injuries, compound fractures, and penetrating injuries of the chest, abdomen, oropharynx, esophagus, central nervous system, and eye. The choice of agent or agents is dependent upon the bacterial flora expected to be encountered.

Regardless of the indication, the dosage of the antibiotic selected should be adequate to produce the desired antibacterial effects in the blood and in the extracellular fluids. The duration of therapy should be sufficiently long to permit the natural defense mechanisms of the body to eradicate the inhibited organisms in the lesion; on the other hand, unnecessarily prolonged therapy is unwise and may be harmful. After 72 hours the antibiotic therapy program should be reviewed, reevaluated and changed as indicated (Table 6-1).

Penicillin. This is still the most widely useful and effective of the antibiotics. It is effective against most of the gram-

positive cocci that produce purulent infections in ambulatory patients: streptococcus and staphylococcus. It may be given to ambulatory patients by repeated intramuscular injection, but oral administration is generally more convenient. In tablets of buffered potassium penicillin G, penicillin G, or penicillin V the drug is given in doses of 200,000 to 500,000 units four to six times daily.

Penicillinase-Resistant   Penicillins. These drugs should be used only against known or suspected penicillinase-producing staphylococci. Cloxacillin (Tegopen) or dicloxacillin (Pathocil, Veracillin, Dynapen) are preferred for oral use. Parenteral forms of nafcillin (Unipen), methicillin (Staphcillin), or oxacillin (Prostaphlin) should be used for severe infections.

Other Semisynthetic Penicillins. These drugs are effective against some gram-negative as well as gram-positive organisms. Ampicillin (Polycillin and others) is a much overused "broad-spectrum" antibiotic. It should not be used for the prevention or treatment of infections caused by penicillinase-producing staphylococci, Pseudomonas, or the Klebsiella-Aerobacter group. It is active against many other gram-negative and gram-positive organisms. Carbenicillin (Pyopen, Geopen) is effective against some strains of Pseudomonas and Proteus resistant to other antibiotics. Hetacillin (Versapen) is broken down into ampicillin in the blood and has the same antibacterial spectrum. None of these drugs is recommended for initial use in the treatment of infection in the ambulatory patient, but they may be useful in later situations, depending upon the results of sensitivity testing. All show cross sensitivity reaction in patients allergic to penicillin and should be avoided in such situations.

Tetracyclines. This group of antibiotics includes a large number of derivatives of the basic tetracycline structure which have similar antibacterial spectra. These agents are classified as "broad-spectrum" antibiotics because of their action against a wide variety of gram-positive and gram-negative organisms. Both oral and

Table 6-1. Choice of Antimicrobial Drugs for Organisms Encountered in Surgical Infections[*]

	Penicillin G	Penicillins (Penicillinase-resistant)	Erythromycin	Linocomycin Clindamycin	Vancomycin‡	Ampicillin	Cephalosporins	Tetracyclines	Chloramphenicol‡	Kanamycin‡	Gentamicin‡	Polymyxin‡	Carbenicillin‡
Gram-Positive Cocci													
Streptococcus pyogenes	x		a	a									
† Streptococcus viridans	x(P)		a		a(P)		a(P)						
† Enterococcus	x(P)				a(P)	x(P)				x	x		
† Anaerobic Streptococcus	x(P)		a						a				
† Staphylococcus aureus	x			a	a(P)		a			a(P)	a		
† Staphylococcus aureus (penicillinase-producing)		x		a	a(P)		a			a(P)	a		
Gram-Positive Bacilli													
Bacillus anthracis	x		a				a						
† Clostridium perfringens	x(P)		a(P)				a(P)						
† Clostridium tetani	x(P)						a(P)						
Gram-Negative Bacilli													
Escherichia coli													
community acquired						x(P)	a	a		a(P)			
hospital acquired						a	a			x(P)	a		
† Aerobacter aerogenes								a	a	a	x	a(P)	a
† Proteus sp.								a	a	x(P)	a		a
† Pseudomonas aeruginosa											x	a(P)	x
† Bacteroides			a			a		x	x				

*Adapted from Medical Letter, Vol. 14, No. 2, Jan. 21, 1972
x, Drug of choice; a, Alternative drugs; (P), Parenteral administration advised even if both oral and parenteral forms available.
†Resistance may be a problem—sensitivity tests should be performed.
‡Not indicated for treatment of minor infections.

parenteral forms are available. They are most useful in the ambulatory surgical patient for the treatment of infections suspected of being of mixed gram-positive and gram-negative, or predominantly gram-negative origin, such as perirectal abscesses or urinary tract infections. Although not the primary alternative for the treatment of clinically apparent staphylococcal or streptococcal infections they are often effective against these organisms when the patient is allergic to penicillin. Gastrointestinal side effects are relatively common with this group of drugs.

Cephalosporins. Cephalothin (Keflin), cephaloridine (Loridine) and cephalexin (Keflex) are moderately broad-spectrum antibiotics with activity against most gram-positive and many gram-negative organisms. Some cross sensitivity with penicillin exists and, therefore, patients allergic to penicillin may be allergic to the cephalosporins. Cephalexin is the drug of choice for oral administration, as the others are available only in parenteral form.

Lincomycin and Clindamycin. These are structurally related drugs with an antibacterial spectrum similar to that of penicillin. They may be used for the treatment of susceptible staphylococcal infections in patients sensitive to penicillin. Gastrointestinal disturbances are frequent side effects of oral therapy.

Aminoglycosides. This group includes streptomycin, neomycin, kanamycin, and gentamycin. They are more active against gram-negative bacteria than against gram-positive bacteria. All of these drugs are ototoxic and nephrotoxic. They are most useful in the treatment of serious, hospital-based infections.

Erythromycin. This drug has an antibacterial spectrum similar to that of penicillin and is most useful as an alternative drug in patients with a history of penicillin allergy.

Whereas approximately 70 percent of staphylococcal infections in hospitalized patients prove to be resistant to penicillin, and approximately 40 to 60 percent to chlortetracycline and its analogues, less than 10 percent are resistant to erythromycin. This drug is given orally in doses ranging from 100 to 600 mg. every 4 to 8 hours. Toxic complications have been relatively few and mild, consisting mainly of abdominal cramps and diarrhea in a small percentage of recipients.

Chloramphenicol. This is a broad-spectrum drug which may cause fatal blood dyscrasias. Its use should therefore be limited to serious infections by susceptible bacteria which cannot be treated effectively by other agents.

Other Antibiotics. Many other antibiotics are available to the physician for the treatment of infection. These drugs are rarely necessary or desirable in the treatment of the ambulatory patient. They are used primarily in hospitalized patients but are available if sensitivity tests indicate their use in infections not responding to initial therapy.

SUPPORTIVE THERAPY

Systemic Measures. In addition to the antibiotic program already outlined in the treatment of infections in ambulatory patients, due consideration must be given to various systemic measures which have as their purpose an increase or the main-

tenance of the patient's general resistance. One of these is rest, or at least the avoidance of fatigue. A balanced diet of easily assimilated foods and care to avoid constipation are important. When pain is not controlled by other means, acetylsalicylic acid or codeine may be administered in sufficient quantities to keep the patient comfortable until the wound becomes painless. The reduction of resistance to infection in diabetic and cachectic subjects and in others with poor peripheral circulation is well known, and such conditions must be treated concomitantly with the infection. The popularity of vaccines, toxoids, and other biologicals (except for tetanus prophylaxis) for the purpose of increasing the patient's resistance or response to infection has waned since the widespread use of antibiotics.

BIBLIOGRAPHY

Bauer, A. W., Kirby, W. M. M., Sherris, J. C., and Turck, M.: Antibiotic susceptibility testing by a standardized single disc method. Am. J. Clin. Path., *45*:493, 1966.

Carney, R. G.: Topical use of antibiotics. JAMA, *186*:646, 1963.

Dible, J. H.: Inflammation and repair. Ann. Roy. Coll. Surg. (England), *6*:120, 1950.

Dunlop, D. M., and Murdock, J. McC.: The danger of antibiotic treatment. Brit. Med. Bull., *16*:67, 1960.

Editorial: Prophylactic antibiotics may do more harm than good. JAMA, *188*, (Suppl. 39) 1964.

Finland, M., and Weinstein, L.: Complications induced by antimicrobial agents. New Eng. J. Med., *248*:220, 1953.

Handbook of Antimicrobial Therapy, Medical Letter, Vol. 14, No. 2, January 21, 1972.

Koenig, M. G.: An approach to antimicrobial therapy of common infections. Am. Pract., *13*:453, 1962.

Lepper, M. H.: The use and misuse of antibiotics and other chemotherapeutic agents. Med. Clin. N. Am., *45*:1663, 1961.

Livingood, C. S., and Mullins, J. F.: Management of bacterial infections of the skin. Postgrad. Med., *12*:15, 1952.

Lyman, I. R., Tenery, J. H., and Basson, R. P.: Correlation between decrease in bacterial load and rate of wound healing. Surg., Gynec. Obst., *130*:616, 1970.

Pulaski, E. J.: Common Bacterial Infections. Philadelphia, Saunders, 1964.

Ungar, G.: Inflammation and its control, a biochemical approach. Lancet, *2*:742, 1952.

Weinstein, L., Goldfield, M., and Chang, T.: Infections occurring during chemotherapy, a study of their frequency, type and predisposing factors. New Eng. J. Med., *251*:247, 1954.

Weinstein, L.: The use and abuse of antimicrobial agents. Med. Sci., *14*:34, 1963.

———: Chemotherapy of infection. In Harrison, T. R., *et al.* (eds.): Principles of Internal Medicine. ed. 3. New York, Blakiston-McGraw-Hill, 1958.

Welch, H., *et al.*: Principles and Practice of Antibiotic Therapy. New York, Medical Encyclopedia, 1954.

7

Specific Surgical Lesions

Mark W. Wolcott, M.D.

FOLLICULITIS, FURUNCLES, AND CARBUNCLES

Stages of Infection. Folliculitis, furuncles, and carbuncles are the names applied to local staphylococcal infections of the skin and the subcutaneous tissues. Each begins as an infection of a hair follicle or of a sebaceous gland and progresses to produce a small area of induration with central necrosis known as a pimple or a pustule. By further extension, the infection involves the underlying subcutaneous tissues, and a single area of central necrosis surrounded by a well-formed area of redness and induration is formed; this is called a furuncle or a boil. In areas in which there are dense fibrous septa extending from the skin to the underlying fascia, as in the back of the neck, the infection may extend from one area of subcutaneous tissue to another without effective walling off of the process, thus attaining a considerable size. This lesion is known as a carbuncle. It may be noted, therefore, that these lesions must be looked upon as progressive stages of the same process, and the variations in progress may be considered, in part, to be indicative of the patient's general and local "resistance" to the staphylococcal infection and of the architecture of the infected tissues.

Predisposing Factors. In many instances the recognition and the appropriate management of predisposing factors may be as important as the administration of specific measures. Therefore, it is essential to keep in mind the following recognizable local and systemic factors which determine the degree of "resistance" of the skin to pyogenic infection: (1) trauma of any form, which includes exposure to irritants, deodorants, and defatting agents; (2) poor hygiene; (3) local causes of pruritus, such as insect bites and pediculosis capitis; (4) excessive sweating, especially of intertriginous sites, hands, and feet; (5) climatic factors; (6) diabetes; and (7) blood dyscrasias. In order to treat these infections effectively, it is essential for the physician to recognize and correct these predisposing factors whenever they are present.

Location and Description. These lesions may occur on any part of the body, but the most frequent sites are the face, the back of the neck, the axillae, the groins, the buttocks, the arms, and the proximal phalanges of the fingers.

The earliest lesion is characterized by a small reddened firm mound of induration, which is itchy and tender and in a few days shows a central yellow point. This furuncle, or pimple, may extend no farther, and the process may subside with

72

the discharge of a drop or two of pus or may simply "dry up." Frequently, however, there is a deeper extension, with gradual enlargement of the area of inflammatory induration. Pain, which is a common manifestation, is present and increases with motion. In this case the area of inflammation has extended beyond the skin into the subcutaneous tissues, and, in the untreated lesion, the protective wall of inflammatory induration usually takes from 4 to 6 days to become well formed. By this time the central necrotic core, with serosanguineous pus, is prominent, and drainage of pus and necrotic material may occur spontaneously or after surgical incision. As soon as drainage is established, tension is relieved, pain decreases in severity, and the process subsides when the necrotic material has all been evacuated.

In the carbuncular type of infection, most often seen on the back of the neck or on the dorsum of the hand, the walling-off process does not seem to keep pace with the tendency of the infection to spread in the poorly resistant fat lobules lying between the fibrous tissue septa beneath the skin. As a result, the encircling inflammatory wall of induration is frequently wide in diameter, and pointing takes place at multiple sites in the skin over the underlying necrosis. An elevated temperature and evident "toxemia" as a result of absorption from the area of infection usually are present.

The prognosis depends on the clinical type of infection, the site of involvement, the predisposing factors, the duration of infection, and the nature of the causative organisms. Superficial pustular folliculitis and furuncles tend to have a more or less self-limited course and to clear up readily with various types of therapy. In some cases furuncles are recurrent. A dominant etiologic factor may be an underlying dermatitis, in which case proper treatment of the dermatitis may result in a permanent cure of the furunculosis. Through the process of auto-inoculation, staphylococci may be carried from a lesion and infect other parts of the body.

Unless suitable precautions are taken, the micro-organisms are conveyed by fingers or handkerchief to other parts of the body, such as the nose, the eyes, and the external ear, where they are liable to persist. Recurrent infection in the axilla, a warm, moist hairy area with apocrine glands, is readily understandable. All physicians recognize that furuncles and carbuncles in the center of the face may give off small emboli and give rise to cavernous sinus thrombosis, septicemia, or metastatic infection at some distance away from the original infection. Also, it is well known that the staphylococcal infections in the newborn and in children may lead to serious sequelae, such as osteomyelitis. Appropriate antibiotic therapy has significantly reduced the mortality and the morbidity from these serious complications of cutaneous infections.

In general, cutaneous pyogenic infections of brief duration are more amenable to therapy than are those that are chronic. The causative organism also influences the prognosis. If the offending *Staphylococcus aureus* is sensitive to the antibiotic selected, institution of adequate effective local therapy as quickly as possible after the infection becomes apparent is likely to result in prompt resolution of the infection.

Treatment. The treatment of established local staphylococcal infections still rests chiefly on the surgical principles of rest, elevation and heat, and drainage when pus has formed. Scrupulous cleanliness, is the first principle of management. For the smaller furuncles and carbuncles, effective treatment further consists in protecting and immobilizating the area with an adhesive cone over an application of neomycin or other antibiotic ointment at the site of pointing. The area around the furuncle or boil is shaved, and, after the necrotic bleb has been removed with a needle or forceps, a small dot of ointment is placed at the point of the lesion. A circle of adhesive, cut along one radius, is placed to cover the entire area of induration in the form of a cone (Fig. 7-1). In many cases, the infection

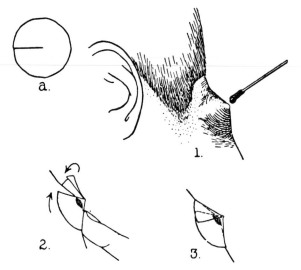

Fig. 7–1. Adhesive-cone dressing for small furuncle.

may be aborted by this treatment; in others, the use of 95 percent phenol, cautiously applied with a toothpick swab to enlarge a small sinus or to open an abscess near the surface which is pointing, is still good practice. After two or three days, the area of central necrosis may be lifted out with a sterile forceps or mosquito hemostat. This treatment is continued until all the central slough has liquefied and drained away.

In some boils, when movement of a part prevents an effective walling off of the process and when there is an associated cellulitis of the adjacent tissues, as, for instance, in furuncles on the dorsum of the proximal phalanx of the finger, the application of splints and dry heat is beneficial.

Parenterally administered penicillin or one of the other antistaphylococcal antibiotics is given to hasten localization of the infection process. Under this regimen the cellulitis surrounding the lesion will subside in 36 to 48 hours, and, with localization of the process, there will be a discharge of the central necrotic area followed by rapid healing. Incision in such cases is not performed until localization has taken place, and usually by this time spontaneous drainage will begin. It may be necessary to incise this drainage site slightly.

The use of penicillin and other antibiotics has revolutionized the treatment of this condition. When antibiotics are administered early and in sufficient dosage, they aid the body defenses in bringing under control the general and the local manifestations within a period of 48 to 71 hours, and they have so modified the subsequent course that both mortality and morbidity are reduced significantly.

Since the invasive qualities of this lesion now are so effectively controlled by antibiotics, radical excision has become obsolete. Instead, limited surgical intervention is recommended when indicated; this consists of incision and drainage of abscesses when they occur during therapy, and excision of tissue hopelessly devitalized by suppuration and necrosis. Penicillin or one of the newer synthetic penicillinase-resistant drugs is administered in adequate doses, either intramuscularly or by mouth. Patients with extensive carbuncles and systemic manifestations are usually best treated in a hospital until localization and adequate drainage has been obtained.

In some cases, furuncles are recurrent. Usually, this is due to one or more of the predisposing factors previously listed, although in some instances the most exhaustive studies do not reveal any apparent cause. The most thorough attention to skin hygiene and to the nutrition and the general health of the patient is important. Trauma, such as that due to the pulling of hairs from the nares, the wearing of chafing, dirty clothes, or the rubbing or the fingering of the lesions, is avoided. The possibility of an underlying allergic dermatitis should be borne in mind, and, if it is present, it should be suitably treated. Sugar metabolism should be investigated and controlled if abnormal. A restriction of carbohydrates, even in the absence of demonstrable elevation of the blood sugar, may be beneficial. It is difficult to evaluate the utility of toxoids and vaccines. Of all these preventive measures one may state that they are certainly not uniformly successful but that in some cases they seem to be effective in checking recurrence.

It is now recognized that in chronic furunculosis the upper respiratory tract, particularly the anterior nares, even though apparently healthy, is often colonized with *Staphylococcus aureus*. Occasionally, instead of the nose, the eye, the ear, the axilla, or some other region is the reservoir from which infection continues to be distributed. Infection also persists in the neighborhood of a lesion until it is completely healed.

LYMPHANGITIS

Etiology and Symptoms. Acute lymphangitis is an infection which extends along the lymphatic vessels. It frequently originates from a superficial wound, which may be small, such as a pinprick, and spreads proximally through the lymph channels to the lymph nodes. A hemolytic streptococcus is the most common causal organism. Lymphangitis of the upper extremity often arises from a hand infection due to a puncture wound caused by a needle, a pin, or a wire, or due to a blister or an infected incised wound. Lymphangitis of the lower extremity may arise from an infected blister, callus, or toenail, or from an interdigital fungous infection or the numerous scratches or bites on the legs of children.

A patient suffering from lymphangitis will generally give a history of having suffered one of the foregoing wounds of entry for the microorganisms, but he may not remember having sustained such a wound. The limb is swollen and painful, though the initial edema does not pit on pressure, as in thrombophlebitis. It is tender to palpation, particularly along the course of the affected lymphatics. The latter may be recognized by their giving rise to *red streaks* which run up the extremity. These red streaks are tender to palpation, as are the regional lymph nodes.

The general condition of the patient may be one of malaise or of prostration. There may be a chill if the infection is severe, and the temperature and the pulse are both elevated. As in any infection, the severity will vary according to the virulence of the organism, the degree of contamination and inoculation, and the resistance of the patient. The onset of symptoms and the systemic reaction will be more fulminating in the severe infection, and the local signs will develop more rapidly in those cases. Injudicious incision or other trauma, neglect or continued functional use of the part favors rapid spread and complications such as septicemia and even death. There is little tendency for abscesses to form. When local breakdown of tissue does occur, it is characterized by either gangrene of the overlying skin or the development of thin, watery pus.

Treatment. Much of the fear of lymphangitis has been dispelled by early proper treatment with antibiotic drugs. Their extraordinary efficacy in combating these infections has been proved beyond question. Thus, the treatment of acute lymphangitis consists primarily in the control of its invasive characteristics by antibiotic therapy, rest, and heat, and secondarily in incision and drainage of collections of pus and necrotic tissue should they present themselves. Penicillin is the drug of choice in hemolytic streptococcal lymphangitis. One of the "broad-spectrum" antibiotics may be employed if allergy or resistance to penicillin exists. With therapy, usually the lymphangitis will subside in 24 to 48 hours, but the treatment should be continued for 2 or 3 days after the inflammatory process has disappeared. Of equal importance in treatment are rest, heat, and elevation of the part infected, and it is usually advisable, even in the less severe cases, to confine the patient to bed during the acute phase of the infection. In mild cases, enforced bed rest may seem to be drastic treatment from the patient's viewpoint, but a safe and a rapid recovery is thereby ensured. Application of heat may be instituted for the comfort of the patient, though this is no longer as essential to resolution of the infection as it was in the prechemotherapy era. When the infection is in the leg, the arm, or the hand, the immobilization accomplished by elevating the part on several pillows is sufficient. After control of the invasive characteristics of the infection by penicillin or one of the other chemotherapeutic agents, drainage of the local lesion may be instituted in the event that pus or necrotic tissue has formed, which is rare.

CELLULITIS

Etiology. Cellulitis is a diffuse inflammation of the tissues caused by pyogenic bacteria. It differs from lymphangitis in that it is not limited to the lymphatic vessels. As does lymphangitis, cellulitis arises from an infected wound, which is usually superficial, and the offending organism is again, most often a hemolytic streptococcus, although a staphylococcus or mixed flora may be involved. The portal of entry may be an obvious open laceration, ulcer, callus, or blister; or it may be a small invisible puncture wound or abrasion. The spread of infection is usually less rapid than it is in acute lymphangitis, and the systemic reaction is not as severe. It is true that a cellulitis may initiate a lymphangitis if it is not promptly treated.

Diagnosis. Increased heat of the affected part, diffuse redness, slight pain and tenderness, and a soft edema of the skin and the subcutaneous tissues are characteristic of cellulitis. Care must be taken to differentiate between a primary cellulitis and the indurated skin over a deep abscess which has become localized and is pointing toward the surface. Timed incision and drainage are indicated in the latter case, whereas conservative therapy is advisable in cellulitis.

Treatment. Rest, elevation of the part if an extremity is involved, and the application of heat constitute the essential local therapeutic measures in the treatment of cellulitis. Penicillin usually produces a rapid control of the infection and resolution of the inflammatory process. Not uncommonly, however, the infection will become localized, and a discrete abscess will form. When induration has diminished and the abscess has become fluctuant and well walled off, incision and drainage will facilitate recovery. No clinical response after 48 hours of penicillin and supportive therapy should lead to the suspicion that penicillin-resistant organisms are the cause of the infection, and change to another antibiotic may be advisable.

ERYSIPELAS

Symptoms. Erysipelas is an acute infectious disease of the skin or, more rarely, of the mucous membranes, due to infection of the superficial lymphatics, particularly in the corium, by the hemolytic streptococcus. If often originates in a wound. For some reason, erysipelas is rarely seen today. It occurs most frequently in individuals past midlife, and, in the absence of prompt adequate specific therapy, there is a definite tendency to recurrence of the infection. The infection seems to have seasonal variation, appearing most often during the fall and the spring. The disease is characterized by an abrupt onset of systemic symptoms, usually with a chill, headache, severe malaise, and fever. The local lesion, which occurs about the face or the forehead in the majority of cases, is distinctive. The skin becomes hot, red and indurated and has a well-defined, palpably raised, and sharply demarcated margin. The burning local pain and redness that occur may precede the systemic reaction, although the skin lesion usually does not appear until 6 to 12 hours after the onset of the symptoms. The redness and the induration spread by direct continuity from the periphery, often quite rapidly and vesicles or even large blebs may form in the area of earlier involvement as the lesion progresses.

Treatment. The treatment of erysipelas usually cannot be carried out in the ambulatory patient, although mild cases without marked systemic symptoms may not require hospitalization. A brief discussion of the present-day therapy of this disease is especially indicated, as erysipelas in its milder forms or earlier stages may be seen first in the physician's office or in the outpatient clinic, and abortive treatment may be given.

Antistreptococcal chemotherapy is the most important single agent in the treatment of erysipelas, and it has made older forms of treatment obsolete. Penicillin is considered to be the treatment of choice. It is given intramuscularly, in doses of 600,000 to 1,000,000 units once or twice daily, and it is continued until the patient has been afebrile for at least 3 days. Supportive measures, including the generous administration of fluids, are essential for the comfort and the safety of the patient. Recurrence, which is controlled by additional treatment, is seldom as severe as the original attack; lymphatic damage is often responsible for persistent swelling, especially in the extremities.

Prophylaxis. Disinfection of the hands of attending physicians and nurses and scrupulous care of contaminated instruments are essential. Although strict isolation is not necessary, the care of these patients should not be conducted by those who must simultaneously attend obstetric or surgical patients.

ERYSIPELOID OF ROSENBACH

Etiology. Erysipeloid of Rosenbach, also known as erythema serpens or erythema migrans, is an acute cutaneous infection caused by the organism of swine erysipelas, *Erysipelothrix rhusiopathiae.* This disease has come to be of no small importance in industrial medicine. It occurs most commonly in swine raisers, veterinarians, abattoir employees, and others who handle swine; and in those who handle hides or animal bones. It is also seen not infrequently in those who dress or handle fish or crustacea such as lobsters, oysters, and the like. In an urban practice on the eastern seaboard, erysipeloid of Rosenbach has been observed most commonly as a result of minor injuries of the hand and fingers in veterinary students, butchers, and those cleaning fish and other sea food. It is most often seen in males and in the summer months.

Symptoms. The clinical picture is typical and characteristic, and is easily recognized by someone who has once seen the condition. The first symptom is usually itching, then a burning, throbbing pain at the site of injury, in most cases on the finger. There follow swelling and erythema, which tend to progress to involve the whole finger. The distinctive feature of the infection is the purplish red color of the erythema. The erythema extends slowly from the periphery, forming a sharply defined elevated zone. The areas first involved clear without desquamation or suppuration.

Lymphangitis and lymphadenitis occur in some patients. If the fingers are involved, movement may be difficult, and this stiffness is out of proportion to the degree of soft-tissue swelling. Arthralgia may occur in the fingers, the wrist, the elbow, and even the shoulder joints. Occasionally, this persists for a time after the clearing of the skin lesions. Rarely, there is swelling of the painful joints, and radiographic changes have been reported in cases of longstanding arthralgia.

Diagnosis. The disease is almost always confused with erysipelas, from which it may be distinguished by the purplish-red rather than the fire-red color of the lesion and by the fact that the peripheral zone is never as raised and as

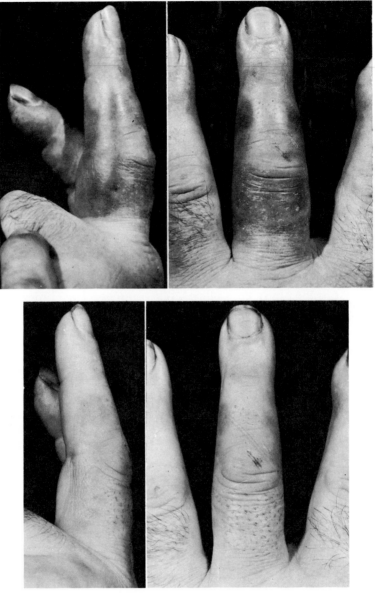

Fig. 7–2. (*Top*) Erysipeloid of Rosenbach in a butcher. (*Bottom*) Appearance after 3 days of penicillin therapy. (Official U. S. Navy photographs)

sharply demarcated as it is in erysipelas (Fig. 7-2). The site of infection, usually the hand, and the lack of severe systemic reaction aid in the diagnosis.

The diagnosis is not difficult to make if the condition is kept in mind as a possibility. A history of contact with fish or animal material should arouse suspicion.

Strict limitation of the process to one location, usually the hand; the erythematous, edematous lesion, with tenderness of the joints on lateral pressure; and the slow progression, limited to the fingers and the hand, should clinch the diagnosis.

Treatment. The causative organism,

Erysipelothrix rhusiophathiae, exhibits relatively uniform sensitivity to penicillin, chlortetracycline, and chloramphenicol. The infection responds rapidly to the injection of 300,000 units of penicillin intramuscularly on 2 or 3 consecutive days. On this regimen over 90 percent of the patients respond satisfactorily, and in most cases the severe deep-seated pain and throbbing disappear in 24 hours.

ACUTE LYMPHADENITIS

Etiology. Lymphadenitis is an inflammatory process of the lymph nodes which is almost invariably due to lymph-borne infections, although occasionally it may result from blood-borne infections or direct trauma. Although any organism capable of producing infection in tissues may produce lymphadenitis, streptococci and staphylococci are most frequently responsible. The infection is usually secondary, but it may be primary or it may be superimposed on primary pathology of lymphatic tissue. Single nodes or groups of nodes may be affected, or involvement may be widespread, depending on the nature of the etiologic agent.

Diagnosis. A regional lymph node or a chain of enlarged nodes often provides a clue to the diagnosis. Thus, acute inflammation of the neck may follow oral sepsis, scalp sepsis, superficial wounds of the head or infections of the tonsils or the respiratory tract. Chronic infectious cervical adenitis may be due to delayed resolution of acute cervical adenitis, or it may be due to tuberculosis, syphilis, anthrax, actinomycosis, or other infection.

In the upper extremity, the antecubital and the epitrochlear glands may be involved early in infections involving the ulnar side of the hand. In infections of the radial side of the hand, the axillary glands are first to be involved. Infections of the middle finger may drain into either the antecubital or the axillary glands, but in some instances they drain directly into the supraclavicular glands.

Enlarged inguinal nodes occur in sepsis of the lower extremity; e.g., in interdigital infection, infected varicose ulcers, and cellulitis or infection in the rectal or the genital area.

Ulcerating lymph nodes, regardless of their location, suggest tuberculosis, tularemia, anthrax, actinomycosis, specific venereal disease, or malignancy. Differentiation between infection and malignancy is important and necessary.

Course. The course of the inflammatory process within the lymph nodes may vary greatly, depending particularly upon the virulence of the invading organism, the nature of the primary infection, the resistance of the patient, and the management of the lesion. As a rule, the primary lymphadenitis appears in the neck, the axilla, or the groin at the height of the primary infection. There is often no evidence of intervening lymphatic involvement. The lymph nodes become tender, hard, and enlarged. In the majority of cases, bacterial lymphadenitis will quickly subside when the primary infection has been adequately controlled. In some cases the primary area of infection may have healed, so that retreatment of the primary lesion is not helpful. In some instances, necrosis and abscess formation will result. The infection may extend beyond the lymph nodes and involve adjacent tissues, thus producing a spreading cellulitis.

Treatment. The treatment of lymphadenitis must be directed primarily toward the treatment of the original portal of infection. This holds true whether the lymphadenitis is of a fulminating, suppurative type or of a low-grade smoldering type. The management of the primary lesion will, of course, depend entirely upon its nature.

Rest is important during the acute stages. In severe infections, rest in bed with elevation of the affected part, if the primary lesion involves an extremity, is advocated. Immobilization with dressings, splints, or even plaster affords a means of complete rest for an affected extremity in an ambulatory patient. Heat applications are indicated, as they are for any acute inflammation. Antibiotics, usually penicillin given intramuscularly in doses of 500,000 to 1,000,000 units daily,

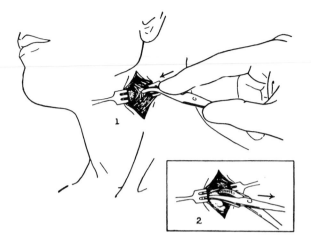

Fig. 7–3. Method of opening suppurative adenitis with a hemostat. After incising the skin, the closed hemostat is plunged through the wall of the abscess, the index finger guarding the tip so that the hemostat does not pass too deeply, when the abscess cavity is entered, the blades are spread apart and the hemostat is withdrawn, the opening in this way being enlarged bluntly.

are indicated. In the early stages the infection may be aborted; in the later stages, even if fluctuation is present and incision is indicated, the antibiotics hasten healing.

When suppuration occurs, as evidenced usually by fluctuation of the node, incision and drainage are necessary. Incision too early, however, will tend to spread the infection. It is best to delay incision until the induration has practically disappeared and a localized abscess has formed. In the neck, it is frequently difficult to demonstrate fluctuation in the enlarged deep nodes. However, a lymphadenitis that persists as an enlarged, hard swelling for 10 days or more after an acute infection has subsided usually is found to be the seat of a suppurative necrotic process, and incision is indicated.

In incising a lymphadenitis, it is best to make a small incision over the most prominent part of the mass and then to enter the suppurative process with a closed blunt hemostat. When pus is found, the hemostat is removed with the blades open, thus enlarging the wound (Fig. 7-3). The wound is then explored with a curved hemostat or a probe, and the incision is enlarged in the direction of the longest diameter of the abscess, the edges of the wound being held open with rake retractors or Allis forceps. When the

abscess is completely open, the lips of the wound are filled loosely with gauze which is to be removed in 24 hours; otherwise it may prevent drainage. In suppurative lymphadenitis of the neck, the same method of opening the abscess is used, but frequently it is inadvisable to enlarge the opening to the full extent of the abscess because of important structures which must be protected against trauma. In such cases, the wound is prevented from closing too rapidly by means of a double-barreled rubber tube (Fig. 7-4). This tube keeps the wound open and permits drainage until it is removed.

Penicillin is usually the drug of choice in pyogenic infections, with chlortetracycline, chloramphenicol, and oxytetracycline as alternatives. Streptomycin is specific therapy for tuberculosis and for tularemia; chlortetracycline or oxytetracycline, for lymphopathia venereum. Penicillin, chloramphenicol, or the tetracycline antibiotics may be used with benefit in actinomycosis.

ABSCESSES

Etiology. Superficial or deep local abscesses are the residual complications of such infections as lymphadenitis, cellulitis, erysipelas, and suppurative thrombophlebitis. Occasionally, an abscess re-

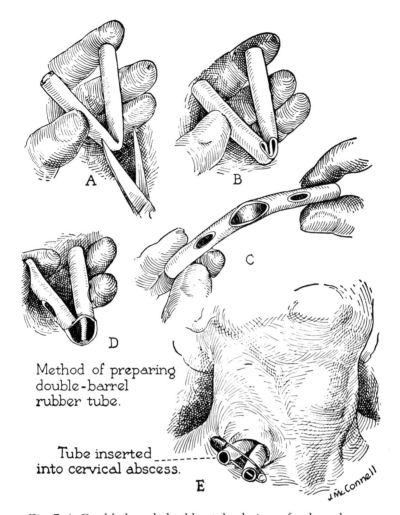

Method of preparing
double-barrel
rubber tube.

Tube inserted
into cervical abscess.

Fig. 7–4. Double-barreled rubber tube drainage for deep abscesses.

sults from contamination at the time of a direct penetrating wound.

Treatment. Incision and drainage, after localization, are the only adequate treatment. A liberal incision, so placed as to afford direct drainage, is advocated. The direction of the incision should also be so chosen as to avoid injury to important adjacent structures and to prevent disabling or disfiguring scars. In deep abscesses that extend along a fascial space, an accurate anatomic knowledge of the part is required to obtain adequate drainage without injury to important structures or impairment of function. The advantages of a bloodless field, easily obtained with an inflated blood-pressure cuff, should be remembered when deep infections of the extremities are being incised.

Drain material, such as plain fine mesh gauze, that favors and does not prevent escape of wound secretions and that can easily be removed is advocated. Gauze drains aid in securing hemostasis and in keeping the lips of the wound open until inflammatory induration establishes an adequate drainage tract. They should be

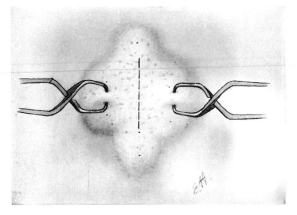

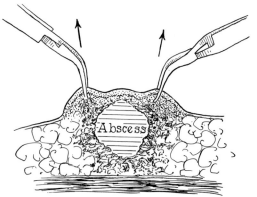

Fig. 7–5. Method of incising a superficial abscess under local infiltration anesthesia. The skin and the superficial tissues overlying the abscess cavity are infiltrated in the usual manner. Towel clips are inserted into the anesthetized skin on either side of the proposed line of incision. An assistant lifts up the towel clips as the incision is made into the cavity. In this way, pressure on the abscess by the knife during the incision is avoided, as is also the severe pain that accompanies such pressure. Following incision of the abscess, the towel clips on the wound edges may be used as retractors to aid in exposing the cavity.

removed within 48 hours. By that time they have served their purpose and, once removed, need not be replaced. Prolonged maintenance of gauze drains may block drainage.

The choice of anesthesia for incision and drainage will depend upon the site and the size of the abscess, the equipment available, and the mental make-up of the patient. Superficial abscesses, furuncles, and suppurative lymph nodes may often be incised in the office or the clinic under local skin infiltration. An 0.5 or a 1.0 percent solution of procaine is injected into the skin along the line of the proposed incision. It must not be diffusely infiltrated into the normal tissues about the abscess for fear of spreading the infection. The anesthetized skin is then grasped with a towel clip, or between two clips, and lifted up while the incision is made. Deep pressure over the inflamed

area is thus avoided and painless incision can be performed (Fig. 7-5).

Occasionally a short-acting general anesthetic is necessary. Several such agents are available (see Chapter 3).

TETANUS

Tetanus is an acute disease caused by the action on nerve tissue of a diffusible exotoxin produced by *Clostridium tetani*. The portal of entry may be located in any part of the body, but most often tetanus occurs in wounds of the feet, the calf, the thigh, the buttock, or the axilla. The patient gives a history of a wound of entry for infection, and usually there is physical evidence of such a wound. Nail-puncture wounds, splinter injuries, cartridge or other burns, and traumatic wounds are common portals. Superficial suppuration under a gauze dressing or a crust provides

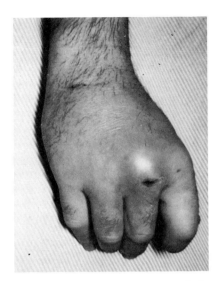

Fig. 7–6. Cellulitis around human bite over metacarpophalangeal joint.

sufficiently anaerobic conditions for the tetanus bacillus. The incubation period varies from 4 days to 3 weeks, depending somewhat upon the character, the extent, and the location of the wound.

Surgical Prophylaxis. The surgical prevention of tetanus is based upon the fact that *Clostridium tetani* is a strict anaerobe, which means that its spores can germinate and give rise to actively growing, toxin-producing bacilli only in an environment free from oxygen. It follows that all open wounds due to violence must be carefully debrided, all necrotic tissues and foreign bodies being removed with as little trauma as possible. If the tissues in the wound following débridement have an adequate blood supply, then all parts of the wound may be considered to be sufficiently oxygenated, and tetanus spores, even if they are present, do not find conditions suitable for germination. Conversely, if débridement has not been adequate, if the wound contains foreign bodies, blood clot, and areas of necrotic tissue, or if the blood supply is precarious, then conditions readily become suitable for the germination of spores and the production of toxin. Puncture wounds, particularly if contaminated, may require incision.

Immunoprophylaxis. See A Guide to Prophylaxis against Tetanus in Wound Management in Chapter 5.

HUMAN BITES

Definition. Human bites are traumatic wounds inoculated with the organisms found in the mouth. The most common site for the lesion is over the metacarpophalangeal joint on the dorsum of the hand, when the clenched fist of one combatant strikes the teeth of his opponent (Fig. 7-6). Sometimes the injury is intentional. Bites acquired by attendants caring for psychiatric patients and by policemen bringing in prisoners are not an uncommon occurrence. Finally, the injury may occur as a result of accidental puncture by utensils (forks) or instruments (dental) contaminated with human saliva. The aerobic and the anaerobic cocci, fusiform bacilli, and spirochetes present in the mouth are thus transferred to a broken area of the skin, into which may also enter any or all of the bacteria present on the skin when the wound was incurred. Anaerobic streptococci seem to be the most important of these microorganisms, although, because all act in synergism with each other, none can be ignored. The spread of infection is by way of the tissue planes contaminated by the injury. The lesions include soft-tissue necrosis, cellulitis, abscess formation, tenosynovitis, thenar and palmar space infections, and dorsal subcutaneous and subaponeurotic space infections.

Prophylaxis. These are potentially dangerous injuries, especially when they are ignored or treated incorrectly. The general lack of comprehension of the pathologic process, combined with outright mismanagement, accounts for a major portion of the poor results which follow them. In the preantibiotic era, mutilating surgery and amputation of digits, or even of an extremity, were sometimes performed, and an occasional fatality occurred.

Ideal prophylaxis in human bites of the hand begins with cleansing the part for at least 10 minutes with soap and water or with some detergent. Strong antiseptic solutions are never used. An atraumatic technique is used, and the depths of the wound receive special attention. Only after careful and thorough cleansing are the depth, the extent, and the characteristics of the injury determined. Needless to say, this entire process must be performed with good anesthesia of the affected part and gentle handling of the tissues. Débridement is carried out if gross devitalized tissue is present. It is never advisable to attempt primary closure of these wounds, and tightly packed gauze in the wound is avoided. The hand is splinted in the position of function, whether or not surgery is indicated. In any event, penicillin therapy is begun as soon as the patient is seen, and all surgery is performed under its protection. There are no reported cases of tetanus resulting from human bites; however, tetanus immune globulin or toxoid is given.

Treatment. If, as often happens, the victim is not seen until the infection is established, the affected part resembles an ordinary cellulitis, with or without lymphangitis and constitutional symptoms, and is very painful, especially on movement. There is a slight-to-moderate discharge, which frequently has a foul odor. The infection spreads progressively with time.

In the treatment of the infected human-bite wound, the main reliance is on chemotherapy based on culture and sensitivity of the organism. The part is cleansed and swathed in dressings, and, if it is the hand that is involved, it is splinted in the position of function and kept elevated. Incision and drainage are resorted to after localization has occurred. Necrotic tissue, if it is not extruded spontaneously, is meticulously debrided. Physical therapy, repair of severed tendons, etc. are delayed until after the infection has resolved and the wound has healed.

ANIMAL BITES

Treatment. Bites inflicted by dogs, cats, and other domestic animals, although usually limited to minor abrasions, may result in lacerated or penetrating wounds which are usually badly contused. Such wounds demand the careful immediate care given any potentially infected contused wound. In addition, the possible transmission of rabies, a specific infectious disease of mammals, always must be considered in the treatment of animal bites.

The first step in the treatment of a bite wound should be careful cleansing of the wound and the surrounding skin area. Good anesthesia, with either an adequate local or regional block, or with general anesthesia, is essential. All badly traumatized and nonviable tissue should be debrided. Primary suture of the wound usually is not advisable. If the animal concerned is rabid, has suggestive symptoms, or cannot be identified, it is recommended that the wound be treated as if rabies might result.

RABIES

Rabies, or hydrophobia, is an encephalitis, usually fatal, due to a neurotropic virus acquired from the saliva of a rabid animal, usually as a result of a bite. Although rabies is now well under control in regions in which public health service programs are in operation, sporadic outbreaks do occur from time to time. Dogs are most commonly responsible for transmitting the virus to men, although other mammals may do so on occasion. Bats are an important reservoir in the western hemisphere. Although most human cases occur during hot weather, the disease affects lower animals in all seasons.

Prophylactic Treatment. Prevention and control of rabies entail the impounding of stray ownerless dogs and the restraint of other dogs by their owners. In most communities, mass immunization of the canine population population is required on an annual basis. The principle threat in the United States now comes from skunks, bats, foxes, and raccoons.

In dealing with bites from animals suspected of having rabies, all factors of the case should be considered in order to make a decision concerning the administration of anti-rabies vaccine. When the animal responsible is known to have rabies, or cannot be examined, immediate immunization is indicated. Otherwise, a veterinarian should observe the dog for 14 days. If the dog was infective at the time of the bite, it will die during this period, and immunization of the patient must then be started. However, since rabies due to bites about the face and the neck tends to have a shorter incubation period, it may be advisable in such cases to begin immunization at once and to continue it until a full course of vaccine is given. The incubation period varies from 10 days to 12 months and depends largely on the amount of virus introduced and the severity of the laceration.

Rabies Antiserum. For the most serious types of exposure, passive immunization with rabies antiserum is available. Because of the possibility of a very serious type of reaction to the equine serum, a careful history of allergy and of possible sensitization to serum by previous injections should be obtained and tests for sensitivity should be carried out. (As a precaution against a severe anaphylactic reaction it is well to have at hand a syringe containing 1 ml. of 1:1000 epinephrine for immediate use should the occasion arise.) The dose of antiserum given is 40 units/kg., and half of it should be given locally into the wound. To be maximally effective the passive immunization with antiserum should be instituted within 24 hours after the bite of a rabid animal. Existing laboratory and human studies support the view that the rabies virus remains at the wound site for probably about 3 days, during which time it is subject to the action of the injected antiserum. After that time it is believed to become fixed in the nervous tissue itself, where it cannot be neutralized by rabies antibody.

All bites inflicted by possibly rabid animals should be treated by copious flushing with 20 percent soap in water, 1 percent benzalkonium chloride, or 43 percent to 70 percent ethanol. Whiskeys of 86 proof or greater can be used in emergencies.

The decision whether to immunize or not should be based upon the local incidence of rabies, the type of animal inflicting the bite, and the circumstances surrounding the incident.

If the biting animal is a domestic one, such as a dog or cat, its behavior during and after the attack is most important. Healthy animals that appear to have been provoked into biting should merely be observed, without treatment of the victim. Animals with signs suggestive of rabies should be sacrificed and their brains examined for rabies infection. Treatment should be started at once and stopped if the laboratory report is negative.

Bites of sylvatic animals, when unprovoked, must be considered contaminated by rabies virus unless the biting animal can be captured and shown to be free of rabies. Rodent bites, such as those inflicted on slum children by rats, or on middle-class children by pet hamsters, ordinarily need no antirabies treatment. However, strains of rabies virus developed for vaccination of dogs, when given to other species, may not be sufficiently attenuated. Rabies can thereby be provoked in the pet rodent, resulting in a hazard for human contacts.

In our opinion, antiserum should be used locally and parenterally, in addition to vaccine, whenever exposure to rabies has been proven or is highly likely. This statement is based on the fact that in the clinical situation it is impossible to estimate the amount of virus introduced into the wound. In infection of guinea pigs with small doses of rabies virus, vaccine alone sufficed for protection, but when moderate doses were given, antiserum was necessary in addition to vaccine. The combination of antiserum and vaccine provides an immediate rise in the level of antibody, which should result in the maximal neutralization of the virus while it is still susceptible to the action of antibody. A single dose of antiserum (40 units/kg.) followed by vaccine immediately gives detectable circulating antibody, which persists through the period of 10 to 14 days before a response due to vaccine takes place. This therapy is a double-edged sword, however, because even one dose of antiserum may slightly suppress the response to vaccine unless the latter is given in adequate antigenic mass.

Antirabies Vaccine. The vaccines available are of three main types:

1. Simple type, made of the suspension of the brain tissue of rabid animals, the virus being killed with phenol.

2. The irradiated type, in which the virus in the brain suspension is killed by ultraviolet radiation.

3. Duck embryo inactivated vaccine. (This vaccine is believed to contain less of the factors which produce post-vaccinal allergic encephalitis.)

Vaccine, whether duck embryo or simple type, must be given daily for at least 14 days. Some authorities recommend 21 daily injections, but there does not seem to be good evidence that 21 are superior to 14. The inoculations cannot be given over a shorter period of time or in larger volume less frequently; daily stimulus is necessary. In order to insure that antiserum does not suppress the active antibody response, booster doses of vaccine must be administered 10 days and 20 days after the last injection of the initial series.

BIBLIOGRAPHY

Treatment of Local Infections

Altemeier, W. A.: Chemotherapy in surgery, *In* Carter, B. N.: Monographs on Surgery, New York, Nelson, 1950.

Altemeier, W. A., and Giuseffi, J.: Treatment of surgical infections in the ambulatory patient. Surg. Clin. N. Am., 1259, 1951.

Koch, S. L.: Boils and carbuncles, Surg., Gynec. Obstet., *117*:231, 1963.

Pulaski, E. J., and Shaeffer, J. R.: The background of antibiotic therapy in surgical infections. Int. Abstr. Surg., *93*:1-20, 1951.

Pulaski, E. J.: Treatment of soft-tissue infections, Antibiot. Med. Clin. Ther., *4*:657, 1957.

————: Surgical Infections, Prophylaxis, Treatment, Antibiotic Therapy, Springfield, Ill., Thomas, 1954.

Sanford, J. P., Prendergast, B. S., Balch, H. H., and Hughes, Carl W.: An experimental evaluation of the usefulness of antibiotic agents in the early management of contaminated traumatic soft tissue wounds. Surg., Gynec. Obstet., *105*:5, 1957.

Erysipeloid

Gregory, P. O.: Erysipeloid, a method of treatment, J. Maine Med./Assoc., *44*:1, 1953.

Tetanus

Carter, W. S., and Holder, T. M.: Correct use of tetanus prophylaxis, Mod. Med., 184, 1964.

Ipsen, J.: Changes in immunity and antitoxin level immediately after secondary stimulus with tetanus toxoid in rabbits. J. Immun., *86*:50, 1961.

McComb, J. A., and Dwyer, R. C.: Passive-active immunization with tetanus immune globulin (human). New Eng. J. Med., *268*:857, 1963.

McDonald, R. T., Kirtland, H. B., Jr., Brown, R. G., and Gibson, R.: Rapid immunization with tetanus toxoid with antitoxin titer assay, Surg., Gynec. Obstet., *119*:81, 1964.

McDonald, R. T., Kirtland, H. B., and Brown, R. G.: Tetanus prophylaxis in the unimmunized; administration of oxytetracycline and intradermal toxoid, with restricted use of tetanus antitoxin, Calif. Med., *96*:257, 1962.

Skudder, P. A., and McCarroll, J. R.: Current status of tetanus control. JAMA, *188*:625, 1964.

Stafford, E. S.: Active immunization against tetanus. Arch. Environ. Health, *8*:742, 1964.

Human Bites

Boyce, F. F.: Human bites. A study of a second series of 93 (chiefly delayed and late) cases from charity hospital of Louisiana at New Orleans, Southern Surg., *14*:690, 1948.

Mason, M. L., and Koch, S. L.: Human bite infections of the hand, with a study of routes of extension of infection from the dorsum of the hand. Surg., Gynec. Obstet., *51*:591, 1930.

Rabies

Dean, J. D.: Treatment of rabies. Mod. Med., (April 13) 140, 1964.

Habel, K.: Rabies (hydrophobia) *In* Conn, H. F., ed.: Current Therapy 1953. Philadelphia, Saunders, 1953.

Hildreth, E. A., Jr.: Treatment of rabies. Penn. Med. J., *67*:44, 1964.

Hildreth, E. A., Jr.: Prevention of rabies, or the decline of Sirius, Ann. Int. Med., *58*:883, 1963.

8

Snakebites and Insect Bites

C. C. Snyder, M.D.

SNAKEBITES

The poisonous snakes of medical significance native to the United States are known as rattlesnakes, cottonmouth moccasins, copperhead moccasins, and coral snakes. The first three belong to the family Crotalidae, which is represented by 210 species and subspecies. They have a heat sensitive organ, called a "pit", below and in front of each eye; hence the name pit vipers. Coral snakes, which do not have this pit feature, are members of the Elapidae family and are represented by 87 species and subspecies. The largest of the domestic serpentine venomers is the *Crotalus adamanteus* (eastern diamondback rattlesnake). The *C. adamanteus, C. atrox* (western diamondback rattler), and *C. scutulatus* (Mohave rattlesnake) are responsible for the most critical bites in the United States. These are followed, in sequence of serious envenomation, by the *Agkistrodon piscivorus* (cottonmouth water moccasin), the genera *Micrurus* and *Micruroides* (coral snakes), and the *Agkistrodon mokeson* (copperhead moccasin).

Snakebite deaths, throughout the world, happen more frequently than most doctors realize, estimates of 15,000 to 20,000 annually being far too low. Recent indications, as determined by perusal of the literature and physicians' reports, are that the total is 75,000. This does not include an untold number of bites which are never treated or reported. The University of Utah-V. A. Hospital team has treated 114 human snakebites, and Findlay Russell of California has treated more than this amount. The majority of snakebites in the United States have been recorded in the southern states. A poisonous snake is endowed with a pair of specialized glands, relatively comparable to the parotid salivary glands of humans in size, contour, and position, but variable in that the serpent's gland comprises in addition a venomous glandular portion. The principal salivary duct empties its contents into the hollow fang on the anterior surface at its base. This injecting apparatus is a specially constructed, canalized tooth, which serves to expel the toxin.

Protein fractionation of poisonous venom discloses a diversity of active principles, the names and descriptions of which are dependent upon the interpretations of individual investigators who sometimes are not in agreement. Regardless, it is the concensus that Elapidae venom contains potent neurotoxins and respiratory toxins but only mild hemolytic and cytolytic enzymes. These factors account for the extreme systemic reaction, yet rather mild local reaction, observed in Elapidae (cobra and coral) envenomation. In comparison, Crotalidae venom is mildly neurotoxic, but, due to powerful hemolysins, cytolysins, and coagulant factors, it produces severe proteolysis, necrosis, and slough of tissue at the bite site. Venom from the Viperidae simulates many of the actions of Crotalidae poisoning.

An early correct diagnosis of envenomation is important because immediate therapeutic procedures can be lifesaving. In contradistinction, vigorous therapy with horse-serum antivenom for misdiagnosed poisonous serpent bites may terminate in misfortune. If possible, the venomer should be retrieved and taken to an authority on herpetology for identification. The presence of fang marks in the skin is diagnostic of venenation. There may be only one fang mark, two fang marks, three marks, four marks, or even six marks. Pain is the most common symptom in cases of Crotalidae and Viperidae bites, the average onset occurring within 10 minutes. The discomfort may be only slight, moderate, or severe. Local erythema becomes evident and is progressive. Edema usually appears in a few minutes and is definitely progressive. The bites of Elapidae (coral and cobra) snakes usually are painless and initially without swelling; edema usually starts an hour or so after the bite and reaches a plateau in 24 to 48 hours; other signs are eyelid ptosis, hemoptysis, and incoagulable blood. The victim may worsen and exhibit symptoms of shock (weakness, syncope, hypotension), become nauseated, vomit, exhibit urinary and fecal incontinency, begin to twitch, and not respond to external stimuli. If the patient becomes moribund, the pupils dilate, respiration is difficult, the pulse is hardly palpable, and unconsciousness follows. Following snakebite without venenation, none of these symptoms occur routinely, nor do they occur in this sequence. Reid reported recently a most important observation: that it is incorrect to assume that all venomous snakebites are fatal and to assume that snakebites that do not produce symptoms of poisoning are always inflicted by nonpoisonous snakes; that 53 percent of the victims of "lethal" viper, cobra, and sea-snake bites escape with mild or no poisoning; and that more than half of the bites inflicted by poisonous serpents do not produce serious envenomation. In summary, he says that snakes bite humans strictly as a defensive mechanism and that little venom is injected; "therefore poisonous snakebite is not synonymous with snakebite poisoning."

Because the effects of snakebite differ in their severity, their treatment should also be varied. Therefore, snakebites should be classified, and a simple method is:

1. MILD: scratch marks, no pain, minimal swelling.
2. MODERATE: fang marks, pain, local swelling, no systemic symptoms.
3. SEVERE: fang marks, immediate excruciating wound pain, progressive swelling, cyanosis, bullae, and systemic symptoms.

For the mild type of envenomation, the wound should be cleansed with soap and water or alcohol, and dressed if necessary. Incisions and antivenin are not indicated. For moderate envenomation, the fang marks should be incised and antivenin given. The severe effects of snakebite should be treated vigorously by applying a tourniquet, excising the fang-mark area, giving antivenin, and hospitalizing the patient (Fig. 8-1).

Treatment for venomous snakebite is divided into (a) immediate (first-aid) treatment in the field and (b) hospital therapy. Snake-infested areas, occult foliage, old logs, caves, and dens should be avoided. Keep a vehicle near for emergencies. Carry a snakebite kit (a flat tourniquet—25¢, two alcohol-prep sponges—10¢, a disposable scalpel in sterile foil—20¢, Wyeth polyvalent antivenin—about

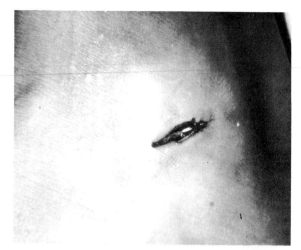

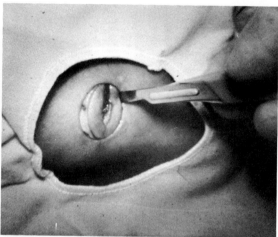

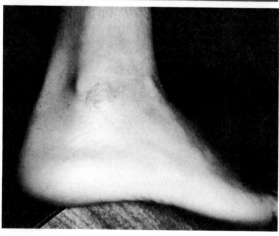

Fig. 8–1. (*Top*) Rattlesnake bite inflicted at the lateral malleolus; treated by linear incision and sction, but edema continued progressively. (*Center*) Elliptical excision and venom retrieval proved to be more efficacious. (*Bottom*) Small skin graft a week later afforded desired result.

$10, a 100-mg. vial of Solu-Cortef—75¢, a disposable syringe—8¢, and a 100-ml. vial of normal saline solution with tubing—90¢) and know how to use it.

FIRST-AID TREATMENT

1. *Incarcerate the antigen*, using a flat tourniquet applied between the bite and the heart; this should be tight enough to

impede the superficial venous and lymphatic return, but not so tight as to obstruct the arterial supply or produce ischemia. The tourniquet should admit a finger beneath it easily and should *not* be removed and reapplied at short intervals because this perpetuates the spread of the venom. Every effort should be made to avoid elevation of blood pressure by activity or acceleration of circulation with stimulants or drugs. The affected area should be kept at heart level, without elevation or dependency. The victim should be taken to the nearest physician or hospital as soon as this is feasible. The snake should be slain and its carcass retrieved for identification.

2. *Retrieve the antigen,* after cleansing the wound with the alcohol sponges, by making only one linear incision (not cruciate incisions) through the fang marks with the disposable scalpel. The incision is extended one-fourth inch beyond the punctures and should avoid vital structures, such as nerves, tendons, and large vessels. Cruciate incisions are condemned, as they macerate, necrose, and harbor anaerobes. Digitally express or mechanically suction the wound for 20 to 30 minutes, but avoid trauma to the soft tissues. Oral suction is not advocated, as it introduces bacteria into the wound.

3. *Neutralize the antigen,* using Wyeth's polyvalent antivenin. It is. disadvantageous to inject the antivenin into the snakebite area, where edema reigns and inhibits absorption of the antivenin. It is also difficult, when the antivenin is given in this way or intramuscularly, to retrieve the antivenin or to treat the victim if he is allergic to the antivenin. It is permissible for the laity to inject the antivenin intramuscularly to achieve faster absorption. (Intravenous and intra-arterial administration are discussed below.) Never inject antivenin into the base of a digit because this may obliterate the vessels by causing pressure or spasm and may result in loss of the digit.

HOSPITAL TREATMENT

1. The physician or his nurse should immediately become acquainted with the traumatic incident by recording a *rapid history.* If the victim is a former patient, the doctor will know whether or not the patient has allergic manifestations, and, if he does, he will proceed cautiously.

2. With the tourniquet still in position, the *fang marks should be excised,* the excision extending one-half inch beyond each fang mark and down to the vital structures beneath the skin.

3. If the victim is not allergic to horse serum, one vial of polyvalent antivenin should be administered intravenously or intra-arterially to effect rapid neutralization. These two methods of therapy produce immediate allergic phenomena, if such are bound to happen, and the allergic reaction can be counteracted rapidly via the same route. The antivenin is diluted by adding it to 100 ml. of isotonic saline to which has been added 100 mg. of Solu-Cortef, and it is given over a period of 20 minutes, propelling the solution by means of a rubber bulb. The author favors the intra-arterial route in preference to the intravenous route because by the former route the antivenin reaches, contacts, and neutralizes the venomous antigen faster. If the patient is known to be allergic or if the skin test is positive, and, therefore, host desensitization is required, the dosage of antivenin must be tempered to the severity of the snakebite. The initial dose given subcutaneously may be 0.1 ml. of a 1:10, 1:100, or 1:1000 dilution of the antiserum, and subsequent doses should be doubled and given every 15 minutes until 1 ml. of undiluted serum is accepted by the host without reaction. The rest of the material is then administered subcutaneously, where it may be excised if a reaction ensues.

Hypersensitivity reactions range from local urticaria and generalized erythema to full-blown anaphylaxis with bronchocongestion and vascular collapse. Immediate. therapy includes epinephrine, corticosteroids, and antihistamines. None of these agents should be used for snakebite in the absence of hypersensitivity reactions. It has been proved that some antihistamines act synergistically with snake venom, and these drugs are therefore contraindicated in snakebite therapy. The tourniquet should be removed if the extremity is ischemic or cyanotic; otherwise, tourniquets are left in position for two hours if necessary, but must be loosened in relation to the ensuing edema. Children, because they have less blood volume and, thus, greater venom concentration, need more antivenin than do adults. If more than one vial of antivenin is necessary, it should be administered without hesitation. In 15 canines and 41 humans, only 1 vial of antivenin per patient, given intra-arterially, was necessary to neutralize *C. adamanteus* or *A. piscivorus* antigen successfully.

4. Cryotherapy is beneficial when it is used to decrease metabolic processes in the area of the bite. Frostbite induced by extensive ice application and superimposed upon a snakebite, modifies a serious condition into a critical one. Therefore, cooling this inflammatory process with mild hypothermia is beneficial, but freezing it is detrimental, because of local tissue damage and the increased escape of venom when the ice is removed. One scientist (Stahnke, 1969) will take issue with this approach.

5. *Ancillary therapy.* Steroid treatment, at one time recommended, is now believed to be of value only to counteract allergic manifestations of the horse-serum antivenin. Several clinicians and investigators have come to the conclusion that ACTH, cortisone, hydrocortisone, and also procaine neither effect absolute recovery nor prevent tissue damage and inflammation. A recent conversation with Herbert Stahnke revealed that he has not been impressed with alcohol ingestion during snake envenomation. Our experiments revealed that alcoholic beverages are contraindicated because they accelerate circulation and camouflage important symptoms when respiratory depression is present. Tetanus antitoxin or booster, antibiotics, analgesics, oxygen, transfusion, calcium, tracheostomy, fascial incisions, and hemodialysis certainly must be utilized when indications are presented. All victims of venomous snakebite should be closely observed for 72 hours following the snakebite.

HYMENOPTERA

This order includes bees, wasps, hornets, ants, and other insects of which the venomers are the females. The venom is expelled via an ovipositor which has the dual purpose of injecting poison and depositing eggs. Some ovipositors are smooth and others are barbed; the former type may sting repeatedly, whereas the latter type hooks into the victim and tears from the insect, causing its death. The lancet deposited in the victim adds antigens to the bee venom. Responses in the animal victim may range from only a slight histamine wheal to a dramatic, fatal anaphylactic shock. The interval between the envenomation and death is usually rapid—less than an hour. Drop for drop, the venom of the bee is just as potent as is that of the rattlesnake. The usual symptoms are pain at site of the sting, swelling, erythema, intense heat, arthralgia, pruritus, and urticaria. If allergic systemic symptoms ensue, the venom's hemolytic and neurotoxic effects appear, with the development of petechial hemorrhages, malaise, weakness, nausea, vomiting, abdominal cramps, dyspnea, vascular collapse, and death.

The treatment for severe hymenopterous envenomation must be prompt. If indicated, establish an open airway, start oxygen and artificial resuscitation, and prepare an intravenous infusion of 3 to 4 mg. of Benadryl per kilogram of body weight, followed by 10 ml. of 10 percent calcium lactate or gluconate solution. Immediate *but* slow injection of 0.8 ml. to 1.0 ml. of 1:1000 epinephrine into the vein may be lifesaving. Other antihistamines or adrenal corticoid, or steroid therapy may be of benefit. Cold packs and local applications of antihistamine ointments are adjunctive treatment. Emergency kits for treating allergic reactions to insect stings should contain: a tourniquet to be used for extremity bites, thumb forceps to remove the stinger, a disposable syringe for epinephrine injection, and antihistamines. A significant desensitization may be achieved by using a polyvalent antigenic preparation made from the antigens of bees, wasps, hornets, yel-

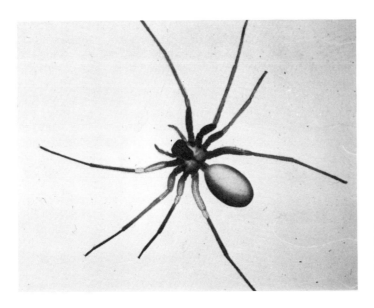

Fig. 8–2. Brown recluse spider, also known as the fiddler because of the dark guitar- or violin-shaped insignia on its back.

low jackets, and ants. It is suggested that, for adequate protection, this material be taken for three years.

SPIDERS

All spiders are venomous. There are two groups of poisonous spiders in the United States, *Latrodectus* (widow spiders) and *Loxoscelus* (brown spiders). Black widow spiders are found in all the states, and bites have been reported from most of them. There are three species of *Latrodectus* in America: *L. geometricus, L. mactans,* and *L. curadaviensus.* Spiders propagate the poison from their venom glands via a pair of appendages near the mouth. The venoms of the black widow spider are histolytic and systemic, and 23 protein fractions have been found. There have been thousands of clinical cases and many deaths have been reported, but these represent only a fraction of the true number, because many cases have been misdiagnosed and many other patients never reported for treatment. A most popular spider to receive current medical attention is the *Loxosceles reclusus* (brown recluse spider) (Fig. 8-2). This drab fellow is found throughout the south central United States and sports a dark fiddle-shaped insignia on the dorsal cephalothorax.

The major symptoms of black widow spider bite are severe pain, cramps, and muscle spasm that eventually affect the whole body. Misdiagnoses include intra-abdominal emergency, coronary thrombosis, lobar pneumonia, and tetanus. There is a specific antivenom for *Latrodectus* envenomation. Although calcium gluconate has been used in the past as a muscle relaxant, methocarbamol (Robaxin) is the present choice. Analgesics, cardiotonic agents, and antihistamines are used for symptom relief. Pain and discomfort usually persist for 24 hours and then decrease by the next day. Death due to latrodectism is uncommon.

Arachnidism due to the brown recluse spider is exhibited by anorexia, apathy, and dehydration during the first 8 hours postbite. The bite site becomes erythematous and then forms a blister surrounded by a halo of ischemia. In a week or so, the central area becomes depressed and necrosed (Fig. 8-3). The necrosis spreads and forms an ulceration. Systemic reactions consist of chills, fever, nausea, vomiting, arthralgia, and a petechial eruption within 24 hours after envenomation. A diagnosis of loxoscelism is only presumptive if the venomer has not actually been seen. Patients have been protected against brown spider venom injections with methyl prednisolone.

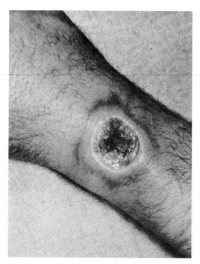

Fig. 8–3. Brown recluse spider bite, exhibiting the typical result of an ulcer with an elevated periphery and an umbilicated center.

Total excision and primary closure of the site are recommended in human cases. Skin grafts to the ulcer take poorly.

SCORPIONS

All scorpions are venomers, and instead of biting they inject their venom via a tail stinger. Some produce a local reaction, whereas others produce a systemic effect. Scorpions found in Arizona and the Southwest are known to be potentially lethal (Fig. 8-4). In Arizona, there are twice as many deaths from scorpion venom than there are from all other venomous animals. Scorpion venom seems to produce its effects through increased amounts of circulating catecholamines, which cause myocardial damage and cardiac failure. The lethal species of scorpions found in the areas mentioned above are *Centruroides sculpturatus* and *Centruroides gertschi.* Symptoms include copious salivation and chaotic convulsions. Hypothermia has been suggested as a means to prevent rapid absorption and should be initiated immediately after the sting. The severe pain that accompanies the sting is said to be dramatically relieved by the local injection of emetine hydrochloride in a concentration of one grain (65 mg.) in one ml. of solution. Evidently emetine is a direct antagonist of the poison. Antivenin is available to Arizona physicians and has probably been helpful in the treatment of human cases. Morphine and demerol are contraindicated and may convert a sublethal to a lethal envenomation.

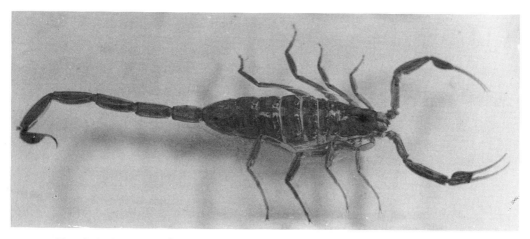

Fig. 8–4. Scorpions do not bite, but inject their venom through a tail stinger.

BIBLIOGRAPHY

Andrews, C. E.: Venomous snakebite committee annual report. J. Florida Med. Assoc., *55*:308, 1968.

Arbesman, C. E.: The allergic response to stinging insects; IV—Cross-reactions between bee, wasp, and yellow jacket. J. Allergy, *36*:147, 1965.

Bogen, E.: The treatment of spider bite poisoning. *In* Buckley, E. E., and Porges, N. (eds.): Venoms. pub. 44, p. 101. Washington, D. C., Am. Assoc. Advance. Sci., 1956.

Davidson, T.: Inside the world of the honey bee. Nat. Geographic Mag., *154*:188, 1959.

Dillaha, C. J., Jansen, G. T., Honeycutt, W. H., and Carlson, R. H.: North American loxoscelism—necrotic bite of the brown recluse spider. JAMA, *188*:33, 1964.

Ditmars, R. L.: The Reptiles of North America., p. 119, Garden City, N. Y., Doubleday & Co., 1951.

Ellis, E. R., and Smith, R. T.: Systemic anaphylaxis after rattlesnake bite. JAMA, *193*:151, 1965.

Fardon, D. W., Wingo, C. W., Robinson, D. W., and Masters, F. W.: The treatment of brown spider bite. Plast. Reconstr. Surg., *40*:483, 1968.

Frazier, C. A.: Insect sting reactions in children. Ann. Allergy, *23*:37, 1965.

Grazier, D. B., and Carler, F. H.: Use of the artificial kidney in snakebite. Calif. Med., *97*:177, 1962.

Gueson, M.: Catecholomines and myocardial damage in scorpion sting. Am. Heart J., *75*:715, 1968.

Y., Doubleday & Co., 1951.

Ellis, E. R., and Smith, R. T.: Systemic anaphylaxis after rattlesnake bite. JAMA, *193*:151, 1965.

Fardon, D. W., Wingo, C. W., Robinson, D. W., and Masters, F. W.: The treatment of brown spider bite. Plast. Reconstr. Surg., *40*:483, 1968.

Frazier, C. A.: Insect sting reactions in children. Ann. Allergy, *23*:37, 1965.

Grazier, D. B., and Carler, F. H.: Use of the artificial kidney in snakebite. Calif. Med., *97*:177, 1962.

Gueson, M.: Catecholomines and myocardial damage in scorpion sting. Am. Heart J., *75*:715, 1968.

Holmes, M. McA.: Scorpion bites. Brit. Med. J., *2*:353, 1957.

Horen, W. P. Arachnidism in the United States. JAMA, *185*:839, 1963.

Jensen, H., and Westphal, U.: Chemical structure and interrelationship of toad poisons. *In* Buckley, E. E., and Porges, N. (eds.): Venoms. pub. 44, p. 75. Washington, D. C., Am. Assoc. Advance. Sci., 1956.

Kennedy, C. B.: Insect stings and bites; diagnosis, treatment, and prevention. Postgrad. Med., *37*:193, 1965.

Levi, H. W.: The number of species of black widow spiders Theridiidae Latrodectus. Science, *127*:1055, 1958.

McCollough, N. C., and Gennaro, J. F.: Evaluation of venomous snakebite in the southern United States from parallel clinical and laboratory investigations; Development of Treatment. J. Florida Med. Assoc., *49*:959, 1963.

———: Evaluation of snakebite. J. Florida Med. Assoc., *69*:965, 1963.

O'Connor, R., and Erickson, R.: Hymenoptera antigens: an immunological comparison of venoms, venom sac extracts, and whole-insect extracts. Ann. Allergy, *23*:151, 1965.

Parrish, H. M., and Scatterday, J. E.: A survey of poisonous snakebites among domestic animals in Florida. Vet. Med., *52*:135, 1957.

Reid, H. A.: Symptomatology, pathology, and treatment of land snake bite in India and Southeast Asia. *In* Bücherl, W., *et al.* (eds.): Venomous Animals and Their Venoms, p. 611, New York, Academic Press, 1968.

Shaffer, J. H.: Stinging insects—a threat to life. JAMA, *177*:473, 1961.

Snyder, C. C.: A.A.H.A. Scientific Presentations, *61*:65, 1963.

Snyder, C. C., and Knowles, R. P.: Snakebite! Consultant, July-August, 1963.

———: Pathogenesis and treatment of poisonous Snakebites. J. Am. Vet. Med. Assoc., *151*:1635, 1967.

Snyder, C. C., Knowles, R. P., Pickens, J. E., and Emerson, J. L.: Snakebite poisoning. *In* Catcott, E. J. (ed.): Canine Medicine, p. 253. Wheaton, Ill., Am. Vet. Pub., Inc., 1968.

Stahnke, H. L.: Hypothermia and scorpion venenation. Southwest. Med., *46*:285, 1965.

———: The Treatment of Venomous Bites and Stings. p. 21. Tempe, Ariz., Arizona State University Bureau of Publications, 1966.

———: Personal interview, Jan., 1969.

Stahnke, H. L., and Stahnke, J.: The treatment of scorpion sting. Arizona Med., *14*:576, 1957.

9

Burns and Frostbite

Mark W. Wolcott, M.D.

BURNS

Burns are the destructive changes occurring in tissue due to excessive heat, chemicals, ultraviolet irradiation and other agents. For descriptive purposes, burns are classified into degrees. A first-degree burn is characterized by superficial erythema; a second-degree burn, by vesiculation and bleb formation; and a third-degree burn, by destruction of the entire thickness of the skin and, perhaps, involvement of the underlying structures. This classification considers only the depth of tissue involvement, whereas an equally important factor in determining the seriousness of a burn is the extent of body surface involved. Burns that involve more than 10% of the body surface in children, or 15 percent in older adults, must be regarded as serious; and the person should be hospitalized. A rough estimate of the involved body surface may be obtained if the entire body surface is divided into thirds—the legs and the buttocks constituting one third, the trunk and the neck one third, and the arms and the head one third. The necessity for prompt hospitalization of young children with burns of as little as 5 percent of the body surface should be stressed.

In the consideration of burns in ambulatory patients, one must of necessity consider only relatively minor burns, that is,

minor as regards the extent, degree, and location. A patient with a third-degree burn of only 5 percent of the body surface should be hospitalized, whereas one with a first- or second-degree burn involving 10 to 15 percent of the body surface may just as well be treated on an ambulatory basis. Those with burns about the eye or in flexion creases, even if these are of relatively minor extent, should probably be hospitalized, at least initially. In addition, one must consider the first-aid treatment of all burns. The more serious aspects of burns—the shock, hemoconcentration, and other serious disturbances of fluid balance—are not complications which can well be taken care of in the ambulatory patient.

FIRST-AID TREATMENT OF BURNS

The first-aid treatment depends somewhat upon the extent, the location, and the degree of the burn. In first- or second-degree burns, almost any form of treatment which combines protection of the lesion with relief of pain will give good results. In more extensive burns of second or third degree, however, primary treatment is of particular importance because it may influence the ease with which subsequent treatment may be given. Most burns, by their very mode of causation, are primarily sterile. If the entire epidermis is not destroyed, they will heal rapidly if infection does not enter the picture. The organisms that cause troublesome infections are most often those from the nose, the throat, and the hands of the patient himself or of his attendant; hence the importance of an early protective dressing. A thorough washing with soap and water followed by a simple petrolatum dressing applied with firm pressure is probably all that need be done for most minor burns. For patients with more extensive burns, which are associated with shock, hemoconcentration, and other physiologic disturbances, hospitalization is necessary. In such cases, first aid consists of the application of a simple protective dressing, the relief of pain by giving morphine, and the institution of an intravenous solution, such as saline or Ringer's lactate, leaving the definitive treatment for the better facilities afforded by the hospital.

Prevention of infection should include tetanus prophylaxis. However, the prophylactic use of antibiotics given parenterally is not indicated for the burn itself. The use of 10 percent Sulfamylon cream (alpha-amino-para-toluene sulfonamide) topically is recommended and it should be applied once daily when used. It is not necessary in first-degree burns or in most small second-degree burns.

Treatment of First-Degree Burns

In first-degree burns the tissue damage is minimal; there is an erythema resulting from superficial capillary dilatation, and there are also capillary changes of mild degree in the outer layers of the skin in which transudations and effusion have not developed. These burns result mostly from contact with hot fluids or from exposure to sunlight or an ultraviolet lamp, but occasionally are flash burns due to an explosion. When they involve a considerable surface of the body, they give marked pain and may produce systemic symptoms, such as nausea, vomiting, headache, and malaise. As a rule, however, patients recover within 24 to 48 hours without marked systemic disturbances. Various antiseptic and anesthetic ointments have been recommended and used for years. The oily ointments that exclude the air from the burned area give considerable relief. It is questionable whether the anesthetic incorporated in the ointment is of any particular value, and it can be toxic if large areas are treated.

Treatment of Second-Degree Burns

In second-degree burns there is a more marked local tissue disturbance, with capillary wall destruction resulting in edema and bleb formation. These burns are by far the most frequent in number. They may be due to scalding, flame, or the touching of hot objects. When they are seen by physicians, usually numerous blebs have already formed, but others may form during the subsequent days. Numerous local applications have been suggested and used in the treatment of such burns. Tannic acid and other eschar-producing drugs fell into disfavor during wartime experience with burns. This occurred for various reasons, but chiefly because better results could be obtained with other local applications. The best results can be obtained by the following treatment:

1. Wash the area with white soap and water.

2. Do not break blisters or otherwise debride the wound.

3. Cover with fine mesh gauze impregnated with petrolatum or Sulfamylon cream.

4. Apply over this a firm dressing bulky enough to keep dirt away from the injury.

This treatment is probably as satisfactory as any. Whether or not blisters should be broken is a minor debatable question; blisters will usually break anyway if a firm pressure dressing is applied, and the protection afforded by an intact blister is questionable, since bacteria invade it from surrounding skin. In addition, many blisters are already broken by the time the patient reaches the surgeon for treatment.

The important points in the care of a limited second-degree burn are:

1. To do all that is necessary in the way of cleansing and preventing infection at the primary dressing.

2. Not to re-dress the burned area, except to change the outside dressings, until the burn is healed; unless, of course, there are complications, i.e., infection.

The importance of not re-dressing a small second-degree burn for from 10 to 14 days cannot be too strongly stressed. If the primary dressing has been adequate, most second-degree burns will be entirely healed when the dressing is removed.

TREATMENT OF THIRD-DEGREE BURNS

In third-degree burns there is destruction of tissue involving not only the skin but also the underlying tissues. If these burns are small in area, the patient can be kept ambulatory, but in the case of third-degree burns of any extent hospitalization is recommended. In the local treatment of these areas, the preparations described for second-degree burns are used and the principles of treatment are the same. No effort is made to excise the burned areas. When the burn is first re-dressed on the 10th to the 14th day, the destroyed tissue can be lifted off with forceps and scissors. An ulcer with a granulating tissue base remains; this must heal, either by secondary intent or by skin grafting. The latter method definitely is preferable and, as soon as clean granulations are formed, either a Thiersch or a Reverdin skin graft may be used to hasten the epithelization. Pinch grafts may be used for ambulatory patients if the part on which the graft is to be placed can be immobilized by splinting.

LATER TREATMENT OF BURNS

The granulation tissue in the area of third-degree burns may become hypertrophic and, instead of appearing as a bright-red, easily bleeding surface, becomes a grayish, gelatinous, unhealthy overgrowth. Healing is very much delayed by this excessive granulation, and the deposition of excessive fibrous tissue produces hypertrophy and unsightly scars, which later may give contractures.

The treatment is to cover the area as soon as possible with epithelium. It is quite difficult for the epithelium, as it grows in from the sides, to cover the granulating area; therefore, nature must be given some aid. The most effective and the most rapid method is by the application of skin grafts, but, before this can be done, it is necessary to remove the excessive granulation, either by actually cutting it away with a razor, scissors, or a knife or by removing it with a preparation of a caustic chemical such as a silver nitrate stick. With the former method, there is usually considerable oozing, which is easily taken care of by pressure; with the latter method, the oozing is usually not so great, but grafts cannot be applied until a day or two later, when the effects of the silver nitrate have disappeared. Occasionally, the same result may be obtained by the use of pressure dressings over the area of hypertrophied granulation. When the granulating area is smooth and even with the surface of the surrounding skin, the epithelium from the sides grows in more rapidly and skin grafts are more likely to "take."

A high vitamin and high caloric diet, fresh air, sunlight, and other such measures of good hygiene should be taken into account in caring for these patients.

FROSTBITE

Etiology. Frostbite is a form of peripheral vascular disease due to cold, which produces peripheral vascular changes that cause the typical symptoms and lesions. There are numerous predisposing factors which may account for the occurrence of frostbite. It is easy to understand how patients with peripheral arterial disease, such as endarteritis, arteriosclerosis, or diabetes, or with circulatory incompetence, as in myocarditis or debility, may develop tissue changes earlier than do patients with a normal peripheral circulation. The wind velocity at the time of exposure to cold is also a factor; the loss of heat produced by the motion of the surrounding air predisposes to the development of frostbite. Another factor of importance is previous frostbite; areas once subjected to it are more readily susceptible to subsequent exposure to cold. Moisture is another factor which predisposes to frostbite. Wet clothing, especially wet shoes and socks, permits chilling by conduction.

Course. On exposure to cold, the capillary bed and other vessels of the exposed parts dilate and produce an active hyperemia. Continued exposure produces a vasoconstriction with, first, cyanosis and, then, blanching of the part due to ischemia. If the application of cold is continued, gangrene may develop due to the prolonged ischemia and anoxia.

Symptoms. The history given by the patient is usually quite characteristic. After exposure to cold the patient notices in hands, feet, ears, or nose at first a sticking, burning sensation and then a definite numbness or anesthesia. The part of the body involved becomes wax-white in color. The numbness should be a warning that further exposure to cold is dangerous. If the patient goes into a warm room, the ischemic area becomes intensely red and edematous and is associated with an itching and tingling sensation. Chilblains may form; these are nodular swellings surrounded by a reddened area of hyperemia or cyanotic flat swellings in the area exposed. Chilblains cause symptoms long after the exposure to cold is over. They are characterized by a painful, tingling sensation, which is aggravated when the part becomes warm. In this stage, complete recovery may follow if the exposure has been of short duration.

If the exposure to cold is continued after numbness appears, more marked tissue changes occur. When the exposure is terminated and the part is warmed, vesicles and blebs form over the exposed part, with marked swelling of the soft tissues and a burning, painful sensation (Fig. 9-1). Prolonged exposure or exposure to marked degrees of cold produces death of the tissues and gangrene (Fig. 9-2).

Treatment. Although for years it has

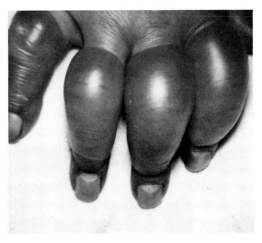

Fig. 9–1. Vesicle formation on fingers early after frostbite.

been taught that rubbing snow on the areas of frostbite is the accepted method of treatment, there is no clinical or experimental evidence to support this therapy. Dry warmth seems to be the most effective treatment, and this is easily obtained by placing the frostbitten parts against warm areas of the body in a room of normal temperature. If blebs have formed, they should be punctured and the part protected with sterile cotton or wool bandaged lightly in place. If areas of cyanosis and anesthesia persist, it is probable that local gangrene will develop.

Conservative therapy is the method of choice in the treatment of peripheral disease due to exposure to cold. If the part can be protected from repeated exposure, frequently an unbelievable recovery takes place. Patients with frostbite of ears, nose, or fingers may be kept ambulatory, but those with frostbite of the feet frequently demand hospitalization.

All patients who have been subjected to frostbite should be warned against further exposure to cold.

BIBLIOGRAPHY

Gage, A. A., Ishikawa, H., and Winter, P. M.: Experimental frostbite and hyperbaric oxygenation. Surgery, *66*:1044, 1969.

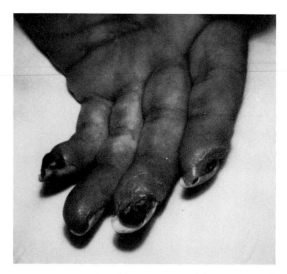 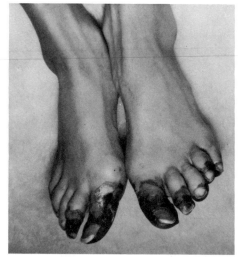

Fig. 9–2. (*Left*) Gangrene of finger tips after frostbite. (*Right*) Gangrene of toes after frostbite.

Hanson, H. E., and Goldman, R. F.: Cold injury in man: a review of its etiology and discussion of its prediction. Milit. Med., *134*:1307, 1969.

Low, M. B.: Tannic acid-silver nitrate treatment of burns in children. New Eng. J. Med., *216*:553, 1937.

Owens, J. C.: The consequences of frostbite. Geriatrics, *26*:82, 1971.

Robinson, D. W., Masters, F. W., and Forrest, W. J.: Electrical burns: a review and analysis of 33 cases. Surgery, *57*:385, 1965.

Shuck, J. M., and Moncrief, J. A.: The management of burns. Curr. Prob. Surg., February, 1969.

Sumner, D. S., Boswick, J. A., Criblez, T. L., and Doolittle, W. H.: Prediction of tissue loss in human frostbite with xenon-133. Surgery, *69*:899, 1971.

Washburn, B. Frostbite. New Eng. J. Med., *266*:974, 1962.

Wilson, O., and Goldman, R. F.: Role of air temperature and wind in the time for a finger to freeze. J. Appl. Physiol., *29*:658, 1970.

10

Foreign Bodies

Mark W. Wolcott, M.D.

GENERAL CONSIDERATIONS

Foreign bodies in the soft tissues present many problems in the treatment of ambulatory patients.

The first problem is infection in the primary wound. Potentially, almost all wounds due to foreign bodies are infected, and, because of the small wound of entrance, tetanus bacilli, as well as the common pyogenic organisms, must be considered as likely invaders. It should be a rule, therefore, in the primary treatment of foreign bodies to give tetanus prophylaxis routinely.

The second problem is whether or not to remove the foreign body. When it has recently entered the tissues, is easily located, and is easily accessible, its removal is usually attempted. If, however, no symptoms are produced and removal would entail an operation which might do more harm than the presence of the foreign body in the tissues, it is usually better judgment to let it remain. Many foreign bodies, especially metallic ones, may become encysted by scar tissue and give no symptoms whatever. At any time, however, due to trauma or latent infection, the encysted body may become painful and demand treatment.

When it is decided to remove a foreign body, the problem of locating it in the tissues arises. This may not be difficult if the object can be palpated or if it is relatively large and the wound of entrance is plainly visible. When the foreign body is small and deeply located in fat or muscle, its removal is difficult, particularly when it cannot be definitely localized in the tissues with reference to some point on the skin surface. This is especially true of small sharp-pointed objects, such as needles or parts of needles, which may move in the tissues as a result of pressure or the movement of tendons and muscle.

In localizing a foreign body in the soft tissues by roentgenograms, a point on the skin which can later be identified is selected. The wound of entrance, if visible, is usually the point chosen, since it will be easily visible at the time of operation. If, however, the wound of entrance has already healed, some other point on the skin in the region in which the foreign body appears to be located may be selected and marked with silver nitrate. This makes a black stain which will last for several days.

The head half of a pin is placed on the skin with a small piece of adhesive, the head being located at the site of the wound of entrance or on the silver nitrate dot. The part is then immobilized with a splint. Wooden splints are the best, since they are not radiopaque. Roentgen films are then made in the anteroposterior and the lateral positions. With such films available, the location of the foreign body in relation to the wound of entrance may be definitely determined, its distance from the skin surface may be seen, and its direction in the tissues may be ascertained. The splint should not be removed while the films are being made; it should be left in place from the time the roentgenogram is made until the time of operation. This is very important, because if movement of the part is permitted, the foreign body may move to a different place in the tissues. Thus, after a roentgenogram of a foreign body in the foot has been made, the patient should not be permitted to walk before the operation.

There are several important aids that should always be employed in the operative removal of a foreign body.

First, the field should be absolutely bloodless. When the foreign body is in an extremity, hemostasis is best obtained by using a tourniquet. The use of an Esmarch bandage prior to application of the tourniquet gives further assurance of a bloodless field. When tourniquets cannot be used, a local anesthetic plus epinephrine aids visualization very materially by keeping the field dry. The tension produced by retraction of the tissues also helps to prevent the slight ooze that may come from the capillaries or the veins.

Second, although absolute anesthesia is usually not necessary in the removal of foreign bodies, adequate local anesthesia is imperative. Block anesthesia is often more helpful than local infiltration because no tissue edema is associated with such an anesthetic; on the other hand, in superficial foreign bodies, local infiltration anesthesia can be used without difficulty.

Finally, the proper selection of the incision is important. The incision must be made in such a way as to permit adequate exposure of the bed and easy removal of the foreign body; also, the underlying tissues must be considered, so that the wound will not be made where it will damage important structures. When possible, the wound is made to cross the axis of the foreign body transversely; this is especially helpful in trying to locate deep foreign bodies in fatty or muscular tissues. If the wound of entrance can be located, it frequently is possible to enlarge it, the direction taken by the foreign body being known from the roentgen film. In many cases of recent entrance of a foreign body, there may be an area of bloodstain which can be traced to the site of the body in the tissues. The procedure at the time of operation will be discussed in greater detail in connection with the various types of foreign bodies encountered.

TYPES OF FOREIGN BODIES

Wood Splinters. Wood splinters are a very common type of foreign body in the soft tissues; they are found in any part of the body, but most frequently in the hands, feet, and buttocks. Most often, the foreign body is a piece of floor or other board that has been exposed to all sorts of bacterial contamination; therefore, the wounds produced are potentially highly infected wounds and the danger of tetanus is especially great. As a rule, the wound of entrance is so large and the pain is so marked that the patient seeks treatment immediately. Roentgenography is usually not employed to locate the splinter because wood is not radiopaque unless it happens to have been painted (Fig. 10-1). Conservative treatment in this type of case is most dangerous. If the foreign body can be removed easily and early and the entire wound excised, the wound can be sutured primarily, and healing with primary union can be expected. If an attempt is made to incise the skin conservatively at the wound of entrance and to pull out the splinter, there is considerable danger that bits of splinter will be left in the wound, with a resulting certainty of prolonged infection. Adequate incision is therefore desirable.

When a splinter is superficial and lies more or less parallel to the skin surface, it is wise to infiltrate the area around the wound of entrance and along the course of the foreign body with procaine solution. The entire wound of entrance is

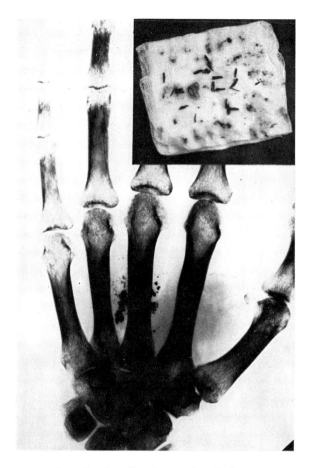

Fig. 10–1. Painted wood produces a roentgen shadow. The removed splinters are shown on the gauze sponge.

excised, and, after the skin is divided over the line of the splinter, good retraction is obtained to permit exposure of the entire foreign body in the tissues. Every part of the bed of the splinter should be visible, and the fatty tissues in which it lies should be completely excised. If this comparatively radical procedure is carried out early, the wound may be irrigated with saline and closed primarily with good prospect that primary healing will occur. In this treatment, of course, the use of tetanus toxoid or tetanus immune globulin (human) as a prophylactic measure must not be neglected.

Splinters under the fingernail are treated by excision of that portion of the nail that overlies the splinter. This can usually

be performed without anesthesia, the scalpel being held almost parallel to the nail and a V-shaped area of nail over the splinter being excised (Fig. 10-2). By this method the entire splinter may be removed and an anaerobic wound converted into an aerobic one. A simple finger dressing is all that is necessary until the wound is healed.

Rees* has reported an ingenious method for the removal of foreign bodies, such as needles, thorns, and splinters, that break off under the dermis at nearly right angles to the surface of the skin. Difficulty in removing such objects is often encountered because the incision may pass on one side or the other of the foreign body, and it is difficult to determine on which side it lies. Rees suggests that the incision be made only through the skin and that the skin then be undercut on all sides for a distance of about

---

*Rees, C. E.: The removal of foreign bodies: a modified incision. JAMA, *113*:35, 1939.

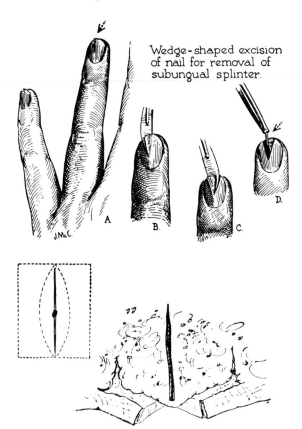

Wedge-shaped excision of nail for removal of subungual splinter.

Fig. 10–2. Excision of portion of nail over a subungual splinter.

Fig. 10–3. Removal of foreign body by the method of Rees. After an incision through the wound of entrance, an area of skin is undermined and pressure is made on the sides of the wound. The fat containing the foreign body thus is made to protrude into the wound. Rees advises removal of the fatty tissue round the foreign body, as well as the foreign body itself.

¼ inch. In this way, the fatty tissue in which the foreign body lies is not disturbed, and by exerting pressure upon the sides of the wound, the fat may be extruded into the wound, bearing the foreign body with it (Fig. 10-3). He advises excision of the fat containing the foreign body rather than simply removing the object. When the foreign body projects at the skin surface, he makes an elliptical incision centered on the wound of entrance. The removal of the elliptical piece of skin in the center then shows the exact location of the foreign body, which may be removed as described above (Fig. 10-4). In such exploration for foreign material, he advises that local anesthesia be produced not by infiltration but by means of a field block around the area in which the foreign body is believed to lie. In this way, the thickening of the tissues by edema is avoided.

Steel Splinters. Steel splinters are fre-quently seen in those who have been hammering on chisels or other metal objects. These splinters may enter the tissues at any point and, because of their small size, are often unnoticed by the patient, except for a slight sting at the time of wounding. Later, some bleeding may be observed, and this calls the patient's attention to the tiny wound. When such a history is obtained, one can be almost certain that there is a small foreign body embedded in the tissues, and a roentgen film will demonstrate it. Metal splinters entering the tissues in this way may be embedded very deeply, and they are especially difficult to find. Furthermore, the heat that is generated by the pounding may render them fairly sterile and the question arises as to the advisability of attempting to remove them. Occasionally, when a splinter lies deeply, it may be better surgical judgment to leave it; on the other hand, if the splinter

Fig. 10–4. Removal of contaminated foreign body by the method of Rees. First an elliptical incision is made round the wound entrance. After undermining the wound, the elliptical piece of skin is excised, showing the location of the foreign body in the subcutaneous fatty tissues. The foreign body and surrounding fatty tissues are excised, and the wound is sutured primarily.

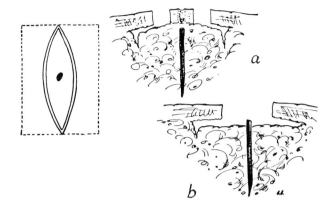

lies superficially under the skin and its removal is easy, an operation for its extraction should be performed. A lesion due to this type of foreign body should be examined for injuries to important structures, that is, for severed tendons, nerves, and so forth; frequently, though the skin opening is relatively minor, rather serious difficulty may be produced in the deeper tissues.

Cinders, Coal, and Stone. Cinders, bits of coal, stone, and other similar materials are foreign bodies commonly found in the tissues in accidental wounds, especially in children. Often their presence is not recognized at the time the primary wound is treated and, as a result, they lie embedded in the tissues for a considerable period of time. As a rule, they are not embedded very deeply, but, because they carry with them considerable amounts of infective material, they almost always set up local infections. Although the primary wound apparently has been treated adequately, the embedded foreign body produces a chronic draining sinus. This is so common that we have come to suspect that any traumatic wound that continues to drain septic material over a period of time has a foreign body embedded in it. Investigation of such a wound with a needle or other searching object will frequently locate the embedded cinder. When the wound is incised and the foreign material is removed, healing takes place rapidly.

Clothing. Bits of clothing may frequently be foreign bodies. They have the same potentiality for causing infection as do other foreign materials. A possibility that often is overlooked is that clothing may have become embedded in the tissues. Cloth is not radiopaque; hence roentgenograms will not reveal its presence.

Sutures. In the case of surgical wounds which become infected and from which there is a small draining area, the possibility must be borne in mind that a suture is acting as a foreign body. Silk sutures are the worst offenders, and the next are large catgut knots. The search for possible sutures may be facilitated by the use of a small crochet hook, sterilized and inserted into the wound. It is often possible to catch the offending suture with the hook and draw it out of the wound. Healing then takes place. Here is another instance of a chronic draining wound caused by the presence of a foreign body.

Glass. Broken glass is a common foreign body; it is seen most frequently in the hands and the fingers, having occurred from the breaking in the hands of a glass object. In automobile accidents, glass from the shattered windshield may be found anywhere in the body, frequently in the forehead and the face. Glass is often a foreign body in the feet. Difficulties often arise in making the diagnosis because the patient does not know whether the glass has simply cut him or has remained embedded in the tissues. Palpation of the wound frequently gives no indication in this respect. It is usually worthwhile to have a roentgen film made when embedded glass is suspected; many types of glass will show on the roentgen film, especially glass from a windshield. When there is uncertainty as to the presence or the absence of glass in the tissues, it usually is wise to treat the wound primarily as a laceration, unless the glass can be seen or palpated or demonstrated on the roentgen film. After healing has occurred, glass will make itself evident by the pain produced by pressure upon it; an incision can then be made over the painful spot and the glass removed. In an operation for the removal of bits of glass from the tissues, absolute hemostasis must be obtained because even at best glass is seen with a great deal of difficulty.

Fish Bones. Fish bones and the bony parts of fins are frequently embedded in the tissues. Potentially they are highly infective, and their removal should be attempted as soon as possible. The danger from such foreign bodies is not only the usual type of infection but also the erysipeloid of Rosenbach. These bodies are radiopaque and can, therefore, be demonstrated on the roentgen film. They usually are not deeply embedded in the tissues and almost invariably are in the hands or the fingers. Their removal is usually easy because they can be well localized. It is wise not to attempt to suture the wound but to leave it open and treat it as a primary infection.

Needles. Needles or parts of needles of various sorts are common foreign bodies in the hands and the feet.

These foreign bodies are among the most difficult to localize, because they are so small and because, in the feet at least, they are frequently deeply embedded in the fatty adipose tissue. Accurate localization is the secret of their removal. They are best located through an incision which is designed to cross transversely the long axis of the object. Most needles, after they have been in the tissue for any period of time, become oxidized and black and, therefore, are seen fairly easily

if the field is bloodless. It has been found that if the incision is made along the line of entrance of the needle, there is frequently a dark-stained area of hemorrhage which can be followed.

We have rarely found it necessary to use the fluoroscope in locating needles in the hands or the feet, where they are most commonly embedded. The occasional needle embedded in other parts of the body, however, is removed with a great deal of difficulty. Fluoroscopic visualization is a considerable aid in this respect.

Not infrequently, hypodermic needles are broken off in the subcutaneous tissues. The danger from this type of foreign body is not great, because most of the needles are sterile when inserted; nevertheless, their removal is usually attempted if it is possible to do this easily. Patients who are diabetic and give themselves their own insulin often break needles in the thigh. These are removed with a great deal of difficulty unless they can be well localized in the soft tissues. It may be wiser to leave them in place rather than to attempt their excision.

Bullets. Various types of bullets are often embedded in the tissues. In most cases of shot of very large caliber, the foreign body has penetrated so deeply and has caused so much damage that the patient should be admitted to the hospital for care. On the other hand, small shot (BB or bird shot) may be only superficially embedded in the tissues, and the patient may be ambulant. These foreign bodies are radiopaque, and their localization by roentgen examination is, therefore, comparatively easy. Fortunately, in many cases, the heat generated by the firing of the gun and by the passage of the bullet through the air renders such foreign bodies relatively sterile, so that, when they are inaccessible, their removal may be delayed until it is seen whether or not infection takes place.

Fishhooks. Fishhooks are occasionaly embedded in the soft tissues, usually in the fingers. Because of the barb, their removal is difficult, but this may be accomplished by pushing the point through the remaining portion of the soft tissues, cutting off the barbed portion of the hook

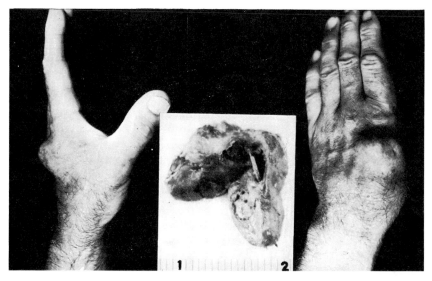

Fig. 10–5. Foreign body granuloma on the dorsum of the hand. This was thought to be a fibroma, but on opening the tumor, an encysted splinter was found. The patient then recalled that a splinter had entered the hand many years before.

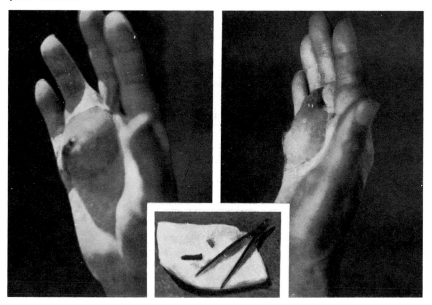

Fig. 10–6. Photograph of foreign body described in the text. A small piece of file was removed from an area of spontaneous drainage in the center of the granulomatous mass. The entire process subsided following removal of the foreign body.

with pliers, and then withdrawing the hook in the direction from which it entered. Such wounds can be treated with hot moist dressings until the danger from infection is past.

LATE TREATMENT OF FOREIGN BODIES

Foreign bodies left in the tissues for a considerable period of time may become encysted by fibrous tissue and give no symptoms (Fig. 10-5). At times the irritation produced by them causes a granulomatous swelling which may be so hard and firm as to be mistaken for a tumor growth (Fig. 10-6). One such case occurred in the author's experience. A piece of a file became embedded in the hand of a woman when she was 19 years old; she appeared for treatment when she was 83 because of a swelling of the hand, which was mistakenly diagnosed as a sarcoma. Because it was thought that the sarcoma arose from the bones of the hand, a roentgen examination was made; this disclosed the true state of affairs—the presence of the foreign body. Through a small incision in the center of the granulomatous area, the piece of file was removed, and the granuloma promptly disappeared. In a few patients, the same reaction has been caused by silk sutures in a wound. The knowledge that this type of reaction occurs and that the removal of the foreign body results in prompt healing is useful on occasion.

11
Cysts and Tumors

Mark W. Wolcott, M.D.

SEBACEOUS CYSTS (WENS)

Etiology. Sebaceous cysts are common examples of a retention type of cyst, in which the outlet to the duct is blocked, usually by secretion; the gland continues to secrete, producing a dilatation of the duct and the gland. The cysts are found anywhere on the skin surface, but mostly on the scalp, the face, the ear, and the neck.

Diagnosis. Very frequently the cysts are multiple. They may occur at any age, but they are seen most often in adults past midlife. As a rule, they may be diagnosed on simple inspection, but occasionally they have to be differentiated from dermoid cysts, neurofibromas, and lipomas. The fact that they are always attached to the skin at the outlet of the duct is a helpful diagnostic point in this respect. Frequently, the duct is seen definitely as a black depression in the skin, and occasionally it is so dilated as to permit the sebaceous contents to be expressed from the cyst by pressure. On the scalp, the cysts may become large in size, sometimes as large as a small orange (Fig. 11-1).

Symptoms. Sebaceous cysts cause few symptoms except disfigurement or the discomfort caused by their presence in areas in which pressure may be exerted upon them, as on the scalp. Frequently they are complicated by infection. This adds the symptoms of pain and rather rapid enlargement of the cyst area. When infection makes its appearance, the increase in the swelling is due to a rupture of the cyst wall, with the formation of a pocket of pus in the area of the cyst. The previously hard or doughy mass now may become definitely fluctuant.

Treatment. The treatment of sebaceous cysts is excision. The operation can usually be performed under local anesthesia: the cyst is exposed by a simple incision of the skin over it, and frequently the duct entrance on the skin surface is removed with the cyst. If the cyst is ruptured during its removal, its wall can easily be identified and removed after evacuation of its contents (Fig. 11-2).

Two variations in the treatment of sebaceous cysts have been suggested. Their advantage is that suture of the wound is not needed and, therefore, a less formal procedure is necessary. After infiltration around the cyst with procaine solution, make a small incision through the overlying skin and the cyst wall with the needle electrode of an electrosurgical unit. Express the contents of the cyst. The area containing the cyst is then kneaded between the thumbs and the fingers of the two hands until the edge of the cyst wall protrudes at the stab wound. This is grasped with a toothed forceps or a hemo-

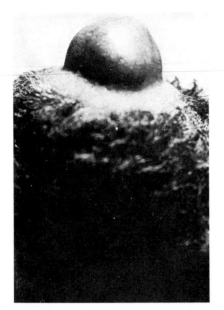

Fig. 11–1. Large sebaceous cyst of scalp.

stat, and, with gentle traction and continued kneading, the entire wall of the cyst can usually be delivered. Almost no bleeding is encountered. A pressure dressing is applied.

Danna suggests a method that is especially good for the treatment of multiple cysts of the scalp, but of course it may be used wherever multiple cysts are to be treated. A needle is inserted into the most prominent area over the cyst, preferably near the duct opening. The tip of the needle should barely protrude into the cyst cavity. A whitish eschar is produced around the needle tip by touching the needle with a diathermy electrode (unipolar current). The very weak current used produces only a momentary stinging sensation, and, as a rule, anesthesia is not necessary. In 5 to 8 days a button of necrotic skin comes away, leaving a large opening into the cyst cavity. "In the course of the next 3 to 6 weeks, the cyst gradually empties itself; the cavity gets smaller and smaller till the bottom of the cavity finally presents on the surface." This "soon levels off in a straight line with the surrounding skin. There is no drainage of any consequence during this time."

When the cyst is infected, simple incision and drainage are indicated. Occasionally, the cyst wall may lie free in a pocket of pus, in which case the cyst itself may be removed. No extensive dissection of the cyst wall should be performed in cases of infection, first, because there is the danger of spreading the infection, and second, because the dissection is difficult and one cannot be sure that the entire cyst wall has been removed. Furthermore, infection may result in a cure of the cyst after a simple incision.

IMPLANTATION CYSTS

Etiology. These cysts appear as a result of an injury, usually caused by a blunt object, in which a bit of epidermis is driven beneath the skin surface. When healing takes place, the displaced epidermis acts as a skin graft and grows to form a subcutaneous cyst, the cyst resulting from the distention of the implanted skin due to desquamated epithelium and sebaceous material.

Diagnosis. Implantation cysts are almost always seen on the palmar surface of the hands and the fingers or on the feet, areas in which ordinary sebaceous cysts are not usually found. As a rule, a history of an injury is obtained, and a scar may be visible over the cyst swelling. Usually, the implantation cyst is attached to the undersurface of the skin at the site of the scar. Except for their being disfiguring or inconvenient, these cysts cause no symptoms. Occasionally, because of trauma due to their exposed position, they become painful.

Treatment. The treatment is simple excision; usually these cysts do not shell out from a well-defined capsule as do the sebaceous cysts. The operation can be performed under local anesthesia without difficulty.

CUTANEOUS TUMORS

CUTANEOUS HORNS

Cutaneous horns are hard, hornlike projections extending above the level of the skin; they develop due to a marked

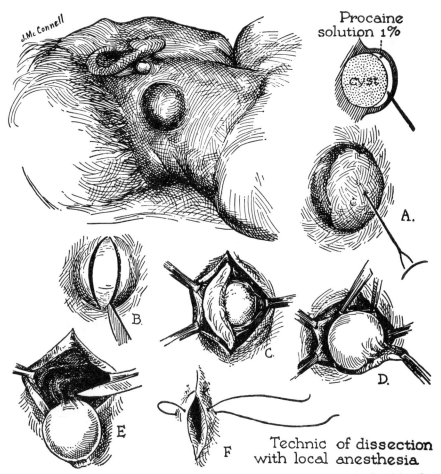

J.McConnell

Procaine
solution 1%

cyst

A.

B.

C.

D.

E.

F

Technic of dissection
with local anesthesia

Fig. 11–2. Excision of a sebaceous cyst of the neck. Procaine hydrochloride solution, 1 percent, is infiltrated over the cyst (*A*). It is frequently possible to insert the solution between the cyst capsule and the surrounding tissues so that the dissection may be partly performed by the local anesthetic injection. When the cyst is so large that the skin is stretched over it, an ellipse of skin may be excised with the cyst (*B*). If the lips of the wound are kept on tension by finger pressure or by grasping the edges of the wound with Allis forceps (*C*), the dissection may be partly accomplished without manipulation. The tissues under the cyst are dissected bluntly with a curved hemostat (*D, E*). The wound is closed with vertical mattress sutures, the deep portions of which grasp the bed of the cyst (*F*).

keratosis of the horny layer of skin, which fails to be discarded. The skin surrounding the base of the horn is usually normal in appearance. As time goes on, these lesions may grow to considerable size (Fig. 11-3). They may occur anywhere on the body, but most often they appear on the head, the back, and the extremities.

They are frequently found in older people and should really be regarded as a type of senile keratosis. Their danger lies in the fact that approximately 12 percent of them become malignant. They may be removed easily by surgical excision under local anesthesia. All should be submitted for histologic examination.

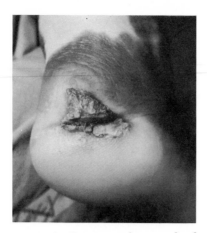

Fig. 11–3. Cutaneous horn on heel.

PAPILLOMAS

Small papillary growths occur on the skin in many areas. The lesion consists of a layer of skin covering a central stalk of fibrous tissue, which contains a nutrient artery and vein. These tumors appear often on the back and in the axilla and occasionally on the neck. They give no symptoms unless they are traumatized, at which time they become edematous and somewhat painful. Occasionally, trauma produces thrombosis of the central vessel supplying the papilloma and dry gangrene occurs.

Treatment may be by one of several methods. The papilloma may be easily removed by ligation of the base with a silk thread. This shuts off the blood supply, and the portion of the papilloma distal to the ligature becomes gangrenous and falls off. Another method is excision by electrodesiccation after injection of the base with a small amount of local anesthetic. When the papilloma is especially large, it is perhaps better to excise it under local anesthesia, closing the wound with one silk suture.

WARTS OR VERRUCAE

A wart, or verruca, is a benign epithelial growth formed by hypertrophy of the papillae. It may occur at any location on the cutaneous or mucous-membrane sur-faces. These lesions are caused by a filtrable virus that belongs to the papovavirus group. They are autoinoculable and can be transferred from one person to another by inoculation. They have been given names according to the shape or the location of the wart.

Verruca Vulgaris (Seed Wart). The ordinary common warts are seen more often in children, but they are also encountered in adults. They occur most commonly on the hands and the fingers; however, they may appear at any place on the skin or the mucous membrane. They may be single or multiple. These warts cause few symptoms, except disfigurement. Occasionally, because of trauma, they will bleed or become infected. Those which are found underneath the nails or on the plantar surface of the foot may cause discomfort due to pressure.

In discussing the treatment of common warts, it should be pointed out that these lesions may disappear spontaneously or with relatively simple types of treatment; on the other hand, they may be so recalcitrant as to defy almost any method of therapy.

In some cases these lesions may be treated by the injection of sclerosing solutions into the base of the wart. This is done without anesthesia, a tuberculin syringe and a fine-gauge needle being used. Any of the solutions used for the injection of varicose veins, such as sodium morrhuate solution, may be used. The heavier solutions appear to have a distinct advantage in that they remain localized at the point of injection. Only a few drops are injected. After a few days, the wart becomes dry and hard, and, after 10 to 14 days or longer, depending upon the size of the wart and the thickness of the surrounding skin, the wart comes off or can be trimmed off, leaving a practically normal skin underneath.

The pedunculated type of wart may be removed easily, simply by clipping it off with scissors after a local anesthetic has been injected at the base. The remaining tiny wound is treated by application of a simple pressure dressing or by superficial electrodesiccation.

Surgical excision of these common warts is an excellent method of treatment, depending upon the site of the lesion. If the lesion is located where it can be excised, and the remaining wound sutured without difficulty, this is probably the most rapid and the surest method of treatment. When the wart is located over an articulation, however, or when the skin is tense, excision is not indicated.

Most dermatologists depend upon electrodesiccation for removing warts. The needle is inserted into the wart several times, a very mild current being used. The dehydrated wart is then removed either with scissors or a sharp curetter, care being taken that the "core" is removed. The base is then very mildly and superficially desiccated, leaving a dry scab. No further dressing is necessary. Some authors use another method of desiccation: with a very fine spark, the verruca surfaces are seared lightly. This procedure is repeated at weekly intervals, and involution and desquamation of the lesion occur within 6 weeks. This method is recommended for verrucae which do not respond to the usual methods of treatment.

Roentgen or radium irradiation of warts is a well-recognized method of therapy, but it should be applied only by a dermatologist or a radiologist who is familiar with the technique. This therapy is of particular value for warts that occur at the side of, or underneath, the nails, because it is so difficult to treat warts at these sites by other methods. It is also excellent for treating multiple warts in a localized area. It should be used as a last resort.

Various local applications also have been useful in the treatment of verrucae. Fuming nitric acid has been used for many years, the application being made with a wood swab stick after the area surrounding the wart has been protected with petrolatum. Several applications, at intervals of from 5 to 7 days, may be necessary. More recently, bichloroacetic acid has been used in the same way. These applications cause the warty growth to become hard and black. This dead tissue must be removed with a scalpel or a curette before the subsequent application of cauterizing solution. Usually, not more than two or three applications are necessary.

Cryotherapy, using either liquid nitrogen or solid carbon dioxide, is another effective way of treating warts, especially the common warts on the fingers, face, penis, vagina, and anus. It is also excellent for treating subungual warts; here, finger block anesthesia can be used. When liquid nitrogen is used, a wisp of cotton on the end of a wooden applicator is dipped in the liquid nitrogen, and the chemical is carefully painted on the wart. Care should be taken not to freeze normal tissue. It is applied long enough to turn the wart white. Several applications, several days apart, are usually necessary. A blister forms and then dries, and the wart can then be peeled off.

Solid carbon dioxide is easier to use and more readily available. A pencil-sized piece of solid carbon dioxide is shaped and held briefly in contact with the wart until it turns white. The operator holding the carbon dioxide must take care to protect his hands. Several applications are usually necessary. Several portable cryosurgical machines that are quite satisfactory are on the market (see Chapter 12).

Verruca Plana Juvenilis. This is the term for the small, flat, skin-colored or light-yellow lesions; they occur chiefly on the face, neck, and hands. They are smooth, only slightly raised, and are not warty to the touch; they are seen most often in children, but they also occur in adults, and they are multiple. Probably the most effective method of removing such lesions is either by excision under local anesthesia or by electrodesiccation.

Verruca Plantaris and Verruca Acuminata. These lesions will be discussed in detail in the chapters on surgery of the feet and of the anal region.

MESODERMAL TUMORS

KELOIDS

Etiology. Keloids are irregular overgrowths of fibrous tissue occurring in

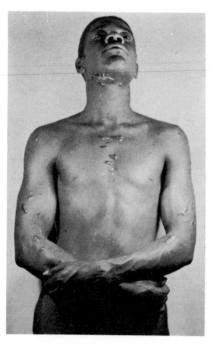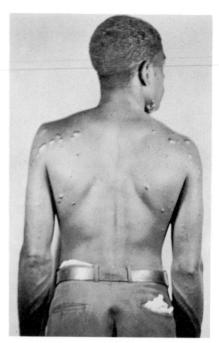

Fig. 11–4. Multiple keloids in a Negro. Every slight injury to the skin in this patient had resulted in a keloid growth.

scars. They are raised above the surrounding skin and frequently become almost pedunculated. They always result from some injury to the skin or the deeper tissues, although the injury itself may be minor in nature, such as a mosquito bite or an acne furuncle. In the Negro race there is a definite predisposition to the formation of keloids (Fig. 11-4); in the white race it is sporadic. In the Negro race this predisposition appears to be present in adult life, whereas in the white race it is more likely to be present in childhood.

Treatment. The treatment of keloids varies somewhat according to the stage at which the lesion is seen. While they are forming, during the first 6 months, irradiation with radium or roentgen rays appears to give fair results. This treatment is given at intervals of from 4 to 6 weeks over a period of several months. In the case of large old keloids, which are often radioresistant, surgical excision is recommended, with irradiation to be begun in divided doses as soon as the sutures are removed.

Some authors have used steroids to treat keloids. Bernstein uses intramuscular depot glucocorticoids (Depo-Medrol, 40 mg. every week, or Aristocort suspension, 25 to 40 gm.) in a series of weekly or fortnightly injections. A response is usually seen within a month. The response of most keloids to systemic steroid therapy is complete regression. The size of other keloids may be reduced by 25 to 50 percent by this therapy, after which the injections may be made into the lesion itself (Fig. 11-5). Maguire injected the steroid triamcinolone acetonide (Kenalog) directly into the keloid with excellent results; 2 ml. of a solution composed of equal parts of triamcinolone (10 mg./ml.) and 1 percent Xylocaine were used.

LIPOMAS

Lipomas are tumors composed of adipose tissue. They may appear in almost any location in the body, but are most commonly seen in the subcutaneous tissues of the neck, the back, and the but-

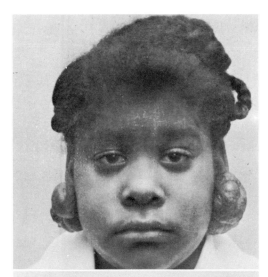

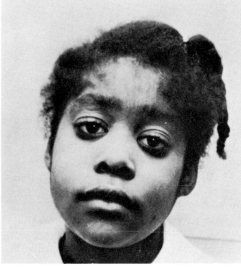

Fig. 11–5. (*Top*) Large keloids of the ear lobes in 8-year-old girl. Unsuccessful attempt to treat by excision and x-ray therapy at age of 5, with large recurrences. (*Bottom*) Treatment by excision, followed in 7 days by intramuscular depot injections of glucocorticoids. Result after 12 months. No evidence of recurrence. (Bernstein, H.: Angiology, *15*:253, 1964)

tocks and in the proximal portions of the extremities. They may appear at any age, but are rare in children as compared with the incidence in adult and late life. They vary greatly in size—from the size of a hazel nut to that of a baseball, or even larger (Fig. 11-6, left). They also vary greatly in consistency, depending upon the amount of fibrous tissue in them and upon the tissue in which they are found. The lipomas of the side of the neck are soft, almost fluctuant (Fig. 11-6, right); they are easily movable in the tissues and have no very definite encapsulation. On the other hand, tumors of the back of the neck and the forehead and the multiple tumors of the arms usually contain a large amount of fibrous tissue, are hard masses that lie in a fairly well-formed capsule, and are fixed to the tissues by fibrous septa which traverse them (Fig. 11-7). Frequently the soft, fluctuantlike tumors must be differentiated from cysts, whereas the harder, firmer tumors must be distinguished from fibromas, sebaceous cysts, and sarcomas.

Symptoms. The symptoms caused by lipomas are few: the masses produce disfigurement, and, rarely, following trauma, they become painful or tender.

Diagnosis. There are several points which are helpful in distinguishing lipomas from other superficial tumors. The soft type of lipoma is definitely attached to the skin by fibrous-tissue bands, so that pressure upon the tumor produces an orange-peel-like surface. The skin surface over large lipomas appears to be cooler than the surrounding skin. The absence of the symptoms of acute inflammation and the long duration of the swelling make the diagnosis between lipoma and abscess a relatively simple one. Lipomas rarely develop malignant change, but their removal is indicated because of the disfigurement or the discomfort produced by them.

Treatment. Almost all lipomas may be removed under local anesthesia in ambulatory patients. The operation is performed under field block or local infiltration, and in most cases the line of cleavage between the tumor and the surrounding fatty tissues is easily demonstrated. Tissue tension produced by firm retraction is of value in reducing the amount of bleeding and in permitting more rapid dissection. Often, lobules of the tumor lie in pockets formed by fi-

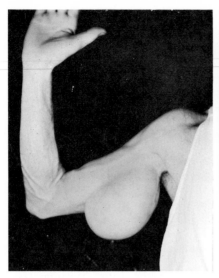
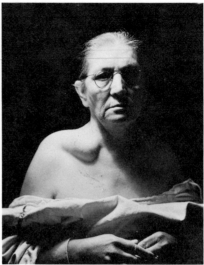

Fig. 11–6. (*Left*) Large lipoma of the upper arm. (*Right*) A typical lipoma of the lower neck. These tumors are so soft that they frequently appear to be fluctuant.

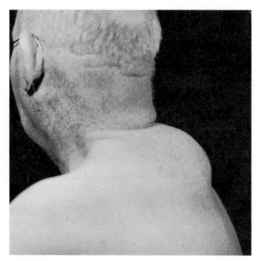

Fig. 11-7. A typical lipoma of the back of the neck. These tumors are relatively hard, firm, fixed masses due to fibrous-tissue bands which extend from the underlying fascia to the under-surface of the skin.

brous-tissue septa, and retraction will permit these lobules to be withdrawn with the tumor. The blood supply of the tumor usually enters it from below, and this is the only area which needs clamp-ing and ligation. After removal of the tumor, it is important that the dead space remaining be obliterated with interrupted buried sutures. Mattress sutures should be used in the skin. A pressure dressing is applied to prevent the accumulation of blood or serum in the wound.

Multiple fibrolipomas occur frequently on symmetrical portions of the arms and the body. These appear as hard, smooth masses in the subcutaneous tissues and are frequently somewhat tender and pain-ful. The tender tumors may be removed as desired by the patient.

FIBROMAS

Fibromas (Fig. 11-8) are hard, rounded, movable, slow-growing, noninflamma-tory tumors. They are found usually in adults, in the skin or the subcutaneous tissues almost anywhere on the body. On section, they are composed of bundles of connective tissue which are almost carti-laginous in their hardness.

Fibromas usually cause no symptoms, except disfigurement or, occasionally, slight pain due to trauma. On palpation they are sometimes very similar to seba-ceous cysts and must be distinguished

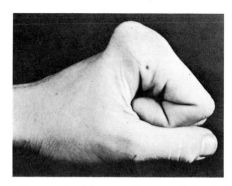

Fig. 11–8. Fibroma, dorsum of hand.

from them. Sebaceous cysts are always attached to the skin at the exit of the duct, whereas the skin moves over fibromas, which in turn are usually movable over the underlying tissues.

Fibromas almost never undergo malignant degeneration.

Treatment. When, for any reason, it seems to be desirable to remove a fibroma, excision may be performed under local anesthesia without much difficulty.

VASCULAR TUMORS

HEMANGIOMAS

It is now generally believed that hemangiomas represent malformations rather than neoplasms. They are the most common tumor of childhood and are present at birth in 83 percent of the cases. The remaining 17 percent almost invariably appear before the patient is 3 years old. They may appear in any location of the body and in any tissue, but they occur most often in the skin and in the subcutaneous tissues, although hemangiomas of the mucous membranes and of the muscles are not uncommon. The fact that they appear frequently on the skin of the face makes them disfiguring blemishes, which is one reason for their early treatment. As a rule, hemangiomas are benign in nature. They are not definitely encapsulated, but are usually well demarcated from surrounding tissues. Occasionally the growths spread rapidly and take on malignant character-

istics, and, very rarely, they even metastasize.

Capillary Hemangiomas

Nevus Flammeus (Port-Wine Stain). The port-wine stain is the simplest of these vascular lesions. It consists of an increased number of dilated capillaries and venules in the deeper layers of the skin, over which the epidermis may be very thin and frequently has a velvety surface. It appears as a poorly defined, irregular reddish or purplish area not raised above the skin; it occurs most commonly on the face or about the neck, but it may appear anywhere on the skin surface. This hemangioma does not tend to spread. In rare instances, the lesion disappears spontaneously. This is most likely to take place in the bright-red telangiectatic dilatations that appear on the back of the neck and over the forehead.

The treatment of nevus flammeus is somewhat difficult. The object of the treatment is to remove the disfiguring blotch either by excision or by closure of the dilated vessels which produce it. For small tumors, excision, with or without skin graft, may be the preferred method of therapy. However, other methods of treatment are available. Irradiation, either with roentgen rays or radium, is particularly effective in the first year of life. As the child gets older, these tumors become more radioresistant. The application of carbon dioxide snow with firm pressure for 10 to 20 seconds may result in thrombosis of the superficial capillaries and the disappearance of the purplish color. Both irradiation therapy and carbon dioxide snow may produce a blanching of the area, which often becomes pearly white and smooth due to atrophy of the underlying tissues, so that successful treatment may substitute a white scar for the discolored area.

Strawberry Hemangioma (Hemangioma Simplex). The strawberry mark (Fig. 11-9), probably comprises the largest group of these tumors. It is slightly raised above the skin and is lobulated. It is either a reddish or a bluish color, depend-

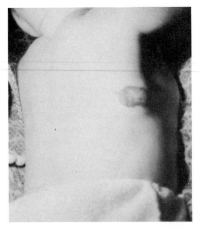

Fig. 11-9. Hemangioma simplex (strawberry hemangioma) of chest wall.

ing on the amount of arterial or venous blood in it. There is great variation in size, but the majority are relatively small in diameter. They occur anywhere on the skin but are found most commonly on the face and the head. They are composed of widely dilated capillaries and venules with very little perivascular connective tissue. The true skin and subcutaneous tissues are displaced by masses of endothelial cells. Not uncommonly, there may be palpated in the subcutaneous tissues a mass which extends out beneath the surrounding normal skin.

Treatment of Strawberry Mark. Richardson believes that no treatment should be given for strawberry hemangioma until the child reaches 5 years of age. He claims that the hemangioma "involutes" and may entirely disappear if the parents can be persuaded to withhold treatment. If there is a residual disfiguring lesion, this can be better treated in the older child than in infancy.

Margileth and Museles are of a like opinion. In their experience, more than 90 percent of congenital cutaneous hemangiomas disappear spontaneously. In spite of the fact that hemangiomas may increase in size during the first months of life, they report that strawberry, cavernous, and mixed hemangiomas begin to regress during the last 6 months of the first year of life. At this time the brilliant strawberry

redness begins to be replaced by a dull redness. Small grayish foci appear. These gray areas increase in size and coalesce. Tumorous areas soften and decrease in thickness during the second and third years of life, with very little change in the surface area.

The chief difficulty with conservative treatment is to convince parents that the hemangioma will disappear spontaneously. Probably the most convincing method is to show before and after photographs of other children, and to make a photographic record of their own child to show by measurement the spontaneous involution over a period of time (Fig. 11-10).

During the period of spontaneous involution, there are occasionally some alarming complications which can usually be treated by simple methods. The most common of these are ulceration, bleeding, and infection. Compresses of warm moist saline solution are usually applied, and an antibiotic ointment is used as needed. Bleeding is usually of only a few drops of blood and is easily controlled by pressure. Strangely enough, bleeding and even secondary infection seem to exert a favorable effect upon the involution process. There is rarely any residual scarring, and if there is scarring it is less conspicuous than the original hemangioma.

Not all hemangiomas will disappear spontaneously. For those showing rapid or atypical growth, or those showing no regression by 5 years of age, some other form of treatment must be selected.

Surgical excision may be employed if the lesion is small and in an area where excision can be done. MacCollum found that in only about half of 418 cases were the lesions of the proper size or position for excision to be deemed advisable.

Other methods of therapy are the local application of carbon dioxide snow and irradiation by radium or roentgen rays. Brown and Byars have implanted radon seeds into the hemangioma. Kaessler, who used 20 percent quinine dihydrochloride and urethane, diluted with equal parts of 2 percent procaine hydrochloride with epinephrine, and Macomber and

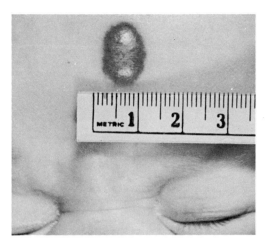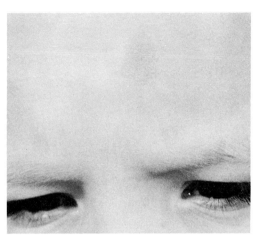

Fig. 11–10. Strawberry hemangioma. (*Left*) At birth. (*Right*) At 3 years of age. The lesion was not treated. (Margileth, A. M., and Museles, M.: Pediatrics, *36*:410, 1965)

Wang, who used sodium morrhuate, have reported on injection methods. These authors attempt to produce thrombosis of the hemangioma by depositing sclerosing solutions into or around the vascular spaces of the lesion. There is usually considerable reaction—redness, swelling, tenderness, and occasional blistering—but this subsides after one to two weeks, leaving a blanched area which gradually becomes soft and smooth. It may be necessary to repeat the injections at intervals of 4 to 6 weeks.

Cavernous Hemangiomas

The cavernous hemangioma consists of large blood spaces or sinuses lined with endothelium. These vary greatly in size, and there is considerable variability in the amount of connective tissue which lies between the sinuses. This lesion may be found not only in the subcutaneous tissues but also in the mucous membranes and, less frequently, in the muscles and the deeper organs. On the skin, the cavernous hemangioma appears as a definite swelling with a bluish or a reddish blue tinge transmitted through, rather than being in, the skin; the swelling is compressible and may be emptied by pressure or by elevation, depending upon its location. Conversely, straining or crying may make the tumor become tense and larger. This characteristic often makes the lesion a terrifying one for the mother, who notices the definite enlargement when the child cries. The lesion usually is present at birth and gradually increases in size until puberty. Very frequently it is combined with a lymphangioma.

Treatment. The treatment of cavernous hemangioma varies in different hands. Here again, surgery is recommended when the lesion is in such a situation that it can be excised safely. MacCollum has used carbon dioxide snow in a few cases, but, in most instances in which surgical excision cannot be performed, he treats the lesion by endothermic coagulation. This operation is performed under general anesthesia and should probably be done in the hospital or in a surgicenter. The principle of the treatment is to pass a coagulating current of low intensity through a needle inserted into the hemangioma until the tumor tissue immediately adjacent to it becomes blanched. The needle is then reinserted at intervals of about 1 cm. and the procedure is repeated. Care must be taken that too vigorous coagulation does not result in a slough. In the treatment of these lesions, Peyton and Leven have used sclerosing solutions with more satisfactory results. These authors inject a solution of 7 percent sodium

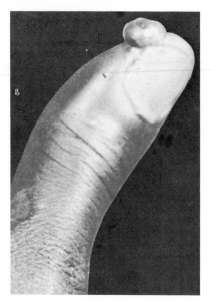 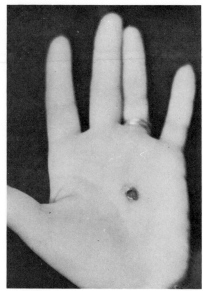

Fig. 11–11. Granuloma pyogenicum (infectious granuloma). Both of these lesions appeared in the hand following subcutaneous infections. Both responded to cauterization with silver nitrate stick.

morrhuate, introducing the needle into the vascular spaces and withdrawing it until blood is obtained by suction. The amount injected varies from a few drops to about 2.5 ml. Manual compression is maintained until a rubber-sponge pressure bandage has been applied over the area. At the time of injection, a stinging or burning sensation is experienced by the patient. This lasts only a short time and is followed by a definite painful sensation that lasts for an hour or more. Moderate compression reduces the amount of discomfort experienced. There follows in the next day or two a definite swelling, with discoloration and edema, which eventually subsides as the vessels in the hemangioma become thrombosed. Spontaneous resolution of the cavernous hemangioma may occur, and a period of waiting is usually indicated. Protection of the lesion from trauma is important, since infection and ulceration can occur.

Granuloma Pyogenicum

Diagnosis and Symptoms. Granuloma pyogenicum should really be classified as an infection of the skin, but, because of its tumorlike form and because it must be differentiated from tumors, it will be discussed here. This lesion is a reddish, wartlike, often pedunculated, tumor of the skin. It is usually characterized by a surrounding collar of thickened, bluish white, macerated epithelium. In the author's experience, it practically always follows some local injury, which becomes the site of a low-grade infection. The infection remains localized, but granulation tissue continues to pile up at the site of the local area of injury. The maximum size of these tumors is about that of a pea, and the chief symptom is bleeding, which occurs on the slightest trauma. Most often, the granulomas are found in those areas in which injury is frequent, as, for instance, in the hands and the fingers (Fig. 11-11); less often they are found on the lips and the face. Patients usually seek treatment because of the marked bleeding, and a diagnosis has been made of a malignant tumor because of this symptom. Furthermore, there is sometimes a tendency to recurrence if the entire granulating area is not removed. The differentiation from carcinoma is easily made, however, because of the lack of invasion of the surrounding tissues and because of the history of local injury.

Treatment. The treatment of granuloma pyogenicum is relatively simple, the chief objective being to destroy completely the hypertrophic granulation. This may be done most simply by excising the tumor with scissors under local anesthesia. Considerable bleeding may follow this procedure, but it can be controlled by pressure, or, if the tumor mass is in a position such that a tourniquet can be applied, this should be done before excision. After the granuloma has been removed, the base should be cauterized with a silver nitrate stick. A simple pressure dressing may then be applied. This method offers the simplest and the most rapid method of treatment in these cases. The tumor may be destroyed by electrodesiccation in the same manner and with the same results.

GLOMUS TUMORS

Pathology and Etiology. The neuromyoarterial glomus is a normal structure found in the fingers, the nail beds, the toes, the feet, and perhaps elsewhere in the skin. It is probably a peculiar type of arteriovenous anastomosis; the blood vessel is usually twisting or S shaped, is thin walled, and is surrounded by a rich network of sympathetic nerve fibers and nontypical muscle fibers. It is believed that the normal physiologic function of these organs is the maintenance of a constant capillary pressure and the control of peripheral temperatures. This normal structure may become a tumorlike mass and give very definite symptoms. The cause of the enlargement or the development of the tumor appears to be trauma in about one half of the cases; or, at least, there is a history of injury in this proportion of cases.

Symptoms and Diagnosis. Local hyperplasia of the glomus is characterized by the appearance of a small, exquisitely tender, bluish or reddish blue nodule, often only a few millimeters in diameter. Clinically, the tumor is associated with paroxysms of extremely severe pain localized in the region of the glomus or, at times, radiating from it. The pain may be induced by pressure or other slight trauma and, at times, by changes in temperature. Frequently there is localized sweating associated with the paroxysms.

On examination, the tumors are found to vary in size and appearance according to their location. One common type is found under the nails of the fingers and toes. Here the lesion appears as a small purplish area which is excruciatingly painful when even the slightest pressure is aplied to the nail. There may be some slight deformity of the nail distal to the tumor and some pressure atrophy of the distal phalanx. Elsewhere in the skin, the tumor varies according to its deep or superficial location. Arising as it does from the glomus situated in the reticular area of the skin, the growth may expand superficially to lie immediately under the superficial layers of skin, and, in such cases, it appears as a purplish or a reddish dot which, when touched, gives extreme pain. The hyperplasia may also extend downward and project into the subcutaneous tissues, in which case there may be no discoloration of the skin and no visible or palpable evidence of its location. When the tumors are located in the soft tissues, they are slightly larger than the subungual lesions and are usually slightly raised, elastic, movable nodules in the subcutaneous tissues.

Treatment. The treatment of glomus tumor is excison; by its removal the painful symptoms are relieved immediately. At operation, at which there may be more difficulty than usual in obtaining good local anesthesia, a bluish red, usually encapsulated, tumor is found attached to the skin in the soft tissues. This can be shelled out without difficulty. If the lesion is subungual, it is recommended that the entire nail be removed and that the tumor be excised rather than that an attempt be made to excise it through a small opening in the nail. There is usually no tendency to recurrence after excision. Glomus tumors are radioresistant and should never be treated by irradiation.

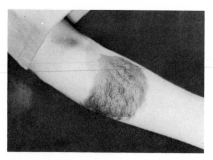

Fig. 11–12. Pigmented nevus of the pilose type. This nevus was removed by multiple operations. Part was removed at one time and the wound was sutured; then more was excised at a later date. It is perhaps better to excise the entire nevus and apply skin grafts.

PIGMENTED NEVI AND MELANOMAS

Terminology. The confusion in the nomenclature of the pigmented lesions of the skin is matched only by the controversy with regard to their origin and the best methods of treatment. The general trend is to include under the term *benign pigmented nevus* or *mole* the host of common and widespread benign pigmented lesions. The terms *melanoma, malignant melanoma, melanosarcoma,* and *melanocarcinoma* are reserved for those rare but highly malignant pigmented lesions which usually develop from a pre-existing nevus.

Benign Pigmented Nevi

The variety of lesions included under the term *nevus* is great. The simplest is the pigmented macula, nevus spilus. This is the common and widespread brownish mole. Some of them cover large areas of the body. Frequently, the mole contains hair; this type is known as pilose nevus (Fig. 11-12). Some forms are raised and flat; others are papillomatous or wartlike in character. It must be realized, however, that a nevus may be superimposed on another lesion, such as a wart or a papilloma.

The amount of pigmentation varies greatly. Some are poorly pigmented and inconspicuous. At the other end of the scale is the highly pigmented, blue-black or slate-colored, smooth, rounded, shiny mole.

The nevus is the most frequent growth in man. Few individuals, if any, are entirely free from such lesions. Probably the average person has at least 20 pigmented moles. They are found most frequently on exposed areas—scalp, face, chest, back, and extremities. They are congenital in origin but may not be apparent at birth. The sexes are involved equally.

The nevus that is considered to be premalignant is the junction nevus. This receives its name from the fact that the nevus cells grow actively at the dermoepidermal junction. It is flat and smooth, usually hairless, and from light-to-dark-brown color. The common mole is the intradermal nevus. It is flat or raised and may contain hairs. Usually it does not have malignant potentialities, but the junction nevus may appear in combination with the intradermal nevus to form the compound nevus, which may therefore be premalignant.

Since malignant melanomas are so rapidly fatal, and since it is so difficult, if not impossible, to determine clinically the presence of malignant change, it is only logical to consider the excision of moles as a prophylactic measure. The moles which should be looked upon with suspicion and which demand prompt action are those which show (1) increase in size or in pigmentation; (2) itching or pain; (3) irritation and discomfort; (4) infection; (5) bleeding, ulceration, weeping, or crusting; or (6) elevation and enlargement of a flat lesion. Moles which are especially prone to become malignant are those appearing in blond individuals with pale soft skin. Moles located on the feet, on the genitals, and under the nails are considered to be extremely dangerous.

There appears to be good evidence that at least 50 percent of malignant melanomas arise from pre-existing junction nevi. It is also recognized that chronic irritation, infection, and trauma seem to play a definite role in the production of malignant melanomas from pre-existing moles. Chronic irritation and trauma may consist of any of the following: irritation from shoes, collars, corsets, suspenders, brassières, corn plasters, trauma from fingering because of habit, combing of hair, repeated pulling of hairs, scratches, lacerations (shaving). Moles subjected to these forms of chronic irritation or trauma should be removed as a prophylactic measure.

Most authors agree that wide excision of the mole is the only adequate treatment. The excision should include a good margin of surrounding normal skin and the underlying fat.

Since nevi are radioresistant, they should never be treated by x-ray or radium irradiation. There is also a definite danger in treating moles by electrocautery or electrodesiccation, since the nevus cells may not be completely destroyed and the irritation of the electrocautery may induce the remaining part of the tumor to grow more rapidly and even to become malignant.

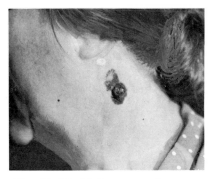

Fig. 11–13. Malignant melanoma resulting from a pre-existing benign nevus.

Melanomas

Melanoma is the most malignant of all skin tumors and one of the most malignant of all tumors. It constitutes about 1 percent of all malignant tumors and causes from 0.5 to 1 percent of all deaths due to malignancy. Though this tumor may be found in a wide range of ages, it is most common in middle-aged individuals. There is no significant difference in incidence between the sexes. The areas of predilection are the head and the lower extremities, especially the feet.

Etiology. The varied microscopic picture which may be presented has been mentioned. The origin of most of these tumors is a pre-existing junction nevus, and in many of the remaining cases, the patient may simply not have been aware of the existence of the original mole. Because melanoma usually develops from a pre-existing nevus which may have been present for years without giving trouble, the patient frequently delays seeking medical advice until the lesion is far advanced (Fig. 11-13). Melanoma may be quiescent for years, and moles, apparently benign, which are removed by chance, may show localized malignant changes. However, once the melanoma begins to extend, the prognosis is poor, and most patients die within 3 years. Rarely, a type of melanoma is seen which has very little pigment; this is called achromic melanoma.

Once melanoma has developed, the prognosis is poor, especially if the regional nodes are involved. Therefore, one should not temporize with doubtful nevi or with those subject to trauma. The occurrence of any of the gross changes listed previously as evidence of malignancy means that the melanoma is already well on its way toward extension and that hope for cure is slight. Indeed, metastatic spread may occur without local evidence of malignant change.

The treatment of a recognized melanoma should not be attempted on an ambulatory patient. Because melanomas are often not recognized before surgery, wide excision of all nevi is mandatory.

CANCER OF THE SKIN

Basal Cell Cancer

Basal cell cancer, or rodent ulcer, is a malignant growth arising from the basal layer of the skin. It appears most commonly in individuals past midlife. It is

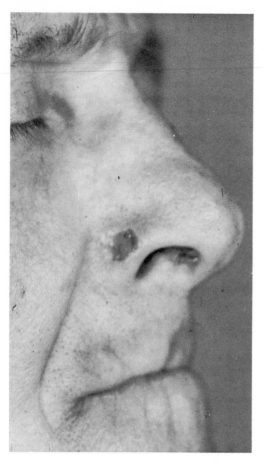

Fig. 11–14. Basal cell carcinoma in a typical location. (Carmen Thomas)

development of this type of lesion. It is found much more frequently in those who live in the country than it is in those who dwell in the city.

Prophylaxis. In considering basal cell carcinoma, attention should be directed to its prophylaxis by removal of these precancerous lesions at an early stage. Excision under local anesthesia with primary suture of the wound, especially in older people, may be regarded as wise prophylactic therapy.

Diagnosis. The basal-cell carcinoma occurs most often on the nose (Fig. 11-14), the cheeks, the outer canthus of the eye, and over the temples. Occasionally, it occurs on the forehead, the ears, or the trunk. The appearance of the growth may be flat, nodular, ulcerative, or annular. Characteristic of all the lesions, however, is the hardness of the edges, which gives them a raised, heaped-up effect. The ulcers are covered with yellowish crusts or scabs, and there is an exudation of yellow, serous material; bleeding in small amounts is not at all uncommon, especially following slight trauma. Any shallow, bleeding ulceration which persists for several weeks on the face of one past midlife is, in all probability, a basal cell carcinoma.

Symptoms. Symptoms produced by basal cell cancer are relatively trivial; occasionally, there is some itching or irritation, but most often patients seek treatment because of the ulceration, which refuses to heal. The progress of the growth is usually slow, and metastasis is rare, if it occurs at all; for these reasons this tumor is a relatively benign type of carcinoma. However, should it invade bone or cartilage, the difficulty of cure increases tremendously, and it becomes an invasive, destructive lesion which, even if cured, leaves marked deformity.

Treatment. The average early basal cell carcinoma can be cured if it is completely destroyed; it is important, however, that this complete destruction occur at the time of the primary treatment. It makes little difference whether the treatment is irradiation with roentgen rays or radium, electrocoagulation, or surgical excision so

relatively rare in the Negro race, but it is not uncommon in the white.

Etiology. This lesion practically always arises from some precancerous dermatosis, the most common of which is the seborrheic wart, or senile keratosis, frequently seen in elderly people. These warts develop slowly and are slightly raised yellow-black areas covered with a greasy-appearing scale which is extremely adherent. They appear most often on the face, the neck, the back, and the extremities, especially on the hands and the arms. These lesions are believed by many to be caused by exposure to sunlight and wind; hence there is a predisposition in carpenters, sailors, and farmers, who are much in the open, to the long as the lesion is completely destroyed or removed. Many of these tumors can be handled in ambulatory patients by relatively minor procedures, such as excision, electrocoagulation, or irradiation. Excisional therapy is probably the best, except in areas where the skin is tight, as over the nose or ear. If electrodesiccation or roentgen therapy is elected as the method of therapy, a biopsy for tissue diagnosis is most desirable.

SQUAMOUS CELL CANCER

Etiology. Squamous cell arises from the squamous cell layer of the skin. It is believed to arise almost exclusively from chronic injury to previously normal or abnormal tissues. It may result from injuries, various types of dermatoses, scars, or ulcerations, and there now is definite information pointing to the possibility that various chemicals are etiologic factors in this type of cancer.

Diagnosis. Squamous cell cancer occurs most frequently on the face, the ears, the scalp, the extremities, and the genitals. Clinically, it appears in two forms: the ulcerative type, characterized by an indurated ulcer with raised edges and a necrotic base; and the cauliflower form, which presents a fungating, granulomatous, or papillary appearance. The ulcerating type, although less malignant, has great destructive properties; it spreads from the periphery, the indurated edges breaking down to form a necrotic base. The edges are frequently undermined, and the tumor may spread from its undersurface as well as along its edges, thus invading deeper structures. The cauliflower type is less destructive, but it has greater malignant tendencies; metastasis and recurrence are more frequent. This is especially true when it occurs in the extremities. Metastasis of both the ulcerative and the cauliflower types occurs late.

Treatment. Treatment of squamous cell carcinoma of the lip is discussed in Chapter 14. In the extremities, surgical removal or irradiation is the treatment of choice, depending upon the age and the physical status of the patient and upon the size and the type of the lesion. A combination of irradiation and surgery may also be advisable. It is wise for the surgeon to consult with the radiologist in deciding upon the method of treatment for the individual lesion.

GANGLIA

Pathology. A ganglion may be defined as a cystic swelling surrounded by a fibrous tissue wall and occurring in the vicinity of joint capsules and tendon sheaths. The cause of the appearance of a ganglion has never been absolutely determined. For many years ganglia were thought to be herniations of tendon sheaths; but there is more widespread acceptance of the theory that ganglia arise as a result of a degenerative process in the mesoblastic tissue surrounding joints and tendon sheaths and elsewhere in the body.

Incidence. Ganglia appear about three times as often in females as in males. The majority of the cases appear in the second and third decades of life and comparatively few in the later decades. The relation of trauma to the etiology of ganglia has not been definitely determined.

Ganglia appear most commonly on the anterior surface of the wrist (Fig. 11-15), but they may arise from any of the connective tissues in the body. They are not at all uncommon on the palmar surface of the wrist, along the flexor tendon sheath in the distal palm and the proximal portion of the finger, over the dorsal surface of the distal phalanx of the finger and the toe, along the tendons inserting on the head of the fibula, on the dorsal surface of the foot, and, relatively more uncommon, in the connective tissue of the scalp, of the tendons themselves, and along the nerves.

Symptoms. The symptoms produced by ganglia vary considerably with their location. The most prominent and constant symptom is the presence of the mass; this is easily visible when it appears subcutaneously on the wrist or the finger. It can be further demonstrated by flexion or extension of the wrist, depending on

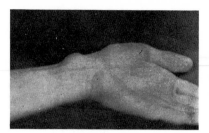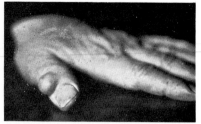

Fig. 11–15. (*Left*) Ganglion of the anterior surface of the wrist. (*Right*) Ganglion or mucoid cyst of the dorsal surface of the distal phalanx of the thumb. (DeOrsay, R. H., Mecray, P. M., Jr., and Ferguson, L. K.: Am. J. Surg., *36*:313, 1937)

which surface is involved. At times the swelling is a smooth rounded mass; at other times, it is multilocular. The ganglia vary in consistency; they usually are hard and firm, and are frequently diagnosed as bony or cartilaginous lesions, but they may be cystic and definitely fluctuant. This probably depends upon the stage of development at which the ganglion is seen. The size of the lesion often varies increasing after excessive movement or use of the part and decreasing with rest.

Pain is frequently a symptom; it may be dull and constant in character, or it may appear following the use of the affected part. Pressure upon the ganglion may give definite sharp pain. This is particularly true of ganglia appearing on the flexor tendon sheaths in the palm, where grasping a hard object causes extreme pain. There may be an associated weakness of the area involved by the ganglion, such as the wrist, the finger, or the toe.

Treatment. The indications for treatment of ganglia are three in number: (1) the desire of the patient for removal of the unsightly mass produced by the ganglion; (2) relief of the feeling of weakness of the part; and (3) relief of the pain or the soreness.

Four methods have been used in treating ganglion—rupture, aspiration with or without injection of sclerosing solutions, excision, and hydrocortisone injection.

Rupture. Although in the past rupture of the ganglion by striking it with a heavy book or sharp finger pressure was dramatic, the permanent cure rate is quite low,

and this technique is no longer recommended.

Aspiration. Treatment by aspiration of the ganglion contents has been disappointing. In many cases the contents of the ganglion are of such a firm, jellylike consistency that aspiration is unsuccessful. In other cases, the multilocular character of the ganglion has made it difficult to be certain that the contents were entirely evacuated, even though some of the gelatinous material could be removed. When aspiration is attempted, a largebore 14-gauge 1-inch needle should be employed. Attempts to remove the gelatinous material with smaller needles are usually unsuccessful.

After all the material has been aspirated, the syringe is removed and the needle may be left in place for injection of a sclerosing solution. Some authors inject sodium morrhuate; usually 1 or, at most, 2 injections are required. The injections produce moderate pain and local edema that last a day or two, but the therapy usually is not disabling. Personal experience with aspiration and injection has not been favorable.

Excision. The most successful method of treatment has been careful dissection and excision of the ganglion (Fig. 11-16). Whenever possible, a tourniquet is used to produce a bloodless field. This permits a more rapid and accurate dissection. The operation may be performed under local infiltration anesthesia. With strict aseptic precautions and retraction to keep the sides of the wound on tension, the gan-

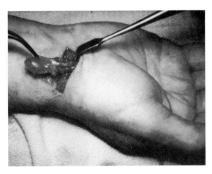

Fig. 11–16. Excision of ganglion of flexor surface of the wrist.

glion is separated from the surrounding tissue by blunt and sharp dissection. At its base, it is wise to excise a fairly generous amount of the surrounding tissue. This is the best insurance against recurrence.

If the capsule of the joint or the tendon sheath is opened, no effort is made to close it. After the closure of any dead space, the skin is sutured with vertical mattress stitches. A firm compression bandage is applied, and the part is splintered when possible. The patient is ambulatory throughout treatment.

It is wise not to promise that there will be no recurrence after the removal of a ganglion. Even wide excision of the surrounding tissues may not prevent the same process from recurring, with the formation of another ganglion.

Hydrocortisone has been used in the treatment of ganglia. Hydrocortisone in saline solution, 25 mg. per ml., is injected in amounts of from 0.3 to 0.5 ml. directly into the swelling, without anesthesia or aspiration. A single treatment is successful in most cases, but 2 or 3 injections at weekly intervals may be necessary.

BIBLIOGRAPHY

Cysts, Sinuses

Anderson, N. P.: Cysts, sinuses, and fistulas of dermatologic interest. JAMA, *135*:607, 1947.
Danna, J. A.: The treatment of sebaceous cysts by electrosurgical marsupialization. Ann. Surg., *123*:952, 1946.

Domonkos, A. N., and Andrews, M. D.: Diseases of the Skin. Philadelphia, W. B. Saunders, 1971.
Erich, J. B., and Johnsen, D. S.: Congenital dermoid cyst. Am. J. Surg., *85*:104, 1953.
Kanee, B.: Simple technic of cyst removal. Canad. Med. Assoc. J., *85*:1350, 1961.
New, G. B., and Erich, J. B.: Dermoid cysts of the head and neck. Surg., Gynec. Obstet., *65*:48, 1937.
Nicholl, R. B.: A variation of surgical technic in the removal of the sebaceous cysts of the scalp. J. Am. Osteo. Assoc., *44*:396, 1945.

Hemangioma

Bowers, R. E., *et al.*: The natural history of the strawberry nevus. Arch. Derm., *82*:667, 1960.
Brown, J. B., and Byars, L. T.: The interstitial radiation treatment of hemangiomata. Am. J. Surg., *39*:452, 1938.
Kaessler, H. W.: Vascular birthmarks: treatment with injection of sclerosing solution. JAMA, *110*:1644, 1938.
MacCollum, D. W.: Treatment of hemangiomas. Am. J. Surg., *29*:32, 1935.
Macomber, W. B., and Wang, M. K. H.: The hemangioma. G. P., *8*: 41, 1953.
Margileth, A. M. and Museles, M.: Current concepts in diagnosis and management of congenital cutaneous hemangiomas. Pediatrics, *36*:410, 1965.
Peyton, W. T., and Leven, N. L.: Hemangioma and its treatment. Surgery, *3*:702, 1938.
Prouty, J. V.: Treatment of hemangiomas with roentgen rays. Am. J. Roentgen., *54*:172, 1945.
Young, F.: Vascular birthmarks: diagnosis and treatment. J. Pediat., *14*:671, 1939 (Abstr. in Digest Treat., *3*:245, 1939).
Zarem, H. A., *et al.*: Induced resolution of cavernous hemangiomas following prednisolone therapy. Plast. Reconstr. Surg., *39*:76, 1967.

Keloid

Bernstein, H.: Treatment of keloids by steroids with biochemical tests for diagnosis and prognosis. Angiology, *15*:253, 1964.
Conway, H., and Stark, R. B.: Corticotropin (ACTH) in the treatment of keloids. Arch. Surg., *64*:47, 1952.
Maguire, H. C.: Treatment of keloids with triamcinolone acetonide injected intralesionally. JAMA, *192*:325, 1965.
Robinson, D.W.: Hypertrophic scars and keloids. Am. Surg., *19*:90, 1953.

Warts

Blaney, D. J.: Warts and host defence. Cutis, 5:588, 1969.

Goldman, L.: Warts: are they here to stay? Consultant, 4:36, 1964.

Hollander, L.: Treatment of warts. G. P., 5:55, 1952.

Kent, H.: Warts and ultrasound. Arch. Derm., 100:79, 1969.

Massing, A. M., and Epstein, W. L.: Natural history of warts. Arch. Derm., 87:306, 1963.

Sutherland-Campbell, H.: Common warts: effective treatment. Arch. Derm. Syph., 30:821, 1934.

Glomus Tumor

Kolodny, A.: Glomus tumor; glomangioma. Ann. Surg., 107:128, 1938.

Laymon, C. W., and Peterson, W.: Glomangioma (glomus tumor). Arch. Derm., 92:509, 1965.

Ganglion

Barnes, W. E., Larsen, R. D., and Posch, J. L.: Review of ganglia of the hand and wrist with analysis of surgical treatment. Plast. Reconstr. Surg., 34:570, 1964.

DeOrsay, R. H., Mecray, P. M., Jr., and Ferguson, L. K.: Pathology and treatment of ganglion. Am. J. Surg., 36:313, 1937.

King, E. S. J.: The pathology of ganglion. Aust. New Zeal. J. Surg., 1:367, 1932.

McEvedy, B. V.: Simple ganglia. Brit. J. Surg., 49:585, 1962.

Sarma, P. J.: The injection treatment of ganglions and bursae: indications and limitations. Surg. Clin. N. Am., 20:135, 1940.

Nevi, Melanoma

Jennings, W. K.: The pigmented nevus. G. P., 5:35, 1952.

Knutson, C. O., et al.: Melanoma. Curr. Prob. Surg., December 1971.

Lockhart, C. E.: Excision of pigmented skin lesions. Am. Surg., 23:229, 1957.

McNeer, G., and Gupta, T. D.: Differential diagnosis of melanoma. CA, 15:120, 1965.

Mundth, E. D., Guralnick, E. A., and Raker, J. W.: Malignant melanoma. Ann. Surg., 162:15, 1965.

Pack, G. T., Davis, J., and Oppenheim, A.: The relation of race and complexion to the incidence of moles and melanomas. Ann. NY Acad. Sci., 100:719, 1963.

Peterson, R. F., Dykes, E. R., and Anderson, R.: Superficial malignant melanomas. Surg., Gynec. Obstet., 119:37, 1964.

Roys, H. C.: Management of pigmented nevi. Northwest Med., 51:211, 1952.

Cornu Cutaneum

Bart, R. S., et al.: Cutaneous horns: clinical and histopathologic study in 35 patients. Acta Dermatovener., 48:507, 1968.

12

Cryosurgery

Andrew A. Gage, M.D.

Cryosurgery is a method of producing tissue necrosis by freezing in situ. It is an excellent method for the local destruction of lesions, and its applicability using local anesthesia makes it very suitable for the ambulatory patient and the high-surgical-risk patient.

Since 1965, the uses of cryosurgery have expanded, to a limited extent, into most of the specialties of surgery. Its acceptance has developed most rapidly for use in those areas of the body which are easily accessible to treatment, either by unaided visual inspection or via endoscopy. For certain uses, as the treatment of tumors, cryosurgery cannot yet be considered a standard method of treatment. It has acquired a firm hold in dermatologic practice but is not yet generally practiced by surgeons, whose caution in quick acceptance of the technique is justified by the realization that tissues resist freezing injury and that cryosurgical technique and equipment need improvement. Still, it appears that the advantages of cryocoagulation exceed those of surgical excision, electrocoagulation, and other methods of local tissue destruction in certain special circumstances. Its special suitability for high-surgical-risk patients,

especially those who have problems which are difficult to manage by other methods of treatment, insures it a place in medical practice. This chapter emphasizes those uses which have found acceptance for the patient who has a disease which may be treated under local anesthesia in the office or outpatient clinic.

CRYOSURGICAL APPARATUS

In response to the differing needs of surgeons in various specialties, many cryosurgical tools have been developed in the past eight years. The surgeon now has a choice of apparatus varying from a simple disposable unit for cataract extraction to the sophisticated apparatus required for neurological surgery. The cryogenic agents, gases in the normal state, commonly used with the apparatus are nitrogen, carbon dioxide, Freon, and nitrous oxide, all of which are nonexplosive. Liquid nitrogen is readily obtainable, easy to handle, nontoxic, and has a boiling point of about $-196°C$ at atmospheric pressure. Its very cold temperature makes extensive freezing possible and makes it the most suitable of the

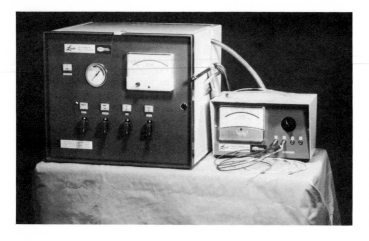

Fig. 12–1. Linde cryosurgical apparatus, Model CE-4, which functions only as a closed system to freeze with the use of cryoprobes. A Linde tissue-temperature indicator and attached thermocouples mounted in needles are also shown.

cryogenic agents for the destruction of large volumes of tissue. On the other hand, carbon dioxide and Freon 22 (chlorodifluoromethane) have wide usefulness in areas where lesser degrees of freezing will suffice. With carbon dioxide, the lowest attainable temperature is $-78.5°C$, and Freon 22 has a boiling point $-40°C$. Liquid nitrous oxide may give a freezing temperature of $-80°C$. These agents permit the construction of easily maneuverable lightweight apparatus with rapid response time in comparison to some apparatus using liquid nitrogen. Details regarding the construction and operation of various types of cryoinstrumentation may be read in the general reference books on cryosurgery.

The choice of equipment depends upon the nature of the lesion being treated. Successful management of large tumors requires the considerable freezing capability of liquid nitrogen units. Some models* may be used either as closed systems, so that liquid nitrogen is not released on the tissue, or to spray liquid nitrogen onto the lesion. The cryogen feedlines are not vacuum insulated, and the probes lack controls for temperature and cannot be heated. Lack of a probe heater is incon-

venient, but, on the other hand, the capability for use as a spray device is of considerable advantage in certain situations. A more efficient unit† (Fig. 12-1) functions only as a closed system, the freezing being done via cryoprobes; liquid nitrogen circulates through the probe tip, and, after change of phase, the gas is returned to the equipment cabinet for venting. The flexible feed shaft is vacuum insulated. Controls on the console make possible reasonably accurate control of the temperature of the probe tip, and, after termination of freezing, the heater in the probe near its tip speeds its release from the tissues. These features make this unit more suitable for freezing via endoscopy than is the apparatus without a heater, but inability to use it as a spray system is a disadvantage. Small tumors, especially if benign, can be treated with a hand-held unit using liquid nitrogen, or, if very small, with a unit using some other type of cryogenic agent. Inflammatory lesions can be satisfactorily treated with units using nitrous oxide, carbon dioxide, or Freon. Apparatus suitable for office or clinic use is available in all cryogenic systems.

TECHNIQUE

Cryosurgical techniques are intended to freeze tissue as efficiently as possible. The technique will necessarily vary in different parts of the body and with different types of lesions. The treatment of

---

*Linde Model CE-8, Frigitronics, Inc., Shelton, Conn.; Brymill Model SP-5, Brymill Corp., Vernon, Conn.

†Linde Model CE-4, Frigitronics, Inc., Shelton, Conn.

malignant tumors is more aggressive than the treatment of benign disease. It will also vary according to the apparatus chosen and, possibly, with the adjunctive use of other methods of treatment. The use of spray apparatus is different from the use of cryoprobes. In general, however, the basic objective is to freeze tissue in situ, without excision and thus avoiding hemorrhage. The devitalized tissue becomes liquified and is absorbed, or sloughs. Healing of the wound follows. Careful application of technique is essential to be sure that the desired result of treatment is obtained.

Freezing with Cryoprobes. The manner of use of the closed systems is to choose a cryoprobe suitable for the size and location of the lesion. Large tumors require large probes for effective freezing. The end of the probe is pressed firmly on the tumor. If contact is poor, as might be the case if the tumor overlies bone, a small amount of water-soluble hospital lubricating jelly is placed about the probe tip. Soft bulky tumors may be penetrated by the cryoprobe in order to obtain greater contact with the tissue and to produce more extensive freezing. Usually, however, surface-contact freezing is preferable because no wound is produced, the chance of bleeding is lessened, the tissue planes are not disrupted, and the chance of dissemination of tumor cells is minimized.

When freezing begins, the probe becomes fixed to the tissue and cannot be moved. Removal of heat from the tissues largely depends on the temperature of the cryoprobe, the area and quality of contact between the cryoprobe and the tissue, and the duration of freezing. The probe is always used as cold as possible because a large probe-tissue temperature gradient is a prime factor in controlling the rate and extent of freezing. The larger the gradient, the more rapid the enlargement of the frozen area. Heat sources and the shape of the cryoprobe also modify the volume and shape of the frozen area. Apparently

identical freezing conditions will yield variation in tissue freezing unless careful attention is given to these factors, especially to the extremely important one of maintenance of good contact between cryoprobe and tissue. When freezing begins, the probe becomes fixed to the tissue and must be held motionless. Even slight movement of the probe can cause fracture in the bond between the tissue and the probe and interfere with heat exchange, with resultant deficient freezing.

The extent of freezing is judged by inspection and palpation as the frozen tissues turn white and hard. With surface-contact freezing, the shape of the frozen area is roughly hemispherical, the depth of the freezing being about the same as the lateral spread of the freezing from the side of the probe. Freezing is allowed to continue until the frozen area encompasses the entire lesion and a reasonable amount of surrounding normal tissue. Most lesions are too large to be frozen in a single application of the probe, and, in such cases, immediate successive applications overlapping the frozen zone are necessary. The tissue is allowed to thaw, and after about 10 minutes the entire area is frozen again.

The duration of freezing time of each application varies and cannot be prescribed beforehand because of the many variable factors involved in treatment. It is not possible to use theoretical calculations of freezing capabilities of probes in clinical practice. Instead it is necessary to develop by experience some knowledge of the characteristics of each cryoprobe in order to determine how large a frozen area will form in any chosen time-temperature freezing cycle. For example, a probe commonly used in tumor therapy, a 9.5-mm. cryoprobe,‡ used at $-160°C$, will produce a roughly hemispherical frozen lesion 3 cm. in diameter in 3 minutes (Fig. 12-2). If probe contact is maintained for 5 minutes, the area frozen is about 4 cm. in surface diameter. On continued contact, the ice ball grows very slowly, and later the frozen edge no longer advances. If additional freezing is required, the cryoprobe is moved to a new, unfrozen site.

---

‡PR-5 cryoprobe, Frigitronics, Inc., Shelton, Conn.

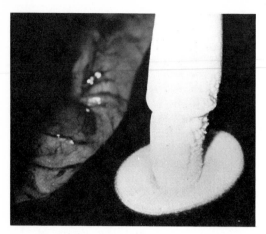

Fig. 12–2. Canine liver being frozen with the Linde PR-5 probe. After three minutes of contact with the probe at −160°C, a white frosted appearance shows the frozen area; the depth of penetration is about the same as the spread of the frost from the side of the probe. With proper technique, the area of necrosis will closely correspond to the visibly frozen area.

Successive adjacent applications widen the frozen area but only slightly increase the depth of freezing. In the tissues adjacent to the probe, tissue temperatures colder than −80°C and commonly as cold as −170°C are reached in less than a minute. An apparatus with a vacuum-insulated feedline functions much better than an apparatus with a less efficient feedline insulation. However, with any equipment, the necessity of freezing large volumes of tissue may pose problems.

Even though the cryoprobe is always used at the same cold temperature, the quality of the contact of the tissue with the probe and variations in heat sources will cause differences in the rate and extent of freezing. With each application, it is necessary to continue freezing until the desired amount of tissue is frozen or until the edge of the frozen area ceases to advance. In the course of treatment, the rate of expansion of the frozen area slows as an equilibrium is established between heat brought to the area by the circulation and heat loss to the cryoprobe. Although, at times, the frozen area may still be

cooling after 10 minutes of treatment, usually, applications of more than 7 minutes are not advisable because the rate of enlargement of the frozen area slows considerably after that time. If the entire tumor area is not included in the frozen area in 7 minutes, the probe is thawed and moved to another site. Treatment is completed when the volume of tissue frozen and refrozen is equivalent to that excised in a conservative local excision.

Liquid Nitrogen Used as a Spray. In this technique, a spray of liquid nitrogen, produced by flow through small apertures in nozzles or needles at the end of a feedline, is directed on the lesion. The liquid nitrogen vaporizes on the lesion and causes freezing. The advantages of using liquid nitrogen as a spray are that the cryogen is being used at its coldest possible temperature and that it can be moved about, so that freezing is extensive and wide rather than deep. Of course, if the spray is directed only at a small area, then deep freezing will be achieved as well. The disadvantage of the spray is that as the tissue freezes it loses its ability to vaporize liquid nitrogen, and runoff of liquid nitrogen occurs. Therefore, the spray is more difficult to control than the closed system. With persistence, it probably is possible to freeze a larger area with the spray than with the probe, but it requires very careful technique.

The choice between the use of liquid nitrogen as a spray and its use in a cryoprobe depends on the lesion and its location. Cryoprobes offer the advantage of more accurate control of freezing, and their use therefore results in a more predictable area of necrosis. They are especially well chosen for the oral cavity or pharynx and are absolutely necessary when freezing is done through endoscopes. Cryoprobes can be used on any skin lesion and also can be used to penetrate tumors for freezing. In general, freezing with cryoprobes has a wider range of usefulness than does the use of spray devices. The use of liquid nitrogen as a spray is best for accessible lesions, such as those in the skin. Superficial lesions are most easily treated, but the spray also has considerable advantage in the extensive freezing required by bulky external cancers.

Use of Thermocouples. Thermocouples must be used whenever possible in order to assess the progress of freezing and to determine the tissue temperature. Thermocouples mounted in needles are inserted into the lesion and at its periphery to be certain that lethal temperatures are reached. They also offer protection against undesired destruction of normal tissue at the periphery of the lesion. A thermocouple placed close to the probe shows the progress of freezing and reveals any fault in heat exchange as early as possible (Fig. 12-3).

A thermocouple shows only the temperature where it is located. The cryosurgeon must use the evidence from one or more thermocouples to help visualize a thermal profile throughout the entire frozen area. Extreme gradients in temperature develop in the frozen area during cryosurgical treatment. The rate of freezing decreases with increasing distance from the probe, and expansion of the frozen area gradually slows. The coldest temperatures and the most extensive freezing damage occur close to the site of the probe-tissue contact. Remote from the probe, freezing is slower, tissue temperatures are higher, and the probability of cell survival increases. The temperature at the border of the frozen zone is about zero, and here cell survival is possible.

The exact lethal temperature is difficult to define. Though ice crystals begin to form in tissue at $-2.2°C$, consistent cell death is said to require temperatures at least as low as $-20°C$ for a minute. With regard to cancer therapy, this temperature will not surely kill all cells. To produce necrosis in a large volume of tissue requires considerably colder temperatures. In freezing animal tissues under cryosurgical conditions, temperatures much colder than $-20°C$ must be achieved in order to produce cell death in single freeze-thaw cycles. Even at temperatures of $-50°C$ or warmer, single freezing episodes are uncertainly destructive. Temperatures of $-60°C$ and colder are certain-

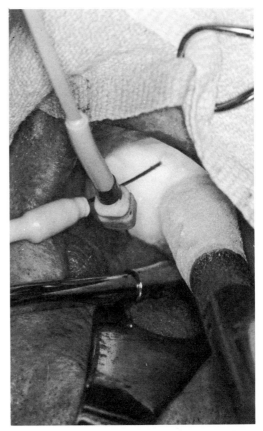

Fig. 12–3. Carcinoma of the palate, being frozen with PR-5 probe. Thermocouples have been placed in the frozen area close to the probe and at the periphery in order to determine that lethal temperatures are achieved.

lylethal, even with single freezing episodes, and predictable areas of necrosis are produced. In cancer cryosurgery, such considerations become important, and emphasis should be placed on producing temperatures at least as cold at $-50°C$ in all of the tumor area, allowing the warmer parts of the frozen area to include apparently normal tissues. Fortunately, repetition of freezing greatly increases the lethality of the freezing process, so that there probably is no cell survival even at $-20°C$. This means that everything visibly frozen will die, excepting only a narrow margin at the periphery.

Since the goal of cryosurgery is the production of a desired area of tissue

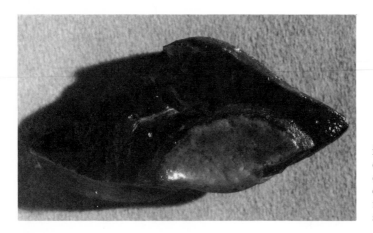

Fig. 12–4. Canine liver, frozen 10 days previously. A cross section shows a typical cryogenic lesion in the form of a sharply circumscribed necrotic area, roughly hemispherical in shape.

necrosis, it is important to use techniques to achieve maximal lethal effect. The important points in technique may be summarized as follows: (1) use a cryogen suitable for the lesion; (2) maintain good tissue-cryogen contact; (3) use cryoprobes as cold as possible; (4) control the freezing procedure with thermocouples; (5) freeze as quickly as possible; (6) thaw slowly and unassisted; (7) overlap frozen areas; (8) repeat freezing after thawing; (9) include a margin of normal tissue.

EFFECT OF FREEZING ON TISSUE

Freezing kills cells. The lethal effects are due to cellular changes such as crystallization of water, toxic concentration of electrolytes within the cells, and irreversible damage to cell membranes. Cell injury is enhanced by the effect of freezing on the circulation. After freezing and thawing, the treated area becomes congested and circulation through small vessels stagnates. Loss of circulation deprives all cells of any possibility of survival.

The cryogenic lesion is characterized by a sharply circumscribed area of necrosis (Fig. 12-4). After thawing, frozen tissue becomes swollen and discolored due to hemorrhage and congestion. A zone of hyperemia develops about the periphery of the lesion. Over the next few days, a sharply demarcated necrosis, corresponding closely to the area previously frozen, becomes evident. In the skin, an eschar forms. In the oral cavity and the rectum, necrotic tissue appears more quickly, and in these environments an eschar does not form, but rather the tissue sloughs or is liquified. The time required for sloughing of necrotic tissue depends in part upon its composition. Tissues rich in collagenous tissue, such as the skin, resist structural change, and complete separation of necrotic tissue requires many days. On the other hand, cellular tissue sloughs very quickly. Major blood vessels resist freezing injury. Experimental work shows that the major change in arteries is a hyperplasia of the intima of the blood vessel, which in small vessels leads to occlusion, but in larger vessels only narrows the lumen until final healing occurs.

The effect of freezing on bone is of particular pertinence to cryosurgery. Experiments have shown that bone devitalized in situ by freezing is slowly resorbed and simultaneously replaced by new bone, a process of repair that requires many months. In the meantime, the devitalized bone continues to maintain form and function during the healing stage. Observations made upon bone in the oral cavity, frozen during clinical cryosurgery, have confirmed experimental work on devitalized bone. Sequestration is uncommon, even though healing requires many months. It is this favorable response that permits extensive freezing of the mandible and the maxilla in the treatment of oral tumors and likewise permits extensive freezing of rodent ulcers and other cancers overlying bone, invading its foramina, or eroding its structure.

DISEASES OF THE SKIN

The present wide use of cryosurgery in dermatologic practice is described fully in the excellent monograph by Zacarian. A large number of benign lesions of the skin are suitable for cryosurgery. Verrucous and keratotic lesions, hemangiomas, and a variety of other benign tumors and inflammatory lesions of the skin are successfully treated. Cryosurgery is the most convenient method of treatment for multiple seborrheic keratoses and for senile and other precancerous keratoses.

Skin Cancer

Skin cancer is easily and efficiently treated by freezing in situ. The histologic type of the cancer is not important, because there is no meaningful difference between the sensitivities of squamous cell and basal cell carcinoma to freezing injury. Melanomas are also easily destroyed by freezing, but primary melanomas are best treated by excision. Excepting melanomas, almost all skin cancers are suitable for treatment by freezing. However, most single skin cancers are small and can be cured easily by surgical excision, which must be the preferred method because histologic examination of the tissue offers some evidence of the adequacy of treatment. Radiotherapy is also effective and is used to treat cancers in locations where excision is difficult, such as around the face, and to treat those lesions which cannot be excised. In many patients with skin cancer, perhaps these time-proven methods should be used, though cryosurgery is a strong competitor. However, the advantages of freezing in situ are ease of treatment, little need for anesthesia, no chance of implantation of tumor cells, and surprisingly favorable healing.

There are some skin cancers which should be considered for cryosurgery preferentially. They are (1) multiple small skin cancers; (2) cancers arising in irradiated skin; (3) cancers located over bone, so that periosteal lymphatics may be invaded or the underlying bone may be eroded by cancer; (4) cancers located about the ear, the eye, or the nose; (5) large cancers, difficult to excise; and (6) cancers which persist after radiotherapy or excision.

Multiple small skin cancers are suitable for freezing because many lesions can be treated on the same visit more quickly than they can by excision. Cancers arising in irradiated skin often are not large but are located in areas about the face, where tissue loss is costly from a cosmetic viewpoint. Freezing permits conservative treatment, with minimal tissue sacrifice in achieving cure (Fig. 12-5, *left* and *right*). If treatment is inadequate the first time, it can be repeated as often as necessary to eliminate the tumor. This is also true of the cancers that are located about the ear, the eye, or the nose.

More difficult problems in treatment are presented by infiltrating carcinomas which have resisted other forms of treatment and which involve deep structures about the nose, the eye, or the ear (Fig. 12-6, *left* and *right*). Such patients may be given palliative treatment on an ambulatory basis, but attempts at cure require hospitalization for general anesthesia. Some cancers persistent after surgical excision or radiotherapy and involving areas about the face, or neglected extensive cancers of the external ear, may be successfully treated by cryosurgery. In some cases, it is advisable to partially excise the tumor in order to facilitate freezing the deeper tissues. In general, the method of using cryosurgery for the treatment of such large tumors is to freeze as much as possible, wait for the necrotic tissue to slough, then biopsy suspicious areas of the wound to guide the repetition of cryosurgery. The wound is not closed, to permit detection of persistent cancer at the earliest possible moment. Facial nerve paralysis commonly occurs after freezing lesions of the ear canal, but function usually returns in several months if nerve continuity is not interrupted. This surprisingly rapid return of function is an

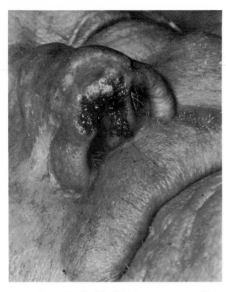
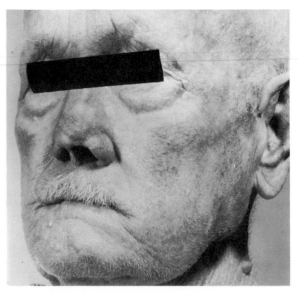

Fig. 12–5. (*Left*), Squamous cell carcinoma of the ala nasi and nasal septum, occurring in skin irradiated years earlier for skin disease. Scars of previous excision are seen. This lesion is ideally suited for conservative cryosurgery. (*Right*) A year later, the cosmetic effect of treatment is excellent. There is no sign of persistent disease.

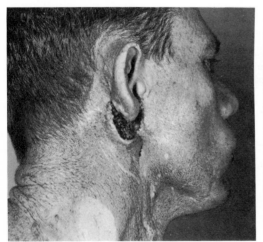
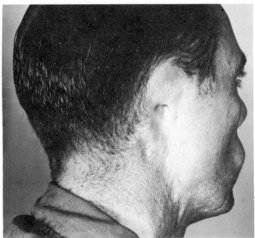

Fig. 12–6. (*Left*) Squamous cell carcinoma of the external ear, growing into the canal, destroying the lower portion of the earlobe, and ulcerating the tissues of the neck. The cancer is persistent after excision and radiotherapy. Treatment will be partial excision and then freezing of the remaining cancer. (*Right*) One year later, the treated area is well healed, and there is no sign of persistent disease. The patient will be given a prosthetic ear.

indication that cryosurgery is the best method of treatment in certain situations where there is risk of undesired major neurologic damage from conventional surgical excision.

Cryosurgery is also useful for the palliation of advanced primary or metastatic cancer of the skin, especially bulky protuberant carcinomas anywhere on the body. Tumor size is easily reduced. Discomfort or pain is relieved and hemorrhage is prevented. The palliation achieved is not lasting, because invasion continues and symptoms recur. Life probably is not prolonged. Repetition of treatment every few months is needed to control growth. Treatment must be given with care to ulcerating tumors of the neck. Although it is well known that normal blood vessels are resistant to freezing injury and that rupture or thrombosis does not occur, these experimental findings do not apply to the blood vessels which are involved in tumor. Therefore, after deliberate or inadvertent freezing of cervical carcinoma which involves the carotid artery, the risk of disastrous hemorrhage during the period of sloughing is considerable. Metastatic melanomas respond very well to freezing. Only the frozen tissue dies, and there is no evidence of any cryo-immunologic response.

TUMORS OF THE ORAL CAVITY

Benign and malignant tumors and precancerous conditions of the oral cavity are well suited to treatment by local freezing. Except for the skin, cryosurgical techniques are more easily used in the oral cavity than in other parts of the body. There are special advantages to its use in oral diseases. First, the oral cavity is easily accessible to treatment. Second, often local anesthesia can be used, so operative risk is reduced. Third, the effect of treatment is readily observed in the postoperative period. Fourth, repetition of treatment, when necessary, is easily done. Fifth, cryosurgery offers the outstanding advantage of permitting local treatment without sacrifice of bone or the oral cavity.

Benign Tumors

Benign tumors of the oral cavity are usually ideal for treatment by cryosurgery. Local or topical anesthesia is adequate for most lesions, and treatment should be conservative, so that normal tissue is not unnecessarily destroyed. Tumors that overlie bone are specially suited for treatment. Cryosurgery offers a considerable advantage over excision in terms of operative blood loss, postoperative pain and risk of infection, and probability of cure. Hemangiomas and mixed tumors of the oral cavity are successfully treated. Most often a cryoprobe is used because it offers better control of freezing than does a liquid nitrogen spray.

Precancerous conditions are easily treated by cryosurgery under local anesthesia. Most such lesions are superficial, so that freezing must be wide rather than deep, sometimes covering large areas. Either the cryoprobe or the spray system can be used. If the cryoprobe is used, multiple applications of short duration are necessary because treatment need be given only to a depth of a few millimeters. Extensive superficial precancerous lesions may be better treated by the use of a spray of liquid nitrogen. Caution must be observed that undesired runoff of droplets of liquid nitrogen into other areas does not occur. Papillary epithelial hyperplasia, hyperkeratosis, and leukoplakia are satisfactorily treated by freezing. Since freezing is superficial, postoperative edema is not troublesome. The patient is able to eat a soft diet, and healing is ordinarily rapid.

Oral Cancer

The usual treatment of oral cancer is surgical excision or radiotherapy, but these commonly accepted methods of treatment are associated with a number of problems related to the effects of treatment or to failure of treatment to cure. Loss of form or function of the mouth and jaws after radical surgery is not to be minimized, and radiotherapy is associated with disagreeable sequelae in relation to radionecrosis of bone. Other patients have problems related to untreated, neglected cancer. Some patients with apparently curable oral cancer are not candidates for surgical excision because of the operative risk imposed by associated disease, and others refuse surgical treatment. These considerations mean that cryosurgery may be used for widely different reasons in oral cancer. The goal of treatment may be palliation of incurable cancer or attempted salvage of localized advanced cancer after failure of other methods of treatment, or cryosurgery may be used as the primary treatment for cancer.

Palliation of Advanced Oral Cancer. Neglected oral cancer causes pain and bleeding. Its growth interferes with mastication and deglutition. Some patients may be incurable because of local spread, while others have rather small primary lesions with extensive metastatic disease. In bulky tumors, the goal of treatment is principally to achieve reduction in size of the tumor. Painful lesions are especially suitable for treatment by freezing, even though small in size. Relief of pain is occasionally immediate and complete, but more often partial. During the first days after the freezing of large bulky tumors, nutrition by nasogastric tube or parenteral route is needed. However, rapid reduction in tumor size usually permits ingestion of food within a few days. Regrowth of the tumor occurs, of course, so ordinarily repetition of treatment is needed in three or four months. Radiotherapy may be used in combination with cryosurgery to produce a longer-lasting effect. The palliative results of cryosurgery for large bulky tumors are often disappointing because the presence of a large volume of necrotic tissue in the oral cavity is often difficult for aged or debilitated patients to tolerate. Therefore, except for the relief of pain, radiotherapy is probably preferable to cryosurgery for large cancers.

Oral Cancer Persistent after Excision or Radiotherapy. In most cases, cancers persistent after treatment are incurable. However, there are patients with a rather small amount of persistent disease after radiotherapy or excision; yet often further surgery is not possible and further radiotherapy is considered inadvisable. Cryosurgery is often an excellent alternative method of therapy and affords some chance of cure. The risk is small in the sense that the usual methods of treatment have failed or cannot be used, so there is good justification for use of a new therapeutic technique. Survival of such patients is an indication of the usefulness of cryosurgery as a method of salvage when disease is persistent after other methods of treatment. Even though cure may not be obtained, striking relief of pain may be achieved.

Primary Treatment of Oral Cancer by Freezing. Certain patients with oral cancer may be treated by freezing in situ in preference to any other type of therapy. This departure from standard methods of treatment requires careful selection of patients in order not to compromise the chance of cure through faulty judgment as to the extent of the disease. Selection of patients is based on the following criteria:

1. The cancer is on or adjacent to bone, so that excision would require removal of a portion of the mandible or palate.

2. The patient has extensive cardiopulmonary disease, so that the risk of extensive operation is prohibitive.

Either one of the reasons is sufficient to select a patient for consideration of cryosurgery. In addition, cryosurgery may be offered to patients who refuse suggested radical excision or radiotherapy or who are not suitable for such treatment for a variety of reasons.

It is better to select patients with small cancers rather than large ones because the chance of cure is increased and because large cancers tax the capabilities of cryosurgical apparatus to achieve lethal temperatures. Cryosurgery is more likely to cure small tumors than large ones, but of course that is true of any other treatment method also. Advanced cancers of the oral cavity, especially those of the floor of the mouth, the base of the tongue, and the pharynx, are probably not curable by cryosurgery, and the technique should not be used for extensive cancer unless necessitated by the general condition of the patient.

It is best to select patients who do not have enlarged cervical lymph nodes at the time of examination. Suitable for office treatment or clinic treatment under local

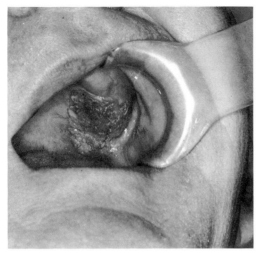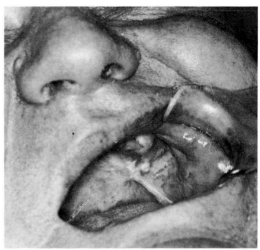

Fig. 12–7. (*Left*) Squamous cell carcinoma of the upper alveolar ridge and adjacent palate. Deep penetration is limited by the underlying bone. This is an ideal case for cryosurgery. (*Right*) A year after treatment, the treated area is well healed with some fibrosis. There is no tumor in the treated area (now three years after treatment).

anesthesia would be only those patients who have small to moderate-sized lesions without enlarged cervical lymph nodes. However, there are certain patients who are high surgical risks who may be best managed by cryosurgery to the local intra-oral lesion followed by· radiotherapy to the neck nodes. Cryosurgery is particularly well suited for tumors overlying the palate or mandible because invasion of tumor is limited by the bone (Fig. 12-7, *left* and *right*). The lethal effect of freezing extends into the bone and destroys any tumor which may be there. Cancers of the tongue and the floor of the mouth are not as suitable for cryosurgery as cancers overlying bone because infiltration of the tumor may be surprisingly deep, invasion via lymphatics may be early, and the risk of failure is higher than with lesions overlying bone. On the other hand, small to moderate-sized cancers in the anterior portion of the floor of the mouth are acceptable for treatment because of easy accessibility and because the extreme disability caused by resection of the anterior part of the mandible encourages acceptance of the risk of cryosurgery. Conservation of the bony structure of the oral cavity is the outstanding

reason why cryosurgery deserves a place in the surgical management of oral cancer. In selected cases, a survival rate comparable to that afforded by surgical excision can be achieved, and this result can be achieved at less cost to the patient in terms of operative mortality and postoperative functional disability.

Postoperative Care and Complications. Patient care following intra-oral freezing is ordinarily simple. Most problems are related to the edema, which begins to form after thawing and increases to a maximum within a day, interfering with deglutition to some extent, depending upon the amount of swelling in the area frozen. Oral secretions are copious. The tongue after freezing becomes remarkably edematous. Such patients are not suitable for treatment on an ambulatory basis because they probably will need a nasogastric tube or intravenous feeding. Lesions in the posterior portion of the oral cavity are not suitable for freezing in a clinic because edema is a potential threat to the airway. In such patients, often a tracheostomy is done at the time of freezing in order to avoid any difficulty in the postoperative period.

Postoperative pain is usually minimal,

and only analgesics are required for the discomfort caused by swelling of the tissues in the oral cavity. Since some fever and leukocytosis always develop, a broad-spectrum antibiotic, such as ampicillin, is given prophylactically for several days after treatment. Over several days, the previously frozen tissue becomes necrotic, and a mass of malodorous tissue develops in the oral cavity. The use of pleasant-tasting mouthwash is helpful during this period. The partially necrotic, liquifying tissue sloughs in small pieces over a three-week period, until the wound has a clean granulating base. Separation of the necrotic tissue may be aided by careful débridement during this period. About 3 weeks are required for the wound to become sufficiently clear of necrotic tissue to permit close examination of the base and rebiopsy of suspicious areas. In cases where tumor is still present, cryosurgical treatment is repeated. Most soft-tissue wounds heal surprisingly well in about 4 weeks. However, if the bone is exposed by slough of the soft tissue, then healing is prolonged and may not occur for a year or two. Devitalized bone in the treated area requires as long as two years for completion of repair.

Complications of freezing oral lesions are related to the mass of necrotic tissue that develops after treatment. There may be obstruction to deglutition or danger to the airway. Later complications are paresthesias, trismus, hemorrhage, and sequestration of bone. Paresthesias usually subside within a few days, but occasionally sensory loss over the lip and chin and part of the tongue may persist for a month. Fortunately, nerves commonly regenerate after freezing injury, so numbness and paresthesias are rarely a serious long-term problem. About 7 to 10 days after freezing, when the necrotic tissue begins to slough, hemorrhage sometimes occurs from previously frozen lesions of the floor of the mouth and the tongue and less commonly from elsewhere in the oral cavity. Bleeding is controlled by suture-ligature or by electrocoagulation. Although it is well known that large vessels resist freezing injury, whenever necrotic tissue due to any cause begins to slough,

there is risk of hemorrhage. Trismus is a serious postoperative problem. It occurs after the freezing of tumors in the retromolar area and apparently is due to edema and, later, fibrosis of the pterygoid muscles. Exercise of the jaw during the postoperative period is a partial solution to this problem. Devitalization of bone occurs during the freezing of tumors overlying the mandible or the palate, but only minor sequestration has occurred, even though bone repair may require as long as two or three years, depending upon the volume of bone frozen. It appears evident that the effect of freezing on bone is less deleterious than is that of radiotherapy.

GYNECOLOGIC DISEASE

Chronic Cervicitis. Benign cervical lesions, such as chronic cervicitis, endocervical polyps, leukoplakia, and condylomata acuminata, are also easily treated by cryosurgery. Its principal use is for chronic cervicitis. The extent of the disease must be carefully evaluated and the possibility of invasive carcinoma excluded. The extreme temperature gradient necessary for the treatment of carcinoma is not needed for the treatment of inflammatory disease, so apparatus using carbon dioxide or Freon is satisfactory. To avoid freezing the cervix during pregnancy, treatment is best given within two weeks of the last menstrual period. Cryosurgical treatment can be performed in the physician's office or in the outpatient clinic without need for anesthesia. The probes have special shapes that are designed to fit within the cervical canal for a short distance. Apply the probe at room temperature and in good position and then initiate freezing. Treatment can be conservative, and it is only necessary to freeze about 2 or 3 mm. beyond the edge of the obviously diseased area. In order to cover the entire area, repeated applications may be necessary in some instances. If the disease is minor, only a single application is necessary. In unusual cases, to achieve a greater degree of tissue necrosis and deeper penetration, freezing is repeated immediately after thawing.

However, a double freeze-thaw cycle is rarely needed in the treatment of benign cervical disease.

In the postoperative period, some patients have mild intermittent cramps, which may be treated with aspirin or similar analgesics. Immediately after treatment, some patients have described headaches, dizziness, and flushing; this is a vasomotor reaction and soon disappears. Usually, a heavy, clear, watery vaginal discharge develops and lasts about 10 to 14 days, gradually lessening as healing occurs. Slight bleeding may occur during the slough of necrotic tissue, but severe hemorrhage is unlikely. Because of the possibility of causing bleeding from the cervix due to trauma, abstinence from sexual intercourse for about three weeks is advised. Healing occurs in about 8 to 10 weeks. Cryosurgery appears to be somewhat better than electrocauterization because patient discomfort is less and healing time is shorter. In terms of complications, there are no serious problems with either technique.

Cervical Carcinoma. Cryosurgery may prove to be ideal treatment for preinvasive cervical carcinoma. In choosing patients, exclusion of invasive carcinoma of the cervix by cell smears and biopsy must be certain. In carefully chosen patients in whom invasive carcinoma of the cervix is not present, excellent results can be achieved by cervical cryosurgery. In such cases, later examinations at intervals must be carefully done. Cryosurgery should not be used for the primary treatment of invasive cervical cancer. It can be used for palliation of advanced incurable cervical malignancy. The benefits include decrease in tumor bulk, discharge, and bleeding as well as some relief of pain.

Diseases of the Vulva. A wide variety of vulvar diseases may be treated by freezing in situ. Benign tumors and small cutaneous malignant tumors may be frozen. Vulvar condylomata acuminata, treated by a variety of therapeutic methods with imperfect results, may be treated by cryosurgery as well. Freezing offers a number of advantages when compared to electrocoagulation or excision. Only local anesthesia is needed, and all the lesions may be treated in one visit to the clinic. Good visual control of the freezing process is possible, and treatment should include about 2 mm. of normal tissue beyond the lesion. In cases with extensive involvement of the vulva with condylomata acuminata, it is prudent to stage the freezing over several visits in order to avoid excessive vulvar edema.

DISEASES OF THE ANUS AND RECTUM

Anal and rectal diseases are a prime area of usefulness for cryosurgery. In general, any local lesion which can be excised or treated by electrocoagulation can also be treated by freezing in situ. At times cryocoagulation is preferable because little anesthesia is required, there is no bleeding, and the amount of subsequent necrosis is predictable. At times it cannot compete with established methods of treatment, either because a tissue specimen is needed for histologic examination or because lack of vision does not permit adequate control of the freezing process. In the anal region, there is little difficulty with determining the extent of disease, but in the rectum, adequacy of visualization of the lesion may be a problem. Good treatment can be given in the anus and lower rectum through a large-diameter proctoscope, but vision through a sigmoidoscope is poor when a large-diameter cryoprobe must be used in its lumen.

HEMORRHOIDS

Cryohemorrhoidectomy is a practical conservative method of treating any type of hemorrhoidal tissue, from irritating external skin tags to large edematous prolapsing hemorrhoids in high-surgical-risk patients. Its major usefulness may be in office practice, perhaps as an adjunct to the injection treatment of hemorrhoids. Treatment is done under local anesthesia. A clamp is applied to the hemorrhoidal tissue, and the cryoprobe is applied to the tissue within the clamp. Freezing is allowed to extend to include the entire hemorrhoidal area, and it is not repeated.

Treatment can also be given without use of the occluding clamp. As freezing begins, the adherent cryoprobe is used as a retractor to lift the hemorrhoidal tissue away from the underlying sphincter. Rubber band ligature of the hemorrhoid has been combined effectively with freezing in situ. Placed just before freezing, the rubber bands occlude the circulation and encourage thrombosis and necrosis.

In the days after freezing, a serous discharge may be copious while the hemorrhoid undergoes necrosis. Gradually the necrotic tissue separates to leave a clean granulating wound in about 5 to 10 days. Mucosa grows over the wound to complete healing, which is somewhat delayed, as is true with all cryosurgical procedures, because the necrotic tissue must be eliminated before wound healing can occur. Healing is generally complete in 3 weeks. During this time there is little discomfort and the inconvenience of the discharge. Sitz baths and, occasionally, the use of Xylocaine ointment ease postoperative discomfort.

Other types of inflammatory or nonneoplastic diseases of the anal canal may be treated also. Anal papillomas or polyps can be cured easily. Condylomata acuminata are more difficult to treat successfully because the disease is often so extensive and often extends into the anal canal. Still, the variety of treatments advocated for condylomata acuminata attest to the limited effectiveness of any one method. When cryosurgery is used, careful follow-up observation is required to treat the lesions missed or inadequately frozen on the first occasion. In freezing, care must be taken to encompass the entire lesion and to include about 2 mm. of normal skin. Postoperative discomfort is relieved with sitz baths and Xylocaine jelly.

VILLOUS ADENOMA

Benign polypoid tumors of the rectum respond extremely well to freezing because their lack of dense fibrous tissue facilitates quick sloughing and avoids delay in healing. Adenomatous polyps probably are not best treated by freezing because the commonly used snare-and-fulguration technique affords a specimen for histologic examination. However, cryocoagulation may be used instead of fulguration to destroy any residual cells which may be in the base. Freezing will perform this task better than electrocoagulation, but it does not control bleeding as well.

Villous tumors of the rectum are nearly ideal for cryocoagulation. Because they grow superficially, freezing is easily done, though the extent of the tumor may be great. The tumor sloughs readily after freezing. In comparison with electrocoagulation, often used for this tumor, freezing affords the advantages of careful control of the treatment process and avoidance of hemorrhage. Either technique has the shortcoming that biopsy shows only the nature of the tissue removed, and malignant degeneration may exist elsewhere in the specimen. This risk must be assumed when any treatment method short of total excision is used. After treatment, the patient is examined periodically, and treatment is repeated as often as needed to eliminate the disease. Extensive lesions commonly require repetition of treatment.

COMPARISON WITH OTHER METHODS OF TREATMENT

The advantages of cryosurgery may be summarized for comparison with other methods of local treatment. Its merit lies in simplicity of use, rather little need for anesthesia, lack of hemorrhage, and few complications in the postoperative period. These advantages are related to the fact that nothing is excised, but rather the tumor is allowed to become necrotic and slough. Healing, especially of bone, has been remarkably favorable, and bone conservation has been possible.

The limitations of the technique are several. Only local treatment is given, so lymphadenopathy must be managed by an alternative treatment method. There is difficulty in evaluating the extent of freezing, especially when treatment is given via endoscopy. Determining depth of freezing is a problem even when vision is good. Another problem is the difficulty in freezing large volumes of tissue, even though liquid nitrogen is used as the cryogenic agent. Improvements in cryosurgical apparatus are needed in order for the technique to achieve greater therapeutic usefulness.

As a method of producing local necrosis of tissue, it must be compared with other physical and chemical methods of producing similar effects and with conservative local excision of tissue. Perhaps the closest comparison must be with electrocoagulation, which commonly is used as a means of excision and may be associated with considerable bleeding, which does not occur with cryosurgery. A more competitive electrosurgical technique is the use of electrocoagulation to slowly cook tissue rather than attempt excision at the same time. Still, cold is more easily controlled than electrocautery, and the depth of treatment is more predictable. The use of heat for the destruction of tissue is more painful than is the use of cold, so increased anesthesia is needed. Explosion hazards must be considered in electrocoagulation but not in cryocoagulation. Healing of bone and soft tissues is better after freezing than after cauterization. With cryosurgery, scar formation is often surprisingly little. Local surgical excision cannot compete successfully with cryosurgery in selected cases. Surgical excision requires more anesthesia, causes bleeding, and cannot deal satisfactorily with lesions overlying bone unless the bone is removed.

BIBLIOGRAPHY

General

Cahan, W.: Cryosurgery of malignant and benign tumors. Fed. Proc., 24:S241, 1965.

Cooper, I. S.: Cryogenic surgery: a new method of destruction or extirpation of benign or malignant tumors. New Eng. J. Med., 268:743, 1963.

———: Cryogenic surgery for cancer. Fed. Proc., 24:S237, 1965.

Gage, A.: Cryosurgery for cancer; an evaluation. Cryobiology, 5:241, 1969.

———: Cryosurgery for diverse human tumors. Panminerva Med., 13:475, 1971.

Haschek, H.: Latest developments in cryosurgery. Proceedings of the International Congress of Cryosurgery, Vienna, June, 1972. Verlag der Weiner Medizinischers Akademie, Vienna, 1972.

Meryman, R. T.: Cryobiology. New York, Academic Press, 1966.

Rand, R., Rinfret, A., and Von Leden, H.: Cryosurgery. Springfield, Ill., Charles C. Thomas, 1968.

Von Leden, H., and Cahan, W.: Cryogenics in Surgery. Flushing, N. Y., Medical Examination Publishing Co., 1971.

Effects of Freezing on Tissue

Carter, D., Lee, P., Gill, W., and Johnston, R.: The effect of cryosurgery on peripheral nerve function. J. Roy. Coll. Surg. Edin., 17:25, 1972.

Cooper, I., Samra, K., and Wisniewska, K.: Effects of freezing on major arteries. Stroke, 2:471, 1971.

Cooper, T., and Trezek, G.: Rate of lesion growth around spherical and cylindrical cryoprobes. Cryobiology, 7:183, 1971.

Gage, A., Fazekas, G., and Riley, E.: Freezing injury to large blood vessels in dogs, with comments on the experimental freezing of bile ducts. Surgery, 61:748, 1967.

Gage, A., Greene, G., Neiders, M., Emmings, F.: Freezing bone without excision; an experimental study of bone-cell destruction and manner of regrowth in dogs. JAMA, 196:770, 1966.

Gaster, R., Davidson, T., Rand, R., and Fonkalsrud, E.: Comparison of nerve regeneration rates following controlled freezing or crushing. Arch. Surg., 103:278, 1971.

Gill, W., DaCosta, J., and Fraser, J.: The control and predictability of a cryolesion. Cryobiology, 6:347, 1970.

Neel, H., Ketcham, A., and Hammond, W.: Requisites for successful cryogenic surgery of cancer. Arch. Surg., 102:45, 1971.

Skin Disease

Gage, A.: Deep cryosurgery. *In* Epstein, E. (ed.): Skin Surgery. pp. 551–577. Springfield, Ill., Charles C. Thomas, 1970.

Grimmet, R.: Liquid nitrogen therapy: histologic observations. Arch. Derm., 83:563, 1961.

Torre, D.: Cryosurgery of premalignant and malignant skin lesions. Cutis, *8*:123, 1971.

Zacarian, S. A.: Cryosurgery of Skin Cancer and Cryosurgical Techniques in Dermatology. Springfield, Ill., Charles C. Thomas, 1969.

Tumors of the Oral Cavity

Chandler, J., Hiott, C.: Cryosurgery in the management of tumors of the head and neck. Southern Med. J., *64*:1440, 1971.

Emmings, F., Gage, A., and Koepf, S.: Combined curettage and cryotherapy for recurrent ameloblastoma of the mandible: report of case. J. Oral Surg., *29*:41, 1971.

Emmings, F., Koepf, S., and Gage, A.: Cryotherapy for benign lesions of the oral cavity. J. Oral Surg., *25*:320, 1967.

Emmings, F., Neiders, M., Greene, G., Koepf, S., and Gage, A.: Freezing the mandible without excision. J. Oral Surg., *24*:145, 1966.

Gage, A.: Cryotherapy for oral cancer. JAMA, *204*:565, 1968.

————: Cryosurgery for oral and pharyngeal carcinoma. Am. J. Surg. *118*:669, 1969.

————: Cryosurgery for oral and pharyngeal carcinoma. Panminerva Med., *13*:488, 1971.

Gage, A., Koepf, S., Wehrle, D., and Emmings, F.: Cryotherapy for cancer of the lip and oral cavity. Cancer, *18*:1646, 1965.

Goode, R. and Spooner, T.: Office cryotherapy for oral leukoplakia. Trans. Am. Acad. Ophthal. Octolaryng., *75*:968, 1971.

Hansen, J.: Cryosurgical therapy of benign lesions of the skin and mucous membranes. Int. Surg., *56*:401, 1971.

Henderson, R.: Cryosurgical treatment of hemangiomas. Arch. Otolaryng., *93*:511, 1971.

Miller, D.: Three years experience with cryo-surgery in head and neck tumors. Ann. Otol. Rhinol. Laryngol., *78*:786, 1969.

Sako, K., Marchella, F., and Hayes, R.: Evaluation of cryosurgery in the treatment of intra-oral leukoplakia. J. Cryosurg., *2*:239, 1969.

Von Leden, H.: Cryosurgery of the head and neck. Texas Med., *68*:108, 1972.

Gynecologic Diseases

Collins, R., Golab, A., Pappas, H., and Paloucek, F.: Cryosurgery of the human uterine cervix. Obstet. Gynec., *30*:660, 1967.

Ostergard, D., and Townsend, D.: Malignant melanoma of the female urethra treated by cryosurgery with radical vulvectomy and anterior exenteration. Obstet. Gynec., *31*:75, 1968.

————: The treatment of vulvar condylomata acuminata by cryosurgery. Cryobiology, *5*:340, 1969.

Ostergard, D., Townsend, D., and Hirose, M.: The treatment of chronic cervicitis by cryotherapy. Am. J. Obstet. Gynec., *102*:426, 1968.

————: A comparison of electrocauterizaton and cryosurgery for the treatment of benign disease of the uterine cervix. Obstet. Gynec., *33*:58, 1969.

Diseases of the Anus and Rectum

Lewis, M., De LaCruz, T., Gazzaniga, D., and Ball, T.: Cryosurgical hemorrhoidectomy: preliminary report. Dis. Colon Rectum, *12*:371, 1969.

Strauss, A., Appel, M., Saphir, O., and Rabinovitz, A.: Immunologic resistance to carcinoma produced by eleetrocoagulation Surg., Gynec. Obstet., *121*:989, 1965.

13

Access Routes for Hemodialysis

Mark W. Wolcott, M.D. *and*

J. Gary Maxwell, M.D.

The need for access routes for intermittent chronic hemodialysis for "end stage" renal disease or for dialysis in the shorter-term acute renal failure case has existed since the first perfection of successful equipment for large-scale hemodialysis by Kolff and Berk[12] in 1944. The first artificial kidney was introduced by Abel, Rountree, and Turner[1] in 1913. Quinton, Dillard, and Scribner[16] in 1960 developed the first successful arteriovenous shunt, thus making this life-saving technique available for the first time to large numbers of patients with irreversible renal failure.

Several changes in material and techniques have improved the duration of, and modified the problems with, the arteriovenous shunt. In 1966, Brescia[6] created a surgical arteriovenous fistula. With this anastamosis, usually between the radial artery and an adjacent vein, venous blood flow in the forearm increases to the point where flow rates of 200 ml. per minute can be delivered with a blood pump to the artificial kidney through a simple venipuncture and returned through another venipuncture. In some situations, in which the single-needle technique of Kopp[13] can be used, only a single venipuncture is necessary.

In both arteriovenous shunts and fistulas, the increase of 10 to 15 percent in cardiac output has been well tolerated.

In the remainder of this chapter the technique and location of arteriovenous shunts and fistulas, and the management of complications and suggested means of minimization of these will be described.

All of these procedures can be carried out on ambulatory patients quite successfully, although some of the patients may be hospitalized because of the severity of their renal disease or other diseases at the time an access route is to be created.

The importance of careful attention to technique and to details of management cannot be overstressed.

ARTERIOVENOUS SHUNTS

Although internal arteriovenous fistulas have been a great advance, they do require a blood pump. Many patients are still trained using arteriovenous shunts. Occasionally *venipuncture* for a home dialysis patient cannot be accomplished for one reason or another. The external arteriovenous shunt therefore is still a major access route for chronic hemodialysis.

For acute dialysis, the arteriovenous shunt remains the primary route, since

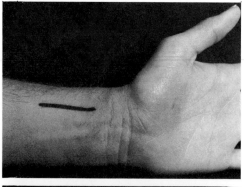

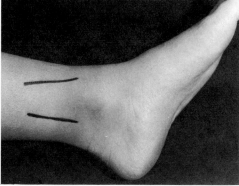

Fig. 13–1. (*Top*) Mark on wrist showing position of skin incision for wrist shunt. (*Bottom*) Marks on leg showing positions of skin incisions for leg shunt.

the surgically constructed arteriovenous fistula usually requires several weeks to mature before being ready for use.

Usually, the shunt is established between the radial artery and an adjacent vein in the forearm. The site is usually at the wrist but may be higher up the forearm, to an inch or so below the flexion crease at the elbow. Above this point, there will be occlusion and thrombosis of the shunt caused by bending the elbow.

The ulnar artery can be used in place of the radial artery, but care must be exercised if the radial has already been used and has become occluded, since insufficient blood supply to the hand is a great danger. In addition, the ulnar artery is usually quite small.

The anterior or posterior tibial artery and the adjacent saphenous vein can be used in the lower leg. Leg shunts are not as successful as arm shunts because of excessive motion, danger of bumping, and, perhaps, poorer flow and greater risk of infection.

TECHNIQUE FOR EXTERNAL ARTERIOVENOUS SHUNT

Figure 13-1 shows the usual site for the establishment of an external shunt in the forearm (*top*) and in the leg (*bottom*). Rarely, the profunda femoris artery and the saphenous vein in the groin may be used.[4] The anesthesia may be either local infiltration or axillary block in the arm, local or low spinal for leg shunts.

In the forearm, an incision 4 to 6 cm. long is made about 3 to 5 cm. proximal to the flexion crease at the wrist and 2 cm. lateral to the radial artery impulse. The subcutaneous tissues are bluntly separated down to the antebrachial fascia, beneath which lies the radial artery. The radial artery is exposed by carefully incising the antebrachial fascia in a longitudinal manner. The artery is carefully dissected from its accompanying venae comitantes and approximately 4 cm. of artery is carefully freed, any small arterial branches being ligated with 5 - 0 nonabsorbable suture material. The freed section of artery is carefully wrapped with a small piece of gauze soaked in 1 percent papaverine hydrochloride while search for a suitable adjacent vein is carried out. The cephalic vein usually is available 2 to 4 cm. lateral to the radial artery in the subcutaneous tissues at the level of the incision. It is dissected out, care being taken not to traumatize it and to ligate small branches. It, too, is bathed with a sponge soaked in 1 percent papaverine.

Once the artery and vein are ready for cannulation, (Fig. 13-2), the positions of the cannulae are assessed, and stab wounds are made distally for the exit of the Silastic tubing. These should be in line with the respective artery and vein.

The Teflon tips for the artery and vein are carefully selected. The largest tip compatible with the vessel into which it is to be inserted is used, but care must be taken that it not be too large or tear of the

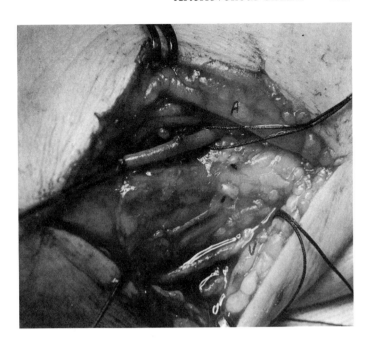

Fig. 13–2. Radial artery (*A*) and cephalic vein (*V*) ready for cannulation.

vessel intima may occur, and this has been shown to be a major cause of later thrombosis at the cannula tip. When the proper tips for the artery and the vein have been selected, each tip and its attached Silastic tubing are filled with a heparinized saline solution (10,000 units to 100 cc. saline), and a small atraumatic bulldog clamp is placed on the end of the tubing.

The vein is cannulated by first ligating it as far distally as it has been freed and then making a longitudinal incision, 3 to 4 mm. long, a little proximal to this ligature. Back-bleeding is prevented by lifting up gently on a 3 - 0 ligature previously passed around the proximally freed vein. The vein is gently flushed with heparinized saline, and the tip of the cannula is gently inserted into the lumen, fine forceps being used to hold the incision open. Occasionally the vein is still in spasm, and it may be gently dilated with a curved fine mosquito hemostat prior to inserting the tip. The Teflon-tipped cannula is advanced for the full length protruding from the Silastic tubing and is tied in place with the 3 - 0 nonabsorbable tie. A second tie is placed around the Silastic cannula and the vein. The cannula and vein are now flushed with 5 to 10 cc. of heparinized saline and the bulldog clamp is reapplied to the cannula.

The artery is now cannulated in a similar manner, except that we like to place three 6 - 0 atraumatic sutures through the proximal edge of the arterial incision, which is made in a transverse manner. We believe this helps to prevent peeling back of the intima, which occasionally may occur on insertion of the Teflon cannula tip. As in the case of the vein, gentle dilatation of the artery using a small mosquito hemostat will often facilitate placement of the cannula tip. Once in place, the cannula is fixed in the same manner as is the venous cannula. The cannula is flushed with heparin and the bulldog clamp reapplied.

We are now ready to bring the two cannulae through the stab wounds previously placed and to connect them. To pull the cannula through, one can pass a thin clamp from the skin side through the stab wound into the incision, grasp the end of the Silastic cannula, and pull it through. Once both cannulae are pulled through their respective stab wounds, the ends are connected by a short Teflon tube and the bulldog clamps are removed, permitting flow of arterial blood into the vein (Fig. 13-3).

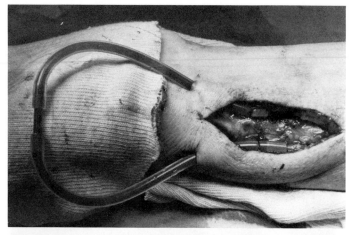

Fig. 13–3. The cannulae in place and connected.

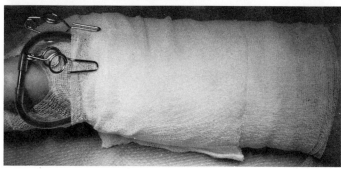

Fig. 13–4. Bandage of shunt in place. Note the two clips attached to gauze for occluding the cannulae arterial and venous catheters should they come apart.

The wound is closed using a few interrupted nonabsorbable 5 - 0 sutures in the subcutaneous tissues and either a subcuticular or interrupted 5 - 0 nonabsorbable suture in the skin.

A water-soluble antiseptic ointment containing neomycin and polymyxin is placed about the exit sites of the two cannulae. A light sterile dressing split to lie about these and over the wound is next placed, and then a soft circular dressing is applied (Fig. 13-4). In a child or a noncooperative adult, a light splint may be applied from hand to elbow for a day or so.

Aftercare is most important and will be discussed later under complications.

Other vessels in the forearm may be used, and various combinations of arteries and veins are possible. Often the basilic vein in the mid-forearm is more available than the cephalic vein. Separate incisions are then necessary—one for the arterial limb and one for the venous.

Placement of a leg shunt follows the same principles as in the arm. Either the anterior or posterior tibial artery may be used in combination with the saphenous vein.

Occasionally use of a Thomas shunt[21] is required if all other access routes have been exhausted. This is a hospital procedure and will not be described here.

ARTERIOVENOUS FISTULAS

A most significant addition to the methods of treatment of the patient needing long-term hemodialysis has been the development of the internal, surgically created, arteriovenous fistula.[10] Usually the radial artery and an adjacent vein are used. More recently, the use of the saphenous vein, divided and connected in situ to the superficial femoral artery,[20, 8] has been described. Also the use of a length of a saphenous vein placed in the forearm between the cephalic vein and the radial or the ulnar artery [15] as a substitute vein for those persons no longer with useable arm veins has been successfully carried out. Still more recently, the use of homologous vein segments as substitutes for nonexistent adequate veins for construction of internal arteriovenous fistulas has been described.[2]

None of these latter procedures are considered to be ambulatory procedures, but they are mentioned for completeness.

We will describe the construction of the usual arteriovenous fistula at the wrist, which is an ambulatory procedure.

TECHNIQUE FOR ARTERIOVENOUS FISTULA AT THE WRIST

The anesthesia is either local infiltration or axillary block. The incision is the same as for placement of a shunt at the wrist. Once the radial artery and the cephalic vein have been located and mobilized, the arteriovenous fistula can be developed in one of several ways.

It is most important to free an adequate 3 to 5 cm. of both artery and vein so that no tension exists at the suture line and so that excessive angulation of the vessels is not produced.

The vein is carefully dissected free of all adventitia to permit its dilatation once arterial flow is established. The artery is likewise carefully freed up, and all small branches are ligated. Wrapping both artery and vein for 5 to 10 minutes with a gauze sponge soaked in 1.0 percent papaverine is most important to manage spasm.

The arteriovenous fistula may be constructed side to side, artery to vein; or end to side, vein to artery; or end to end, artery to vein.

Control of blood flow is by use of Rummel tourniquets of 3 - 0 silk placed proximally and distally on the artery and on the vein. A small piece (1 cm.) of plastic tubing in place of the rubber tubing permits occlusion of the vessels with small hemostats. After these tourniquets are tightened down, incisions are made in both artery and vein 1.0 cm. long and opposite each other, (for side-to-side

anastamosis). Before beginning the anastamosis, 5.0 cc. of heparin solution (5000 units in 50 cc. of saline) is injected both proximally and distally into both artery and vein.

The anastamosis is done with 6 - 0 or 7 - 0 double-armed atraumatic nonabsorbable suture material. Great care is necessary in suture placement to assure catching all layers of both vessels. Be sure to place sutures carefully at both corners. We prefer interrupted sutures, although in large vessels continuous sutures may be permissible. The back wall is usually done first, and then the front wall, although this is a matter of individual preference (Figs. 13-5 and 13-6).

Once the occluding tourniquets have been removed, light application of a dry gauze sponge for 3 to 5 minutes will control the modest ooze at the suture line.

Closure of the wound is the same as for arteriovenous shunts. Great care to prevent compression or kinking must be observed. The dressing should be light, and the use of a splint is advisable for a day or so.

Several other variations of arteriovenous fistulas in the arm have been described and are feasible if the radial artery-cephalic vein fistula fails or is not available. Among these are the transpalmer fistula between the distal radial artery stump and a small vein in the forearm[14] or between the ulnar artery and the basilic vein[11] or proximally between the cephalic vein and the brachial artery.[7]

Marked dilatation of the veins occurs a few weeks after the establishment of an arteriovenous fistula.

MANAGEMENT AND COMPLICATIONS

Meticulous care of the arteriovenous shunt is mandatory. Careful cleaning about the exit sites of the cannulae is done on a daily basis. General cleanliness is necessary, and protection of the shunt area with sterile dressings and soft stretch-gauze wrapping must be done daily. The patient must at all times avoid hitting the shunt.

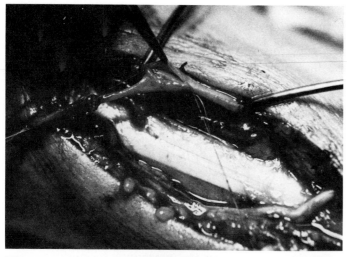

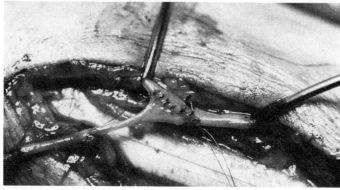

Fig. 13-5. (*Top*) Beginning suture of vein to artery, end to side, using 7 = 0 nonabsorbable suture material placed by interrupted technique. (*Bottom*) Completed arteriovenous fistula.

In the case of the internal arteriovenous fistula, much less care is necessary once healing has taken place. However, prolonged pressure over the fistula site may lead to occlusion, especially if this occurs in the first few weeks.

The problems associated with the external arteriovenous shunt include infection, clotting, and bleeding. Septicemia with or without endocarditis can occur. Thrombosis may be associated with repeated pulmonary embolism.

The problems of revision of shunts may try the very best in a surgeon.

For prompt delineation of early shunt problems the technique of shunt angiography has proved most useful.[5, 18]

Infected shunts should be removed because they may lead to septicemia. Low-grade local infection about the point of emergence of the cannulae in itself does not indicate removal. This can be treated by local cleaning and antibiotics.

Bleeding usually necessitates prompt removal. In the case of clotted shunts, initial declotting can be performed by aspiration of the clot by syringe followed by flushing the venous line with a heparinized saline solution. The passage of a balloon catheter can often be used to remove clots from the artery or the vein. If care is used, this can be done under local anesthesia. (Urokinase, 5000 Plough units per ml., is used in England.[17] Two to three ml. of this solution is instilled into the limb of the shunt. If only one limb is clotted, the other limb is filled with heparinized saline and the shunt tubing is clamped for 2 to 4 hours, following which the clot is aspirated and the cannula is irrigated with saline. Urokinase is not yet available in the United States.)

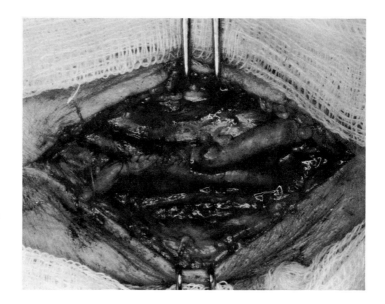

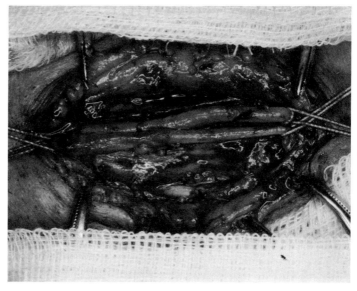

Fig. 13–6. (*Top*) Side-to-side arteriovenous fistula showing position of artery and vein. (*Bottom*) Side-to-side arteriovenous fistula completed. In this case, a continuous suture of 7 = 0 nonabsorbable material was used.

In patients who are shunt clotters, oral use of aspirin,[3, 9] 10 mg. 4 to 6 times a day; and of dipyridamole, 50 mg. 3 to 4 times a day, seems to be of benefit. Antacid therapy should be used concomitantly. Surgical correction of the shunt should be undertaken if efforts to declot are unsuccessful or if angiography shows angulation of the tip of the cannula or stricture of the vessel just distal to the tip.

In recent months, the use of the arteriovenous shunt as an access route for long-term total parenteral nutrition has been described.[19] Its role is to be evaluated.

REFERENCES

1. Abel, J. J., Rountree, L. G., and Turner, B. B.: The removal of diffusable substances from the circulating blood by means of dialysis. Trans. Assoc. Am. Physicians, *28*:51, 1913.
2. Abu-dalu, J., Urea, I., Zonder, H. B., and Rosenfeld, J. B.: Hemodialysis treatment by means of a cadaver arterial allograft. Arch. Surg., *105*:798, 1972.

3. Andrassy, K., Ritz, E., Schoeffner, W., Hahn, G., and Walter, K.: The influence of acetylsalicylic acid on platelet adhesiveness and thrombotic fistula complications in hemodialysis patients. Klin. Wschr., *49*:166, 1971.

4. Belzer, F. O., and Kountz, S.L.: Arteriovenous Quinton-Scribner shunt with the profunda femoris artery and saphenous vein. Surgery, *70*:443, 1971.

5. Berne, T.V., Turner, A.F., and Barbour, B. H.: Angiographic evaluation of Quinton-Scribner shunt malfunction. Surgery, *69*:588, 1971.

6. Brescia, M.J., Cimino, J. E., Appel, K., and Hurwich, B. J.: Chronic hemodialysis using venipuncture and a surgically created arteriovenous fistula. New Eng. J. Med., *275*:1089, 1966.

7. Cascardo, S., Acchiarda, S., Beven, E. G., Popowniak, K. L., and Nakamoto, S.: Proximal arteriovenous fistulae for hemodialysis when radial arteries are unavailable. Proc. Europ. Dial. Transplant Assoc., *7*:42, 1970.

8. Firlit, C. F., and Canning, J.: Saphenofemoral shunt. Arch. Surg., *104*:854, 1972.

9. Harker, L.A., and Slichter, S. J.: Platelet and fibrinogen consumption in man. New Eng. J. Med., *287*:999, 1972.

10. Johnson, B.: Reduction of dialysis complications with arteriovenous fistula. Surg. Advances, *3*:2, 1972.

11. Kinnaert, P., Vereerstraeten, M. G., and Toussaint, C.: Ulnar arteriovenous fistula for maintenance hemodialysis. Brit. J. Surg., *58*:641, 1971.

12. Kolff, W. J., and Berk, H. T. J.: Artificial kidney, dialyzer, with great area. Geneesk. Gids, *21*:214, 1944.

13. Kopp, K. F., Gutch, C. F., and Kolff, W. J.: Single-needle dialysis. Trans. Am. Soc. Artif. Intern. Organs, *18*:75, 1972.

14. Morgan, A. P., and Bailey, G. L.: The transpalmer fistula for hemodialysis. Arch. Surg., *104*:353, 1972.

15. Mozes, M., Hurwich, B. J., Adar, R., Eliahous, H. E., and Bogokowsky, H.: Arteriovenous vein graft for chronic hemodialysis; A preliminary report. Surgery, *67*:452, 1970.

16. Quinton, W., Dillard, D., and Scribner, B. H.: Cannulation of blood vessels for prolonged hemodialysis. Trans. Am. Soc. Artif. Intern. Organs, *6*:104, 1960.

17. Robinson, P. J., Glanville, J. N., Smith, P. H., and Rosen, S. M.: Management of clotting in arteriovenous cannulae in patients on regular dialysis therapy. Brit. J. Urol., *42*:590, 1970.

18. Schreiber, M. H.: Angiographic demonstration of the causes of external arteriovenous hemodialysis shunt failure. Clin. Radio, *22*:210, 1971.

19. Scribner, B. H., Cole, J. T., Christopher, G., Vizzo, J. E., Atkins, R. C., and Blagg, C. R.: Long-term total parenteral nutrition. JAMA, *212*:457, 1970.

20. Sheil, A. G. R., Storey, B. G., May, J., and Rogers, J. H.: Use of the saphenous vein for arteriovenous shunts in the upper thigh. Med. J. Aust., *2*:1241, 1970.

21. Thomas, G. I.: Large-vessel appliqué arteriovenous shunt for hemodialysis: a new concept. Am. J. Surg., *120*:244, 1969.

14
Scalp, Face, and Salivary Glands

C. C. Snyder, M.D.

SCALP

OPERATIVE ANATOMY

The scalp is that soft tissue which blankets the skull and extends from the supraorbital ridges anteriorly to the external occipital protuberance posteriorly and blends bilaterally with the temporalis fascia. The scalp is layered, which is quite important to the patient and profoundly advantageous for the surgeon. The outermost layer of the five strata is the *skin* (Fig. 14-1), which is unequaled in thickness anywhere else in the human body. The skin is so firmly adherent to the next two underlying layers, the superficial fascia and the galea aponeurotica, that surgically the three must be considered as one. This intimate soft tissue intertexture is responsible for the limited gaping of superficial scalp wounds and the restricted spread of infections; whereas the infinitesimal degree of blood vessel retraction from these wound edges, and the prolonged patency of the severed blood vessel ends, are to blame for the profuse hemorrhaging from simple scalp lacerations.

The second layer, or *superficial fascia,* is remarkably inelastic because it is composed of short fibrous septa which hold it firmly to the skin above and the galea below. Any swelling immediately below this dense layer, such as hematoma, exu-

date, or edema, becomes incarcerated and compresses the adjacent sensory nerves, inducing an aggravating pain. If the material becomes offending, it must be released externally.

The *galea aponeurotica,* the third layer of the scalp, is the conjoined aponeurosis for the scalp muscles. This glistening helmet of fibrous protection is loosely attached to the periosteum by an intervening layer of subaponeurosis.

The fourth layer, or *subaponeurotic layer,* consists of loose areolar connective tissue. The surgeon should consider this stratum the "danger layer", because it contains the emissary veins, which empty into the venous sinuses of the cranial hemispheres. Lacerations involving this scalp stratum are surgical emergencies, as they gape widely, remain open, and afford direct portals for bacteria to the meninges and intracranial sinuses. These wounds should be cleansed thoroughly, debrided, and closed loosely.

The fifth and deepest scalp layer is the *periosteum,* which is surprisingly thin to be such a tenacious structure. One can strip it easily from the skull, merely with the finger, except where it attaches to the dura mater at the suture lines. Bone in any part of the body needs coverage, and the skull bone is similar in this respect. Therefore the periosteum, being the last line of defense for the skull, should remain intact. Split-thickness skin grafts

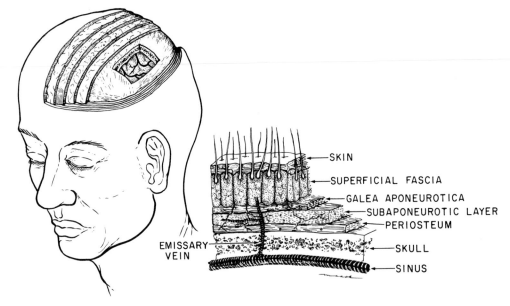

Fig. 14–1. Anatomy of scalp.

take well on periosteum, but live with difficulty on bare bone.

The vascular anastomoses of the scalp are so profuse that fresh wounds heal readily and serious infections are rare when proper surgical care is provided (Fig. 14-2). Hinge and trapdoor scalp flap wounds produced by trauma usually remain viable because of the abundant circulation supplied by the temporal, supraorbital, suptratrochlear, posterior auricular, and occipital blood vessels. Unfortunately, hematomas are common because of this vascular abundance, but usually they are confined to a single skull bone by the adherent periosteum at the suture lines.

Most of the venous tributaries of the

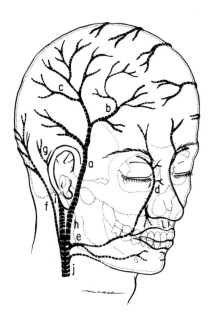

a - SUPERFICIAL TEMPORAL
b - FRONTAL
c - PARIETAL
d - FACIAL
e - MAXILLARY
f - OCCIPITAL
g - POST AURICULAR
h - EXTERNAL CAROTID
i - INTERNAL CAROTID
j - COMMON CAROTID

Fig.   14–2. Arteries of scalp and face.

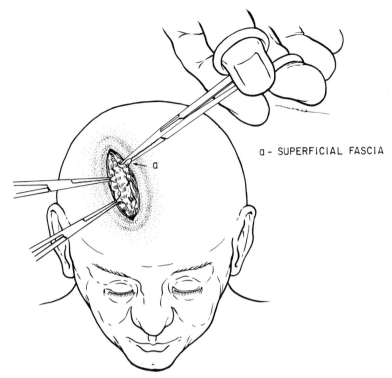

a - SUPERFICIAL FASCIA

Fig. 14–3. Control of hemorrhage from scalp wounds.

scalp terminate in the external jugular veins; but the emissary vessels, empty into the superior sagittal sinus, and the frontal and supraorbital veins, contribute to the cavernous sinus via the ophthalmic veins. The lymph drainage of the scalp is important both in acute and chronic disease and should be inspected with each patient examination. The frontal scalp lymphatics empty into the submaxillary nodes, the posterior scalp vessels into the occipital nodes, and the lateral scalp channels into the posterior auricular nodes. Knowledge of these lymph pathways becomes important when examining head malignancies.

LACERATIONS OF THE SCALP

All cranial trauma regardless of the extent demands neurological evaluation. This may be achieved quickly, but must be noted in writing in the patient's chart.

Local infiltration of 1 percent Xylocaine with epinephrine will suffice for shaving, cleansing, débridement, and wound closure. If scalp hemorrhage is a problem, the superficial fascia is grasped with hemostats and pulled over the bleeding vessels temporarily (Fig. 14-3). The wound edges are debrided of nonviable tissues in such a manner that the margins can be approximated without tension. Then stent sutures of medium-sized stainless-steel wire are positioned and the scalp edges coapted. The stent wire sutures are tied over a bandage as though around a package (Fig. 14-4). When the wound is too large for primary closure, parallel relaxing incisions may be indicated (Fig. 14-5). The open donor sites may be grafted or left to granulate. Surgical alternatives to this closure are a variety of local skin flaps; scalp arteries are always used as a nutritive source. Partial avulsions of the scalp occur daily in industry, on the highways, and on the ski slopes.

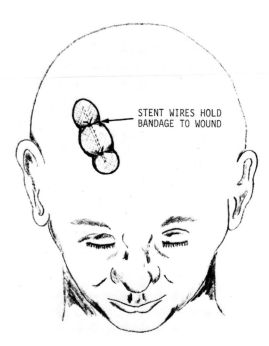

STENT WIRES HOLD
BANDAGE TO WOUND

Fig. 14–4. Stent wire sutures.

INFECTIONS

All traumatic wounds of the scalp must be considered contaminated, because bacteria accompany the traumatizing agent and pieces of dirty skin and clothing into the wound. If the wound margins become devitalized, a favorable medium for the bacteria is furnished, thus permitting a contaminated wound to become an infected wound. As long as the wound is only contaminated, that is, the bacteria remain on the skin surface, prevention of infection is possible by cleansing with soap and water combined with surgical débridement. Once the wound is infected by penetrating bacteria, cleansing and excising may result in the sacrifice of vital structures. Obviously, the period of contamination (preinfection period), which averages 6 to 8 hours post-trauma, is the ideal time to treat a wound. Determinants which alter the period of contamination are: the patient's general condition, the type of wound (clean incision, laceration, contusion, puncture), circumstances at the time of injury, and the efficacy of the first-aid treatment. In the treatment of all

potentially infected wounds, it is essential to remember that the healthy living cell is the best of all antiseptics and better than any antibiotic; therefore, as many living cells must be saved as possible for better wound healing.

CELLULITIS

Diffuse inflammation of the scalp usually begins as a local infection (folliculitis, puncture, or abrasion), and initial attention should be focused on this primary lesion with fomentations, incision, or excision. The secondary reaction, consisting of erythema, edema, and pain, is given the usual hygienic care. If a definite organism is responsible, and this is substantiated, it is treated with specific antibiotic therapy. Circumscribed purulent lesions such as furuncles are shaved of surrounding hair, incised, and drained. Invasive furuncles, such as carbuncles and subaponeurotic abscesses, are treated more vigorously because of the possibility of extension of the infection into intracranial venous sinuses. The causative organism is determined, and the infection is treated locally as well as systemically. Local therapy includes a liberal incision and débridement of necrotic tissue, packing with iodoform gauze, and the use of a rubber tissue drain or continuous wet dressings with an antibiotic solution. A systemic broad-spectrum antibiotic is administered orally or parenterally.

DERMOID CYSTS

These are congenital and may be seen at birth, although 60 percent are diagnosed between the ages of 15 and 40 years. They are found at various suture lines, but are most common at the lateral end of the supraorbital ridge (Fig. 14-6) and the frontonasal plate (50 percent of the cases). They are also seen in the palate and the floor of the mouth (25 percent) and the ventral-dorsal body midline (15 percent). The dermoid cyst appears as a painless, round, encapsulated mass, deep to the skin and attached at its base to the

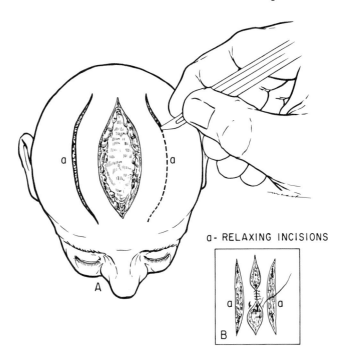

Fig. 14–5. Parallel relaxing incisions.

skull suture line or adjacent tissue. When
it is removed and examined, its wall is
found to be thick and lined with a skin-
like membrane containing hair follicles,
sweat and oil glands, and squamous cells,
but the layers are in reverse order, the
horny layer being toward the center. The
cyst contains a caseous matrix of dead
epithelium, hair, sebum, and, occasionally, vestigial remnants of other germ layers
(bone, cartilage). Dermoid cysts of the
mouth floor may simulate cystic hygroma,
thyroglossal duct or branchial cysts, lipoma, mucoceles, or salivary gland tumors. It makes little difference because all
these lesions are treated identically—
surgically. Sialograms are useful in estab-
lishing a diagnosis. Dermoid cysts should
be removed because they interfere with
function, may cause deformity, undergo
infection, and occasionally become malignant (1 to 3 percent). In infants, when
the stalk is connected intracranially, surgery may be delayed until after puberty,
as sometimes skull growth obliterates the
opening. In older children, or in the event
of intervening infection before puberty,
the cyst may be incised, drained, and later
removed. When elective surgery is done,

the skull opening, if present, may be
closed by a splinter bone plug, rotating a
small periosteal flap, or cauterizing the
foramen.

For the removal of dermoid cysts, general anesthesia or local infiltration anesthesia may be used. An incision is made
over the cyst: for supraorbital cysts, incisions are made in the eyebrow; cysts in
the floor of the mouth (Fig. 14-7) are
enucleated through incisions in the gin-
givobuccal sulcus; and for other cysts,
incisions are made in the flexion creases

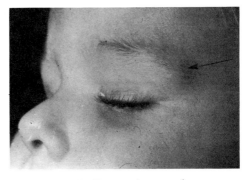

Fig. 14–6. Dermoid cyst of supraorbital ridge.

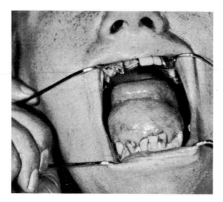

Fig. 14–7. Dermoid cyst in the sublingual area. (Shore, B. R.: Ann. Surg., *108*:305 1938)

of the skin. When the cyst is behind the ear, excision of the cyst is best performed through an incision parallel to the cephalic border of the ear. A cleavage line is established and the cyst is excised by blunt dissection. Sometimes it is necessary to incise the cyst wall and empty the contents so the cavity lining will reveal the extent of the lesion. With a finger or an instrument in the cavity, the lesion is easily removed by dissecting close to the external wall of the cyst. To inhibit recurrence the entire cyst should be extirpated. The wound is closed using stent sutures.

SEBACEOUS CYSTS

Because oil glands are numerous in the scalp and face, sebaceous cysts are common in this area.

Surgical intervention is achieved under local anesthetic infiltration between the cystic mass and adjacent tissues. After the area of the cyst has been shaved and prepared, an elliptical incision of the skin surrounding the duct orifice is made, and this island of tissue is elevated with a skin hook. The cyst is freed along a cleavage line by combined sharp and blunt dissection. After the lesion has been removed, the wound is closed by stent and skin sutures, the former tied over a cotton bolus to obliterate dead space, eliminate hematomas, reduce edema, and fix the bandage without tape, gauze, or collo-

dion. If the sebaceous cyst is on the face, the treatment of choice is to excise the ductal orifice through an elliptical incision, empty the contents by digital expression, grasp the cyst wall with a mosquito hemostat, and deliver it through the skin incision. The wound is closed with one stent and one or two skin sutures. Multiple adjacent sebaceous cysts behind the ears should be excised as a group and the skin closed. Less than 1 percent of sebaceous cysts become malignant.

THE FACE

OPERATIVE ANATOMY

Like the scalp, the cheeks are composed of five layers. The outermost is the skin, and the next is a superficial fascia layer; a modest muscular layer follows, and the inner layers are the submucosa and mucosa. The remaining portions of the face lack the last two layers. The facial skin contains sweat and oil glands and hair follicles. The epidermis follows the ducts of the glands and the shafts of the hair deep into the dermal area. This is a most important anatomical feature, because when the skin is burned or the top layer is abraded, these downgrowths of epithelium furnish islands of new epidermal replacement. Hair shafts grow at an angle, and when transplanting hair follicles for eyebrows, it is necessary to design the surgical incisions respecting this angle. The skin is composed of reticular fibrous bundles containing elastic tissue fibers, which keep the skin in a state of tension and also facilitate the construction and transfer of surgically formed skin flaps. It is this same elastic tissue which upon degeneration releases the skin tension. This skin hypotonicity, associated with aging and shrinking of the underlying musculature, produces excessive skin folds which are commonly known as wrinkles (Fig. 14-8). The successful surgical closure of a large defect is dependent upon separating or undermining the superficial skin from the underlying short facial muscles, and upon stretching the remaining elastic fibers.

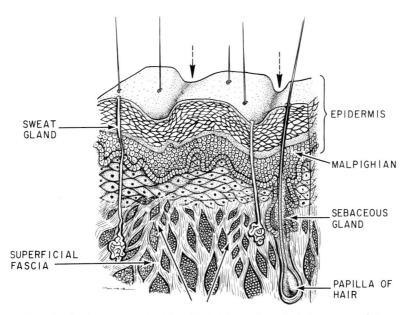

Fig. 14–8. Anatomy of skin. Shrinking of underlying musculature produces skin folds (wrinkles).

In 1861, Langer punctured the skin of a freshly deceased human body with an auger and watched the round holes become eliptical, the long axis of the puncture wound being parallel to the lines of skin tension. Wounds that are parallel to the lines of tension (flexion creases) tend to become narrower and to heal readily; whereas wounds at right angles to the lines of tension tend to gape open and to heal slowly, with the formation of heavy scars. Elective incisions should be positioned parallel to these lines of tension for fast healing and less scarring (Fig. 14-9). When a scar has contracted across a flexion crease, it may be released and corrected by Z-plasty (Fig. 14-10).

The blood vessels of the face form a network which is abundant everywhere but in the avascular epidermis. The vascular mesh is particularly dense in the lips, auricle, and nasal mucosa membrane. The larger blood vessels are the basis for designing skin flaps (Fig. 14-11). Branches of the external carotid artery, such as the occipital, external maxillary, and superficial temporal arteries, will maintain a satisfactory vascularization to a variety of skin flaps. As the matching of skin color on the face is the difference between a good and a superb result, skin flaps from the face to the face are preferred.

SOFT TISSUE INJURIES

Soft tissue wounds are corrected as early as possible. Washing the wounded area with a mild soap and irrigating with sterile saline or water is less damaging to the exposed wound depth than the use of tinctures or strong antiseptics. A local nerve block, or infiltration with an anesthetic, permits the clamping of bleeding vessels, débridement, and repair. While this is being done, the nurse or attendant should administer antitetanus therapy as described elsewhere (see Chapter 5).

Primary Repair of Lacerations. After the wound is free of contaminants and devitalized tissue, stent sutures of 5-0 stainless-steel wire are positioned to obliterate dead space, render hemostasis, reduce edema, decrease tension on the wound edges and hold the bandage to the wound (Fig. -4). Subcutaneous sutures of

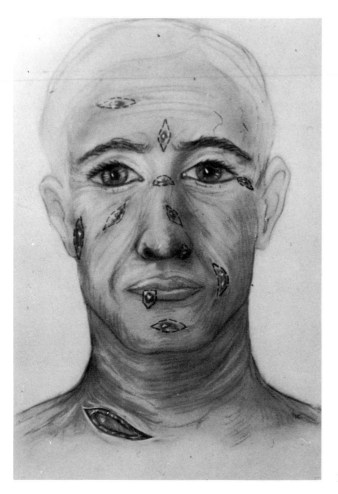

Fig. 14–9. Excision of lesions parallel to flexion creases.

5-0 clear nylon, either as a continuous pullout or interrupted subcuticulars, are used to coapt the dermis. An occasional skin suture of the same size nylon, or paper adhesive strips, will complete the epidermal closure. The steel stent sutures are then tied over a bandage. This eliminates taping and head bandages.

Primary Repair of Avulsions. Early skin replacement, by means of free grafts or attached flaps, is possible because of the abundant network of facial blood vessels. That sound surgical judgment is necessary before initiating repair is axiomatic; and this is dependent upon experience. All completely detached skin parts are inspected, and if they are not macerated severely, they are transformed into full-thickness grafts by resecting the adipose tissue and replanting the skin over the cleaned wound. Tie-over sutures of nylon immobilize the bandage over the skin graft (Fig. 14-12). If the avulsed soft tissue remains attached to the host by a pedicle, it deserves defatting, revising, and replacement into the recipient bed (Fig. 14-13). Half-buried mattress sutures of 5-0 nylon reattach the dermal flap.

Eyebrow trauma is common in facial injuries. Lacerations through the eyebrow need close approximation and on occasion may benefit from Z-plasty (Fig. 14-14). There are instances when a whole eyebrow or parts of an eyebrow must be reconstructed, and the procedures used differ with the individual patient. The hair-bearing free graft is taken from the scalp in an area where the hair follicles

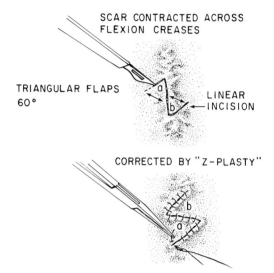

SCAR CONTRACTED ACROSS
FLEXION CREASES

TRIANGULAR FLAPS
60°

LINEAR
INCISION

CORRECTED BY "Z-PLASTY"

Fig. 14–10. Z-plasty. The angles at the apices (*a* and *b*) of the triangular flaps should be about 60°. If they are less than 60°, the vascularity of the flap is endangered; and if they are more than 60°, the rotational mobility becomes less. All the incisions should be through the depth of the scar and should include a portion of subcutaneous fat.

are plentiful and the hair shafts are parallel. The free graft must be thick enough to include the follicles and wide enough to incorporate three rows of hair shafts. The eyebrow graft is sutured into its bed with fine nylon, and a light compressive bandage is applied. There is usually a shedding of the shafts during the next two months, but regrowth takes place. Sometimes a second free graft must be added to achieve the desired result. The superficial temporal artery flap insures a complete brow restoration as well as surgical satisfaction. It is an island flap attached to the branches of the superficial temporal vessels. It is tunneled subcutaneously through the scalp to its recipient supraorbital area (Fig. 14-15).

Facial Nerve Injury. Whenever facial lacerations are deep, the wound should be inspected for injuries to nerves and to Stensen's duct. Any severed portion of the facial nerve may be satisfactorily repaired if the two cut ends can be brought together. The monosuture technique (Fig. 14-16) is adaptable to small peripheral branches. A 5-0 black nylon suture is introduced through a small button of fascia from the wound (or a piece of silicone), and then is passed intraneurally through both cut nerve ends. The nerve is reefed for close approximation, and the suture is tied over another button of fascia. Larger severed nerves are repaired by the epineural cuff method (Fig. 14-17). The two cut nerve ends are placed end to

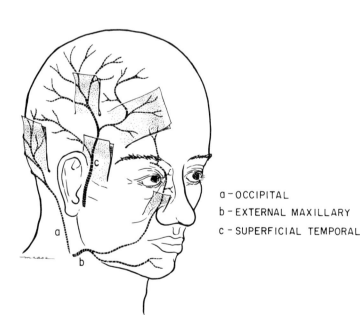

a – OCCIPITAL
b – EXTERNAL MAXILLARY
c – SUPERFICIAL TEMPORAL

Fig. 14–11. Satisfactory vascularization to a variety of skin flaps.

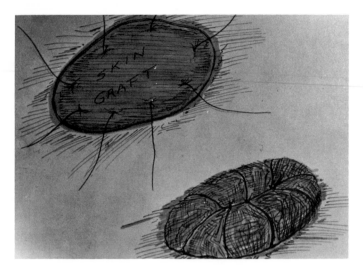

Fig. 14–12. Stent tie-over bandage.

end, and one end is pared, saving the epineurium, the most tenacious part of a peripheral nerve. The epineurium is pulled over the other cut nerve end and sutured. This enhances a closely approximated covered repair. A silicone wrapping for further protection may be added if desired.

Stensen's (Parotid) Duct Injury. This structure is located in the vicinity of the intersection of a straight line drawn from the middle of the upper lip to the auricular tragus with an oblique line parallel to the anterior border of the masseter muscle (Fig. 14-18). The buccal branch of the facial nerve crosses Stensen's duct as it emits from the parotid parenchyma. The syndrome of facial injury, scar, swollen face, and numbness is pathognomonic of a leaking Stensen's duct or a parotid

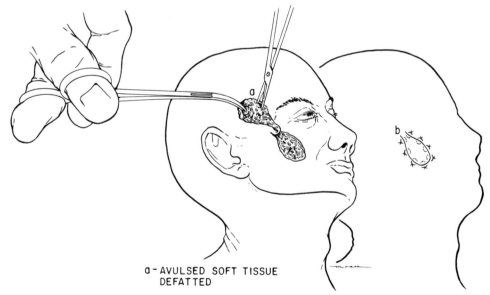

a - AVULSED SOFT TISSUE DEFATTED

b - HALF-BURIED MATTRESS SUTURES (5.0 NYLON) REATTACH THE DERMAL FLAP

Fig. 14–13. Primary repair of avulsions.

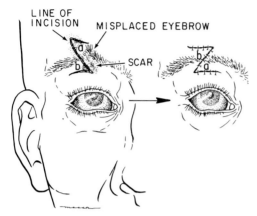

Fig. 14–14. Repair of lacerations through eyebrow (Z-plasty).

gland laceration. The various treatments for early duct injury are: (a) direct anastomosis, (b) ligation of the proximal end, or (c) create a mucosal fistula with the proximal end. Repair is facilitated by threading a polyethylene catheter through the duct ends (Fig. 14-19). The catheter should remain in the duct for one week and then be retrieved.

TEMPOROMANDIBULAR JOINT DISLOCATION

The temporomandibular joint is one means by which the mandible is attached to the skull. The only one other joint in the primate similar to it is the sternoclavicular joint. Acute luxation of the condyle is usually anterior; if it luxates medially or laterally there usually is an associated fracture. Failure to reduce the dislocated condyle results in a chronic problem, due to deformity and poor function. To treat an acute dislocation, the physician stands either in front or back of the patient, who is sitting. The thumbs are positioned bilaterally on the molar area, and the remaining fingers grasp the mandible extra-orally. Thumb pressure is exerted downward and finger pressure upward. This allows the condyle to glide over the tubercle and into the glenoid fossa of the temporal bone. If the infiltration of a local anesthetic into the joint capsule does not afford muscle relaxation, then the reduction should be done under general anesthesia. The patient always feels better if a head-jaw bandage is used to hold the mandible closed and a small

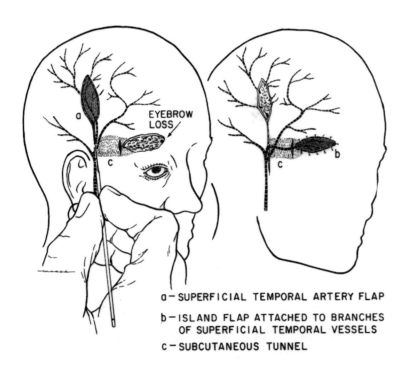

a – SUPERFICIAL TEMPORAL ARTERY FLAP

b – ISLAND FLAP ATTACHED TO BRANCHES OF SUPERFICIAL TEMPORAL VESSELS

c – SUBCUTANEOUS TUNNEL

Fig. 14–15. Island flap for repair of laceration of eyebrow.

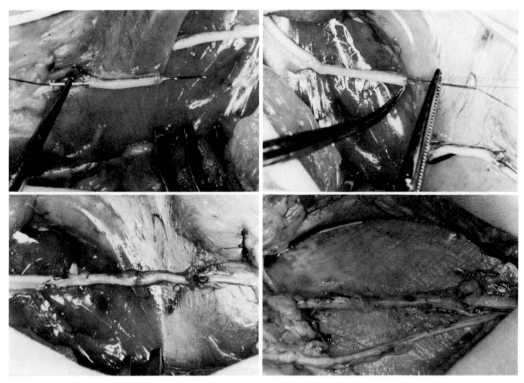

Fig. 14–16. Monosuture neurorrhaphy. *(Top left)* Single intraneural suture through the proximal nerve end. *(Top right)* Continuation of single suture through the distal nerve end. *(Bottom left)* Nerve ending reefed for close approximation, and single suture tied over a small piece of fascia. *(Bottom right)* Appearance 8 weeks postoperatively.

ice pack is placed over the temporomandibular joint area.

NOSE

OPERATIVE ANATOMY

The surgical approach to nasal trauma, infections, and tumors is through a thorough knowledge of anatomy. The nose is the most prominent and conspicuous part of the face and is a common recipient of violence. The *skin* covering the root or base of the nose is thin and loose, and offers itself for easy repair. However, the skin over the remaining nose is thick, taut, and adherent and contains many sebaceous glands, all factors challenging the physician. When sections of nasal tissue are lost from the distal half, due to avulsion or surgical removal, re-

pair by primary closure is difficult. Infected lesions of the nasal skin do not swell much but are exquisitely tender and painful from pressure upon the nerves. The nasal *mucosal lining* is extremely vascular and intimately attached to the cartilage and bone; therefore most nasal fractures are compound.

The *circulation* to the nose is through the internal and external maxillary and the ophthalmic arteries, which end as plexuses in the skin and mucosa. The blood vessels of the skin communicate freely with those of the mucosa. These anastomoses are responsible for the spread of infectious processes from the nasal fossa to the skin, and are also the reason that external nasal surgery must be delayed until internal inflammations subside. Yet, this abundant vessel network affords the advantages of prompt healing,

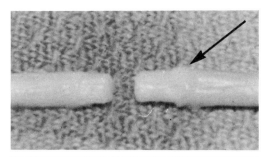

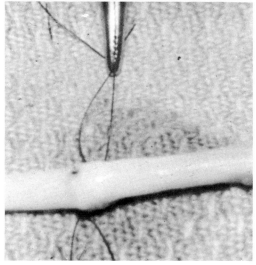

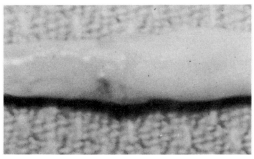

Fig. 14–17. Epineural cuff neurography. (*Top*) Epineural cuff on right; single suture in place. (*Center*) Epineural cuff turned back over apposed nerve ends. Interrupted fine suturesin epineurium only. (*Bottom*) Completed anastomosis with silicone sheeting wrapped around suture line.

less danger of tissue slough, and less conspicuous scarring.

The innervation to the nose is mainly sensory, as the only motor supply needed is a branch of the facial nerve to the alar muscles. The supratrochlear nerve sup-

plies sensation to the nasal root; the external nasal branch of the ophthalmic, to the nasal tip; and the infraorbital branch of the superior maxillary, to the sides of the nose. The mucosa is furnished sensation through the nasopalatine, olfactory, and anterior ethmoidal nerves. Complete anesthesia of the entire nose is easily achieved by injecting less than 8 ml. of Xylocaine into the circles as diagrammed (Fig. 14-20). The sphenopalatine ganglia may be blocked with a Xylocaine or cocaine intranasal pack.

The osseous scaffolding of the nose comprises two nasal bones: the perpendicular plate of the ethmoid and the vomer. The remaining architecture is cartilaginous and includes the superior and inferior lateral cartilages, occasional alar or sesamoid cartilages, and the septal cartilage.

FRACTURES

This mosaic pyramid of bone and cartilage is more subject to trauma than are neighboring solid facial structures. Through direct or glancing blows, the bones lend themselves to unilateral, bilateral, linear, comminuted, depressed, or superimposed fractures—which are nearly always compound (Fig. 14-21). Unfortunately, fractures of the nose usually receive trivial care by attendants who are not acquainted with the anatomy, or who are too busy to devote the necessary attention, and severe complications usually ensue. Diagnosis may be difficult, but there is always a history of trauma and, usually, epistaxis, orbital ecchymosis, pain, crepitation, deformity, and swelling; and x-ray films reveal the break. The two most frequently observed fractures are the bony tip fracture and the lateral in-out fracture. In the case of the former, the fractured tip is either depressed or elevated. The lateral in-out type exhibits a concavity on the side of impact and a convexity on the contralateral side. Roentgenograms sometimes are unsatisfactory; a lateral view is more demonstrative than is an anteroposterior film. When a definite diagnosis is in queestion, treat

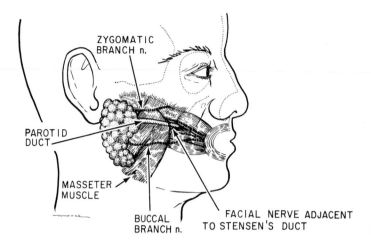

ZYGOMATIC
BRANCH n.

PAROTID
DUCT

MASSETER
MUSCLE

BUCCAL
BRANCH n.

FACIAL NERVE ADJACENT
TO STENSEN'S DUCT

Fig. 14–18. Location of Stensen's duct.

the injury as a fracture regardless, because of the serious sequelae which may result. Due to the excellent vascular supply, fractured nasal bones ossify incredibly rapidly; within two weeks a strong callus has united the broken edges, and in another week they are solid. Therefore displaced nasal fractures should be corrected as soon as possible.

First-aid attention is focused on control of the hemorrhage, which usually is arrested by ice, digital pressure, or intranasal tampon. One percent Xylocaine with epinephrine is used for anesthesia and also assists in hemostasis. Fracture reduction is better accomplished when the patient is free of pain and the area is tidy.

Nonimpacted fractures may be successfully treated with closed reduction by simple digital force. If this cannot be achieved, then an Asche, Walsham, or Kelly forceps serves well. The forceps blades are padded with gauze or rubber tubing, and, with one blade on the inside and the other on the outside, the fracture

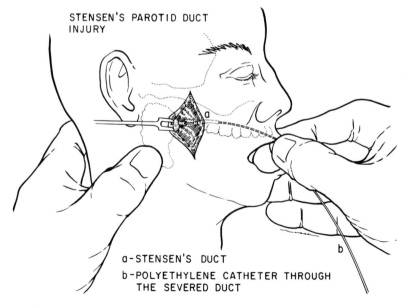

STENSEN'S PAROTID DUCT
INJURY

a–STENSEN'S DUCT
b–POLYETHYLENE CATHETER THROUGH
THE SEVERED DUCT

Fig. 14–19. Repair of Stensen's duct using polyethelene catheter.

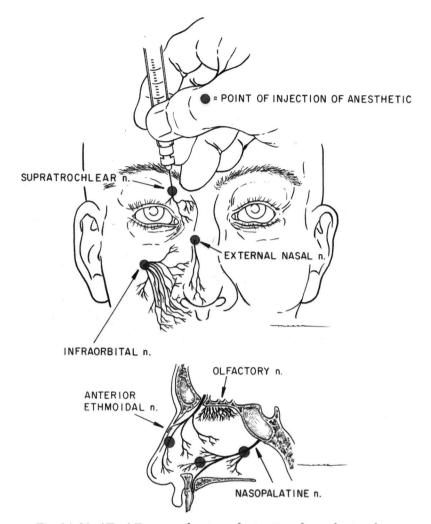

= POINT OF INJECTION OF ANESTHETIC

SUPRATROCHLEAR n.

EXTERNAL NASAL n.

INFRAORBITAL n.

OLFACTORY n.

ANTERIOR
ETHMOIDAL n.

NASOPALATINE n.

Fig. 14–20. (*Top*) Extranasal points of injection of anesthetic solution.
(*Bottom*) Intranasal points of injection.

is elevated and repositioned. Nasal tip fractures are corrected with a blunt instrument and force (Fig. 14-22). Unlike long bones, nasal bones are not influenced by muscle action (flexion and extension), and therefore it is not for this reason that immobilization is used. Immobilization for at least 4 days is necessary to prevent hemorrhage, hematoma, and edema, and to protect the patient from accidently reinjuring the nose. An intranasal packing of Vaseline gauze enclosed in a Surgicel wrapping is inserted, and counterpressure is applied externally by means of a splint of dental compound or metal, and adhesive strips (Fig. 14-23). Ice packs made with a wash cloth, ice chips, and rubber bands are used postoperatively on the eyes and nose (Fig. 14-24). The splint and packings may be removed in 2 to 7 days, depending upon the patient's original trauma and his convalescent progress.

FOREIGN BODIES

Children are the common recipients of these in the form of peas, beans, beads, small coins, buttons, and various types of insects. If the object is not too large, a

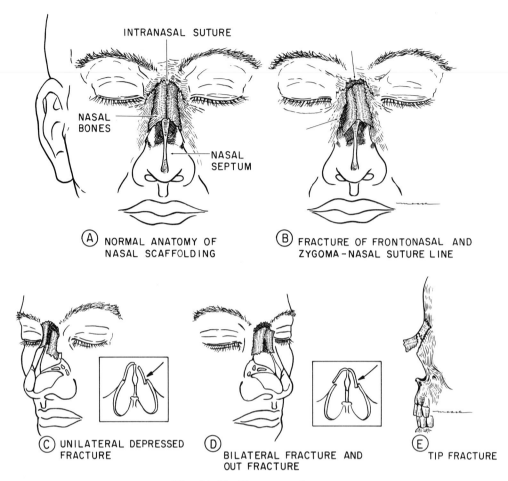

Fig. 14–21. Fractures of nose.

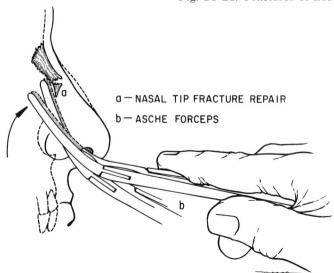

Fig. 14–22. Repair of nasal tip fractures.

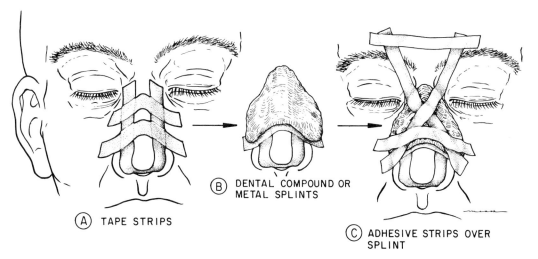

(A) TAPE STRIPS

(B) DENTAL COMPOUND OR METAL SPLINTS

(C) ADHESIVE STRIPS OVER SPLINT

Fig. 14–23. Immobilization of fractures of nose.

cotton applicator or hemostat may be used to push it into the posterior pharynx, from which it is easily retrieved. Objects that are fixed in the mucosa and will not budge may be retrieved by a skin or dural hook, or by splitting the object into small portions. It is not inconceivable, when other methods fail, to fenestrate the septum or surgically separate the ala for more room. Neosynephrine or ephedrine nasal drops will shrink the mucosa, which helps open the passageway. Although syringe irrigation is contraindicated in the treatment of foreign bodies in the nasal vestibule, this is a choice method of removing objects from the ear canal.

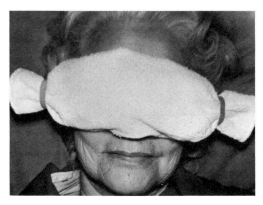

Fig. 14–24. Ice pack in place.

THE EAR

FOREIGN BODIES

Mismanagement of foreign objects in the ear may lead to deafness, and because these emergencies occur frequently, good judgment is important. These foreign bodies may be alive and very active, or inanimate. The former group includes ants, flies, gnats, bees, and larvae; the latter includes peas, beans, hairs, pieces of matches, toothpicks, pencils, and chips of stone or metal.

The object of therapy is to remove the offending agent, and there are various approaches to be entertained. It may be advisable to use a general anesthetic in small children. If the offender is an active insect, it should be killed promptly by instilling into the ear a nonirritating oil, such as olive oil, followed by syringing with boric acid, salt, or any mildly antiseptic solution. If this method is unsuccessful, a small forceps, a metallic hook, or a wire loop should be used to retrieve it. Sometimes a cotton applicator with glue on the end will adhere to the foreign body and retrieve it. If all other approaches have been unsuccessful, it may be necessary to partly detach the external auricle and cartilaginous canal through a

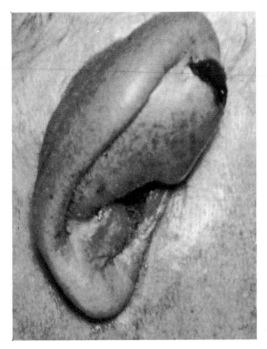

Fig. 14–25. Hematoma of ear.

posterior approach, allowing the object to be removed from the edematous passage.

LACERATIONS

Injuries that expose the ear cartilage should be treated as soon as possible to prevent chondritis and suppuration. The exposed cartilage should be trimmed sufficiently to afford satisfactory skin approximation. The wound edges are coapted with 5-0 nylon sutures, loosely enough to permit serum drainage. The dressing should not be tight, but occlusive and absorptive. Such dressings should be inspected in 24 hours, and if free of infection, allowed to remain in place another 4 days, unless local pain or other evidence of infection makes redressing imperative.

HEMATOMAS

Hematomas of the ear occur daily in athletes such as boxers and wrestlers, although they are also observed as a result of contusions from any cause (Fig. 14-25).

The fluctuant swelling that appears beneath the skin on the anterior surface of the ear, if untreated and not infected, undergoes organization and secondary fibrosis. The ear becomes noticeably thickened and misshapen, resembling a cauliflower; therefore, the terminal deformity in cases of repeated hematoma is spoken of as a "cauliflower ear."

The treatment of auricular hematoma is early drainage of the blood and serum found between the skin and the cartilage; this is best performed within 24 to 48 hours after the injury. Although it is enticing to aspirate the liquid collection by introducing a large needle through a wheal of local anesthesia, it is better judgement to make a small incision at the most dependent part of the hematoma and provide a drain to inhibit recurrence. A moderate pressure dressing must be applied immediately, using a sponge, gauze padding, or a stent suture tied over a bolus of cotton. The dressing is held in place by a circular bandage involving the head and the ear. This dressing may be left in place for 5 to 6 days, when it may be removed without danger of recurrence of the hematoma.

Occasionally, a patient with an old hematoma of the ear may wish to have the deformity removed. In such cases, the fibrous tissue producing the deformity may be excised under local anesthesia. The skin is separated from the underlying scar tissue along one of the natural creases of the ear, and the excessive fibrous tissue is excised down to normal cartilage. The skin then is replaced in its normal position and the wound is sutured with fine nylon. A mold of wet cotton is fitted to the ear to form the future normal contour, and a pressure bandage is applied.

CONGENITAL PREAURICULAR SINUS

This anomaly is seen in the helix, in front of the helix, and as far medially as the cheek. It results from a faulty closure of the first branchial cleft and consists of a sinus tract, composed of squamous epithelium, hair follicles, and other elements of normal skin, that leads to a blind pouch lined with columnar epithelium. The sinus opening may become occluded and then abscess formation results; this requires incision and drainage. The non-infected preauricular sinus requires careful dissection and excision of the entire sinus tract. The optimum time to operate is before infection appears, and the operation is usually performed under local anesthesia.

EARLOBE PUNCTURE

Puncture of the earlobes for the wearing of earrings is commonly requested. It is performed under local anesthesia after symmetrical points in the centers of the earlobes have been marked. A 20-guage hypodermic needle is used to make the tunnel. The purpose is to form an epithelial-lined tract through the lobe. A wire of gold, silver, or steel is placed through the puncture wound and is moved back and forth the next few days. The earlobe is cleaned daily with alcohol. All patients, but especially Negroes, must be warned of the possibility of keloid development.

MOUTH AND TONGUE

MUCOCELES

A mucocele is a retention cyst of the mucous glands within the mouth. It is commonly found on the inner surface of the cheek, in the line of occlusion of the teeth. It may even occur on the dorsum of the tongue. Distention of the ducts of the glands of Blandin beneath the tip of the tongue may cause a swelling of considerable size. This cyst occurs most frequently on the lower lip and appears as a soft, regular, bluish swelling, which frequently varies in size, periodically discharging its contents into the mouth (Fig. 14-26). It produces symptoms due to its presence on the lip, causing a thickness and protrusion, and not infrequently it is bitten inadvertently by the patient. It causes no pain and almost never becomes infected.

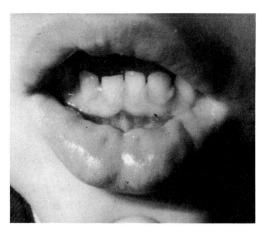

Fig. 14–26. Mucocele of lower lip.

The only indications for treatment are the inconvenience and the disfigurement which it produces.

Treatment. The mucocele may be treated by excision. This operation may be performed under local anesthesia.

After infiltration with 0.5 percent procaine-epinephrine solution around and underneath the cyst, an assistant should evert the lip and hold it firmly on each side between his thumbs and index fingers. A vertical incision is then made over the surface of the cyst and, if this is carefully performed, the mucous membrane may be divided without cutting the cyst wall. Allis forceps may then be placed on the mucous membrane on each side of the incision, and, with the tension produced, the cyst wall can be separated from the surrounding tissues by gentle dissection. The deeper portions of the cyst are somewhat more adherent to surrounding structures, but by careful dissection the cyst may be removed intact. If rupture occurs, it usually takes place in the deepest part of the cyst, a considerable amount of thick, tenacious mucus being evacuated. When this has been wiped away, the remaining portion of the cyst may be removed by sharp dissection.

The wound should be closed with several interrupted sutures of fine silk, so placed as to catch the whole circumference of the wound. The sutures may be removed in 5 to 7 days.

TONGUE LACERATIONS

Lacerations of the tongue may occur due to bites incidental to falls, convulsions, and so forth; or, in the case of children, to falls sustained when they have an object in the mouth. As a rule, small simple lacerations which do not pass through the tongue or do not involve the edge of the tongue may be treated conservatively. Suture is rarely necessary except to control bleeding. Lacerations which involve the edge of the tongue, so that a flap of tongue substance is formed, are best treated by suture. The sutures may be inserted after infiltration with procaine-epinephrine solution. They are placed with small curved cutting-edged needles and should include one half of the thickness of the tongue. This means, therefore, that corresponding sutures should be inserted on the upper and the lower surfaces of the tongue and on the edge of the tongue. They should be of fine silk. In spite of the abundant bacterial flora of the mouth, wounds of the tongue usually heal primarily when sutured. Mouthwashes are useful during the first few days after the insertion of the sutures, which may be removed when they become loose, often as early as the third or fourth day.

TONGUETIE

A congenital shortening of the frenum of the tongue is a rather uncommon but easily treated abnormality. This deformity is usually noted in infancy or childhood. The parents become aware of it because of the inability of the child to stick out his tongue or because of an impediment in his speech.

On examination, the short lingual frenum is at once apparent. Often the tongue cannot be protruded beyond the teeth and during efforts to extend it, the tip is pulled down and the body bulges upward in the mouth.

Treatment. The treatment of tonguetie is incision of the shortened frenum. This operation may be performed in infants without anesthesia, but in older children local infiltration anesthesia is advisable. The infiltration should be made toward the floor of the mouth. Using the broad end of an ordinary grooved director as a retractor, the frenum may be slipped into its central slot and so isolated as to make it easily visible. It is then divided with scissors, care being taken not to carry the incision too far backward because of the danger of injuring the frenal artery. The small amount of bleeding which occurs usually stops without active treatment.

EXOTOSES

Exotoses, or dense bony excrescences, are found in both jaws.

Torus Palatinus. This is an exostosis of the hard palate in the midline, and it presents as a hard oval swelling which varies in size and may be smooth or nodular. It is often mistaken for an osteoma. It is present normally in a certain percentage of people, most of whom never know that it is there. It is painless, does not grow, and should be removed only when it interferes with the fitting of a denture or when the overlying mucous membrane becomes irritated.

Torus Mandibularis. This is an exostosis found on the lingual surface of the mandible, usually bilaterally, in the region of the canines and the premolars. The indications for its removal are similar to those in the case of torus palatinus.

Exostoses may be found frequently in the region of the tuberosities of the maxilla and occasionally in other areas. If removal is indicated, the bone may be trimmed away with bur and chisel under a mucoperiosteal flap.

LEUKOPLAKIA

Leukoplakia, white patches in the mucous membrane resembling white enamel paint (Bloodgood), is a very common precancerous lesion of the mouth (Fig. 14-27). It represents a piling up of the outer layers of the epithelium and is almost invariably caused by the excessive use of tobacco. It may be smooth in the early stages, but in more severe cases it be-

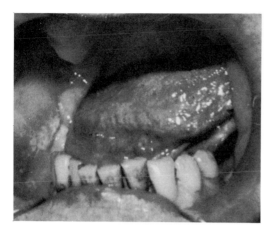

Fig. 14–27. Leukoplakia of mouth.

comes very thick and rough, with fissures and induration at the base.

Treatment. The application of any irritants to these lesions is contraindicated. Smoking should be prohibited and the lesions watched at regular intervals. If they become hard and fissured, they should be excised with an electrosurgical knife or with actual cautery, and the tissue should be examined under the microscope. Otherwise, they should be left alone. They may disappear following the removal of the cause, or they may remain dormant and harmless.

It should be recognized that leukoplakia is definitely a premalignant lesion, and when there is not a definite tendency to regression or when the patient cannot be observed frequently, excision is the safer treatment. Leukoplakia and carcinoma in situ of the lip are removed by a lip shave and, possibly, wedge resection, which is actuated by excising the mucosal surface and replacing it by advancing the labial mucous membrane to the skin margin (Fig. 14-28).

CARCINOMAS

Tongue and Mouth

Most carcinomas of the mouth arise from the pavement epithelium of the buccal cavity. They are called epitheliomas or epidermoid carcinomas. They appear much more frequently in men than in women, and this is believed to be due largely to the frequency of smoking in males.

Etiology. It is estimated that from 50 to 75 percent of carcinomas of the tongue could be prevented by vigorous elimination of precancerous conditions. Leukoplakia is believed to account for 35 percent of all buccal cancer. Destruction of these areas is probably the most important single prophylactic measure against lingual malignancy. Papillomas, ulcers, and fissures are other premalignant lesions of the tongue. These are usually overlooked or disregarded by the patient or by the examiner who sees them at this stage. Nevertheless, vigorous early treatment may prevent subsequent development of cancer. Many of these lesions may be excised, either with a knife or with an electric needle, during the precancerous stages, and in most instances the operation may be performed under local anesthesia in the ambulatory patient.

Diagnosis. At times there is doubt as to the nature of a lesion which appears on the tongue or in the mouth. The diagnosis often can be made on simple inspection and palpation if it is borne in mind that most malignancies of the buccal mucosa are characterized by an indurated ulcer. Sometimes the growth may be more papillary in character, and occasionally it appears as a hard nodular growth which involves the mucous membrane secondarily. An exfoliative cytologic smear is useful as a diagnostic method before biopsy.

Usually, a correct diagnosis can be made clinically, but at times it may be difficult to distinguish between carcinoma and a luetic lesion, either gumma or sclerosing glossitis. Especially is this true if a positive history of syphilis or a positive Wassermann reaction is obtained. The important differential point is that carcinoma usually occurs as a single lesion, situated most often at the border of the tongue, whereas in the case of gumma, there are multiple lesions, which may be at any site on the tongue. Furthermore,

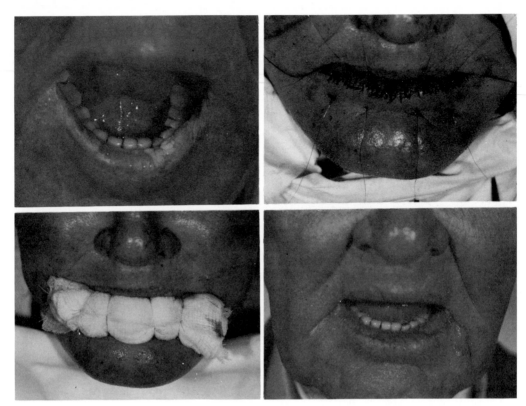

Fig. 14–28. (*Top left*) Several areas of leukoplakia on the lower lip. (*Top right*) The surface of the lip has been removed by sharp dissection, and the raw surface covered with mucous membrane of the mouth advanced to the anterior edge or the lip, by undermining the buccal mucosa. (*Bottom left*) Role of gauze tied in place by four steel wires placed through the lip. This gives firm pressure. (*Bottom right*) The lip ten days later.

the carcinomatous ulcer is usually painful and bleeds easily, whereas the gumma is not particularly painful, nor does it bleed readily.

Tuberculosis of the tongue is seen occasionally, and this also must be distinguished from carcinoma. The tuberculous lesion appears almost invariably in an individual who has pulmonary tuberculosis. It may occur as a superficial or a fairly deep ulcer, and it usually appears at the tip of the tongue. The lack of induration surrounding the ulcer is a diagnostic point.

In making a diagnosis, the removal of biopsy specimens is perhaps the most conservative method. This can be accomplished very frequently in ambulatory patients. A topical application of cocaine solution, 10 to 20 percent is used; it is held in place on a pledget of gauze from 1 to 3 minutes. Excision biopsies, with a knife, a biopsy punch, or the loop electrode, may be done using this type of anesthesia (Fig. 14–29). In removing tissues for biopsy examination, it must be remembered that the tissue at the edge of the ulcer gives the most characteristic appearance under the microscope. The necrotic, fungating material at the base of the ulcer may be nothing but chronic granulation tissue or necrotic cells and of no help in making the diagnosis.

Treatment. For the treatment of carcinoma of the mouth, especially of the tongue, hospitalization is advised. How-

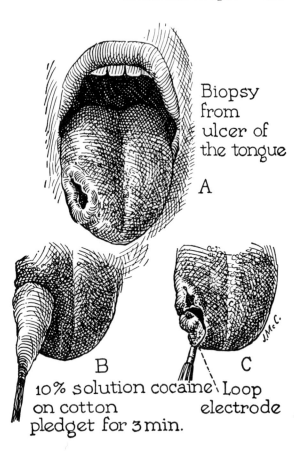

Biopsy
from
ulcer of
the tongue

A

B
10% solution cocaine
on cotton
pledget for 3 min.

C
Loop
electrode

Fig. 14–29. Biopsy of an ulcer of the tongue following local application of 10 percent cocaine solution. The cutting current with a loop electrode is an excellent method of removing such biopsies.

ever, in some instances, irradiation therapy may be carried out with the patient ambulatory throughout his period of treatment. Irradiation is the treatment of choice for the invasive posterior group, whereas surgery plus irradiation benefits

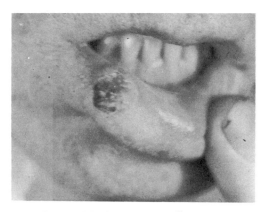

Fig. 14–30. Squamous cell carcinoma of the lip.

the greater number of patients with cancer of the anterior tongue.

Lip

Almost all that has been said concerning carcinoma of the tongue may be repeated with regard to the lip. There is, however, a characteristic difference between these two tumors in that carcinoma of the tongue is a lesion that grows rapidly and is fatal because of early metastasis to regional lymph nodes. Carcinoma of the lip is a comparatively slow-growing ulcer with a fairly good prognosis if it is seen in the early stages. It appears almost invariably as an ulcer and most frequently in the lower lip (Fig. 14–30). Many believe that chronic irritation is a definite factor in its causation. The ulcer refuses to heal, and this is a diagnostic point in differentiating it from other ulcerative lesions of the lips. Any ulcer which persists

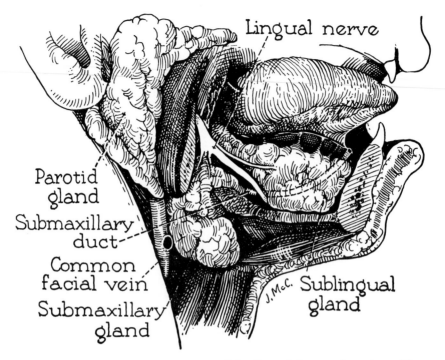

Fig. 14–31. Anteroposterior section of the floor of the mouth as viewed from within. Note the relation of the sublingual gland to the mucous membrane of the mouth and the position of the submaxillary gland as it folds around the mylohyoid muscle. The submaxillary duct is long and extends forward, mesially, and upward.

and does not show progress in healing in a period of 2 weeks should be strongly suspected to be carcinoma.

Treatment. The treatment of carcinoma of the lip has progressed greatly with the advent of new methods of irradiation therapy. A combination of surgical excision and irradiation is used in many clinics. No attempt will be made here to outline the therapy since this is not an area for ambulatory surgical care.

SALIVARY GLANDS

ANATOMY

The salivary glands of chief concern are the sublingual, the submaxillary, and the parotid. The sublingual and the submaxillary glands are located in the sublingual region in the floor of the mouth. The sublingual glands are the smallest of the

salivary glands and lie just behind the symphysis of the mandible, one on each side of the midline, on the mylohyoid muscle. The submaxillary glands are larger and lie behind and lateral to, and both above and below, the edge of the mylohyoid muscle. The secretion is carried to the mouth by a relatively long submaxillary duct (Wharton's duct) (Fig. 14-31). The sublingual gland has several minor ducts, but the main one enters the floor of the mouth with the submaxillary duct at the sublingual caruncle. This caruncle is easily noted, one on each side of the midline of the underside of the tongue, as a small projection containing an opening at its tip.

RANULAE

The term *ranula*, though rather loosely applied to all forms of retention cysts that appear on the floor of the mouth beneath

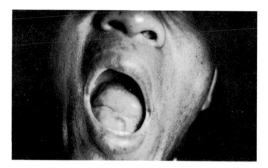

Fig. 14–32. Ranula. In this patient, the ranula recurred following marsupialization and was cured by injections of sclerosing solution.

the tongue, should properly be limited to a retention cyst of the sublingual salivary gland. Most observers believe that it occurs from an obstruction of the sublingual duct, although some believe that it is due to a myxomatous degeneration of a mucous gland. Wharton's duct is not involved in ranulae, and may often be seen as an opaque strand near the cyst. In true ranulae this duct is always patent, and there is no swelling of the submaxillary gland.

Diagnosis. The cyst begins as a small domelike swelling in the floor of the mouth beneath the anterior surface of the tongue. The mucous membrane is stretched tightly over the cystic swelling, which is soft and whitish or bluish gray (Fig. 14-32). The cyst gradually increases in size and elevates the tongue. It is invariably unilateral, but it may extend to the opposite side by expansion. There is an absence of any inflammatory symptoms, and the swelling is painless unless it assumes considerable size, when it may become annoying. The larger cysts are apt to interfere somewhat with speech. Not infrequently, the obstruction to the outlet of the duct may be intermittent, and the ranulae may therefore vary in size, a salty mucuslike material appearing in the mouth as it empties periodically.

Treatment. The treatment of ranulae may be marsupialization, excision of the enlarged duct, or, occasionally, excision of the duct and the sublingual gland. Simple incision or the insertion of a seton

to permit drainage of the contents almost invariably results in recurrence.

The operation of marsupialization may be performed easily on an ambulatory patient under local anesthesia. After a local infiltration with procaine-epinephrine solution over and around the cystic swelling, the mucous membrane is divided and retracted gently with silk traction sutures to expose the dome of the cyst. When the dissection has been carried downward to the level of the floor of the mouth, the projecting portion of the cyst is excised. A thick mucuslike material will escape from the cyst. It is well, in excising the dome of the cyst, to catch the lining membrane with several fine silk sutures which pass through the cyst wall and the adjacent mucous membrane of the floor of the mouth. The entire circumference of the cyst wall thus is sutured to the mucous membrane bit by bit as the projecting portion of the cyst is excised. Sutures are placed about 1/8 inch apart, and they should be left long in order to serve as tractors until all the sutures have been placed. During the operation, a small suction apparatus is of great help in keeping the field free of blood and saliva. Usually, little bleeding is encountered, and the only postoperative care necessary is the use of warm saline mouthwashes.

The prognosis must be guarded, even in cases in which a large opening seems to have been left after marsupialization, for ranulae recur frequently.

SALIVARY CALCULI

Etiology. Calculi occur frequently in the submaxillary gland ducts, but rarely in those of the parotid and the sublingual glands. Calculi may be present in both the gland and the duct. The cause of the calculus formation has been ascribed to inflammation or infection.

Symptoms. The symptoms of a stone in the submaxillary duct are typical and characteristic, but, in spite of this, the patient is often treated for long periods for toothache, lingual neuralgia, lymphadenitis, or malignancy. The presence of the stone causes an intermittent, or often a

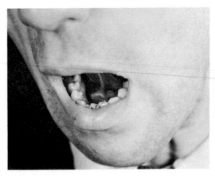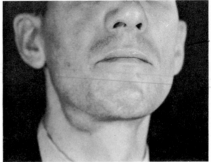

Fig. 14–33. Calculus of the submaxillary gland. Note swelling beneath angle of the jaw.

complete, obstruction of the duct. The result is a painful swelling in the region of the submaxillary gland just below the angle of the jaw (Fig. 14-33). The symptoms are most marked at mealtimes, when physiological engorgement occurs and back pressure on the gland increases. When the obstruction is intermittent, the patient often notes the discharge into the mouth of a salty material, with subsequent relief of pain in the gland.

On examination during an acute attack, a tender edematous swelling may be noted along the course of Wharton's duct on the involved side. At times the stone may be associated with a purulent infection of the duct. In such cases, the outlet of the duct may be reddened and pus may be expressed from it.

Diagnosis. In the majority of cases, the stone lies in the anterior two thirds of the duct, and usually it may be palpated along the course of the duct with one finger in the mouth and another under the chin. In a few cases, the stone may be found presenting at the orifice of the duct. If the stone cannot be palpated, a roentgen examination frequently will reveal its presence and location. Occlusal bite films will show the stones in the submaxillary duct to best advantage, whereas stones in the gland proper are shown by lateral film exposures.

Treatment. The treatment of submaxillary calculus is removal of the stone. This is a relatively easy procedure if the stone is large and lies in the anterior two thirds of the duct. Several procedures may be followed.

In incision, under local infiltration or mandibular or lingual block anesthesia, the mucous membrane is divided over the calculus, exposing the duct. Incision of the duct permits removal of the calculus. When the stone is small and movable, Ivy and Curtis recommend the insertion of a fine silk suture around the duct behind the calculus. Traction upon the suture closes the duct and prevents the calculus from slipping back toward the gland during the operation. The suture is removed after it has served its purpose.

Immobilization of the duct may be obtained by inserting two silk traction sutures through the orifice of the duct. These may be held by an assistant, or they may be hooked between the teeth so as to convert the duct orifice into a fairly large slit. The duct is then cut open until the stone is reached. This technique is most valuable for stones in the anterior one third of the duct.

After removal of the stone, the mucous membrane may be closed with fine silk sutures or it may be left open. Usually, no sutures are inserted if there has been an associated infection of the duct, and the postoperative oozing may demand a small pack in the wound. Postoperatively, hot mouthwashes are of value for several days. For the first 24 hours, a sedative may be necessary, although usually relief of pain and discomfort is almost immediate after removal of the calculous obstruction.

When the calculus lies in the posterior one third of the duct or at its junction with the gland, hospitalization is advised; usually the gland, as well as the calculus, has to be removed through an external incision. It is a more formidable procedure because of the important anatomic structures surrounding the gland.

Dilatation of the duct is another method of treatment. Ballon and Ballon have reported cases in which they were able to dilate the submaxillary duct enough to allow the calculus to be extruded through its orifice. They recommend this procedure when for some reason operation is inadvisable or will not be permitted by the patient.

PAROTITIS

Etiology and Symptoms. The gland becomes infected usually through an ascending spread of organisms along the duct. The most common form of parotitis is the acute pyogenic type, which often follows operation or debilitating disease. This type of parotitis is not under discussion for the ambulatory patient. There is, however, a type of recurrent chronic parotitis which may be seen and treated in office practice. It is characterized by a swelling of the parotid gland which may last several hours, days, or even weeks. In some instances, the swelling may be present in the morning and disappear after eating. The secretion from the gland may not be altered, although some patients may occasionally note an excessive discharge of pus and saliva from the infected gland. Often the discomfort occasioned by the swelling may be relieved by pressure over the gland or the duct. There is usually no febrile reaction and no impairment of the general health.

Apparently, there is no definite cause for this chronic parotitis, although cases are reported which would suggest that dental infection, tonsillitis, sinusitis, or the inadequate cleansing of dentures may be predisposing causes.

Diagnosis. On examination, the involved gland is found to be enlarged, firm, often nodular, and usually slightly tender to pressure. Pressure along the duct or over the gland may often produce a discharge of cloudy saliva, a mass of thick mucus, fibrin, or even pus. It is important to be sure that no stone is obstructing the duct. The diagnosis of calculus may easily be made by roentgenography.

Treatment. The treatment of chronic recurring parotitis consists in attempting to obtain a free flow of saliva by stimulation of the glands and by gentle dilatation of the ducts. In addition, attention must be paid to the eradication of any focal infection in the mouth. Infected teeth and tonsils should receive appropriate treatment. In many cases, simple massage of the gland and stimulation of the salivary flow by mastication or by taking a small amount of lemon juice in the mouth will be sufficient to prevent obstruction of the duct and to produce a subsidence of the symptoms. In most cases, dilatation of the duct is advisable. This may be accomplished by the insertion of small filiforms of gradually increasing size. The cheek is grasped with gauze and the orifice of Stensen's duct is located opposite the upper second molar tooth. A filiform then is inserted through the meatus into the duct until it is stopped by the edge of the masseter muscle. If the cheek then is pulled forward, the duct straightens out and the filiform can pass backward to the gland. By the use of larger filiforms, the duct is dilated gradually. Usually, little pain is caused by this maneuver.

The antibiotics, usually penicillin, give excellent results in controlling both the acute and the chronic forms of parotid infection.

MIXED TUMORS OF THE SALIVARY GLANDS

Mixed tumors are a peculiar group of tumors which occur chiefly in the parotid region and less often in the other salivary glands, in the palatal region, and in the lip. They are considered to be benign;

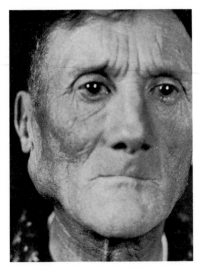

Fig. 14–34. Mixed tumor of the parotid gland.

there is a definite tendency for local recurrence, though only rarely with malignant degeneration.

Etiology. Most likely, mixed tumors arise from malformations and displacements that occur during embryonic life, and they are probably epithelial in origin, the cells arising from the ducts or the secreting portions of the gland. They often contain mucoid material which is considered to be a true secretion of mucin from the tumor cells. For a time, cartilage was believed to be present in these tumors, but Fry's studies have shown that this is not so. The substance that was mistaken for cartilage is, in reality, mucin that has lost its fibrillar appearance and its characteristic of deep staining in microscopic sections.

Diagnosis. These tumors may occur at any age and in either sex. They are more apt to appear before the age of 40. The tumor is seen over the parotid gland, or below and behind the angle of the jaw, as a slow-growing, hard, often nodular, swelling (Fig. 14-34). As a rule, little or no pain is experienced by the patient.

A differential diagnosis must be made between mixed tumors and carcinoma or sarcoma. Most of the latter tumors can be differentiated by the rapidity of their growth; they reach a fair size in a period of months rather than years. Pain is a much more common symptom in the true malignant tumors.

Treatment. Patients usually seek treatment because of the appearance of the swelling in front of or below the ear, and, in cases of typical mixed tumors, removal of the tumor is the most effective treatment.

The excision of a mixed tumor of the parotid can be performed easily under local anesthesia in an ambulatory patient, preferably in the hospital ambulatory care unit, where all supportive facilities are available should the tumor prove to be more extensive than originally thought. In such operations, the course of the facial nerve must be borne in mind; careful enucleation of the tumor in its capsule will prevent injury to it.

A transverse incision is usually made through the skin and the subcutaneous tissues overlying the tumor mass. After the tissues over the capsule have been divided, the dissection is carried on bluntly until the mass is shelled out. When the tumor is small, the operation is relatively easy to perform without rupture of the tumor. In larger tumors, cystic softening may result in easy rupture of the tumor capsule. In such cases, the material which spills from the tumor into the wound must be carefully removed, and, after enucleation of the tumor, the wound should be flushed with saline to remove any bits of tissue which might reseed the tumor cells. The wound cavity is obliterated with several layers of fine sutures, and the skin is closed with silk sutures. No drain is inserted into the wound. The chief postoperative complication to be feared is a facial nerve paralysis. This is easily avoided if the dissection is performed bluntly and is carried carefully around the capsule of the tumor. After operation, the patient should be inspected for evidence of paralysis, which most often appears at the angle of the mouth, usually at the outer portion of the lower lip. As a rule, this immediate paralysis is due to a block of the lower branches of the facial nerve by procaine.

This disappears with the loss of anesthesia.

Although the patient may have no paralysis immediately after operation, an almost complete facial paralysis may appear during the first 24 hours. Most often this is due to the pressure of retraction at operation and the subsequent edema in the wound. In every case in which paralysis has occurred in the author's experience, spontaneous recovery has taken place in a relatively short period.

Prognosis. The prognosis of mixed tumors is good, but cure is not always certain. Recurrences may take place any time up to 30 years after operation (McFarland), and the rate of recurrence may be as high as 20 to 40 percent. On the other hand, recurrences are usually local. Trueblood, State, and Ariel, Jerome and Pack believe that all mixed tumors are potentially malignant and that the parotid gland should be subjected to radical extirpation, the facial nerve being preserved. This would appear to be more radical therapy than the danger of malignancy warrants, and the danger of facial paralysis is great. In the author's experience, mixed tumors have nearly always been benign.

BIBLIOGRAPHY

Salivary Gland Tumors

Ariel, I. M., Jerome, A. P., and Pack, G. T.: Treatment of tumors of the parotid salivary gland. Surgery, *35*:124, 1954.

Beahrs, O. H., Devine, K. D., Woolner, L. B., and Bulbulian, A. H.: Tumors of the parotid gland—their surgical management. Arch. Surg., *79*:900, 1959.

Brohm, C. G., and Bird, C. E.: Primary repair of severed parotid duct. JAMA, *104*:733, 1935.

Furstenberg, A. C.: Diseases of the salivary glands. JAMA, *136*:1, 1948.

Grage, T. B., Lober, P. H., and Shahon, D. B.: benign tumors of the major salivary glands. Surgery, *50*:625, 1961.

Hurwitz, A.: Bilateral ligation of the parotid ducts to prevent salivary incontinence. Ann. Surg., *141*:412, 1955.

Martin, H., and Helsper, J. T.: Spontaneous return of function following surgical section or excision of the seventh cranial nerve in the surgery of parotid tumors. Ann. Surg., *146*:715, 1957.

————: Supplementary report on spontaneous return of function following surgical section or excision of the seventh cranial nerve in the surgery of parotid tumors. Ann. Surg., *151*:538, 1960.

McFarland, J.: The mysterious mixed tumors of the salivary glands. Surg., Gynec. Obstet., *76*:23, 1943.

————: Three hundred mixed tumors of the salivary glands, of which sixty-nine recurred. Surg., Gynec. Obstet., *63*:457, 1936.

Nanson, E. M., Watson, T. A.: Tumors of the salivary glands. Surg., Gynec. Obstet., *114*:718, 1961.

Rawson, A. J., Howard, J. M., and Royster, H. P.: Tumors of the salivary glands: a clinicopathological study of 160 cases. Cancer, *3*:445, 1950.

State, D.: Superficial lobectomy and total parotidectomy with preservation of the facial nerve in the treatment of parotid tumors. Surg., Gynec. Obstet., *89*:237, 1949.

Sumner, W. C.: A clinical approach to parotid gland tumors. Ann. Surg., *149*:852, 1959.

Trueblood, D. V.: Clinical observations and surgical experiences with parotid tumors. Western J. Surg., *52*:109, 1944.

Vellios, F., and Shafer, W. G.: Tumors of the intraoral accessory salivary glands. Surg., Gynec. Obstet., *108*:450, 1959.

Winsten, J., Gould, D. M., and Ward, G. E.: Sialography. Surg., Gynec. Obstet., *102*:315, 1956.

Salivary Calculi

Ballon, H. C., and Ballon, D. H.: Salivary calculi: their treatment by catheterization and dilatation of duct. Surg., Gynec. Obstet., *64*:226, 1937.

Ivy, R. H., and Curtis, L.: Salivary calculi. Ann. Surg., *96*:979, 1932.

Ranula

Crile, G. Jr.: Ranulas with extension into neck (so-called plunging ranulas). Surgery, *42*:819, 1957.

Tongue

Livingston, E. M., and Lieber, H.: Surgical aspects of the treatment of carcinoma of the tongue. Am. J. Surg., *30*:234, 1935.

15
Neck

Mark W. Wolcott, M.D.

INJURIES

LACERATIONS

These may occur as a result of automobile accidents, fights, or, occasionally, self-inflicted wounds.

Treatment. In spite of the profuse hemorrhage, which comes almost always from the superficially placed external jugular vein, the probability of serious wounds in these patients is not great. It is seldom that the deep vessels are involved in the laceration or are cut. Such superficial wounds are comparatively easy to take care of by simple ligation of the severed vessels and primary suture. It is not even necessary for the patients to be admitted to the hospital when the lacerations are small. In cases of deeper incisions or of blows, the complication which is most likely to occur is an injury to the trachea or the larnyx. This is associated with definite signs—the spitting of blood and, often, subcutaneous emphysema, dysphonia, and so forth. It is wise to admit such patients to the hospital because of the danger of more serious complications and the necessity for close observation for a period of time because of possible increasing edema and respiratory distress.

WHIPLASH INJURY OF THE NECK

Whiplash injury is a term applied to that injury of the neck sustained by an occupant of an automobile when it is struck by another car, usually in a rear-end collision. As a result of the collision, the victim's head is pitched backwards to an extreme position, then forward to an extreme position, and then back to a normal position. This mechanism of the "whiplash" effect has been reproduced experimentally in controlled investigations. The relaxed motorist, such as one waiting for traffic and not forewarned of an impending rear-end collision, is the one most affected, which accounts for the fact that the passenger rather than the driver may be most exposed to this injury.

The symptoms of whiplash injury vary greatly. Most often the patient complains of very little pain in the neck at the time of the accident. Between 12 and 24 hours after the accident, or later, the patient will experience pain in the neck, frequently associated with headache. Discomfort in the neck and limitation of motion of the head on the shoulders are. characteristic. The pain is usually poorly localized, but is most often occipital or interscapular. These symptoms may persist for a period of weeks or months, and may disappear only to recur.

In addition to these local symptoms it is not uncommon for patients to develop profound emotional reactions, such as nervousness, anxiety, nervous tension, insomnia, sweating of the hands, etc. It is believed by some that the persistence of many of these psychosomatic symptoms may be the result of litigation incidental to the accident, and that they are often finally resolved to a great extent by settlement of the litigation.

In most cases there is little or minor evidence of trauma. On examination, there is tenderness on pressure at the back of the neck, at times with spasm of the cervical spinal muscles. Often, the muscle spasm is more prounced on one side than it is on the other; this accounts for the tilting of the head forward or to one side. X-ray examination is usually negative, but positive findings may range from a straightening of the cervical curve, to signs of disc pathology, to various degrees of vertebral subluxation. Previously present asymptomatic changes in the vertebral bodies, such as lipping or spurring, may be noted. These may become symptomatic in patients in the older age group following a whiplash injury and may account for the persistent symtoms.

The pathologic consequences of whiplash are variously explained. Some authors believe that there is no major tearing of ligaments or other soft tissue structures at the time of injury. The symptoms are explained as a muscle soreness such as is seen in any muscle after heavy exercise. Others feel that there is definitely stretching of the muscles and ligaments of the neck, with possibly some edema, hemorrhage, and even direct trauma to the cervical nerve roots. In more severe cases there may be injury to the intervertebral disc or secondary fibrosis involving the vertebral joints.

Treatment. In severe cases of whiplash injury, hospital admission is advised. However, in less severe cases treatment may be given on an ambulatory basis, or even at home. The halter type of traction given in the horizontal position can be rigged at home (Fig. 15-1). Traction of 5 to 15 lb., depending on the patient, is given for 30 minutes at a time, two to three times a day, until the acute symptoms subside. Drugs such as the salicylates, barbiturates, and meprobamate are useful as sedatives and to relieve pain. Hot moist packs are helpful in relieving the muscle spasm and soreness. A wraparound collar made of a folded towel helps to hold the neck in extension and is an inexpensive substitute for a cervical collar (Fig. 15-2) in minor cases.

Most of these patients have relatively minor injuries that, with conservative treatment, disappear in a few days or weeks. Others with more severe injuries may have symptoms that persist for months.

Brachial Plexus "Wrench"

Etiology. In severe injuries of the neck, especially in those in which the shoulder is driven down and away from the neck, the brachial plexus may be injured by a sudden pull upon its roots.

Symptoms. The symptoms of brachial plexus "wrench" are extreme tenderness and pain over the entire shoulder and, often, down the arm. The muscles of the shoulder region, especially the trapezius, are frequently in painful spasm. The most marked tenderness is along the sides of the neck. The pain becomes worse on bending the head toward the opposite side and is relieved somewhat by bending it toward the site of injury. A roentgen examination should be done to rule out lesions of the vertebrae, the shoulder, and the acromioclavicular joints.

Treatment. It is imperative to relieve the shoulder of the weight of the arm. This may be done by placing the arm in a triangular sling supported by the uninjured shoulder or in an abduction cast or splint. This is especially necessary if muscular paralyses appear in the arm or the shoulder. In most cases of brachial plexus injury, the prognosis for eventual recovery is good if adequate early treatment is given. In a few cases, infiltration of the scalenus anticus with procaine has produced dramatic relief of pain.

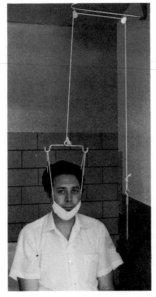

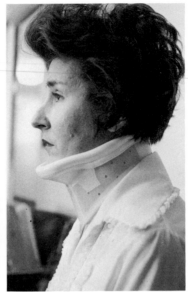

Fig. 15–1. Halter traction for treatment of whiplash injury.

Fig. 15–2. Cervical collar in place.

INFECTIONS

FURUNCLES

Etiology. Furuncular infections are very common in the neck, especially in the hairy portions at the sides and the back. It is probable that the rubbing of shirt and coat collars is an exciting factor, especially in men. The infecting organism is the *Staphylococcus aureus*, and experience seems to point to an individual susceptibility to this infection.

Treatment. The furuncles begin with a sense of itching and slight burning, and may immediately regress without causing further symptoms and without treatment. More commonly, they progress to form a raised, reddened, tender mound of induration, which seems to be pressed upon with every movement of the head. At this stage, it is occasionally possible to abort the infection by the use of antibiotics. Penicillin is usually chosen and, as a rule, controls the infection at once. If resistant organisms are encountered, as determined by sensitivity tests, the appropriate drug is used.

BOILS

Frequently, an infection which begins as a small and innocent-looking furuncle will progress and form a large area of infection, commonly described by the laity as a "boil." The infected area becomes larger and more painful as the wall of inflammatory induration advances in the dense tissues of the neck. The tenseness of the lesion makes every movement torture.

Treatment. Intensive antibiotic therapy—penicillin or erythromycin—usually will result in rapid subsidence of the inflammation and control of the infection.

When the pain is intolerable or when the induration appears to be spreading, a cruciate incision to provide drainage is necessary. This is best made under a short-acting general anesthetic. Hot moist dressings of saline or boric acid solution should be applied until the slough liquefies and separates. A packing of plain or iodoform gauze may be used to control oozing at the time of incision, but, after its removal on the second or the third day, none should be reinserted. The hot wet dressings are discontinued when the slough has been discharged, and a simple dry dressing is applied.

CARBUNCLES

Course of Infection. In the dense tissues of the back of the neck, the furuncular infection often progresses laterally and deeply instead of to the skin surface. The necrotizing action of the staphylococcal toxin attacks especially the fatty tissue lying in the interstices between the fibrous septa that extend from the deep fascia to the skin. The fibrous tissue then succumbs to the necrotoxin, so that eventually a large area of subcutaneous necrosis, which involves not only the subcutaneous fatty tissue and its fibrous septa but also the dense underlying fascia, forms. Numerous sites of pointing appear on the skin in the center of an extending area of tense induration. Not infrequently, the infection extends from one side of the neck to the other.

Symptoms. Besides the local symptoms of intense throbbing pain and excruciating tenderness, there often may be enough absorption of toxic products from the infection to produce fever and leukocytosis. When large carbuncles appear in patients of middle age or beyond, the possibility of their being associated with diabetes must be considered. Determinations of blood and urine sugar should be made.

Treatment. In the care of patients with carbuncles, hospitalization is often preferable, and, for those who are diabetic, it is imperative. However, many patients with a carbuncle of the neck can be kept ambulatory during treatment. This is especially the case when penicillin is used as described above.

The treatment of carbuncles which appears to give the best results in relief of pain and rapidity of healing is radical incision and drainage. The operation is performed under general anesthesia; either a short-acting inhalation anesthetic or an intravenous anesthetic is used. In small carbuncles, a cruciate incision is best (Fig. 15-3). This should reach the full depths of the necrotic tissue and should extend throughout the length of the carbuncle in each direction. Each quarter segment is grasped by an Allis forceps and undercut to the full extent of the necrotic tissue. The period of healing is shortened if the corner of each segment is cut away and if as much necrotic tissue as possible is also removed. This is not sacrificing any viable tissue, and recovery is hastened by excising tissue which would otherwise have to undergo liquefaction necrosis and be discharged as slough or pus. Bleeding is sometimes rather brisk, but ligatures are never necessary, as hemorrhage can be controlled by a snug packing of plain or iodoform gauze and a pressure bandage.

In larger carbuncles, the central core comprising all the draining sinuses should be boldly excised down to the necrotic fascia. Radial incisions are then made through the remaining indurated tissue to the limit of necrosis in all directions. The resulting multiple flaps are then caught with Allis forceps, and each is undercut. With scissors or a knife, all frankly necrotic tissue is excised, especially the dense fascia at the base of the carbuncle. The wound is then held open by traction with Allis forceps and is entirely packed with iodoform gauze in sufficient amount to give pressure. In spite of brisk bleeding, no ligatures are necessary if an adequate pressure dressing is applied.

The most satisfactory dressing is a figure-of-eight bandage for the head and the neck. After the bandage has been applied, the patient is placed on his back for a time, and a pillow is so arranged as to give pressure on the wound. The patient may be allowed to go home after about an hour of rest, but he should be given 5 or 6 tablets of morphine sulfate, $1/6$ gr. (10 mg.), one to be taken every third hour by mouth as needed for pain. The dressing should be inspected before he leaves and, if it is bloody, the outside dressings may be changed and a new bandage applied.

Nothing is done to the wound for the first 12 to 24 hours; thereafter, hot saline or boric acid solution is used to moisten

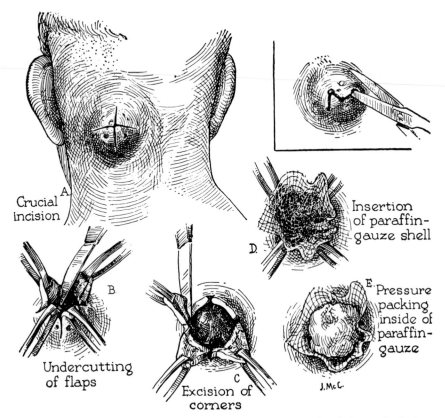

Fig. 15–3. Steps in the incision of a boil or a carbuncle of the neck. (*A*) A cruciate incision is made in the most prominent portion of the induration, and the corners of the incision are caught with Allis clamps. (*B*) Each flap is undercut as far as the necrosis extends. The corners of the flaps are excised (*C*) because these always become necrotic. (*D*) The base of the wound is covered with a paraffin-gauze shell and (*E*) a pressure packing is inserted inside the paraffin gauze. Inset shows conservative method of opening carbuncle when necrosis has progressed to the point at which there are numerous small cutaneous draining points. These may be joined by cutting with scissors without anesthesia.

the dressing 4 to 8 times daily. The dressing is not changed until the third day, when the gauze is removed. No new packing is inserted into the cavity of the carbuncle. The problem then is one of removing the necrotic tissue. No substitute has been found for mechanical measures, that is, scissors and forceps, and wound irrigation.

Healing does not begin until the slough is removed, and sloughing fascia liquefies very slowly; hence the advantage of mechanical excision in clearing the wound of necrotic tissue.

When the wound is filled with clean granulations, the flaps may be replaced, adhesive strapping often being used to advantage. When the flaps have grown into place, the wound will have decreased much in size, but frequently a few pinch grafts may be employed to hasten epithelization and to reduce scarring.

CERVICAL ADENITIS
Acute Cervical Adenitis

Etiology and Symptoms. An acute inflammation of the cervical lymph glands

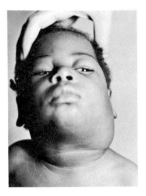

Fig. 15–4. Acute suppurative cervical adenitis in 7-month-old baby following tonsillar infection.

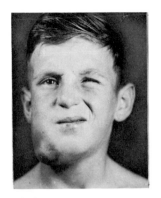

Fig. 15–5. Acute suppurative cervical adenitis 9 days after extraction of an infected tooth.

is always the result of a primary infection somewhere in the area which drains lymph into these nodes. It is not always possible to find the primary source of infection, but, when possible, treatment should be directed not only to the infection of the lymph node itself but also to the primary source of infection, such as an abscessed tooth, infected tonsils, an infected scalp, or a sinus infection (Fig. 15-4).

The infection of a lymph node is usually characterized by swelling of the node and, frequently, of several of the adjacent nodes. This swelling may be somewhat slow to appear and may be characterized only by tenderness. It may arise some considerable time after the original infection has subsided. On the other hand, the infection may develop rather rapidly, with acute swelling, extreme tenderness, and considerable edema and redness of the overlying skin and subcutaneous tissues. This latter type of infection is more likely to occur in children, in whom an acute suppurative lymphadenitis is a relatively common infection. Often the deep nodes underneath the sternocleidomastoid muscle are involved. Frequently, however, the submaxillary glands are also involved, and in children with scalp infections it is not uncommon to see the swelling appear behind the ear in the occipital or the postauricular group of nodes. The infection is usually staphylococcal, but it may be streptococcal, depending on the type of primary infection. In the streptococcal type of infection, there are marked constitutional symptoms and, almost invariably, a rather high fever.

Treatment. Conservatism is the rule in the treatment of acute cervical adenitis. Usually, intensive antibiotic therapy can be counted on to abort an early infection. When the inflammation has progressed to fluctuation, incision and drainage are required. During this period one must not neglect treatment of the primary focus in the mouth, the pharynx, the ear, or the scalp.

Acute Suppurative
Cervical Adenitis

Not infrequently, children are brought to a doctor's office or to a surgical outpatient department after the infection of the cervical glands has gone to suppuration. This progression from acute adenitis to cervical abscess usually takes a period of several days, or even weeks.

Diagnosis and Treatment. When the superficial nodes are involved, the diagnosis of the lesion is evident and the treatment is simple (Fig. 15-5). The process appears as a red, tender, fluctuant area, usually on the side of the neck or underneath the mandible. The pus appears to be just under the skin, and, if an incision is made in the longest diameter of the abscess, this is found to be so. As a rule, adequate incision and drainage of the abscess necessitates the use of a short-acting general anesthetic in children. In adults, a line infiltration in the skin with a local anesthetic is usually adequate. The incision is made through the softest portion of the abscess presenting on the skin surface; this is usually the site at which the abscess is closest to the surface. When the abscess has been incised, the edges of the wound are grasped with Allis forceps, or small rake retractors are introduced, and the abscess is explored gently with the finger or a curved hemostat. After its extent has been determined, the incision is so enlarged as to include the entire length of the abscess cavity. The wound is packed with iodoform gauze and a firm dressing is applied. The packing may be removed after one day and, if the incision has been adequate, the wound edges will gape enough to permit adequate drainage. Simple surface dressings are all that are necessary until healing occurs.

When the deep cervical nodes are involved, the lesion is less easily diagnosed. Because of their deep situation, fluctuation is demonstrated with considerable difficulty, although experienced fingers are often able to determine it when inexperienced ones miss this diagnostic point. One may conclude, however, that if the enlargement of the nodes has persisted for a period of from 10 days to 2 weeks following the subsidence of an acute infection in the mouth or the pharynx, the probability is that suppuration has taken place in the infected gland and incision and drainage are indicated. In the drainage of deep nodes, as in the drainage of superficial glands, a general anesthetic is usually indicated for children, but local infiltration may be employed for adults. The incision is made through the skin and the platysma, and a blunt hemostat is introduced into the most prominent portion of the enlarged lymph nodes. If the proper site has been selected, a flow of pus will immediately follow upon the withdrawal of the hemostat. Often the pus is slight in amount, but it can easily be distinguished in the bloody discharge

from the wound. When pus is found, the instrument should be reinserted into the opening and withdrawn with the blades open; thus the abscess opening is bluntly enlarged without much danger of wounding adjacent structures.

In deep cervical abscesses, because of the danger of injuring important nearby structures, it is inadvisable to enlarge the wound so as to lay open the entire abscess cavity. In such cases, the insertion of a soft sump-type drain into the abscess cavity usually provides adequate drainage, and this tube may remain in place until the suppuration has clearly subsided and all of the slough has disappeared. When the tube has been inserted into the cavity, iodoform or plain gauze packing may be introduced around it for the first 2 or 3 days. The purpose of this packing is to control bleeding and to separate the edges of the wound until such time as inflammatory induration holds the wound open. After removal of the packing, the tube is allowed to remain in place, but packing is not reinserted. At intervals of 3 or 4 hours, the dressings should be moistened with a boric acid or saline solution to prevent the drainage material from drying up and plugging the drainage tract. As soon as the slough has separated from the abscess cavity, the drainage tube may be removed and the wound may be allowed to close; simple sterile dressings are applied.

The application of a dressing which will provide pressure and also stay in place in ambulatory patients is a difficulty frequently experienced in treating cervical abscesses. The dressing should be applied in sufficient amount to permit pressure on the wound by the bandage and to form a good compress for hot moist dressings. The bandage that we have used successfully is illustrated in Figure 15-6. It begins at the back of the neck, is first applied as a circular bandage around the neck for 1 or 2 turns, then is brought under the chin, upward over the head, downward around the occiput to the opposite side of the neck, forward underneath the chin and upward, the part of the bandage from the opposite side being crossed in the midline of the scalp. It is

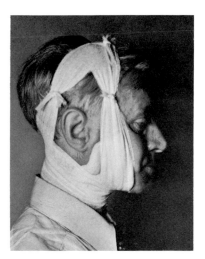

Fig. 15–6. Bandage for lesions of the front and the sides of the neck.

then continued around the opposite side of the occiput, forward around the neck, and is continued in repeated turns as before. The bandage is secured by tightening the bands on either side of the head and over the midline of the scalp with a simple tie of bandage gauze.

TUBERCULOSIS OF THE CERVICAL LYMPH NODES

Etiology. Tuberculous infection of the cervical lymph nodes is seen most often in children and in adolescents. It may, however, appear at any age, and in our experience it is much more common in Negro patients. In the majority of cases, the infection is believed to be of the bovine type. The relative infrequency of the disease now, as compared with the former high incidence, is the result of more careful inspection and testing of milk herds and of the pasteurization of milk. Most authorities agree that it occurs first as an infection of the tonsillar or other lymphatic tissues of the nasopharynx, with secondary extension into the lymph nodes of the neck.

Course and Diagnosis. Usually the infection begins as a discrete enlargement of the lymph nodes of the neck, generally the superior cervical, the upper deep cervical, or the middle superior deep cervical nodes. Bilateral infection is frequent, although not invariable. This finding has often been cited and used as a diagnostic point in differentiating tuberculous enlargements of the nodes of the neck from other enlargements, such as those due to Hodgkin's disease and lymphosarcoma. In our experience, unilateral involvement has not been uncommon. The discrete enlargement of numerous nodes gradually progresses and involves other, adjacent, nodes (Fig. 15-7), and, as the process continues, caseous necrosis may appear, with the production of cold abscesses. As a rule, this stage of the disease is not reached for many months, even years, and nowadays most patients seek treatment long before the cold-abscess stage is reached.

In the diagnosis of tuberculous cervical adenitis, the discrete enlargement of numerous nodes is an important finding. The absence of pain and tenderness, heat, and other signs of acute inflammation is characteristic and helps to rule out the possibility of an acute pyogenic adenitis.

Treatment. The treatment of cervical tuberculous adenitis may be surgical or conservative. The best treatment today is the administration of antituberculous drugs. Isoniazide, 100 mg. three times a day, and streptomycin, 1.0 g. three times a week, and PAS (para-aminosalicylic acid), 1.0 g. three times a day, heal these lesions in 6 months to a year. Therapy should be continued for at least one year. Today, excision is usually done only for diagnostic purposes. Incision and drainage may rarely be necessary in the neglected case which goes on to caseous necrosis and to the development of a cold abscess. In perhaps one quarter of the cases an inadequate response to drug treatment occurs, and en bloc excision is the best treatment.

Prognosis. Statistical studies made of patients with cervical lymphadenitis of tuberculous origin show that its occurrence in children and in young adolescents does not subject them to a greater risk than usual of developing pulmonary tuberculosis. It is even believed that lymph-node tuberculosis that occurs early in life actually serves to immunize the individual against the more lethal forms of the disease. Stanton and Richard, in an investigation of 115 cases of lymph-node tuberculosis, did not find that pulmonary tuberculosis had developed in a single patient in whom the adenitis had appeared in childhood or in adolescence.

Cold Abscesses

Treatment. In the case of patients who present themselves in the late stages of the disease, after having developed a "cold abscess" in the neck, an attempt to remove the involved nodes is somewhat difficult. Excision is much facilitated by treatment with isoniazid and PAS. Many abscesses will resolve almost completely or will become much smaller and less adherent, so that local excision can be readily accomplished. If there are a large number of nodes involved, or if they appear to be deep seated, hospitalization is safer when an en bloc excision offers an excellent chance of cure.

Tuberculous Fistulas

Tuberculous fistulas resulting from rupture of "cold abscesses" are not uncommon, although their occurrence is much less frequent now than formerly. The sinuses appear as small openings that drain a thin fluid containing flakes of caseous material. The sinuses, at first tuberculous, always become secondarily infected, which accounts perhaps for the continued drainage and for the failure of the sinuses to close.

Treatment. In the treatment of tuberculous sinuses, an attempt is made to remove the tuberculous lymphatic tissue. Often, a calcified area of a caseous node may act as a foreign body. The sinus tract should be explored, and the tuberculous node curetted to remove as much as possible of the caseous and calcified material. An iodoform drain inserted into the sinus tract may then promote eventual healing. If this sort of treatment is not successful, a formal excision of the sinus tract and of the involved caseous tuberculous glands is worthwhile.

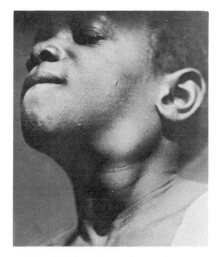 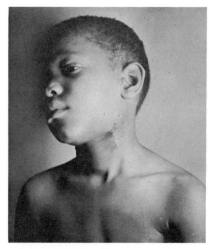

Fig. 15–7. Tuberculous adenitis in a child, excised under local anesthesia. (*Left*) Large mass of tuberculous nodes. (*Right*) Result 1 month later. Patient ambulatory throughout.

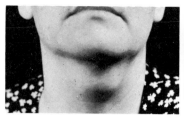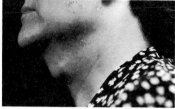

Fig. 15–8. Thyroglossal cyst in usual position in the midline and below the hyoid bone.

CYSTS AND FISTULAS

THYROGLOSSAL CYSTS AND FISTULAS

Etiology. The embryologic development of the median portion of the thyroid gland accounts for the appearance of cysts and fistulas in the midline of the neck. The median anlage of the thyroid is formed at the base of the tongue. It descends rapidly through the tongue and the neck tissues in the early portion of fetal life, and reaches its location anterior to the trachea in the midline. There it joins the two lateral lobes of the thyroid gland. There may be a distribution of some thyroid cells along the line of descent of this anlage. This has been given the name of the thyroglossal tract. Many believe that, in the descent of the thyroid anlage, some of the oral epithelium from the base of the tongue is dragged down with it. This misplaced epithelium may be of the stratified or of the ciliated type, and secretion from it may give rise to the formation of cysts (Fig. 15-8). If the cysts are opened or rupture spontaneously, fistulas are formed. Very rarely, carcinoma may develop from the thyroglossal duct remnant.

Diagnosis and Symptoms. The displaced oral epithelium may produce cysts at any age, but perhaps more often in childhood than in adult life. The cysts appear more often in females than they do in males (about 2 to 1). A swelling appears in the midline of the neck, usually between the hyoid bone and the cricoid cartilage, though it may appear anywhere in the front of the neck, from the hyoid bone down to the sternum. Very often the patient presents himself for treatment after an incision has been made in this swelling, with the result that there is a sinus, or dimple, surrounded by considerable fibrous tissue (Fig. 15-9). This cyst or sinus opening rises on swallowing, due to its attachment to the base of the tongue.

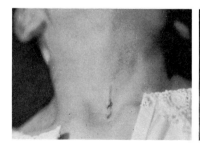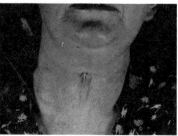

Fig. 15–9. (*Left*) Thyroglossal sinus following incision of an infected thyroglossal cyst. (*Right*) Chronic sinus with deposit of scar tissue following numerous excisions of an infected thyroglossal cyst.

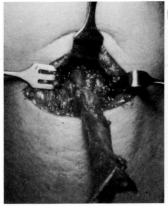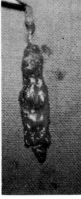

Fig. 15–10. (*Left*) Excision of thyroglossal cyst. Dissection has been carried to base of the tongue. (*Right*) Cyst excised.

This is one of the diagnostic points in differentiating this type of swelling from other midline swellings in the neck. Usually, the cysts are painless and definite fluctuation may be demonstrated. Secondary infection occurs occasionally; in this case, all the signs of inflammation are present, making the diagnosis somewhat more difficult. When a sinus is present, there is a constant discharge of a glairy, stringy, mucuslike material, which causes the patient considerable inconvenience because of soiling. The sinus tract may alternately close and open, closing as the scar tissue at the orifice of the tract contracts, and opening again due to tension in the cyst. If the thyroglossal fistula has been of some duration, it is usually possible to trace the tract to the hyoid bone as a firm tubular structure in the midline of the neck.

Treatment. The cure of thyroglossal cysts and sinuses depends upon the removal of all of the epithelial tissue. This requires a dissection and excision of the cyst or the sinus which extends upward through or under the hyoid bone to the base of the tongue. The operation may be performed under general or local anesthesia in ambulatory patients. The dissection of the superficial portion of the cyst or the sinus is relatively easy, and it is done through a transverse incision, 5 or 6 cm.

long, at the level of the cricoid cartilage.

After separation of the skin and the platysma, the sinus is traced along its path in the median raphe between the sternohyoid muscles up to the hyoid bone. Experience has shown that removing only that part of the tract lying below the hyoid bone almost invariably results in a recurrence of the cyst or the sinus, and that a complete operation usually will entail the removal of the midportion of the hyoid bone and the portion of the tract extending to the base of the tongue. Therefore, with adequate sharp retraction, the hyoid bone is exposed and about half an inch of its midportion is excised. With the finger in the mouth at the position of the foreamen cecum, a tubular portion of the muscles of the tongue is then excised, the excision approaching the finger at the foramen cecum. It is practically impossible to identify the tract in this tissue; therefore, a tubular excision about 6 mm. in diameter is made up to the foramen cecum. When the dissection has reached the mucous membrane of the floor of the mouth, the tract is excised and the cavity is obliterated with interrupted sutures of fine catgut (Fig. 15-10, *left* and *right*).

The operation as described by Sistrunk entails the suture of the divided hyoid bone and the insertion of a drain to the deepest portion of the cavity (Fig. 15-11). The tissues are then closed in layers about the drain. The skin closure may be performed with clips or fine wire sutures. In the experience of the author, a thorough obliteration of dead space along the tract obviates the necessity of introducing the drain. The results of this operation are almost 100 percent cure.

LATERAL CERVICAL, BRANCHIAL OR BRANCHIAL CLEFT CYSTS AND FISTULAS

Etiology. Lateral cervical cysts and fistulae are known to be the result of developmental anomalies that arise in association with the growth processes of the branchial clefts and branchial arches in the embryo.

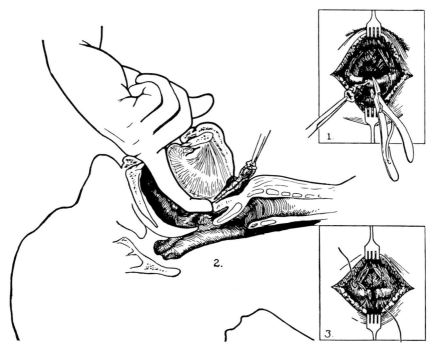

Fig. 15–11. Excision of thyroglossal sinus (Sistrunk). (1) Method of dissecting the sinus tract down to the hyoid bone and excising the mesial portion of the hyoid bone. (2) Excision of the tract above the hyoid to the base of the tongue. (3) Method of uniting the hyoid in the midline after excising the tract.

The embryologic remnants which form the cysts and the fistulas in the neck may communicate with the pharynx, may appear in the neck without any communication with the skin or the pharynx, may appear in the subcutaneous and the deeper tissues and communicate with the skin, or may lead from the skin through an epithelial-lined tract to the pharynx.

The cysts contain the products of epithelial metabolism, and, when there is an external opening, the discharge of these products causes an annoying constant drainage upon the skin surface. The epithelium lining the cyst may vary from the stratified squamous to the columnar type. The cysts at times become infected, often following an acute upper respiratory infection.

Diagnosis and Symptoms. These cysts may appear at almost any age. In the diagnosis of lateral cervical cysts, the following points may be helpful:

They always lie in relation to the anterior border of the sternocleidomastoid muscle. Invariably they are deeply attached, the skin and the subcutaneous tissues moving over them. The only exception to this rule is in the case of infection of the cyst, when the diagnosis is made more difficult because of the inflammatory reaction. The cysts are most often mistaken for cervical lymph node enlargements of either a tuberculous or a chronic inflammatory nature. The differentiation can be made, however, by the absence of any other cervical lymph node enlargements and by the fact that, if the process is inflammatory and of long duration, there would certainly be inflammatory induration that would extend to the subcutaneous tissues and to the skin. Usually these cysts lie rather high in the neck (Fig. 15-12), and this position distinguishes them from cystic hygromas, which almost invariably are found in the lower portion

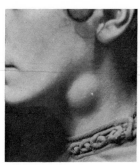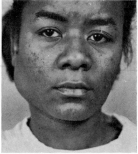

Fig. 15–12. Lateral cervical cysts of the neck, excised under local anesthesia in ambulatory patients.

of the neck. In addition, the hygromas are soft and may be transilluminated, whereas the cervical cysts are firm and can never be transilluminated.

In diagnosing the lateral cervical fistulas, the location of the fistulous opening along the anterior border of the sterncleidomastoid is in itself almost diagnostic. Usually, there is only a single opening. Injection of the tract with Lipiodol, or with some other liquid opaque to roentgen rays, will outline its extent and course very definitely.

Treatment. The treatment of lateral cervical cysts and fistulas is complete excision of the tract. This operation is perhaps best performed under general anesthesia and on a hospitalized patient. However, the discussion is included in this text because of the importance of making a differential diagnosis in these cases. As a matter of fact, some of the smaller cysts may be excised easily enough under local anesthesia in ambulatory patients.

LYMPH NODE BIOPSY

Frequently, the surgeon is called upon the perform a biopsy of one of the lymph nodes of the neck for diagnostic purposes. This operation is easily performed in an ambulatory patient. If possible, a superficial node that is discrete and that is movable in its surrounding tissues is selected. The operation is performed under local anesthesia, usually by infiltration of the skin and the subcutaneous tissues. In operations of this sort, it is important that the surgeon mark the location of the nodule because, after the introduction of the

anesthetic, it is frequently impossible to feel it. Missing the nodule by ½ inch in one direction or another may give the surgeon considerable difficulty. Therefore, as soon as the anesthetic is injected into the skin, it is wise to make a small scratch mark over the center of the nodule which is to be removed. An adequate incision must be made through each succeeding layer of tissue (skin, subcutaneous tissue and platysma) until the nodule is reached. The use of sharp rake retractors in this type of operation keeps the tissues on tension and prevents bleeding, which is troublesome in dissection in a small wound.

When the lymph node has been located, it should not be grasped, but the tissues should be divided and retracted, so that it can be dissected bluntly with a curved mosquito hemostat until it is eventually delivered through the wound. This dissection, without rupturing the node or without touching it, is a work that requires considerable skill. It is most helpful if one corner or one end of the node can first be dissected free; then, with a hemostat grasping the connective tissue over the node, the node can be elevated and dissected from the bottom. The most adherent portions of the node usually contain the vessels, and it is wise to divide these pedicles between small hemostats before cutting them. The hemostat on the portion close to the gland often serves as a good tractor in elevating the node.

When the gland has been removed, the remaining wound is obliterated, buried sutures being used to catch the circumference of the wound; mattress sutures of wire, silk, or cotton are used in the skin. Unless there has been some difficulty with hemostasis, drainage is not necessary, and a pressure dressing is applied.

BIBLIOGRAPHY

Thyroglossal Cysts and Fistula

Baumgartner, C. J.: Branchial and thyroglossal duct cysts and fistulas in children. Surg., Gynec. Obstet., *56*:948, 1933.

Brintnall, E. S., Davies, J., Huffman, W. C., and Lierle, D. M.: Thyroglossal ducts and cysts. Arch. Otolaryng. Chicago, *59*:282, 1954.

Brown, P. M., and Judd, E. S.: Thyroglossal duct cysts and sinuses: results of radical (Sistrunk) operation. Am. J. Surg., *102*:492, 1961.

Judd, E. S.: Removal of thyroglossal duct cyst. Surg. Clin. N. Am., *43*:1023, 1963.

Keeling, J. H., and Ochsner, A.: Carcinoma in thyroglossal duct remnants. Cancer, *12*:596, 1959.

Maxwell, W. T., and Marchetta, F. C.: Papillary adenocarcinoma of the thyroglossal duct tract. Arch. Surg., *80*:224, 1960.

O'Kane, C. R., and Straus, F. H.: Papillary adenocarcinoma arising in association with a persistent thyroglossal duct. Ann. Surg., *138*:805, 1953.

Sistrunk, W. E.: Technique of removal of cysts and sinuses of thyroglossal duct. Surg., Gynec. Obstet., *46*:109, 1928.

Stahl, W. M., Jr., and Lyall, D.: Cervical cysts and fistulae of thyroglossal tract origin. Ann. Surg., *139*:123, 1954.

Stanley, D. G., Robinson, F.W. *et al.*: Thyroid carcinoma in thyroglossal duct cysts: a case report and literature review. Am. Surg., *36*:581, 1970.

Ward, P. H., Strahan, R.W., Harris, P.F. *et al.*: The many faces of cysts of the thyroglossal duct. Trans. Am. Acad. Ophthal. Otolaryng., *74*:310, 1970.

Branchial Cleft Cysts and Fistulae

Bailey, H.: The clinical aspects of branchial fistulae. Brit. J. Surg., *21*:173, 1933.

Baumgartner, C. J., and Steindel, S.: Differential diagnosis between thymic duct fistulas and branchial cleft fistulas. Am. J. Surg., *59*:99, 1943.

Bhaskar, S. N., and Bernier, J. L.: Review of branchial cysts. Am. J. Path. *35*:407, 1959.

Bill, A. H., Jr., and Vadheim, J. L.: Cysts, sinuses and fistulas of the neck arising from the first and second branchial clefts. Ann. Surg., *142*:904, 1955.

Byars, L. T., and Anderson, R.: Anomalies of the first branchial cleft. Surg., Gynec. Obstet., *93*:755, 1951.

Collins, N. P., and Edgerton, M. T.: Primary branchiogenic carcinoma. Cancer, *12*:235, 1959.

Conway, H., and Jerome, A. P.: The surgical treatment of branchial cysts and fistulas. Surg., Gynec. Obstet., *101*:621, 1955.

Gord, D., and Masson, A.: Anomaly of first branchial cleft. Ann. Surg., *150*:309, 1959.

Hoffman, E.: Branchial cysts within the parotid gland. Ann. Surg., *152*:290, 1960.

Huppler, E. G., and Beahrs, O. H.: Hereditary occurrence of branchial cleft fistulas. Surgery, *43*:802, 1958.

Kinder, C. H.: Branchial cyst and lateral cervical fistula, Brit. J. Surg., *42*:53, 1954.

Lane, S. L.: Branchiogenic cyst carcinoma. Am. J. Surg., *96*:776, 1958.

Lyall, D., and Stahl, W. M., Jr.: Lateral cervical cysts, sinuses, and fistulas of congenital origin. Int. Abstr. Surg., *102*:417, 1956.

Meyer, H. W.: Congenital cysts and fistulae of the neck. Ann. Surg., *95*:226, 1932.

———: True branchiogenic cyst and fistula of the neck. Arch. Surg., *35*:766, 1937.

Park, O. K., and Buford, C. H.: Bronchogenic cyst of neck and superior mediastinum. Ann. Surg., *142*:128, 1955.

Skolnik, E. M., Soboroff, B. J., and Fornatto, E. J.: Congenital cysts and fistulas of the head and neck. J. Int. Coll. Surg., *30*:94, 1958.

Tuberculous Cervical Adenitis

Byrd, R. B., *et al.*: The role of surgery in tuberculous lymphadenitis in adults. Am. Rev. Resp. Dis., *103*:816, 1971.

Gillam, P. M. S., and Knowles, J. P.: The treatment of tuberculosis lymphadenitis. Tubercle, *44*:112, 1963.

Mulay, S. G., and Hiranandani, L. H.: A clinical study and the surgical management of two hundred and fifty cases of tubercular cervical lymphadenitis. J. Laryng., *84*:781, 1970.

Reid, R., and Wilkerson, M. C.: Tuberculosis of the cervical lymphatic glands. Brit. Med. J., *2*:740, 1937.

Stanton, E. McD., and Richard, G.: Tuberculous cervical adenitis. JAMA, *102*:1214, 1934.

Whiplash Injury

Braaf, M. M., and Rosner, S.: Whiplash injury of the neck. New York J. Med., *58*:1501, 1958.

Braunstein, P. W., and Moore, J. O.: The fallacy of the term "whiplash injury." Am. J. Surg., *97*:522, 1959.

Erickson, D. J.: The conservative management of cervical syndromes. Postgrad. Med., *36*:194, 1964.

Gotten, N.: Survey of one hundred cases of whiplash injury after settlement of litigation. JAMA, *162*:865, 1956.

McCorral, H. R., Priest, W. S., Compere, E. L., Beattie, E. J., and Buey, P. C.: Neck, shoulder and arm pain. Postgrad. Med., *36*:385, 1964.

Severy, D. M., Mathewson, J. H., and Bechtol, C. O.: Controlled automobile rear-end collisions, an investigation of related engineering and medical phenomena. Canad. Services Med. J., *11*:727, 1955.

Schutt, C. H., *et al.*: Neck injury to women; a metropolitan plague. JAMA, *206*:2689, 1968.

Warsham, R. H.: Acute sprain of the cervical spine. South. J. Med., *56*:252, 1963.

16
Breast

Mark W. Wolcott, M.D.

LESIONS OF THE FEMALE BREAST
CONTUSIONS OF THE BREAST

Contusions of the breast, especially in females, are not uncommon injuries. They may be caused by any blunt object or by kicks from struggling children who are being held. The contused area is painful and tender, and there is sometimes an area of ecchymosis. The injury is frequently a source of considerable concern to the patient because of worry lest it produce a subsequent malignancy. However, there is no evidence to suggest that a single local trauma is a factor in the production of malignancy.

Treatment. Most of the contusions are minor in nature and can be treated easily by supporting the breast. A tight bandage, held firmly in place by adhesive or a tight brassiere, usually gives considerable comfort and relief of the edema which occasionally occurs. After the first 24 hours, hot compresses or heat by application of an electric pad is of value.

SUBCUTANEOUS PHLEBITIS OF THE BREAST AND CHEST WALL (MONDOR'S DISEASE)

This syndrome is occasionally encountered in men, but it occurs in women in about 75 percent of cases. The presenting symptom is a tender cordlike structure appearing just under the skin, extending across the upper outer quadrant of the breast toward the axilla or from the lower inner quadrant of the breast downward toward the epigastrium. The patient will usually notice slight to moderate discomfort, feel the cordlike structure, then examine herself before a mirror. On raising the arm or elevating the breast, she will notice a groovelike indentation or puckering of the skin or a raised strand, which she looks upon as evidence of cancer. Local discomfort is often called to the attention of the patient when the arm is raised, or because of the pressure of a brassière. There are no systemic disturbances, such as fever or general malaise.

The cause of the thrombophlebitis of the breast and chest wall is obscure. In some cases there is a history of injury or of a "strain" of the chest muscles. In others, the lesion may follow an operation of the breast, removal of a fibroadenoma, or biopsy.

The pathology of the lesion is that of an obliterative endophlebitis and periphlebitis. The involved vein lies in the subcutaneous tissue just beneath the skin.

On examination, one finds slight tenderness on palpation and the subcutaneous cord, which can be brought into sharp relief by elevating or depressing the breast, depending on the location of the

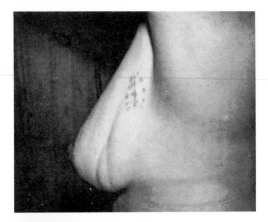

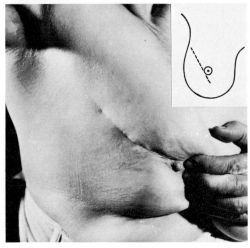

Fig. 16–1. (*Top*) Subcutaneous phlebitis of breast (Mondor's disease) 4 weeks after excision of benign breast mass. Note characteristic skin retraction. (Honig, C., and Rado, R.: Ann. Surg., *153*:589, 1961) (*Bottom*) Subcutaneous phlebitis of breast (Mondor's disease). Note method of demonstrating cord-like vein with depressed skin line due to inflammatory shortening of the skin. (Musgrove, J. E.: Canad. Med. Assoc. J., *85*:34, 1961.)

thrombosed vein. It feels like a uretheral catheter under the skin and is about 3 to 4 mm. in diameter and 15 to 25 cm. in length (Fig. 16-1).

There is little treatment necessary since the condition subsides spontaneously in 6 to 8 weeks. A well-fitted brassiere with good support may be quite helpful. In a few patients, contraction of the cord causes discomfort or apprehension. In such cases, simple division of the cord under local anesthesia will give immediate relief, and the cord will retract like an elastic band. Hot compresses have been used locally. They are of doubtful value. Antibiotics and anticoagulants have been used without demonstrable benefit.

The most important phase in the treatment of these patients is the recognition of the lesion as a benign disease that does not connote systemic disease or malignancy. Assurance of the patient usually relieves all symptoms.

ABSCESS OF THE BREAST

Etiology. Mammary abscess occurs most frequently during the early or the late stages of lactation. It frequently follows a mastitis or ordinary retention of milk secretion; or it may result from an infection which enters the nipple through a fissure or a crack.

Treatment of Superficial Abscesses. Superficial abscesses lie in the subcutaneous tissues, anterior to the breast. They may be subareolar or subcutaneous in position (Fig. 16-2). They appear as superficial reddish, tender, fluctuant areas, and are best treated conservatively by giving antibiotics and by supporting the breast and applying hot moist dressings

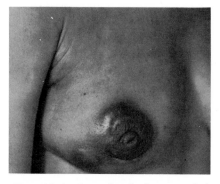

Fig. 16–2. Superficial abscess of the breast. In this case there are 2 abscesses, 1 subareolar and 1 subcutaneous.

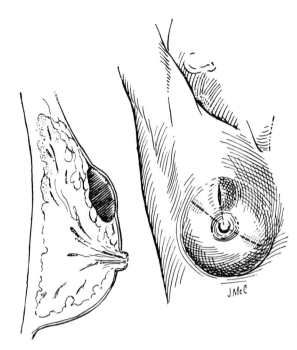

Fig. 16–3. Diagrammatic drawing of superficial abscess of the breast. Note the line of incision radiating from the nipple.

until definite fluctuation occurs. An incision radiating from the nipple is then made under line infiltration of procaine or an equivalent anesthetic (Fig. 16-3). After gently sponging or aspirating the retained purulent material, a small gauze or iodoform pack or rubber dam is inserted for drainage. Support of the breast and hot wet dressings are continued, and the packing is removed on the second or third day. Healing usually takes place rapidly.

Treatment of Intramammary Abscesses. The second type of breast abscess is located in the mammary tissue itself. These abscesses, which almost invariably follow an acute mastitis, make the breast more prominent and cause tenderness on pressure and subcutaneous edema. The tenderness is most marked over the abscess itself. Fluctuation can usually be demonstrated, although this may be more difficult to do than it is in the case of subcutaneous abscesses. With the patient under inhalation or intravenous anesthesia, the incision should be made in a line radiating from the nipple to the periphery over the most prominent part of the abscess (Fig. 16-4). After the cavity has been entered through a small incision, the finger is introduced into the opening and the cavity is explored. Usually, numerous pockets of pus are found; these are divided by septa, which may be broken up by the finger. If the exploring finger demonstrates a more dependent position for drainage, a second radiating incision should be made over that area and drainage instituted through the second wound. Rubber tube drainage is better than the use of gauze packing, although gauze may be used to pack the subcutaneous wound around the tube. Support of the breast and application of hot wet dressings are the immediate postoperative precedures; as soon as the profuse drainage subsides, the tubing may be removed and the cavity permitted to heal.

Treatment of Retromammary Abscesses. Retromammary abscess occurs on the undersurface of the breast in the areolar tissue between the breast and the chest wall. As the abscess is overlain by breast tissue, it is somewhat difficult to palpate it, but the very depth of the tenderness and the lack of definite fluctuation are aids in diagnosis. Drainage of this type of abscess is best accomplished by making an incision along the fold of the breast, usually laterally, between the chest wall and the breast itself (Fig. 16-5).

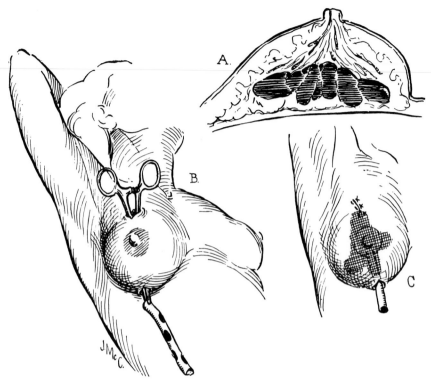

Fig. 16–4. Intramammary abscess; method of drainage with through-and-through tube insertion.

A small incision is deepened until the breast tissue is palpated with the exploring finger; the breast is then raised on the finger and the exploration is carried deeper, to the tissues underneath. When the abscess is reached, the pus escapes and the cavity is explored to determine whether there is a more dependent position for drainage. A counterincision may often be indicated. Rubber tube drainage plus packing in the superficial wound gives good results.

Postoperative Care of Breast Abscesses. All of these types of breast abscess may be taken care of in ambulatory patients. The gauze packs are usually removed on the third or the fourth postoperative day. It is well to instruct the patients to use hot compresses before they present themselves for dressings; this facilitates removal of the packing, after which none is reinserted. The rubber tube is left in place as long as there is much drainage of necrotic material; irrigations through the tube are an effective method of hastening the removal of slough and of obtaining a more rapid cleaning up of the abscess cavity. Incidentally, this method of abscess cleansing is much less painful than that of swabbing with cotton balls. A snug bandage or a tight binder is of great advantage in treating infections of the breast. The edema which occurs in large pendulous breasts often gives more postoperative discomfort than does the abscess itself; this can be largely relieved by effective support. In all of these infections of the breast, antibiotics will aid in the control of the invading organisms, and, if they are given early, may prevent the necessity for incision. If pus is present, however, incision and drainage must be carried out.

Subcutaneous Fat Necrosis of the Breast

Necrosis of the subcutaneous fatty tissue of the breast is mentioned here because it is a benign lesion, and, when a

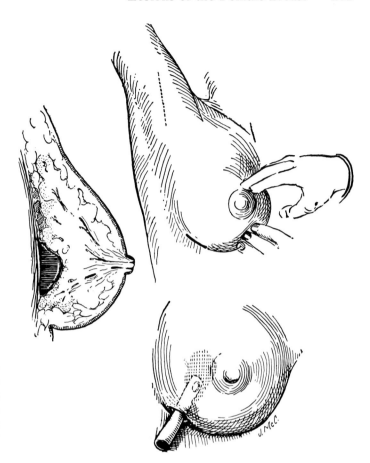

Fig. 16–5. Retromammary abscess diagrammatically shown underneath the breast. Note the line of incision in the fold of the breast and method of drainage by tubes.

definite diagnosis can be made, it can be treated easily in the ambulatory patient. However, its diagnosis often is so difficult that usually it is advisable to treat it only in a hospital or in a surgicenter attached to a hospital. The reason for this is that fat necrosis so closely simulates carcinoma that a diagnosis cannot always be made with certainty until a frozen section is obtained.

Etiology and Diagnosis. Fat necrosis of the breast occurs most often in the adipose tissue of the upper part of the breast. It may occur at any time of life, but it is more common in the fourth and the fifth decades. A history of trauma is not always obtainable, although such a history may be obtained in about 70 percent of cases.

The lesion occurs as an area of edema and eventual necrosis of the subcutaneous fatty tissues; a mass forms and may increase progressively in size. Pain and tenderness usually occur, but not in-

variably. The progressive increase in size, the firmness of the tumor, and the frequency of its adherence to the skin suggest cancer as a diagnosis. Furthermore, retraction of the nipple occurs in about 10 percent of the cases, due to involvement of the fibrous trabeculae that extend to the nipple.

Treatment. Simple excision of the traumatized area of fat and primary suture are all that is necessary if the lesion can be recognized. The extreme difficulty of making the diagnosis in these cases makes it necessary to have facilities for a frozen section at hand during operation and to be prepared for a radical amputation in case carcinoma is encountered; therefore, these patients are best hospitalized for operation. With the development of surgicenters connected to the hospital, one can proceed with this type of case with great safety, knowing that hospitalization is immediately available.

CYSTIC DISEASE OF THE BREAST

Terminology. This condition presents a varied histologic picture and is described under a host of names, the most common of which is chronic mastitis or chronic cystic mastitis. These terms are poor because they imply that the condition is inflammatory in nature, whereas present opinion is that this is not the case in most instances. The more general and descriptive term adenofibrosis is probably better.

This is a benign condition. It is the symptom of pain which focuses the patient's attention on her breast. Often the mass is not symptomatic, but is noted by the patient on breast palpation or accidentally and causes her to fear cancer.

Cystic disease is limited to the age group between puberty and the menopause. An active ovary producing estrogen must be present.

Haagensen has clearly pointed out the necessity of differentiating between gross cystic disease and microscopic cystic disease. As high as 20 percent of all women will have the microscopic changes of cystic disease. Gross cystic disease is just the presence of large and small cysts, and it is important for the surgeon to recognize this and to differentiate it from the normal variable feel of a breast, which often contains fat lobules which the inexperienced may mistake for cysts.

Symptoms and Pathology. A considerable percentage of women experience a premenstrual sense of fullness and heaviness of the breasts, with actual increase in their size. In some women they become quite tender, and shooting, stabbing, or aching pains are felt. Hyperemia of these breasts is indicated by darkening of the areola and dilatation of the superficial veins.

Cyclic mammary pain occurs, which at first is slight and premenstrual in character. It becomes more severe as time passes and finally extends throughout the cycle, though maximum intensity is reached just before the period. In the early stages, the painful, tender area is usually located in the upper outer quadrant of the breast.

The pain frequently is referred to the neck, the axilla, the shoulder, the arm, and the lateral thoracic wall.

On examination, a flat granular or nodular area of increased density can be palpated. This differs from a true tumor in that the margins cannot be felt with the breast pressed flat against the chest wall. However, when the breast is raised, a roughly circumscribed area can be outlined and often involves the whole quadrant. The nodularity at first is more marked before the menstrual period and may be almost undetectable in the interval between periods. Later, however, it persists throughout the cycle. Spontaneous regression of this condition may occur, but frequently, after a period of months or years, it will progress to the formation of cystic disease.

Histologic sections of the areas of increased density may show nothing more than edema of the perilobular connective tissue. In other cases, there is a striking increase in the fibrous tissue. On gross section, the nodular area is firm, white, and glistening. On histologic section, the adipose tissue is practically absent, and the lobules are distorted by the overgrowth of connective tissue; grandular overgrowth is also usually present.

Etiology of Cystic Disease. The etiology of cystic disease is not certain. Inflammation or obstruction of the ducts does not seem to be an adequate explanation of the pain, though the edema of the connective tissue around the lobules and the fibrosis may cause discomfort by creating pressure · and tension. The explanation most widely accepted is that it is due to an endocrine imbalance. Some believe that there is a strong psychological element in this condition.

Treatment of Cystic Disease. There is no accepted method of treatment. Many patients will improve without treatment of any kind, which makes the evaluation of any particular therapeutic measure difficult. Frequently, a well-fitting brassière that gives adequate support to the breast will afford great relief. Taylor and Robertson found that 75 percent of their patients reported improvement or cure when they were given inactive substances or when irrelevant methods of treatment were used.

Testosterone propionate has also been reported to be of value. This form of treatment is not advised since we do not know what we are treating and relief is inconstant and quite probably due to placebo effect.

Cystic disease of the breast is usually a self-limited disease and tends ultimately to regress. There is no reason to operate upon these patients, certainly not to remove the breast. The author has been guilty of removing several of the persistently tender cysts, usually because the patient feared a malignancy. These have invariably been diagnosed as adenosis or chronic mastitis. In a few cases cancer has developed in later life, as often in the opposite breast as in the affected one.

The treatment of choice for larger cysts is aspiration under local anesthesia. It is important to tell the patient that you believe this to be a cyst and that if it proves not to be, surgical excision will be necessary. It is important to tell the patient that she will probably develop new cysts in the same or the opposite breast until she reaches menopause. Because of the apparently modest association of carcinoma (often in the opposite breast) with gross cystic disease of the breast, women with gross cystic disease should be followed on a six-month basis.

ADENOSIS

A component of cystic disease is adenosis. The acini of the gland and the ducts proliferate, invade the breast stroma, and stimulate fibrosis. When adenosis presents as a pure type of epithelial proliferation, a tumor mass that is almost indistinguishable from cancer develops. This is not a common lesion, but it is most difficult to diagnose. It occurs in patients who are 20 to 55 years old. The etiology is probably the same as that of cystic disease.

Treatment. Excision of the mass is all that is required. Because the lesion close-

ly resembles cancer, excision should be done in the hospital, where a frozen section can be done.

CYSTS OF THE BREAST

Description and Diagnosis. Solitary cysts of the breast occur in the late thirties and in the forties, that is, about the time of menopause; this is a point of diagnostic importance. It is generally agreed that single or multiple simple cysts of the breast rarely develop carcinoma. There is evidence that carcinoma may develop in the intercystic portion of the breast tissue, although this rarely ever happens in the area of the original tumor itself. The cysts may appear in any portion of the breast, and, on examination, they are palpated as freely movable, firm, rounded, discrete masses. Depending upon the tenseness of the cyst, fluctuation may be easy or difficult to demonstrate. The finding of definite fluctuation and the absence of inflammatory changes usually make the diagnosis certain. Transillumination is helpful in making a diagnosis, for a cyst is clear like the surrounding breast, whereas solid tumors are dark.

Treatment. Most patients who seek treatment of a solitary cyst of the breast do so because they fear carcinoma. If the diagnosis can be made with a fair degree of certainty, a relatively conservative form of treatment may be carried out, namely, aspiration of the cyst. Aspiration thus is both a diagnostic and a therapeutic measure. It is a perfectly safe office procedure. It spares the patient the uncertainty due to delay in diagnosis, the trouble of hospitalization, and an operation on the breast. If the cyst is entered with an aspirating needle and from 5 to 10 ml. of an opalescent fluid is removed, the diagnosis is made at once, and in the majority of cases the cyst does not reappear. New cysts may appear at other sites in the same or the opposite breast; these may be treated in the same way (Fig. 16-6).

In several cases aspiration is attempted, but no fluid can be aspirated. These patients are sent to the hospital for opera-

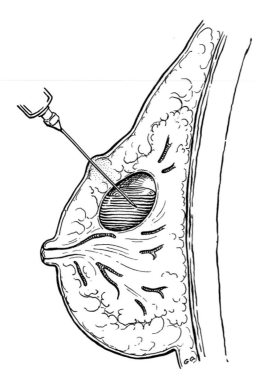

Fig. 16–6. Needle aspiration of discrete breast cyst. After introducing a wheal of cutaneous and subcutaneous local anesthesia, an 18-gauge needle with syringe attached is introduced into the cyst cavity. The cyst should be held in place with the fingers of the left hand as the needle is introduced. Occasionally there is some difficulty traversing the dense breast tissue overlying a deeply placed cyst. The cyst should be aspirated completely.

tion. In most cases the cysts are found presenting on the underside of the breast, but in others the palpable mass is found to be a fibroadenoma.

To aspirate a cyst, a wheal of local anesthesia is made over its most prominent portion, and a small incision is made through the skin with a sharp-pointed scalpel. With the cyst held firmly against the chest wall with the thumb and fingers of the left hand, an 18-gauge needle attached to a syringe is inserted through the skin opening into the cyst. Several types of fluid have been aspirated from breast cysts. If the fluid is straw colored or opalescent, a single aspiration cures the lesion in about 85 percent of the cases. If the fluid is muddy, a single aspiration does not cure nearly as high a percentage of cases. Cysts containing straw-colored fluid with floating flocculi are apt to refill no matter how many times they are aspirated. A cyst containing bloody fluid should be considered carcinomatous.

Any cysts containing bloody fluid, or those cysts which refill promptly, should be treated by more radical operation, for which hospitalization is necessary.

In many cases, because of the tenderness of the cyst and the indistinct conclusions drawn from transillumination, a solitary cyst may be operated upon rather than aspirated. Under local anesthesia, the cyst is exposed after division of the skin and the subcutaneous fatty tissues. It presents usually on the superior surface of the breast as a bluish swelling, and this appearance has given the cyst its common name, blue-dome cyst. It is usually thin walled and, when incised, is found to contain a clear, straw-colored fluid in most cases. Excision of the cyst itself is difficult, but if a small amount of surrounding breast tissue is excised with it, removal is easy. The wound is closed in layers with fine silk or catgut. Skin closure is effected with fine alloy steel wire or other nonabsorbable sutures. If one can be sure that the lesion is a simple blue-dome cyst, incision to permit the escape of the collected fluid is all that is necessary to effect a cure; the wound may then be closed and a pressure dressing applied without further effort at excision.

FIBROADENOMAS

Fibroadenomas of the breast are common tumors in females during puberty or early youth. They appear most commonly in the upper outer quadrant of the breast near the periphery; they are usually hard, freely movable, smooth masses, and, in about one third of the cases, they are painful.

Treatment. Excision under local anesthesia is easily performed. Usually, the tumor may be dissected out of its bed; the resulting dead space is obliterated by placing tiers of fine catgut or silk, and the skin is closed with silk, dermal, or fine alloy steel wire. A pressure bandage is applied. The tissue removed should be carefully examined for malignancy. Although fibroadenomas in young girls rarely show evidence of carcinomatous degeneration, in older women there have been numerous reports of malignant change. This is one reason for removing such lesions.

INTRADUCTAL PAPILLOMAS

Description. Intraductal papilloma is a tumor that usually occurs in the region of the nipple or in the mid-zone of the breast in women who are near the menopause. About half of them are accompanied by a bloody discharge from the nipple. The tumor may also be palpated as a soft, smooth or tense mass, usually freely movable; when transilluminated, it is dark. Ninety-five percent of benign papillomas occur beneath the nipple or in the mid-zone, usually just at the edge of the areola.

Treatment. Excision under local anesthesia is acceptable treatment if the tissue removed can be examined by the pathologist at an early date. Prior to excision, the duct that contains the papilloma is located by palpation, by mammography, or by noting the duct from which the bloody fluid can be expressed. A circumareolar incision extending not more than halfway around the circumference of the areola is placed in the quadrant where the duct is believed to be. Meticulous dissection is required to locate the involved duct, which is usually dilated to 2 to 3 mm. in diameter. Once it is found, it should be ligated and divided. The areolar end should be dissected out to its end in the nipple and then the proximal end followed out 4 to 5 cm into the breast by taking a modest cone of breast tissue along with the duct. After careful hemostasis, closure of the wound with fine nonabsorbable sutures and closure of the skin with fine wire or synthetic sutures complete the operation. This surgery should be done with the patient under light general anesthesia to avoid the distorting effect of a local anesthetic.

PRACTICAL POINTS IN OPERATING ON BENIGN BREAST LESIONS

There are a few practical points which have proven to be valuable in performing breast operations under local anesthesia in ambulatory patients. When the patient has been examined in the erect position, that is, with the breast dependent, it may be somewhat confusing, when the patient lies down, to find that the relative position of the mass has changed. Therefore, before the surgeon starts to scrub up, the patient should be placed on the operating table, with the hand of the affected side under the head, and the site of the tumor should be located definitely by palpation. A nurse or an assistant should hold the breast in the position in which it will be held at the time of operation. A mark in the form of a cross with indelible pencil should then be made directly over the tumor. During the operation, this is of value in locating the site of the tumor when the mass does not appear directly in the wound.

After scrubbing up, preparing the skin, and applying the drapes, the surgeon should again palpate the breast carefully while it is held in the position to be assumed during the operation. It is wise to grasp the nodule between the thumb and the index finger of the left hand while the infiltration of the skin and the subcutaneous tissues over the mass is made with the right. Then, before letting the mass go and before attempting deeper infiltration, two scratches are made on the skin—one longitudinally in the line of the proposed incision and the other transversely at the midpoint of the mass—to mark more definitely the site of the deeper mass. This precaution is taken because, when the edema due to the local infiltration is present, the mass may be less definitely palpable and therefore, more difficult to find and remove.

When the mass does not appear to have a well-defined capsule which permits its easy enucleation, it is wiser to excise the mass than to attempt further enucleation. Although the mass may be, and usually is, benign, local excision is almost as easy as enucleation and is a surer, safer method of attack. It is frequently possible to excise a wedge-shaped area from the periphery of the breast containing the tumor mass. When this is done, the edges of the breast tissue should be caught with Allis forceps as they are incised. This makes it easy to identify them when they are to be united. For suturing breast tissue, fine sutures of catgut or silk may be used on small curved cutting-edged needles; the tissue is brought together in such a manner as to obliterate the dead space left by removal of the tumor mass. Anesthesia is produced by infiltration as the operation progresses, injection being made below and around the breast tissue to block the nerves to the area involved.

Babcock has suggested an ingenious method of removing benign tumors of the breast, without leaving any scars, by making the incision along the edge of the areola. After incising the skin and the subcutaneous tissues, the dissection is carried forward between the breast and the subcutaneous fatty tissues until the tumor is reached. The tumor is then grasped by Allis forceps and brought into the wound, where it is removed by enucleation; the bleeding points are ligated and the wound is closed. This method of removing benign tumors is applicable only to those which are superficially placed and in a position close enough to the areola to permit them to be delivered through an incision at its edge.

After the operation upon the breast, a firm pressure bandage is applied, using gauze held in place by adhesive, and the whole breast is then supported by a snug bandage of gauze which completely surrounds the chest and the back. In this manner, the edema which would otherwise occur is prevented, and this greatly reduces the amount of discomfort which follows such an operation. Usually the patient is provided with from 4 to 6 tablets of morphine sulfate, gr. $1/6$ (10 mg.), to take every third hour as soon as pain appears. The wounds are dressed on the fifth day; the sutures are removed and another pressure dressing is applied. The patient does not require hospital admission.

DISEASES OF THE MALE BREAST

Tumors of the breast in the male, though less common than in the female, also deserve close attention because of the serious character which certain of them assume. Every swelling in the male breast must be treated as carefully as would a swelling in the female breast, and every breast tumor in the male must be regarded as malignant until it is proven otherwise. The male breast is subject to infections of various types and, in addition, to mastitis in all its manifestations. The latter condition is the most common of the male breast lesions.

BENIGN TUMORS

Types. Many types of benign tumors are found in the male breast: fibroma, fibroadenoma, papilloma, papillary cystadenoma, hemangioma, lipoma, sebaceous cyst, and epidermoid cyst.

Description and Symptoms. Of these, by far the most common are the fibrous tissue tumors, fibroma and fibroadenoma. The latter tumor may be either of the pericanalicular variety, in which the fibrosis occurs around the ducts and the acini, or of the intracanalicular variety, in which there is connective tissue proliferation into the lumen of the duct or the acinus. These tumors are rarely multiple and occur most frequently during adolescence and the period of the "male climacteric." They vary in consistency, but tend to be rather firm. On section, they are grayish white in color and fibrous in character. They may show cystic, myxomatous, hyaline, colloid, calcareous, ossific, or even malignant change. The entire breast may be diffusely involved in the fibrosis, or the tumor may be rather well localized, though it is never encapsulated. In most cases, there are no symptoms other than the appearance of a

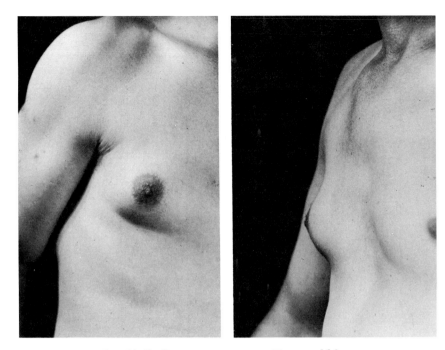

Fig. 16–7. Gynecomastia in an 18-year-old boy.

swelling in the breast. Certain patients, however, complain of a local stabbing or prickling pain and of occasional tenderness.

Diagnosis. In the early stages, the tumor is well defined, smooth, and freely movable. In older people, however, it may become adherent to the skin and surrounding tissues (pseudomalignant fixation), at times with retraction of the nipple and even palpable regional nodes. In such cases, a diagnosis can be made only by biopsy. True "orange-peel" skin is never produced by these tumors. The differential diagnosis between the fibrous tumors and other benign growths also may not be established preoperatively. This is of little consequence, however, since all benign tumors of the breast should be treated alike, that is, by excision.

The other benign tumors are also likely to be asymptomatic except for the appearance of a swelling and, perhaps, slight pain, tenderness, and occasional bleeding from the nipple.

Treatment. The treatment of all benign tumors of the breast is excision because of the fact that early malignant change cannot be determined clinically, and these tumors frequently undergo such change. If the tumor is small and well localized, it may be excised under local anesthesia. Larger and more diffuse growths require simple mastectomy, usually with sacrifice of the nipple. All such tumors should be examined immediately by the technique of frozen section, and radical mastectomy should be carried out promptly if areas of malignant change are found.

GYNECOMASTIA

Description and Etiology. Gynecomastia is a condition in which the male breast undergoes hypertrophy, so that grossly and on microscopic section it resembles the breast of an adolescent girl (Fig. 16-7). In many cases, the onset is at or shortly after puberty; in others, it occurs during senescence. It is seen occasionally in chronic alcoholics with severe

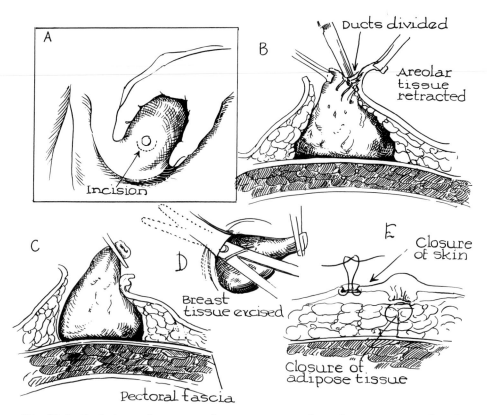

Fig. 16–8. Technique of operation for gynecomastia through an incision at the edge of the areola. (Lynch, R. C.: Plast. Reconstr. Surg., *13*:412, 1954)

liver disturbances and here can be attributed to the inadequate metabolism of estrogen by the liver. It is doubtful if trauma is an etiologic factor in the production of gynecomastia. The condition is sometimes associated with testicular tumors, such as chorionepithelioma or teratoma, and there have been reports of cases following prostatectomy. Frequently, there is atrophy of one or both testes. Some hormonal imbalance is responsible for the hypertrophy, but the exact mechanism is not yet clear.

The hypertrophy may be bilateral or, more often, unilateral. It feels like a "rubbery" button under the areola. It is concentric with the areolar border. Treves points out that this is important to note because cancer of the breast usually forms an eccentric lump.

Minor manifestations of this condition are rather common at the time of puberty, during the phase of adjustment to altered hormonal influences. In the adolescent youth, transient slight enlargement, perhaps with tenderness, frequently occurs. This condition usually disappears promptly. In the rarer, more pronounced cases, such adjustments do not occur and the condition is permanent. The overgrowth may be so striking as to be a source of embarrassment or mental anguish to the patient and may limit his activities. For cosmetic reasons alone, therefore, treatment may be demanded. Gynecomastia in itself is a benign condition, and some consider it harmless. Treves, investigating a large series of patients with gynecomastia, found not a single instance in which breast cancer subsequently occurred. He states, "We think other investigators may erroneously consider gynecomastia a precancerous lesion."

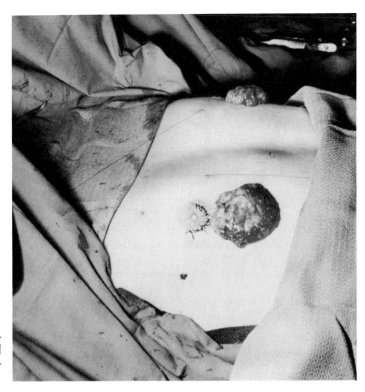

Fig. 16–9. Bilateral gynecomastia treated by removal through a circumareolar incision.

Diagnosis. Gynecomastia must be differentiated from a localized excess of fat or lipoma in the region of the breast. The latter is usually bilateral and soft, with no palpable enlargement of mammary tissue. (It is usually removed surgically for cosmetic reasons.)

Treatment. Treves reports that in 115 patients with gynecomastia complete regression occurred without any treatment. In some cases simple mastectomy has been the method of treatment. The operation may be performed under local anesthesia through an incision made along the lower half of the edge of the areola (Figs. 16-8 and 16-9). This incision may be extended medially and laterally if desired. After separation of the nipple and the subcutaneous tissues from the breast, the breast tissue is brought into the wound from below and is freed from its lateral and mesial attachment as it is turned up from the pectoral fascia. Bleeding is controlled by applying a pressure dressing after suture of the wound. It is wise to introduce a small rubber drain before wound closure.

BIBLIOGRAPHY

Breast Cyst

Farrow, J. H.: Gross mammary cysts. CA, *9*:163, 1959.

Gaspare, M. R.: Aspiration of breast cysts. Calif. Med., *95*:227, 1961.

Hendrick, J. W.: Results of treatment of cystic disease of the breast. Surgery, *44*:457, 1958.

Johnston, J. H., Jr.: Aspiration as diagnostic and therapeutic procedure in cystic disease of the breast. Ann. Surg., *139*:635, 1954.

Rosemond, G. P., Burnett, W. E., Caswell, H. T., and McAleer, D. J.: Aspiration of breast cysts as a diagnostic and therapeutic measure. Arch. Surg., *71*:223, 1955.

Southwick, H. W., Slaughter, D. P., and Humphrey, L. J.: Surgery of the Breast. Chicago, Year Book Medical Publishers, 1968.

Gynecomastia

Lynch, R. C.: An operation for correction of

gynecomastia through an areolar incision. Plast. Reconstr. Surg., 13:412, 1954.

Treves, N.: Gynecomastia, the origins of mammary swelling in the male: an analysis of 406 patients with breast hypertrophy, 525 patients with testicular tumors, and 13 with adrenal neoplasms. Cancer, 11:1083, 1958.

Vernon, S.: Plastic correction of gynecomastia. Plast. Reconstr. Surg., 26:735, 1956.

Moss, N. H.: Cancer of the male breast. Ann. NY Acad. Sci., 114:937, 1964.

Lesions of the Nipple

Atkins, H., and Wolff, B.: Management of nipple discharges. Brit. J. Surg., 51:602, 1964.

Babcock, W. W.: The removal of benign tumors of the breast without visible scars. Surgery, 5:226, 1939.

Copeland, M. M., and Higgins, T. G.: Significance of discharge from the nipple in nonpuerperal mammary conditions. Ann. Surg., 151:638, 1960.

Crile, G., Jr.: Minor surgery for diseases of the nipple and areola. Consultant, 1:24, 1961.

Farrow, J. H.: Benign and malignant lesions of the nipple. Cancer, 8:16, 1958.

Gray, H. K., and Wood, G. A.: Significance of mammary discharge in cases of papilloma of the breast. Arch. Surg., 42:203, 1941.

Hicken, N. F., Best, R. R., and Hunt, H. B.: Discharges from the nipple. Arch. Surg., 35:1079, 1937.

Madalin, H. E., Clagett, O. T., and McDonald, J. R.: Lesions of the breast associated with discharge from the nipple. Ann. Surg., 146:751, 1957.

Taylor, H. B., and Robertson, A. G.: Adenomas of the nipple. Cancer, 18:995, 1965.

Fat Necrosis

Lee, B. J., and Adair, F. E.: Traumatic fat necrosis of the female breast and its differentiation from cancer. Ann. Surg., 71:188, 1920.

Thrombophlebitis of the Breast and Chest Wall

Farrow, J. H.: Thrombophlebitis of the superficial veins of the breast and anterior chest wall (Mondor's disease). Surg., Gynec. Obstet., 101:63, 1955.

Honig, C., and Rado, R.: Mondor's disease—superficial phlebitis of the chest wall. Ann. Surg., 153:589, 1961.

Johnson, W. C., Wallrich, R., and Helwig, E. B.: Superficial thrombophlebitis of the chest wall. JAMA, 180:103, 1962.

Kaufman, P. A.: Subcutaneous phlebitis of the breast and chest wall. Ann. Surg., 144:847, 1956.

Musgrove, J. E.: Subcutaneous phlebitis of the breast (Mondor's disease). Canadian Med. Assoc. J., 85:34, 1961.

Cystic Disease of the Breast

Cutler, M.: The cause of "painful breasts" and treatment by means of ovarian residue. JAMA, 96:1201, 1931.

Goodman, B. A.: Fibrocystic disease of the breast. Arch. Surg., 38:917, 1939.

Lewis, D., and Geschickter, C. F.: Endocrine therapy in chronic cystic mastitis. JAMA, 109:1894, 1937.

Lewis, D.: Ovarian hormones in relation to chronic cystic mastitis. Am. J. Surg., 24:280, 1934.

Nathanson, I. T., Meigs, J. V., and Parsons, L.: Treatment of mammary pain and secretion with testosterone propionate. New Eng. J. Med., 226:487, 1942.

Tumors

Babcock, W. W.: The removal of benign tumors of the breast without visible scars. Surgery, 5:226, 1939.

Geschickter, C. F.: Mammary tumors. Surgery, 3:916, 1938.

Horsely, J. S., Jr.: Benign and malignant lesions of the male breast. Ann. Surg., 109:912, 1939.

Mammography

Gershon-Cohen, J., and Ingleby, H.: Roentgenography of cysts of the breast. Surg., Gynec. Obstet., 97:483, 1953.

Gershon-Cohen, J., and Yiu, L. S.: Mammography of thrombophlebitis. Surgery, 53:657, 1963.

Gershon-Cohen, J., and Ingleby, H.: Roentgenography of unsuspected carcinoma of breast. JAMA, 166:869, 1958.

———: Roentgen survey of asymptomatic breasts. Surgery, 43:409, 1958.

Witten, D. M.: Mammography. Postgrad. Med., 36:242, 1964.

Breast Wounds

Myers, M. B.: Wound tension and vascularity in the etiology and prevention of skin sloughs. Surgery, 56:945, 1964.

17
Abdomen

Luis F. Sala, M.D.

Most surgical diseases of the abdomen are intraperitoneal and require hospitalization for their treatment. However, there are diseases of the abdominal wall or abdomen which can be treated in the ambulatory patient. It behooves one to determine the difference.

CONTUSIONS OF THE ABDOMEN

Etiology and Symptoms. Contusions of the abdominal wall are caused by blows; steering wheels and dashboards are increasingly implicated. Usually the injury is a simple bruise of the abdominal musculature which results in ecchymosis and pain on movement of the muscles, especially on coughing, sneezing, and straining. This may occur without changes in the overlying skin. By itself straining may rupture a muscle, and this may cause much pain and rigidity.

Diagnosis and Treatment. The diagnosis of superficial injuries can easily be made by the tenderness and the pain elicited when the muscles are used against resistance. If all the symptoms are due to simple contusion of the abdominal muscles, the injury may be well treated by adhesive strapping, analgesics, and rest. If soreness persists, infiltration of a local anesthetic often gives a more rapid relief of discomfort.

However, in diagnosing abdominal wall injuries, the examiner must be aware of the danger of concurrent intra-abdominal injury; for this reason, any severe contusion of the abdominal wall is best treated by hospitalization. Pain, particularly pain which increases, distension, nausea, and vomiting are dangerous signs. A rising white blood cell count, lack of peristalsis, and gas not being expelled by rectum also cause concern. A flat plate of the abdomen, taken with the patient erect, for the detection of distended bowel is necessary.

The same observations apply to flank wounds, which may lead to retroperitoneal hemorrhage.

A disturbance that initially seems minor and superficial such as a small stab wound, may be a potentially catastrophic situation.

HERNIA

As a rule, hernia is a lesion requiring operation. Hospitalization is now not always necessary. Many a time, with expert and judicious administration of local or general anesthesia, bed occupation, not necessarily in the hospital as such, may be limited to but a few hours. Hernia repairs in many infants and children, and even selected repairs in appropriately screened adults, may be carried out on a nonhospitalized basis. There are times, however, when operation is contraindicated or when the patient does not wish it. In such cases, ambulatory care may call for truss therapy.

Truss Therapy. A truss is a pad held over the hernial orifice with enough pressure to prevent the abdominal contents from entering the hernial sac. A requirement of the truss is that it keep the hernia reduced through the stresses and strains of ordinary life. The use of a truss should be considered at best a temporary measure in most instances, unless surgery is contraindicated.

The hernias that are most amenable to truss treatment are those of the inguinal type, as they present themselves through an area of the abdominal wall that does not move and at a site where adequate pressure may be applied to maintain reduction.

A truss should not be applied to a hernia that is not completely reducible.

Injection Treatment of Hernia. The injection treatment of hernia is mentioned only to be condemned.

TYPES OF HERNIA

Indirect Inguinal Hernia. This type may appear at any age. The sac of the hernia is the processus vaginalis peritonei, which descends into the scrotum with the testis in fetal life. Normally, this process is obliterated at birth, only the distal portion of it remaining as the tunica vaginalis of the testis. In females, the processus vaginalis descends to the labium majus with the round ligament of the uterus.

In infants and young children, the history (usually given by the mother) is very often the determining factor in the diagnosis.

The mother or the nurse notes the enlargement of the scrotal sac or groin on one or both sides; this is much more evident when the sac is distended by increased abdominal pressure, such as that due to crying. The diagnosis is made by inspection, palpation, and the history. Almost invariably, these hernias are reducible, but they occasionally become

incarcerated. The simple expedient of injecting a small amount of a suitable contrast medium into the peritoneal cavity, holding the infant erect for about five minutes, and taking x-ray films may give positive evidence—by the collection of the radiopaque material in the sac.

If a truss is used, it must retain the hernia under all conditions and must be comfortable, nonirritating, sanitary, and easy to apply correctly.

The treatment of indirect inguinal hernia is surgical. In infants and young children, a high ligation of the sac suffices. Adults require fascial layer reconstruction besides elimination of the sac. Many children and healthy adults with uncomplicated hernias and without complicating factors (obesity, concurrent diseases, etc.) can be operated upon in a minimal-stay facility, which makes the procedure to all effects one of "ambulatory surgery." Their time in this minimal-stay facility is measured in terms of hours, not days. Competency in the management of anesthesia, local or general or both in combination, must be insured.

Direct Inguinal Hernia. These are rarely complicated by incarceration or strangulation, and, if they are without symptoms, no treatment is necessary. If pain or discomfort is a symptom, there usually has been a tear in the weakened transversalis fascia, with the protrusion through this opening of preperitoneal fat. Trusses may be applied for support, but they frequently do not give symptomatic relief. Surgical repair is usually a relatively simple matter and can be accomplished on a nearly ambulatory basis. Relief of urinary obstruction and/or of chronic constipation could well ameliorate the degree of herniation and the symptoms attributed thereto.

Femoral Hernia. Trusses are not advised even as an optional treatment for femoral hernia. Surgery must be performed, and the repair is not an ambulatory procedure. The incidence of complications of this type of hernia is relatively high.

Umbilical Hernia. In infants, such hernias often disappear spontaneously within the first two years of life, without treatment. Those that persist in childhood and in youth, or that are too large from the outset, are best treated by operation. For the acquired umbilical hernia seen usually in late mid-life in obese patients, an abdominal supporting belt with an "umbilical pad" is sometimes used, although it is doubtful if much other than abdominal support is thus accomplished. Surgery is simple and can be carried out under local anesthesia on a nearly ambulatory basis.

Epigastric Hernia. This is the outpouching of a preperitoneal fat through a small stomal fascial defect in the midline. It is mushrooming preperitoneal fat. The repair consists of reduction and/or amputation, hemostasis, and simple fascial closure. There is no peritoneum or sac involved. These hernias are often multiple, and a longitudinal midline incision affords the opportunity for inspection of adjacent midline areas to determine whether other such herniations are present. These hernias may be confused with lipomata and often accompany umbilical hernias. A glob of not-so-normal-looking fat appearing adjacent to an umbilical hernial sac could well be an epigastric hernia.

Incisional Hernia. This lesion is usually a complex surgical problem, the solution of which has been considerably abetted by the advent of nonreactive prosthetic mesh implants. Supporting belts of elastic or webbing, with a pad so placed as to give added pressure over the hernial opening, may afford temporary, symptomatic relief. A longstanding incisional hernia with symptoms of short duration may indicate that disease other than the hernia itself is causing the presenting symptoms. This is not an "ambulatory surgery" situation.

AFTER CARE OF AMBULATORY PATIENTS

After many operative procedures, much of the postoperative care can be given on an ambulatory basis after the patient leaves the hospital. Knowledgeable physicians may thus significantly contribute to shortening hospital stays.

In many cases, removal of sutures, simple inspection of a healing wound, and dressing are all that is required. In other cases, continuing care is necessary, and suggestions are made below for handling such cases.

CARE OF DRAINING ABDOMINAL WOUNDS

After drainage of intra-abdominal sites of inflammation, such as appendiceal abscess or ruptured diverticulum, and after many other abdominal operations, patients who require further care and dressings as ambulatory patients are often discharged from the hospital.

Most of these cases require only simple dressings, wound toilet using sterile gauzes, a protective ointment such as zinc oxide ointment in areas where wound secretions have produced maceration, and an absorbent dressing, thick enough to absorb the wound secretions. Female sanitary pads are most suitable to this end. Skin protectors include the time-tested tincture of benzoin, which, applied to skin, affords not only protection but also, after having been allowed to dry, a base for applying adhesive tape without disturbing the skin itself. Spray-on, silicone-based protectors have also been developed.

Sterile precautions, including the wearing of sterile gloves, are important to the patient and to the physician. Disposable plastic bags can be used to receive and dispose of contaminated material for the sake of sterility, cleanliness, and avoiding offensive odours.

Antiseptic solutions applied locally add nothing, and if noxious to cells may impede rather than hasten healing. In cases in which there are deep drainage tracts or areas of sloughing tissue, mechanical cleansing by scissors-and-scalpel débridement and the use of normal saline irrigations are of value. Plastic bulb syringes are ideal for this purpose. When the wound is free of slough and is healthy, it may be worthwhile to approxi-

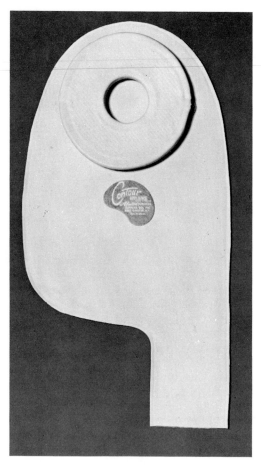

Fig. 17-1. Ileostomy bag showing spoutlike dependent opening for drainage, to be closed with a rubber band when the appliance is worn. This bag has a malleable mesh face plate that can be made to fit irregularities in the abdominal wall. (United Surgical Supplies Co., Inc.)

mate the skin edges with adhesive strips applied to the skin across the long axis of the wound, or even to consider a secondary closure.

It is very important to provide the patient with optimum nutrition at these times. Vitamins, minerals (including zinc), proteins, and calories in abundance are needed. Anabolics may be useful adjuncts.

Foci of infection should be sought and eliminated. The most common source of a persistent infection is the reservoir to which the reduced sinus outlet does not permit adequate free drainage. When this situation is recognized, adequate drainage should be provided. A little local anesthesia and the introduction of a scalpel blade through the sinus should suffice in most instances. Should the sinuses recur, connecting the various stomata present at times becomes necessary. Radiographic visualization of sinuses and recesses is often helpful. Foreign bodies are frequently at fault. Sequestra are in a true sense foreign bodies. Injection of the sinuses at surgery with a dye such as methylene blue has saved the author much time in the identification of errant sinuses, and also much embarrassment.

CARE OF THE AMBULATORY PATIENT AFTER ILEOSTOMY

An ileostomy, to function properly, must project about 2 cm. above the skin surface in the center of a smooth area of skin which will permit the facing of a collecting bag to lie flat upon it. The bag facing is a disc that surrounds the stoma. It is about 3 inches in diameter and is held in place by cement applied to the skin around the stoma and the bag facing. The collecting bag or pouch hangs from the facing, and the whole appliance is held firmly in place with a snug elastic webbing belt, which encircles the body and is attached to hooks on the facing. The usual pouch has a spoutlike opening, which can be closed securely or opened to empty its contents (Fig. 17-1).

The secret of success with an ileostomy is the collection of the secretions from the ileum without leakage. These secretions, which contain digestive enzymes in high concentrations, produce marked excoriation if they are permitted contact with the skin. To avoid leakage, the opening in the disc should fit snugly about the stoma. Its diameter should be about $1/8$ inch greater than the exact diameter of the stoma. This measurement is easily made using the plastic sheet with measured holes provided by appliance manufacturers.

The cement used to hold the disc to the skin adheres only to a clean dry surface.

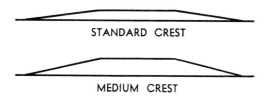

STANDARD CREST

MEDIUM CREST

FLAT PLATE

Fig. 17–2. Types of face plates available for ileostomy bags. The shape is maintained by a thin sheet of brass vulcanized in the rubber facing. (United Surgical Supplies Co., Inc.)

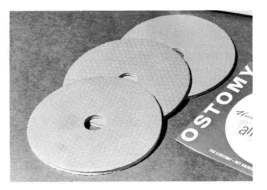

Fig. 17–3. Closed-pore foam rubber pads for use between abdominal skin and facing when the abdominal skin is not flat. (United Surgical Supplies Co., Inc.)

Hence, the skin about the stoma and the bag facing is carefully cleaned and dried before the cement is applied, with the finger, to the skin and the disc in two very thin coats. To avoid irritation from the cement solvent, each coat should dry thoroughly in the air. A thin coat dries more rapidly than a thick coat, and, to form a leakproof bond, the cement should be dry, but sticky. The stoma is then inserted through the opening in the disc, and the facing is pressed firmly in place against the skin. So applied, the bag should form a perfect seal, which should hold without leakage for at least 24 hours. (Many patients wear their appliances day and night without change for 4 to 5 days.) The appliance should be comfortable and should allow complete freedom of movement.

Problems of the Patient with an Ileostomy

Skin Excoriation. If the seal between the facing of the bag and the skin is imperfect, the ileal contents will escape and bathe the skin around the stoma, producing a painful redness and blistering or weeping. This difficulty may be due to several causes.

1. The improperly placed disc may impinge upon the anteriosuperior iliac spine, and the seal is broken by movement of the patient. In such cases, an appliance with a disc of smaller diameter, or one with a flexible rubber disc, should be obtained.

2. The contour of the abdominal wall may require variations in the shape of the disc. Large soft abdomens require a bag facing with considerable convexity to provide the pressure around the stoma which will give a secure and lasting seal. In patients with a thin or a firm muscular abdomen, the facing should have a minimum of convexity or may be entirely flat (Fig. 17-2).

3. When the abdominal skin is not flat, because of scars or for other reasons, pads made of closed-pore foam rubber may be used between the skin and the bag facing. The foam pad, $1/8$ to $1/4$ inch thick, is cemented to the skin about the stoma, and the facing cemented to the pad. The foam pad bends but does not wrinkle, and adapts itself to the contour of the skin to give a secure seal (Fig. 17-3).

4. Difficulties with the placing of the stoma, or its shape, or a fistula through the ileostomy at the skin level, make it difficult for the ileostomy to deliver the intestinal contents into the collecting bag. (The fistula usually occurs as a result of an erosion of the projecting ileostomy by the edge of the disc opening.) A more convex facing and a thin disc at the stomal opening are measures that can be tried to prevent the escape of intestinal contents. In most cases a revision of the

ileostomy is necessary. This requires hospital admission.

Treatment of Skin Irritation. Most patients who have been operated upon for ulcerative colitis come to surgery in a poor nutritional state. The skin is soft and reacts violently to an irritant. Tincture of benzoin is often applied to protect and harden the skin. The irritant most commonly encountered is the hydrocarbon solvent used in the cement that holds the appliance to the skin. If the solvent is not allowed to evaporate completely before the bag is applied, it is trapped between the skin and the bag facing; this causes vesiculation of the skin. If the bag is removed too rapidly or too frequently, the outer layers of the skin may be pulled off, resulting in a red, weeping surface. In this type of weeping skin irritation, the cement will not hold securely, and seepage of intestinal contents underneath the bag facing adds to the irritation. In such cases the skin is cleansed with ether and lightly dusted with karaya gum powder (Pratex, Derma-guard). The karaya powder and the watery exudate or added water form a thin gummy mixture which is densely adherent to the weeping areas. The cement is then applied as usual and the bag put in place. In most cases the skin irritation heals. Some patients use karaya gum routinely. Aluminum hydroxide gel has been used instead of water with karaya powder in a combination known as Neokaraya. It reduces the burning sensation and seems to increase the healing potentialities of karaya, and forms a leathery covering which sticks to the skin as well as does the water-gum mixture. It may be better in those cases who have an allergic reaction to the cement.

In advanced cases it may be wise to stop using the cement for a time, using instead a soothing ointment on the skin (hydrocortisone, Desitin, Kerodex). A thin layer of gauze or a foam pad (see above) is fitted around the stoma. The pouch is then applied and held firmly with a tight belt. When the skin has healed sufficiently, the application of cement may be started again. Adequate nutrition, with emphasis on Vitamin C and zinc, should be provided.

Painful Granulations and Granulomata. Painful granulations may form in the skin under the bag facing. These are especially painful when peristaltic movement pulls upon the skin as intestinal contents are discharged. Electrodesiccation of the granulations after infiltrating a local anesthetic under the skin gives relief of the pain. A karaya powder dressing is then used over the desiccated area until healing occurs (see above). Ten percent silver nitrate solution may be used to control these granulations; the patient himself may apply the silver nitrate on a daily basis.

When the leakage of intestinal contents onto the skin has been neglected over many months, granulomata may form (Fig. 17-4); these prevent the proper application of a collecting bag, so that there is continuous leakage. These patients must be hospitalized for treatment.

Difficulties with the Ileostomy Itself.

1. The appearance of blood on the ileostomy is usually due to irritation of the stoma by its pressing against the bag. This is not serious, and the traumatized mucosa usually heals without treatment.

2. Wartlike granulations may appear about the stoma. These also are due to irritation of the stoma by its rubbing against the collecting bag. They are not important, but their appearance worries the patient. They can be destroyed, without anesthesia, by electrodesiccation or by touching them with a silver nitrate stick. If they recur, it may be well to shift from a rubber bag appliance to one using disposable polyethylene or Saran pouches.

3. Discomfort is caused frequently when the stoma is too long (more than 1 1/2 inches) and presses against the rubber pouch. Here again, a shift to an appliance using polyethylene or Saran pouches is worthwhile.

4. Prolapse of the ileostomy is due to an intussusception of the ileum at the stoma. The prolapse is into the collecting bag, and the gut rapidly becomes edematous beyond the ring of the disc. The

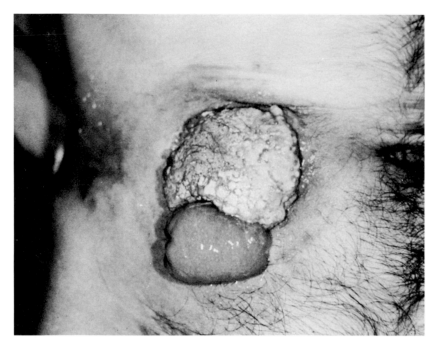

Fig. 17–4. Large granuloma at ileostomy; the result of chronic leakage of intestinal contents onto the abdominal skin.

patient should lie down flat on his back and elevate the bag with its contained prolapse. The prolapse will reduce itself in many cases without further treatment. In other cases the bag can be carefully removed and the prolapse gradually reduced with the fingers.

Once the prolapse occurs, it is prone to recur. An appliance with a flat disc and a tight elastic girdle or waistband over it may be tried as a conservative measure, but experience has shown that once prolapse takes place it most often becomes a chronic disability. The patient should be hospitalized for revision of the ileostomy.

5. Retraction of the ileostomy so that it does not project above the abdominal skin is due to inadequate fixation of the ileum to the abdominal wall and skin. The stoma usually projects when the patient is on his feet, but retracts when he lies down. The retraction makes it difficult for the intestinal contents to enter the bag. If a convex disc does not give a satisfactory result, a revision of the ileostomy will be necessary.

6. Stricture of the ileostomy may be at skin or fascial level. Diligent daily digital dilatation by the patient himself is the best prophylaxis. Slitting the skin and the fascia under local anesthesia remedies more advanced situations. Dilatation by the patient should be taught and established.

7. Hernia may occur about the stoma. This can be often controlled by modifying the ileostomy bag and its support to provide a truss effect. Surgery may have to be resorted to.

Sensitivity. Sensitivity to the compounds of which collecting bags are made or to the rubber in the cement is a difficulty encountered occasionally. In these cases a skin reaction is produced much like that seen occasionally with adhesive. The reaction may outline the shape of the bag where it has come in contact with the skin (Fig. 17-5). A trial with other bags or cements may hit upon a rubber compound which does not contain the chemical irritant to which the patient is sensitive. For those sensitive to the cement the

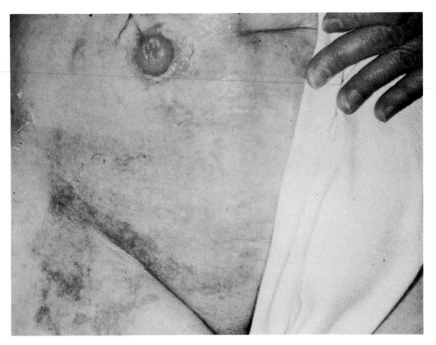

Fig. 17–5. Sensitivity to rubber ileostomy bag. Note outline of the bag on the abdominal skin. This reaction did not subside when the bag was enclosed in a cloth pouch.

use of double-faced adhesive discs of nonirritating material similar to the nonirritating tape produced by the 3 M Company may be of value. A shift to an all-plastic appliance is often the answer.

Odor. The intestinal contents discharged from the ileostomy are at first liquid and then become semisoft as the ileum takes over some of the water-absorbing function of the resected colon. The discharge is relatively odorless. Even the gas which passes from the stoma is practically odorless. It is composed largely of swallowed air. Some foods, such as eggs, fish, etc., may create a stomal discharge which has an unusual and offensive odor. Usually there is no odor from the ileostomy or the appliance that can be detected by others, even those in close contact. This is attested to by the number of patients who hold jobs demanding personal contact, such as hairdressers, bank clerks, salesmen and saleswomen, etc. If odor is a problem with an ileosto-my, it usually reflects a lack of personal hygiene or neglect of bag care. Good care of the appliance is probably the best way to avoid odors. Rubber bags gradually take on an odor if they are not carefully cleaned and dried between applications. Patients who are interested have found ways to remove bag odors. Detergents, scrubbing, and drying answer most of these problems.

Some patients have found that chlorophyll tablets (100 mg.) taken by mouth or, better, inserted into the bag give good control of odor. The number of tablets to be used varies from patient to patient. Some patients use as many as 2 tablets 3 times daily.

Bismuth subgallate has been used effectively to combat ileostomy odor by some patients. About one third of a teaspoon taken at mealtime is the usual method of administration.

Diet. An ileostomy discharges the intestinal contents of the small gut, liquid to semisoft in consistency, and often containing what appears to be undigested food. The undigested foods are mostly vegetables with tough outside skins, such as corn, peas, beans, etc. Soft low residue foods, such as meats, eggs, cheeses of all kinds, sugars, and ground cereals (farina), and liquids are easily digested and absorbed. As a rule, a patient with an ileostomy can eat a rather varied general diet without difficulty. High residue foods can be eaten without restriction if too much is not taken at a time and if they are well chewed. The patient must bear in mind that large masses of undigested high roughage food may have some difficulty passing through the stoma. The patient must experiment with these foods, one at a time, to find out whether or not they can be tolerated.

The patient with an ileostomy usually was maintained on a low residue, high calorie diet for many weeks or months before his operation. After the ileostomy and colectomy, when he finds he can eat a normal diet, he often "goes overboard" on his diet, eats everything in larger amounts, and, as a consequence, gains weight rapidly, so that obesity may become a problem. The physician should aim for a return to a normal nutritional state but should caution against overeating and overweight, as these will affect the ileostomy and the patient.

If an "ostomy" club is available, the patient should be urged to join. The experience and comfort gained will be well worth the effort.

CARE OF THE AMBULATORY PATIENT WITH A LEFT-SIDED COLOSTOMY

Although most patients with a colostomy are taught how to take care of their stoma before they leave the hospital, there are always some minor problems which arise for which the advice of a physician is sought.

The ideal colostomy would be one which evacuates formed feces at a regular time every day or every two days. This ideal situation is occasionally developed by patients who have been taught the physiologic working of the large bowel. There are available teaching guides (Mini-guide, United Surgical Supplies Co. Inc.) which are very helpful in explaining about the anatomy of "ostomies" to patients. Most important, the patient should know that the bowel is evacuated by a rush of peristaltic action which is stimulated by distention of the gut. If the patient understands this mechanism of the normal working of the bowel, he can occasionally so regulate his diet that he can develop a routine for stomal evacuation, much as is possible for rectal evacuation. Each day, usually after breakfast, the patient may, by straining his abdominal muscles as though he were having a normal bowel movement, empty his left colon into a kidney basin. The feces are flushed away in the toilet. This system requires a period of training over several months, and many patients never take the time or effort to develop this type of control.

The patient should further be instructed that the colostomy stoma may tend to constrict if not dilated by finger insertion on a nearly daily basis.

Most patients with a colostomy regulate evacuation of the colon by irrigations. These act as does the common enema to distend the gut, and so stimulate a peristaltic rush which will empty the colon. The aim is to evacuate the fecal material that has collected in the colon. The bulk of the fecal residue (the diet) determines how frequently irrigations should be taken to keep the left colon empty. This varies from patient to patient. Some patients find that daily irrigations are necessary. Others irrigate only at two-day or even three-day intervals. No fecal material should escape from the stoma between irrigations, except for a minimal staining. Colonic mucus which appears at the stoma is a normal secretion of the colonic mucosa. There should be no necessity for wearing a bag.

For irrigations the patient should be seated on the toilet. The apparatus necessary for irrigation has usually been recommended and obtained before the patient leaves the hospital. It usually con-

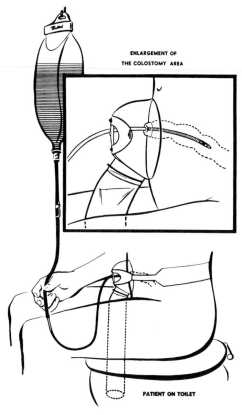

ENLARGEMENT OF
THE COLOSTOMY AREA

PATIENT ON TOILET

Fig. 17–6. Binkley-Deddish type of colostomy irrigation apparatus. This consists of a transparent plastic cup to which a plastic sleeve, which leads into the toilet, is attached. The cup has an opening through which the irrigation catheter can be passed into the stoma. The opening can be closed when the colon empties. The apparatus is held in place with an elastic belt. (United Surgical Supplies Co., Inc.)

should be filled, and the air evacuated from the tubing. The reservoir should be about 24 to 30 inches above the level of the stoma, or about shoulder high when the patient is sitting on the toilet (Fig. 17-6). The #24 rubber catheter, lubricated with soap, mineral oil, or water-soluble jelly, is then inserted into the stoma for a distance of 6 to 8 inches as the fluid begins to run. The height of the reservoir above the stoma regulates the pressure and the rate of flow of the fluid. Too rapid a flow distends the bowel too rapidly and stimulates bowel contractions prematurely, causing cramps and, often, evacuation of a part of the injected fluid before all of it has been given. When a cramp starts to occur, the flow of fluid should be stopped, then slowly continued when the cramp disappears.

The aim is to slowly fill and distend the colon, so that the bowel will be stimulated to produce an evacuation. The colon contents are discharged via the plastic sleeve into the toilet when the bowel feels "full." The irrigation may be repeated until the discharge is fairly clean. The amount of fluid to be used varies from patient to patient as experience dictates; from one pint to one or two quarts is the usual amount. If too much fluid is used, it spills over into the right colon and cecum, where it may be trapped and absorbed; or, later, it may be discharged from the stoma at an inopportune time. To guard against an accident, many patients fold the discharge sleeve and wear it as a pouch for a time after an irrigation, until they are sure further evacuation will not take place.

Irrigation of a colostomy demands a routine that each patient must develop for himself. A regular time should be selected; after breakfast or after dinner at night is the time most frequently chosen. After meals peristalsis is more active, and this may shorten the evacuation time, which usually is from 45 minutes to an hour. After the evacuation of the feces and fluid, there should be almost no discharge from the stoma until time for the next irrigation. A cotton pad or tissue can be placed over the stoma to absorb the small amount of mucus which normally es-

sists of a plastic sleeve that leads into the toilet and is attached to a ring that fits over the stoma; an elastic belt, which holds the ring in place; and a water reservoir, connected by a tube with a shutoff on it to a #24 rubber catheter. The fluid used should be warm and may be tap water, preferably with a teaspoonful of salt dissolved in each quart of water, which renders the water somewhat isotonic. Cardiac patients may have to avoid this sodium ion. The irrigation bag capes. After the irrigation, the skin around the stoma should be thoroughly cleansed with soap and water and protected with a simple ointment. There are ointments especially prepared for this purpose that have proved useful (Uniguard, Fuller Lab.; Ostomy Skin Cream, United Surgical Supplies); these are compounded of petrolatum, stearates, lanolin, and silicone. Waterproof plastic or Saran wrap over the stoma area protects the clothes. This type of dressing is best held in place with an elastic girdle or with the wide elastic band available with some types of jock straps and men's shorts.

Difficulties with Colostomies Seen in Ambulatory Patients

Blood on the Dressing. This is almost always due to rubbing of the stomal mucosa by the dressing. Sometimes some ointment, petroleum jelly or mineral oil, is applied to the dressing before replacing the girdle or belt. If there is more than a minimal amount of blood, or if blood appears with the feces during irrigation, there is cause for concern. Palpation with the gloved finger through the stoma may disclose a polyp or other lesion, or perhaps an endoscopic examination through the stoma after irrigation may visualize a lesion which may demand further operative treatment. Certainly, frank blood appearing at the stoma demands adequate study (x-ray), and usually hospitalization is necessary.

Difficulty Inserting the Irrigation Catheter. This may be due to a blocking of the bowel above the stoma by formed feces. If the tip of the catheter is introduced into the stoma and the stoma is pinched snugly around the catheter with the fluid running, the bowel will distend around the fecal mass. In many cases the catheter may then be advanced; in other cases, the terminal hard fecal mass will be evacuated and the irrigation may then be continued.

Sometimes it seems impossible to pass the catheter because it seems to meet an obstruction. Usually the tip of the catheter is caught in a haustral fold because the direction of the catheter is not in line with the axis of the bowel. It is often possible to determine the direction of the bowel by inserting a finger covered with a rubber finger cot into the stoma. Once the position of the bowel lumen has been determined, it is usually possible to pass the catheter.

Hernia. The area around the stoma appears to bulge when the stoma functions. This is usually due to herniation beside the colon brought out as the colostomy. The contents of the hernia may be the colon proximal to the stoma, or omentum, or small gut. When the colon herniates, it advances from its original position into the subcutaneous tissues between the skin and the fascial layer of the abdominal wall. This may be the cause of difficulty in inserting the catheter. Whether or not operative repair will be necessary depends upon how much trouble such a hernia causes. A firm elastic belt may give the support needed for conservative treatment.

Contracture. The tissues about the stoma have contracted so that the opening is so small it will hardly admit the catheter, and evacuation is difficult. This occurs occasionally in colostomies of some years' duration. Attempts at dilation of the stoma are painful and usually unsuccessful. In such cases, after a thorough cleansing with soap and water, the stoma may be surrounded by 1 percent procaine solution, the skin and the scar being infiltrated. An incision then is made about $1/2$ inch from the stomal opening through the skin and the scar. The cut edge of the skin around the stoma is grasped with Allis forceps and is cut away from the bowel wall. It is important to cut away all of the scar with the skin edge. The end of the colon is grasped with Allis forceps as it is freed from the scar, until the entire end of the colon is free. About 8 sutures are then placed through the skin and the entire thickness of the wall of the bowel. Almost no bleeding is encountered with this operation. A simple dressing is applied. The operation may easily be performed on an ambulatory patient.

Noise, Passage of Gas. The passage of gas at the stoma is often accompanied by a noisy, often embarrassing, episode. The gas passed is largely swallowed air, although certain foods tend to produce an increased amount of gas. There is little that can be done about the passage of gas. Activated charcoal given in generous quantities by mouth may be helpful in reducing the amount of gas passed at the stoma. The usual dosage is 2 capsules 4 times daily, each capsule containing 4 g. of activated charcoal.

Some foods, such as cabbage, peas, cauliflower, and beans, are usually found to produce an increase in intestinal gas. These can be avoided in the diet if experience proves these to be troublesome to the patient. It is probable that the best single factor in the control of gas is adequate irrigation.

The Diet for Patients with Colostomies

The diet of a patient with the usual left-sided colostomy does not have to be restricted. Most patients, by trial and error, find that certain foods do not agree with them and produce either constipation or a loose stool. The diet can be selected to avoid foods which cause difficulty. Constipation is not a bad fault, but loose stools are hard to control. Most patients with colostomies keep some paregoric or some other antidiarrheal mixture at hand for use as the occasion arises.

The foods most often found to give difficulty are onions, cabbage, peas, cauliflower, beans, cucumbers, pickles, and fruits of all types, especially those with bulk and skins. Fried food and an excess of fat in the diet are not well tolerated by some patients. Most of these foods either produce an increase of intestinal gas in their digestion or they add bulk to the fecal mass, both of which factors stimulate colonic peristalsis.

Beer in more than moderate amounts appears to increase colonic activity. Whiskey and wine have less of this effect, although individuals differ in this respect. It may be that the fluid volume rather than the type of drink is the factor. The patient should be taught that a firm stool gives less stomal difficulty than soft or liquid feces, and that the consistency of the stool is the sum of the fecal residue and the fluid intake. Thus, large amounts of high residue foods, (vegetables, fruits, etc.) increase the colonic residue, and fluids in large amounts increase the fluid content of the bowel. The feces proximal to the stoma will tend to be more solid when low residue foods (eggs, cheese, milk, meats, bread, cereals, etc.) are taken and when the fluid intake is curtailed. The food may be regulated to arrive at a desirable diet. With an understanding of the above principles, there need be no restriction of the diet.

Personal Hygiene

One of the real fears of a patient with a colostomy is that of offensive odor. This is usually not a problem if the patient learns to take care of himself by regular and effective irrigations so that he does not have to wear a collecting pouch. The odor associated with a colostomy usually comes from an old rubber colostomy bag which has been poorly cared for. If control of the colostomy has not been achieved by irrigations, it may be necessary to wear a collecting pouch. The most useful are those made of polyethylene plastic; these are disposable and thus do not pick up an odor. Chlorophyll tablets taken by mouth, 2 or 3 tablets per day with meals, are used to reduce the odor of the colostomy discharge. Bismuth subgallate may also be used; one teaspoonful daily should suffice.

Bathing may be carried out normally. Soap and water do not harm a colostomy and are recommended for the skin of the abdominal wall around it. Probably a shower bath is preferable to a tub bath, and immediately after an irrigation is an appropriate time if otherwise convenient.

CARE OF THE AMBULATORY PATIENT WITH A TRANSVERSE COLOSTOMY

For fecal diversion in some patients with diverticulitis of the sigmoid and for

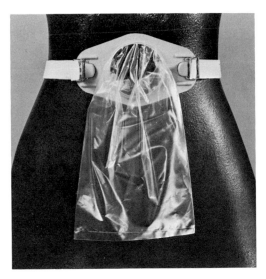

Fig. 17–7. Colostomy device with disposable detachable plastic collection pouches. (United Surgical Supplies Co., Inc.)

decompression of the colon and fecal diversion in patients with carcinomatous obstruction of the left colon, a loop (double-barreled) colostomy is often performed in the right side of the transverse colon. Transverse colostomies are usually temporary, but in some cases are maintained for a period of weeks or months before they are closed. During this period, the patient is ambulatory and will require care in an outpatient department or an office.

The position of the colostomy does not permit enough water to be absorbed from the colonic contents for them to become formed. The result, therefore, is an almost continuous discharge of semiliquid or soft fecal material from the stoma. The patients cannot use irrigations for their colostomy care and, of necessity, must wear a collecting pouch. There are many types available, some made of rubber, others with a plastic facing, and plastic disposable bags. Odor is more of a problem with transverse colostomies. The plastic disposable bags are good because

they can be replaced before they take on an odor (Fig. 17-7).

Care of the skin about the stoma is more of a problem with a transverse colostomy because the fecal discharge is practically constant and the skin is bathed with this discharge. Daily cleansing with soap and water and application of a protective ointment is the best way to prevent or treat the skin maceration that often occurs.

BIBLIOGRAPHY

Colostomy

Golden, T.: Nonirritating multipurpose surgical adhesive tape. Am. J. Surg., *100*;789, 1960.

Grier, W. R., Postel, A. H., Syrarse, A., and Localio, S. A.: An evaluation of colonic stoma management without irrigations. Surg., Gynec. Obstet., *118*:1234, 1964.

McCarty, R. T.: Care of the dry colonic stoma. Surg., Gynec. Obstet., *119*:596, 1964.

Riese, J. A., and Damrau, F.: Use of activated charcoal in gastroenterology; value for flatulence and nervous diarrhea. J. Am. Geriat. Soc., *12*:500, 1964.

Roth, J. L. A., and Bockus, H. L.: Aerophagia: its etiology, syndromes and management. Med. Clin. N. Am., *41*:1673, 1957.

Samp, R. J.: About colostomy management. Ostomy Quart., *1*:87, 1964.

Hernia

Maier, R. L.: The present status of the injection treatment of hernia. Ann. Surg., *122*:85, 1945.

Potts, W. J.: A truss for inguinal hernia in infants. JAMA, *117*:1440, 1941.

Ileostomy

Walker, F. C., and Pringle, R.: Aspects of ileostomy dysfunction; management and adaptation. Brit. J. Surg., *51*:405, 1964.

Wilson, E.; The rehabilitation of patients with an ileostomy established for ulcerative colitis. Med. J. Aust., *1*:842, 1964.

Zetzel, L.: Advice for ileostomy patients. Med. Sci., p. 565, Oct. 1962.

18

Perianal Region, Anus, and Anal Canal

W. A. Shaver, M.D. *and J. R. Groh,* M.D.

DIAGNOSIS OF LESIONS OF THE LOWER RECTUM AND THE ANUS

Symptoms. To treat lesions of the lower rectum and the anal region intelligently, an accurate diagnosis is important. This can be made only if an adequate history is obtained from the patient and a careful examination of the involved area is made. In the history of a patient complaining of anal difficulties, six symptoms are of major significance, and inquiry should be made about them.

The most important of these is bleeding. The appearance of bright blood in the stools signifies an ulceration or trauma to the lower bowel or the anus. It is important to know whether the amount is large or small, whether the blood is mixed with the stool or appears after it, whether the bleeding is in clots or not, and whether it is bright red or dark in color.

The second symptom to be inquired about is pain. It is important to know whether the pain is constant or appears only with bowel movement. Usually, constant pain signifies an inflammatory lesion, whereas pain which appears only with the stool indicates a lesion that is traumatized by defecation. To know the type of pain—whether it is sharp or dragging—and its duration after a stool is helpful in arriving at the diagnosis. Nearly always, pain signifies a lesion of the ectodermal portion of the anal canal, that is, that area supplied by somatic nerves. Even lesions above the pectinate line, such as strangulated internal hemorrhoids, probably produce pain because of the associated edema and inflammatory reaction that appear in the adjacent skin (ectodermal) tissue distal to the pectinate line.

Discharge is another significant symptom. The patient should be asked whether or not the discharge is constant, necessitating the wearing of a pad; whether it is bloody, mucoid, or purulent; and whether or not there is any pain associated with it.

Protrusion at the anus is the fourth symptom and if it is present, the patient should be asked whether the protruded mass disappears after the stool or not and whether it appears only with defecation or also at other times, due to straining.

Itching is a simptom which indicates perianal or anal irritation.

Finally, inquiry should be made about the bowel habits of the patient: has there been any change in the character and the number of the bowel movements, any

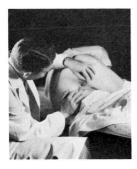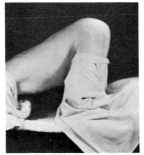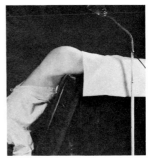

Fig. 18–1. (*Left*) Lateral, or Sims's, position for examination of the anal region and the lower rectum. (*Center*) Knee-chest position for examination of the anal canal and the lower rectum. (*Right*) Position on the proctoscopic table for examination of the anal canal and the lower rectum.

abdominal pain associated with them, or has any increase in the amount of cathartics been necessary?

With this information at hand, one may obtain a fair idea as to the nature of the lesion and as to its location in the anus or, higher up, in the rectum.

Examination of the Patient. No matter how much information may be obtained from the history of a patient suffering from an anal lesion, a diagnosis cannot be made without a thorough examination. The diagnosis of anal lesions across the office desk is inexcusable negligence, because the examination is one which can easily be performed in any office. If a thorough examination is to be made, the patient should cleanse the lower bowel with an enema at least 2 hours before presenting himself at the office. Inspection of the anal canal is possible without preparation, but since an adequate examination usually includes inspection of the lower bowel through the proctoscope, enema preparation is imperative.

The Position of the Patient. To make an examination of the anal region, one of three positions may be used. For older people and pregnant women, the most satisfactory one is probably the lateral, or Sims's, position (Fig. 18-1, *left*). The patient lies on the left side with the left leg extended; the right knee is flexed, and the patient is draped to expose the anal re-

gion. The examiner sits at the side of the examining table.

The knee-chest position is perhaps a more convenient one (Fig. 18-1, *center*) for examination and proctoscopy. The thighs should be perpendicular to the table, the feet extending over the end of the table; the knees should be spread apart, the side of the face placed on a pillow on the table, and the trunk held at an angle of about 45° to the table. This is the only position for the examination of children. It is a difficult position for older patients, and, for that reason, the lateral position is more often used in examining them.

The most satisfactory position for examination and treatment of anal lesions is that obtained on the proctoscopic table (Fig. 18-1, *right*). In this position, the patient leans over the table, which is so tilted that the buttocks and the anal region are easily seen.

The examination of the patient should be carried out in an orderly manner: first, inspection of the anal orifice and the perianal region; second, digital examination of the anal canal and the lower rectum; and third, examination with anoscope and proctoscope of the anal canal, the rectum, and the rectosigmoid.

The inspection of the anal orifice and the perianal region is best done by spreading the buttocks apart, small pieces

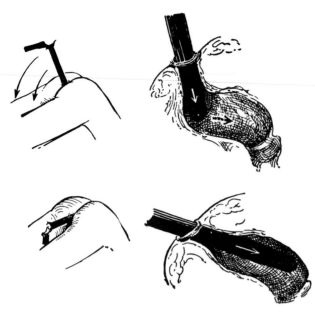

Fig. 18–2. Insertion of the proctoscope. When the patient is in the inverted position, the well-lubricated scope is inserted into the anal canal in an almost vertical direction. After having passed through the anal canal, the outer end of the scope is carried toward the patient's feet to direct the tip along the lower rectum.

of gauze being used to hold the skin under the fingers. The digital examination of the anal canal and the lower rectum is performed with the finger covered with a well-lubricated examining glove or finger cot. The finger should be inserted into the anal canal with the rounded part at the anal orifice; it is then pressed downward along the anterior anal wall until it is inserted past the sphincter muscles into the rectum. If there are painful lesions of this area, the finger should be introduced against the opposite anal wall; in this way, pressure is avoided and pain is reduced to a minimum. Examination should include, first, the region of the anal canal; the finger can then be advanced to palpate the rectum, the coccyx, and, in male patients, the prostate. Palpation of the higher areas of the rectum is carried out first with the hand so directed that the palm is anterior, then with the hand turned over, so that the palm is posterior. Two things to look for in palpation of the anal canal and the lower rectum are, first, areas that are tender on pressure, and, second, masses.

After thorough inspection and palpation, instrumental examination is made,

first of the anal canal and then of the lower rectum. Examination of the anal canal is best made with a lighted anoscope, which may be open at its end or at its side. In its introduction, there must be due regard for painful lesions of the anal canal, and the well-lubricated anoscope should be passed along the anal wall away from the painful lesions. The anoscope permits inspection of the structures of the anal canal, and, with a curved hook, a further examination may be made of the crypts, which are the usual sites of origin of many anal lesions.

All the foregoing examinations may be made without any particular preparation of the patient and without anesthesia.

To complete the examination, a proctosigmoidoscopy should be performed. This entails insertion of a lighted tube through the rectum and rectosigmoid for inspection of the wall of the lower bowel (Fig. 18-2). For this examination, the bowel must be free of fecal material. Occasionally, it is possible to make the examination without previous preparation, but, as a rule, the bowel should be emptied one or two hours before by a cleansing enema.

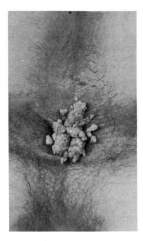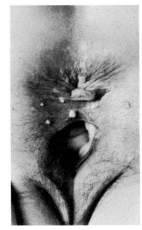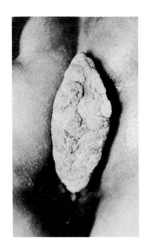

Fig. 18–3. Several varieties of anal warts (condylomata acuminata).

When the bowel has not been prepared for proctoscopy, but it seems desirable to make the examination without delay, the author has employed with very satisfactory results the Fleet enema. This is a solution of 16 g. sodium biphosphate and 6 g. sodium phosphate in a 4½ fl. oz. plastic squeeze bottle with lubricated tip. This is readlily available and easily administered by a nurse and, after about an hour's delay, it permits a complete examination of the anus, rectum, and rectosigmoid at one office visit. There is another commercially available preparation described by Lieberman as microenema (Index). This preparation, also in a plastic squeeze bottle, is a 6 ml. solution containing sodium citrate, sodium lauryl sulfoacetate, sorbital, and glycerine in distilled water. Lieberman states that 84 percent of his patients evacuated the bowel within 10 minutes, and in 84 percent of cases the bowel was clean enough for proctoscopy.

Proctosigmoidoscopy is facilitated considerably by the use of an aspirator to remove liquid fecal material and mucus. In addition, long cotton swabs should be at hand for cleansing as necessary.

At times, after a thorough examination of the rectum and the anus, no cause of the patient's symptoms is found. Adjacent organs may be pressing upon the rectum, thus causing symptoms referred to that area. For this reason, a pelvic examination is important, especially in female patients, in whom rectal pain and discomfort may be due to the pressure of a myoma or a retroflexed uterus.

DISEASES OF THE PERIANAL REGION

CONDYLOMATA ACUMINATA (ANAL WARTS, VENERAL WARTS, ANAL PAPILLOMAS, ANAL VERRUCAE)

Anal warts (Fig. 18-3) appear in the perianal skin and in the skin of the anal canal up to the dentate line. They arise from the papillary layer of the skin and consist of a connective-tissue stalk containing blood vessels and covered with stratified squamous epithelium. There are two chief varieties: one type looks like the usual verruca vulgaris, a wartlike growth in the perianal skin; the other, and more common, type is often spoken of as a "venereal" wart, although there is no relationship between it and venereal disease.

Etiology and Diagnosis. These warts are caused by irritating discharges and may be found associated with hemorrhoids, proctitis, colitis, and, occasionally, with fistulas; in females, they may be due to leukorrhea. They appear as pointed, cauliflowerlike growths, which frequently surround the anal orifice and may extend upward in the anal canal. Usually they are small, but they may attain a very large size. The warts are soft, pale, and bleed readily when traumatized. They may be distinguished from epithelioma of this area by the fact that there is no induration at the base and no ulceration on the surface.

Symptoms. These growths cause considerable irritation of the anal area, often with itching, and, because it is difficult to cleanse them, moisture and excoriation of the perianal skin usually are present. Bleeding may be a symptom, and pain occurs, especially if there is an associated anal lesion, such as a fissure.

Treatment. The treatment of anal condylomas by irradiation has not been too successful, and their removal by electrocoagulation under local anesthesia has been a tedious, time-consuming, and not-always-adequate process. Culp and Kaplan have suggested the local application of a 25 percent suspension of podophyllin in mineral oil to the condylomas. A marked local reaction, with some edema and inflammatory change in the tissues, is produced at the site of application. The condylomas blanch and slough off on the second and the third days after application of the podophyllin, and on the fourth or the fifth day the tissues return to normal, without ulceration or scarring.

Usually the process is painless, but occasionally, if the podophyllin is applied too generously, some sedation may be necessary. If recurrent or new growths appear, they may be treated in the same way. At least a week should be allowed for recovery from one application before another is given.

CONDYLOMA LATUM

Flat condylomas, which occur relatively infrequently, are manifestations of secondary syphilis. Usually, they appear on the perianal skin and often involve the anterior perineum, vulva, and scrotum. They are flat, pearly white, oval or rounded patches, which multiply and often form fungating masses. The edges are sharply defined. They usually cause few symptoms. When they are seen, a diagnosis may be made by a serologic examination. The usual systemic treatment for syphilis will produce a cure. This is the only type of condyloma which is truly venereal.

PRURITUS ANI

Itching of the perianal region and of the anal orifice is one of the most troublesome conditions a physician is called upon to treat. This symptom complex is not uncommon; it appears more frequently in men than in women, and perhaps is seen more often in those who are blond and in those who are obese. It rarely occurs in the Negro race. It is found most often in those between 20 and 50 years of age.

Symptoms. Itching usually begins in a relatively mild form, and the patient tries various proprietary and home remedies in an effort to obtain relief. Lack of success with this therapy may result in more vigorous efforts to obtain relief by the use of anesthetic ointments or other local applications. As a rule, the itching appears first at night and following bowel movements; as time goes on, however, it persists both day and night. Sleeplessness and worry add to the patient's irritability and increase the severity and the prominence of the local symptoms, so that a vicious cycle is established, and the distressing symptoms become almost intolerable.

Etiology. In spite of a very voluminous literature on the subject, the cause of pruritis ani has never been well established. However, several facts are known about its etiology and are helpful in the treatment of the symptom complex. Itching is believed to be a subpain sensation; it travels over the same nerve paths which transmit pain. The impulses of itching arise in the epidermis, and itching is absent when the epidermis is removed or destroyed. Scratching increases the itching. With these facts in mind, one can easily see how minor lesions of the anal canal or of the anal orifice, such as hypertrophied papillae, sentinel piles, skin tabs or cryptitis with edema of the adjacent papillae, serve as sites of an original irritation, which can be increased and spread by scratching.

Many believe that in every case some local pathologic process of the anal canal or of the perianal region can be found to explain the origin of the itching. Others explain the perianal itching as being due to moisture in the perianal region between the buttocks. Lesions of the lower rectum, proctitis, and the retention of large fecal masses are causes of irritating anal discharges.

Another factor that is often cited as the cause of pruritus is local uncleanliness. This factor is a common one and may account for many of the minor degrees of itching. In the more marked cases, however, it is believed by some that there is a sensitization to the bacteria of the stool and of the rectal secretions. The epidermophyton that causes ringworm of the feet and toes is often a primary or a secondary invader. It is thought to be transmitted by the patient from the toes to the perianal region.

There is evidence that venous congestion may cause a mild edema of the skin at the anal orifice that produces secondary itching. This is noted in those cases of pruritus which respond to the injection of internal hemorrhoids. It is more strikingly seen in cases in which itching is associated with thrombosis of a small external hemorrhoid and in cases of edema of the median raphe in females during or immediately following the menstrual period.

Finally, there is a large group of patients in whom there appears to be no demonstrable etiologic factor. These usually are the patients with the most severe pruritus and are, therefore, the most difficult to treat. The inability to find a local cause and the fact that the itching may follow the ingestion of certain foods have suggested an allergic basis for the itching. Tobacco, alcohol, and caffeine are other substances which may bring it on. That there is a marked neurogenic factor in the production of pruritus is shown by the

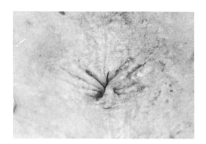

Fig. 18–4. Pruritus ani, showing the thickened perianal skin with deep fissures and furrows between the perianal folds. Note the excoriation due to scratching.

fact that during periods of stress and strain many patients suffer an exacerbation of their itching or have a recurrence of it.

Examination. On examining the patient complaining of pruritus, one may find any of several types of local pathology, depending upon the duration and the severity of the disease. In mild cases, one may be fortunate enough to find a single edematous skin tab or an anterior median raphe which is the local seat of the itching. More commonly, however, the skin around the perianal region appears to be thickened and is grayish pink. The normal radiating folds of the skin at the anal orifice are thickened into rugae, between which may be found deep sulci containing shallow linear ulcers (Fig. 18-4). At times the surface of the skin is thick and sodden. Most commonly, the linear ulcerations are seen in the gluteal fold in the posterior midline, although they may radiate in all directions from the anal orifice. Less commonly, either with or without a previous pruritus, there is an acute process characterized by intense redness of the perianal tissues, often with bleb formation; the process in this stage usually extends forward along the anterior perineum, in females, to the vulva, and in males, to the scrotum. The skin is evidently edematous, and the process is one of an acute dermatitis. In other instances, the skin may be thin and shiny, evidently atrophic; this is considered a later stage of the disease.

Treatment. The treatment of any disease with such an ill-defined etiology as pruritus is at once difficult and unsatisfactory. A carefully taken history may disclose that itching is related to fatigue or nervous upsets, or to the use of alcohol, coffee, or tobacco. Local lesions of the anal canal and the lower rectum should be carefully sought and eradicated. Local anal deformities, such as sentinel piles, fissures, hypertrophic skin tabs, or hypertrophic anal papillae, should be removed as sources of local irritation. If hemorrhoids are present, they should be treated; cryptitis especially should be searched for and, if found, appropriate therapy should be suggested. Regulation of the bowels to prevent accumulation of materials in the lower rectum is worthwhile. Irritating discharges from anal fistulas or, in females, cervical discharges should be given appropriate treatment. In the occasional case of pruritus associated with the menstrual period, there will be discovered a very definite edema of the median raphe, which may be traumatized by the wearing of a sanitary napkin; this factor may be eliminated by the use of a vaginal tampon. Excision of the edematous median raphe has been performed in several cases, with good results.

In some cases of pruritus, there is a tightness of the anal canal, which is believed to be due to the formation of a pecten band—a band of fibrosis in the midportion of the anal canal. This is thought to develop because of chronic congestion in this area and is looked upon by some as a cause of the pruritus. A division of the pecten band under local anesthesia may be easily performed, and in many of these cases it gives almost immediate relief of symptoms.

After eradication of all apparent local causes—and in many cases there are no causes to be discovered—many patients continue to have itching. This is probably due to changes in the skin of the perianal region itself, and, therefore, the itching is no longer initiated by the anal lesion.

The first important measure is to prevent further irritation. This means no further scratching or rubbing of the perianal skin. The patient must recognize that scratching and rubbing with toilet paper increase the perianal irritation and so prolong the itching; therefore, toilet paper should be avoided. Instead, moist warm cotton may be used for cleansing.

The next therapeutic step is an attempt to return the perianal skin to normal. Application of moist heat is the most effective measure. This may be accomplished best by the use of hot sitz baths. There is now available commercially an inexpensive sitz bath for use in the home. The lightweight plastic bowl fits securely in the crockery of the toilet bowl and solves the problem of positioning, and the circulating of fluid from the plastic water bag insures delivery of solution to the bath warm enough and for a long enough period to be effective (Fig. 18-5). Sitz baths may also be taken in a large bowl or a dish pan. (The bathtub is not used because 3 or 4 hot baths daily are quite enervating.) Plain hot water is used in the bath, as hot as can be tolerated comfortably. Sufficient water should be used to cover the perineum. The bath should last about 20 minutes, after which the perineum is dried by blotting it with dry cotton. Instead of using toilet paper, the patient should take a sitz bath after each bowel movement, and he should take at least 4 sitz baths daily, the last one just before going to bed. After the sitz bath, the perianal skin is protected with a mild antipruritic ointment. The author has found that 3 percent ichthyol in zinc oxide ointment is effective in about 90 percent of the cases of mild inflammation.

In cases with more intense inflammation or with lichenification, crude coal tar ointments are used as follows: crude coal tar 8 g., zinc oxide powder 8 g., cornstarch 60 g., and petrolatum 60 g. The ointments prevent maceration of the skin and shield it from discharges from the rectum or the vagina. If this plan of therapy can be followed conscientiously, it will permit the skin to return to its normal texture. In a large percentage of cases, relief of itching will result.

In those cases in which the perianal

some cases the response to such treatment is most dramatic.

Since the advent of adrenal steroids, a new method of therapy for pruritus ani has become available. Hydrocortisone acetate applied locally in a 1.0 or 0.5 percent cream apparently has some local antipruritic effect, although its exact mode of action is not yet well understood. Sarner had better results with the use of fluocinolone acetonide cream, 0.025 percent (Synalar). The perianal skin should first be washed thoroughly with pHisoHex. After this is rinsed off, the skin is blotted dry with cotton, and a pea-sized dab of hydrocortisone cream is applied with the finger and for 5 minutes is massaged into the perianal skin and the anal orifice. This routine is followed in the morning and after bowel movements and at night before retiring. A favorable response should be obtained within 24 to 48 hours. When complete relief of itching is obtained, the treatment may be reduced to once daily and after a month or so, when the skin appears to have regained its normal texture, it may be discontinued. The best results were in cases of idiopathic nonspecific pruritus ani which had failed to respond to other methods of treatment. An excellent protective dressing, which is especially useful when ointments are applied, is made in a butterfly shape to fit in the intergluteal cleft. This is available commercially and is made of absorbent cotton material. It keeps the buttocks separated and remains in place without adhesive tape.

In addition to these more or less conservative local measures, some general instructions and systemic therapy should be given. A bland diet, without stimulants, is prescribed; if any relationship has been noted between the itching and the ingestion of any specific foodstuff or of coffee, the offending substance should be eliminated from the diet. Tranquilizers and sedatives, especially trimeprazine (Temaril), are of value. They should be used with careful supervision of the patient (blood counts, side reactions).

There is some reason to believe that in some cases pruritus may have an allergic

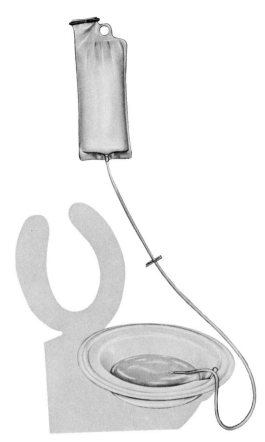

Fig. 18–5. Commercially available plastic "sitz bath" which fits crockery of toilet bowl and is provided with plastic bag reservoir and tube to deliver fluid at the desired temperature. (Sitz-et., Travenol Laboratories)

skin has a moist, soggy appearance, with deep fissures between the rugae, the trichophyton is frequently a secondary factor, and various types of fungicidal ointments may be used. Half-strength Whitfield's ointment often gives relief in such cases. The patient should be warned of some smarting or burning following its application; this is not intolerable, however.

Griseofulvin (Fulvicin) has been used with excellent effect in those cases thought to be due to a fungus infection. Within 3 to 6 weeks, on a dosage of 250 to 375 mg. per day, the itching is relieved. In basis. The author's attention was first drawn to this when a patient with intractable pruritus reported relief of his itching when he was given an antihistaminic drug in the treatment of a nasal allergy. Since that time antihistaminic drugs have been used routinely in the treatment of pruritus ani.

Scratching is strongly interdicted, since little improvement in pruritus can be expected as long as it is continued. If the patient scratches during sleep, cotton gloves should be worn to bed. Instead of toilet paper for cleansing, cotton moistened with warm water and a mild soap or, in acute cases, with oil, should be used, and in no circumstances should there be any vigorous rubbing of the perianal skin. Finally, some provision should be made to ensure the patient's obtaining a good night's rest. Benadryl 50 mg. at bedtime helps to prevent scratching during sleep and is a mild, effective sedative. Barbiturates may be necessary during acute exacerbations of pruritus.

If these measures fail to relieve the patient, more radical procedures must be attempted; for example, various types of injections intended to destroy or to block, temporarily, the nerve pathways from the skin. The injection of alcohol may prove to be an effective procedure. The author first infiltrates the perianal region with 1 percent procaine or 1 percent Carbocaine hydrochloride solution and then injects into the subcutaneous tissues 0.12 cc. of 95 percent alcohol at intervals of about 1 cm., from the anal orifice to beyond the extent of the involved skin laterally, anteriorly, and posteriorly. A fine needle and a vaccine syringe should be used for this injection. Before the patient leaves the office, he should be provided with several tablets of a suitable oral analgesic or narcotic because considerable stinging or burning is present after the procaine wears off. This, however, lasts only a few hours and does not contraindicate the ambulatory care of the patient.

Good relief of itching without any complications has been obtained by means of this therapy, but itching may recur.

Roentgen therapy in the treatment of pruritus ani should be mentioned. In some cases, irradiation gives relief for a period of from 3 to 6 months and sometimes longer. Unfortunately, however, permanent results cannot always be anticipated, and this should be explained to the patient if this form of treatment is to be used.

The prognosis in anal pruritus should be guarded. Relief of the itching is very often followed by recurrence.

DISEASES OF THE ANAL CANAL

HYPERTROPHIED ANAL PAPILLAE

The dentate (mucocutaneous) line in the anal canal is marked by small conical projections from the skin margin; these are called papillae. Normally, they are soft and tend to flatten out as the anal canal is dilated by the passage of the stool mass.

Etiology. The papillae often become hypertrophied as a result of trauma produced by the evacuation of a large hard stool or by repeated spasm of the sphincter in diarrhea. Infectious inflammation plays a significant role in the hypertrophy of the papillae, which is associated with cryptitis and fissure. When hypertrophy occurs, the papillae may easily be identified by palpation as hard teatlike nodules, which are easily movable over the wall of the anal canal. They enlarge, becoming 2 or 3 times their normal size, and they may even assume the proportions of true polyps (Fig. 18-6). Occasionally, a hypertrophied papilla has enlarged to a polypoid tumor the size of a hickory nut (Fig. 18-7).

Symptoms. Hypertrophied papillae produce varied symptoms. Frequently, they are the cause of pain at the time of bowel movements, due to a drag or pull as the stool mass passes over them. Often, bleeding is an associated symptom. They cause anal discomfort by prolapsing during exercise. They may be one of the causes of anal irritability, spasm, and itching.

Diagnosis. The diagnosis is made by

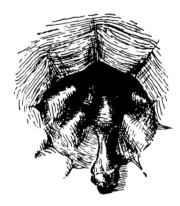

Fig. 18–6. Hypertrophied anal papilla.

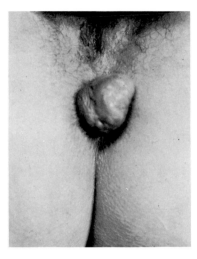

Fig. 18–7. Hypertrophied anal papilla which became polypoid and prolapsed with each bowel movement. This papilla was excised under local anesthesia, and the patient, a hospital employee, lost no time from her work.

palpation and inspection of the anal canal. If the external sphincter is relaxed, the papillae often appear in the anal orifice when the patient strains and the canal is everted by the examiner's fingers. The characteristic nodules are easily recognized by palpation with the finger. They are found within the anal canal, where they arise from a base midway between the sphincters. They can be seen through an anoscope.

Treatment. The treatment is removal of the hypertrophied papillae when they produce symptoms. After local infiltration at the base of the lesions, through an anoscope, the tips of the papillae are caught with an Allis forceps and excised with a cautery or with scissors. The resulting wounds are often painful for a few days, but the discomfort may be relieved by hot sitz baths.

When hypertrophied papillae occur in association with fissures, cryptitis, or hemorrhoids, they may be taken care of at the time of the treatment of the other lesion (Fig. 18-8).

PYOGENIC INFECTIONS
OF THE ANAL CANAL

Almost all the pyogenic infections of the anal canal may be considered to have a common origin in the crypts of Morgagni. These crypts, which may be deep pockets when the anal canal is closed, lie above the dentate line, or mucocutaneous junction. They are lined by mucous membrane, and deep tortuous glands extend from them into the submucosal tissues. In addition, there are patches of lymphoid tissue that lie underneath the mucosa. An infection may extend from the crypt pockets to these glands and the lymphoid tissue, giving no symptoms until it reaches the adjacent skin tissue. Then,

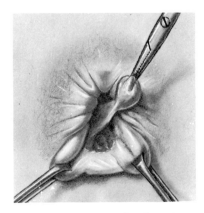

Fig. 18–8. Hypertrophied anal papilla occurring at the upper end of an anal fissure. These 2 lesions are occasionally associated, and, for this reason, every anal fissure should undergo a careful digital examination.

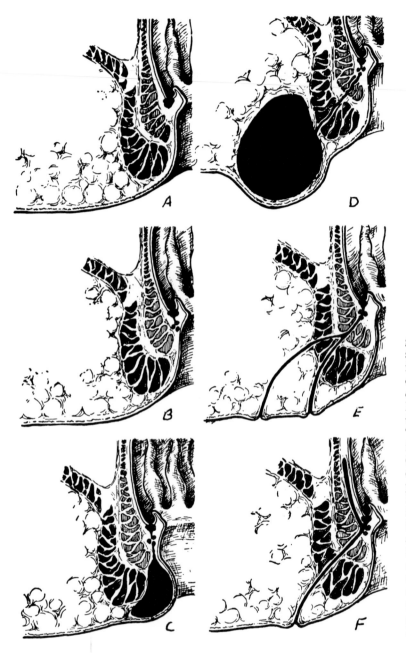

Fig. 18–9. Semidiagrammatic drawings to show the progress of an infection from the anal crypts. (*A*) Infected anal crypt with ulceration. (*B*) Extension of the infection to the deeper glands. These glands may also lie in the muscular tissue. (*C*) Submucous extension of the infection to form a perianal abscess. (*D*) Deep extension of the infection to the fat of the ischiorectal fossa to form an ischiorectal abscess. (*E*) Primary and secondary fistulas extending upward between the circular muscle of the bowel and the mucosa. (Ferguson, L. K.: Surg. Clin. N. Am., *18*:1647, 1938)

because of the inflammatory edema, the overlying papillae become prominent, and pain becomes a symptom.

When an infection in the anal crypts progresses by burrowing, it may extend between the sphincter muscles and the mucous membrane toward the anal orifice to form a perianal abscess, or it may perforate and thus form an ischiorectal abscess (Fig. 18-9).

Cryptitis

Etiology. Normally, the pockets lying between the columns of Morgagni flatten out during the passage of the stool mass.

They are formed by the puckering action of the sphincter muscles and are absent in the cadaver, where the muscle tone is lost. Trauma incidental to the evacuation of large, hard stools in constipation, the frequent anal spasms in diarrhea, the insertion of enema tubes, or the lodging in the crypt of hard foreign materials of the stool permits infecting organisms to gain entrance into the tissues. The relatively deep pocket in the crypt may not drain spontaneously, and the inflammation extends to the lymphoid tissue and the glands underlying its surface. The crypts most often involved lie in the posterior half of the anal ring and, in the majority of cases, at the posterior commissure (Fig. 18-9, *A*).

Symptoms. When confined to the mucous membrane and the submucosal tissue, the infection may produce no symptoms noticeable to the patient. When, however, the inflammation extends to the adjacent papillae, producing an edematous swelling of this sensitive tissue, anal pain and spasm become prominent symptoms. The pain is most acute at the time of, and for a time after, bowel movements, and for this reason cryptitis is often mistaken for anal fissure. As in fissure, constipation is a secondary and aggravating symptom due to the pain associated with bowel movements.

Diagnosis. The diagnosis of cryptitis can be made by digital examination if the gloved finger is inserted carefully into the anal canal. Usually, the edematous, hypertrophied papilla can be palpated, and pressure over the affected crypt gives marked pain. When an anoscope is inserted, the crypt may be entered with a hooked probe (Fig. 18-10). As a rule, except for the edema of the skin edge, few inflammatory signs may be seen. However, the probe inserted into the crypt usually causes definite pain.

Treatment. Treatment of anal cryptitis should err on the conservative side. It does not seem logical to expect any very marked action from topical applications in the crypt, although multitudes of these have been recommended. The problem is one of hastening the subsidence of the

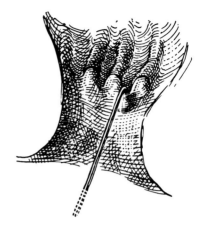

Fig. 18–10. Hooked probe inserted into an anal crypt.

inflammation or, if the inflammation continues because of its deep location, of producing adequate drainage. As an aid in reducing the inflammation, warm rectal instillations are beneficial in keeping the parts clean and the crypts empty. Simple physiologic saline, used in amounts of from 300 to 500 ml., is satisfactory in this regard. Sitz baths may also be used as a method of applying heat. To this therapy should be added instructions as to a bland diet, often with the addition of one of the psyllium seed bowel preparations (Metamucil, Syllamalt) or of Senokot. These soften the stool and give it the necessary bulk to ease its passage. This form of conservative treatment should be given a thorough trial before operation is considered necessary.

When infection has begun to burrow, so that the exploring probe hooks into a deep opening overhung by the tissues at the dentate line (Fig. 18-9, *B*), the treatment indicated is adequate drainage. With a speculum inserted into the anal canal, the pocket of the infected crypt can easily be identified with the hooked probe. Then, with infiltration anesthesia in the tissues overlying the probe, drainage may be obtained by cutting away the hypertrophied papilla and adjacent mucous membrane (Fig. 18-11). This operation is best performed by using the hooked probe as a tractor; the tissues beneath the hook are excised with narrow

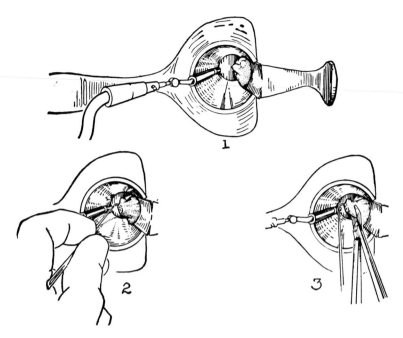

Fig. 18–11. Appearance of an infected crypt through a Brinkerhoff anoscope (1). Using a hooked probe (2) as a retractor, the overhanging skin edge and the edematous papilla are excised with long curved scissors (3).

scissors, and in this way, the deep pocket is converted into an open wound. Bleeding is usually slight and can be controlled by the insertion of plain or petrolatum gauze into the anal canal for a few hours. A small piece of Gelfoam has proved to be even better in the hands of the author. Frequently there is postoperative discomfort lasting for 24 hours; this can be relieved by hot sitz baths and anesthetic ointments. After 48 hours, there is little discomfort except at the time of bowel movements.

Perianal Abscess

When the infection of an anal crypt extends deeply to the perianal lymphatic tissue and then burrows caudally between the mucous membrane and the anal muscles, an abscess forms and presents at the anal orifice; this is called a perianal abscess. This type of lesion appears most often at the midline posteriorly as a painful, reddened swelling (Fig. 18-9, *C*).

Diagnosis. The history given by the patient may often be misleading as to the true course of the infection. There may be no previous history of a painful cryptitis, although there is often a period of several days during which the patient has noted slight discomfort and soreness in the anal canal. The pain then becomes marked and, at the time of bowel movements, almost intolerable; usually it is sufficient to keep the patient awake at night. The systemic reaction is slight. On digital examination, an indurated, rounded, tender mass may be palpated just outside the anal wall, usually in the posterior half of the anal canal and on one side or the other of the midline. The abscess may be situated at the level of the infected crypt or, more commonly, close to the anal orifice. Usually, a tender edematous papilla marks the location of the crypt. When the buttocks are pulled apart, pus may be seen to escape from the anal orifice. An anoscope can be introduced gently without pain if pressure is maintained away from the area of the abscess. The infected crypt can then be identified by the drain-

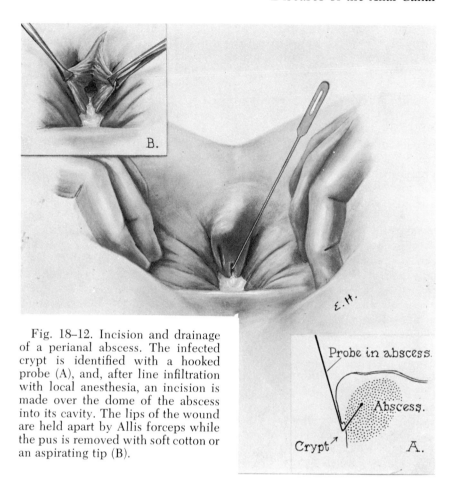

Fig. 18-12. Incision and drainage of a perianal abscess. The infected crypt is identified with a hooked probe (A), and, after line infiltration with local anesthesia, an incision is made over the dome of the abscess into its cavity. The lips of the wound are held apart by Allis forceps while the pus is removed with soft cotton or an aspirating tip (B).

age of pus from it, and the hooked probe will extend through it into the abscess cavity (Fig. 18-12).

Treatment. The treatment of such an abscess is relatively simple and may be carried out without admitting the patient to a hospital. The result is almost immediate relief of pain and discomfort. With the speculum in place and the hooked probe in the infected crypt, anesthesia is produced by infiltration with 1 percent procaine or 1 percent Carbocaine solution. Usually, it is best to infiltrate at the crypt opening first, because edema may obscure this area if the anesthetic is first introduced over the swelling of the abscess cavity. No effort is made to obtain a deep anesthesia. The mucous membrane overlying the abscess is anesthetized from the infected crypt to the far-

thest extent of the abscess cavity at the anal orifice. It is well to carry the infiltration somewhat laterally in order to permit Allis forceps to be applied and to allow the excision of the central portion of skin over the abscess cavity.

A single incision is then made to drain the cavity, and, after removal of the purulent material by suction or gentle sponging, the edges of the wound, including the edematous hypertrophied papilla, are excised. The cavity is then gently packed with petrolatum or narrow iodoform gauze. Care is taken to see that the packing does not lie in the lumen of the anal canal.

The operation as described above is not absolutely painless, but it may be performed with a minimum of discomfort. The sponging of the unanesthetized abscess cavity and the insertion of packing are the procedures which cause pain. If the patient is warned beforehand and if gentleness is used, little difficulty is experienced.

The wound is dressed with gauze held in place with a T-binder. As a rule, incision of the abscess causes almost immediate relief of pain, but it is well to provide the patient with 2 or 3 tablets of a potent analgesic, to be taken by mouth every 3 hours if needed for relief of pain during the first night after operation. A liquid diet may be prescribed for 1 or 2 days. On the third postoperative day, the packing is removed and none is reinserted. Sitz baths of warm water, once or twice daily and after each bowel movement, are used as an easy and efficient method of keeping the wound mascroscopically clean during the healing process. The ordinary sanitary napkin makes a convenient and an easily obtainable dressing after the wound begins to granulate, on about the fifth or the sixth day. No secret is made of the fact that this wound is not and never can be considered sterile, but ordinary cleanliness is advised. Occasionally, drainage from the wound will cause excoriation and chafing of the cheeks of the buttocks. The application of a thin layer of zinc oxide ointment at the site of irritation will give relief from this trouble in 24 hours. Usually, little or no discomfort is experienced after 24 hours, and no restriction in the diet is necessary. The passage of a formed stool is more to be desired than numerous soft or liquid stools. No cathartics are given unless indicated for reasons other than the operative wound.

Ischiorectal Abscess

When an infection from an infected crypt burrows laterally, it may pass between the sphincters or through the fibers of the external sphincter to enter the ischiorectal fossa. This pyramidal space lying between the anal canal and the tuber ischii is filled chiefly with fatty tissue, which offers little resistance to the progress of an infection. Therefore, the abscess may rapidly extend upward along the wall of the rectum or laterally around the anal canal into the fossa of the opposite side.

Symptoms. The rapid necrosis of the fatty tissue does not permit a walling off of the infected process, so that a temperature elevation and other marked systemic changes often result. On local examination, a tense, red area may be seen to the lateral side of the anal orifice. On palpation, either in the anal canal or over the reddened area, acute tenderness is elicited. The area is usually so tender that a demonstration of fluctuation is impossible in the early stages of the process, and it is unnecessary in the later stages, when pus certainly is present. It is often difficult, even impossible, to demonstrate the infected crypt without general anesthesia. In ischiorectal abscess, as in perianal abscess, there often is no previous history which would indicate the presence of a cryptitis. Nevertheless, the almost inevitable development of a secondary fistula after the drainage of an ischiorectal abscess indicates that the origin of the infection is an infected crypt (Fig. 18-9, *D* and *E*).

Treatment. Because of the rapid progress of an infection in the fat of the ischiorectal fossa, incision and drainage at the earliest moment is the indicated treatment. As a rule, general, low spinal, or caudal and transsacral block anesthesia is required and hospitalization is advised, although in a few cases simple incision of the abscess may be performed under local infiltration anesthesia in ambulatory patients, with the knowledge that a secondary fistula will probably result. With the patient in the lithotomy position or in the Sim's position with the involved side down, an infiltration with 0.5 percent procaine or 1 percent Carbocaine is made carefully over the dome of the abscess. When making the infiltration, one must remember that pressure upon an abscess wall, by increasing the tension of the abscess, causes a definite increase in pain. It is imperative, therefore, to make every effort to avoid pressure. The lines of infiltration should be radial and long enough to permit an incision which will open the entire extent of the abscess. Some surgeons prefer a circumferential incision because they believe that drainage is more complete and closure of the wound does not occur too soon. Local anesthesia does not permit a completely painless operation, but the relief of tension immediately following the incision gives such relief to the patient that it may be performed without difficulty under this type of anesthesia. General anesthesia may be used, but unless it is relatively deep, it is difficult to keep the patient in position on the table; thus, local anesthesia is the usual choice for the incision of ischiorectal abscesses in ambulatory patients.

The incision is made after gently inserting the index finger of one hand into the anal canal. Avoiding downward pressure upon the scalpel as much as possible and cutting through the skin and the subcutaneous tissues with sweeping strokes of the knife, the abscess cavity is entered. Frequently, the foul-smelling pus spurts out under considerable pressure, and it is well to hold a protecting sponge to avoid wide scattering of the pus from large abscesses. In the smaller early abscesses, the knife is guided toward the abscess cavity by the finger in the anal canal. In these deeper smaller abscesses, it may be necessary to make deeper infiltration of the subcutaneous fat to obtain anesthesia.

After the abscess cavity is entered, Allis forceps are placed upon the lips of the wound and an exploring finger is inserted gently, bearing in mind that the anesthesia is confined to the wound through which the incision has passed. With the finger in the abscess cavity, it is possible to outline its extent, and the incision should be continued until the entire cavity is laid open.

The wound is then held open with Allis forceps or rake retractors while it is cleaned gently with an absorbent gauze sponge or irrigated with sterile saline. The cavity is then packed with plain or iodoform gauze, a special effort being made not to break any of the vessels that extend like fibrous cords from the lateral

wall of the ischiorectal fossa to the anal canal and the rectum. Dressings are applied and are held in place by a T-binder. The postoperative care is similar to that mentioned for perianal abscess. After removal of the packing on the third day, the wound edges are held apart by the insertion of a simple gauze dressing. Warm sitz baths after each bowel movement and 2 or 3 times daily in addition keep the area clean and permit the mechanical removal of the remaining necrotic tissue. After this type of operation, healing usually takes place in from 2 to 3 weeks.

Antibiotics and Anal Infections

In a general way it may be said that antibiotics are not of great value in the treatment of perianal and ischiorectal infections. These lesions are rarely seen until they are in the abscess stage, and in that stage antibiotics are no substitute for incision and drainage. If adequate drainage is provided, the need for antibiotics is slight and their value is negligible. Rosser believes that they "slow the process, and change the clinical picture, at times sufficiently to confuse the diagnosis or give a false sense of security," even when given early.

Fistula in Ano

Etiology. Fistula in ano is the third type of lesion which may arise from an infected anal crypt. This is a tubular tract, lined with infected granulation tissue, which extends from the infected crypt outward to the skin surface at one side or the other of the anal orifice. This infected tract may appear as a sequela of an ischiorectal abscess. The abscess having been drained by an incision, there still remain the infected crypt and the infected tract leading from it through the ischiorectal fossa. As a result of the incision, the abscess cavity heals by granulation up to and around the drainage tract, which extends to the skin surface at the site of the incision. Sometimes the abscess may heal entirely by granulation and the wound will break open some time later, with the appearance of a fistulous opening. More commonly, however, the fistula appears without any pre-existing acute ischiorectal abscess. In such cases, the organism may be of a lower virulence or the tissues of higher resistance. In any event, the infection extends from the anal crypt across the inner part of the ischiorectal fossa to form a small subcutaneous abscess. This usually ruptures spontaneously, and a fistula remains.

Not infrequently, the fistulous tract is tortuous, and secondary fistulous openings may appear on the skin surface. These secondary tracts arise from closure of the primary tract; the infection burrows through the wall of the original fistulous canal to the surface, and in many cases the tract leads upward along the anal canal and the rectum. Almost always, however, these numerous tracts arise from a single infected crypt (Fig. 18-9, *E* and *F*).

Symptoms and Diagnosis. The symptomatology of fistula in ano is diagnostic. The patient states that he notices a drainage of thick malodorous material from the fistulous opening. The drainage is sufficient to soil the clothing and requires a pad of cotton between the buttocks. For a time, as the scar tissue at the skin opening contracts, the drainage may become less; eventually, the external opening may close entirely, and the patient may consider his fistula healed. Gradually, however, the infected material of the tract produces a small subcutaneous abscess at the site of the former cutaneous opening, and pain and soreness develop. In 2 or 3 days, the abscess ruptures at the scar of the cutaneous opening of the fistula. The pain is relieved, but the drainage becomes apparent again, at first profuse and then, as the acute inflammatory process subsides, less and less until it is reduced to the original amount. This continuous infection produces a fistulous tract lined by infected granulation tissue and having a wall made up of dense fibrous tissue. In a long-standing fistula, the cutaneous opening is easily recognized by its raised circle of scar tissue, from which a drop or two of pus may easily be expressed. By palpa-

tion, the fistulous tract may often be identified as a firm fibrous cord extending toward the anal canal. The secondary tracts usually arise due to the damming up of the infection by a healing over of the cutaneous opening. Most frequently, the secondary opening is found to connect with the original fistula by a subcutaneous tract and may be at considerable distance from the original opening. There may be a large subcutaneous pocket lined by chronic granulation tissue.

A frequently quoted rule for locating the internal opening has been found from practical experience to be very useful: an imaginary line is drawn between the tubera ischii so as to bisect the anal orifice transversely. If the primary external opening of the fistula lies anterior to this line, the internal opening is usually in an infected crypt on a straight line drawn from the external opening to the anal orifice; if the external opening of the fistula lies posterior to this line, the fistulous tract usually is curved and has its origin in an infected crypt at, or just lateral to, the midline posteriorly (Fig. 18-13, *A*). When there are secondary openings, some of which lie anterior to this line, the sinus tract is usually of the posterior type.

Treatment. The treatment of fistula in ano is incision or excision of the fistulous tract from the infected crypt to all the cutaneous openings. When the skin opening of the fistula lies close to the anal orifice and when the tract can be identified easily by palpation or by the gentle insertion of the probe along its course, it is possible to excise the fistula under local anesthesia, and the patient may be ambulatory throughout his period of treatment. With the finger in the anal canal, a probe is introduced through the fistulous tract to emerge at the infected crypt. The end of the probe is then advanced slowly until it appears at the anal orifice. Although this may cause the patient slight discomfort, it is much better to insert the probe before injection of a local anesthetic has caused distortion of the tract (Fig. 18-13, *B*). A local anesthetic is then injected into the tissues above and around the probe; first,

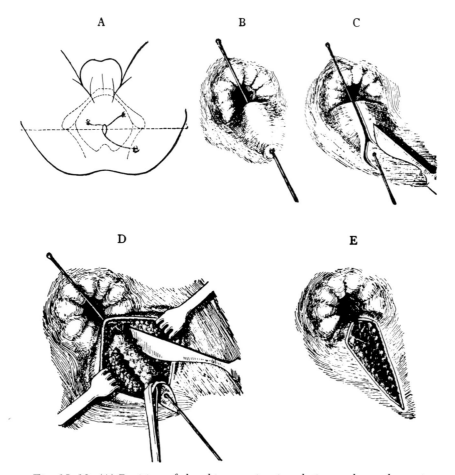

Fig. 18–13. (A) Position of the skin opening in relation to the anal opening of a fistula in ano. An imaginary line is drawn to bisect the anal orifice between the tubera ischii. If the cutaneous opening of the fistula lies posterior to this line, the anal opening is almost invariably at a crypt in the posterior midline. If the cutaneous opening lies anterior to this line, the tract courses in a radial direction to the anal canal.

(B) Short fistula in ano identified with a probe inserted from the cutaneous opening to the infected crypt. Procaine, 1 percent containing epinephrine is infiltrated along the line of the fistula and round the cutaneous opening.

(C) Skin incision for excision of a short fistula in ano.

(D) Excision of fibrous fistulous tract as a cylinder upon the identifying probe.

(E) Wedge-shaped wound resulting from excision of the fistulous tract is packed with plain or iodoform gauze. Healing by granulation is permitted.

an adequate skin infiltration is made, and then the tract is surrounded by a wall of local anesthesia. As a rule, it is best to begin the infiltration at the anal end of the fistula; otherwise, later injections may obscure the internal orifice and an incomplete infiltration will result. The tissues are then incised down to the fistulous tract (Fig. 18-13, *C*). Using sharp rake retractors or Allis forceps, the lips of the wound are pulled apart, and the incision is carried down to expose the tract (Fig. 18-13, *D*).

In a fistula of any duration, the tract has

become so fibrous as to permit its excision intact. If the incision is carried down to the probe and the fistulous tract is laid open, it is wise to excise the cartilaginous-like scar tissue of the fistula. The edges of the wound are excised so as to make a broad V (Fig. 18-13, *E*), and the wound is packed with iodoform gauze, care being taken to see that the packing does not extend into the anal canal. A T-binder pressure dressing is applied, and the post-operative care is similar to that described for perianal abscess.

When the fistulous tract opens at some distance from the anal orifice or when there are multiple openings, the patient is usually hospitalized and operated upon under low spinal, caudal and transsacral, or general anesthesia, although the author has operated upon numerous such cases under local anesthesia in ambulatory patients. With the patient in the lithotomy position, the anal canal is dilated and held apart by four Allis forceps. With a hooked probe, the infected crypt that marks the internal opening of the fistulous tract is then searched for, and, when it is identified, the probe is held in the crypt. In long and tortuous fistulas, it is not always possible to insert a probe throughout the entire length of the tract; therefore, it is imperative that the infected crypt that marks the anal opening of the tract be identified early in the operation. The most important part of the operation is the incision of the crypt, and the frequent recurrences which are seen are mostly due to the fact that the infected crypt was not laid open at the first operation.

In cases of long and multiple fistulas, it is frequently wise to perform a two-stage operation, excising or incising first the portion of the tract farthest from the anal canal and leaving for the second operation the incision of the inner portion of the tract, that is, the portion that passes through the sphincter muscle and the infected crypt. When this type of operation has been decided upon, a probe or a grooved director is inserted into one of the fistulous openings as far as it will pass without force (Fig. 18-14, *A*). An incision is then made in the direction of the probe,

the skin and the subcutaneous tissues being divided down to the tract (Fig. 18-14, *B*). The skin incision is carried around the fistulous opening, and, with Allis forceps and sharp rake retractors holding the skin on tension, the tract may be dissected out intact down toward the anal canal. When secondary tracts leading into the primary fistula are found, these are dissected out in the same manner. As the dissection progresses, the fistulous tract is held taut on the grooved director or the probe with a hemostat. Usually, the director can be passed without any effort along the tract as the latter is dissected free and its curves are obliterated, so that eventually it will emerge in the anal canal at the crypt previously identified by the hooked probe (Fig. 18-14, *C*). When the dissection has been carried down to the anal musculature, the freed portion of the fistula is cut off and drawn off the probe (Fig. 18-14, *D*), and the probe, threaded with a doubled silk ligature, is pulled through the remaining portion of the tract (Fig. 18-14, *E*). The silk thread, which now identifies the mesial position of the fistulous tract, is tied loosely with a triple knot to remain in place as a seton until the time of the second-stage operation (Fig. 18-14, *E*).

When a secondary sinus tract passes upward along the anal canal and the rectum, no effort is made to excise it. As a rule, it is best to lay it open as far as possible without destroying the integrity of the musculature, and the chronic granulation tissue is removed with gauze or a curette. This tract will heal spontaneously if the primary opening at the infected crypt is drained.

In cases in which the tract has been excised as described, in spite of the fact that the wound is definitely infected, primary union may almost always be obtained by suturing if care is taken to obliterate dead space. The wound is irrigated with saline solution before suturing is attempted. The sutures should be of fine catgut and so placed, layer upon layer, as to obliterate the wound left by the excision of the fistula. The inner portion of the wound is not completely sutured, but is packed lightly with iodoform

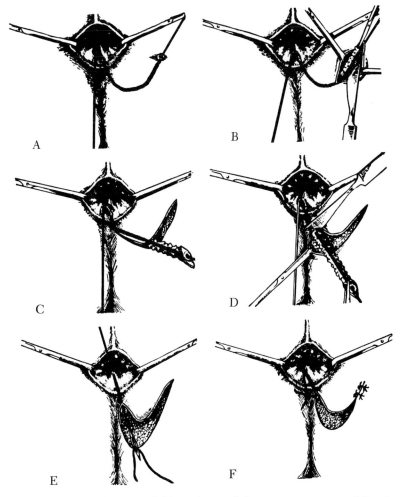

Fig. 18–14. (*A, Top, left*) Technic of the 2-stage excision of fistula in ano; identification of the infected crypt in the posterior commissure and passage of the probe into the external opening as far as the tract will permit.

(*B, Top, right*) Beginning excision of the tract from the external opening, the edges of the wound being kept on tension with retractors or Allis forceps.

(*C, Center, left*) The lateral portion of the tract having been dissected free, the probe may be advanced along its course and the incision continued toward the anal opening.

(*D, Center, right*) The tract is dissected free up to the anal musculature, being kept taut on the probe with a hemostat. When the dissection has reached the anal musculature, the tubelike fistulous tract is divided and the probe is passed onward through the infected anal crypt.

(*E, Bottom, left*) The probe, having been passed through the infected crypt, is threaded with a heavy silk suture, which is drawn through the remaining portion of the fistulous tract and remains as a seton until the second-stage operation.

(*F, Bottom, right*) The lateral portion of the tract is partially closed with buried sutures of fine catgut and silk in the skin. The mesial portion of the tract is packed with iodoform gauze and allowed to heal by granulation up to the seton. When healing has progressed to the seton, the mesial portion of the tract is excised at a second operation.

(Ferguson, L. K.: Surg. Clin. N. Am., *18*:1645, 1938)

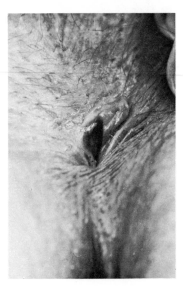

Fig. 18–15. Acute fissure at the usual site at the posterior midline of the anal orifice.

gauze next to the seton. If the subcutaneous sutures are placed sufficiently close to the surface, it is best not to attempt to suture the skin because these wounds often become edematous for a few days, especially when skin sutures have been inserted.

In the postoperative care of these patients, warm moist compresses are applied for 15 minutes every second hour, beginning 24 hours after operation. The packing is removed on the third postoperative day and is not replaced. The moist compresses are continued until the fourth or the fifth day, after which hot sitz baths of physiologic saline solution are substituted. Frequently there is a considerable reaction in these wounds; this will subside without suppuration if hot moist dressings are used.

When the wounds have healed solidly up to the seton, usually in 10 days to 2 weeks, the second stage of the operation may be performed. This may be carried out under local anesthesia and in the ambulatory patient. The tissues included in the seton are well infiltrated with procaine solution, and an incision is made down to the fistulous tract identified by

the seton. As a rule, the edges of the wound are excised and iodoform gauze is inserted. The postoperative care is then as described for perianal abscess (p. 238). With this staged treatment of extensive fistulas, the resulting scar and deformity are minimal, and, as a rule, there is little or no interference with sphincter function.

Fissure in Ano

Etiology. A painful longitudinal ulcer of the anal canal is called a fissure in ano. Most often, this ulceration appears as an infection of a traumatic wound produced by a splitting or a tearing of the skin tissues at the anal orifice by the passage of a large, hard stool. Because of the direction of the anal canal in relation to that of the lower rectum, the stretching and the tearing of the thin skin at the anal margin most often occur at the posterior commissure. There may be a slight amount of oozing incidental to the injury, but in the majority of cases healing takes place without complication. In those cases in which the tear becomes an ulcer, infection occurs, with resulting inflammation of the wound and of the surrounding tissues. The inflammatory reaction frequently produces edema of the papilla at the upper margin of the ulcer and extends by contiguity to the sphincter muscles. The acute fissure is thus produced.

Symptoms. The symptoms produced by acute fissure (Fig. 18-15) are pain and bleeding. The pain occurs characteristically with the stool, and usually it persists for a period of from half an hour to 2 or 3 hours after defecation. Usually, the bleeding is small in amount and may be noticed only as a soiling of the toilet paper or a staining of the clothes. The method by which these symptoms are produced is easily understood if the underlying pathology of the fissure is kept in mind. The trauma to the irritable ulcer due to the passage of the hard stool over it and to stretching of the tissues causes intense pain, which is followed by a spasm of the sphincter muscle. This spasm further traumatizes the ulcer and prolongs the pain for a considerable pe-

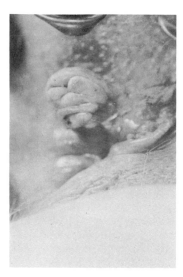

Fig. 18–16. Chronic fissure. Note the hypertrophic skin tissue commonly designated as a sentinel pile.

riod after bowel movements. Defecation is such a painful procedure for these patients that it is often avoided as long as possible, with the result that the stool mass becomes larger and harder as the water is more completely absorbed from it. The following movement is more painful than ever. The dread of a bowel movement results in constipation, and the severe pain during, and persisting after, defecation may so upset an otherwise normal person as to make him a nervous wreck.

As the process continues, scar tissue forms at the edges of the ulcer and especially at the skin surface of the anal orifice, where there are edema and secondary fibrosis, with the formation of a definite overhanging mass of skin and fibrous tissue called a sentinel pile (Fig. 18-16). This is easily noted on inspection and almost invariably lies at the posterior midline, the location of about 90 percent of anal fissures. With the passage of time and the deposit of fibrous tissue in and around the fissure, the symptomatology changes to that of the chronic fissure in ano. The acute pain with persisting spasm is no longer present, and bleeding is rare. The chief symptom is a duller, dragging

pain which occurs at the time of bowel movement and which does not persist for a long period thereafter. The pain in this case is due to the stretching of the ulcer and the underlying fibrosis and also to the dragging of the overhanging sentinel pile, which hangs as a sort of inverted hood at the external extremity of the fissure. In addition, there may be marked pain due to pulling upon a hypertrophied papilla at the upper limit of the ulcer.

Diagnosis. The diagnosis of anal fissure may frequently be made upon the history alone; the pain associated with, and persisting after, defecation, and the appearance of small amounts of bright blood are quite typical. However, one should not rely upon the history; an examination of the anal area must be made. In this examination, the fissure can usually be seen if the buttocks are separated. This may cause considerable discomfort. If the ulcer is extremely sensitive, the pain may be relieved by the application of a swab dipped in 10 percent cocaine solution and inserted gently into the anal canal. The injection of procaine into the sphincter muscles and underneath the fissure is another method of permitting digital and instrumental examination without discomfort. When no anesthesia is used, the index finger should be inserted along the anterior anal wall, with the palm of the hand anterior, and pressure should be made away from the fissure. The finger may then be turned over and the area of the fissure palpated. The ulcer is noted as a depression, and one may feel the dense fibrosis which extends on either side of the fissure, often producing an almost shelflike constriction of the posterior part of the anal canal. This band of fibrous tissue has been named the pecten band. Frequently, an edematous and fibrosed papilla at the upper margin of the fissure can be palpated as a small tender mass. The fissure may be seen with the aid of an anoscope, and, in this examination, one may frequently note a small fistula that leads from the base of the fissure to the skin surface behind the sentinel pile.

Treatment. The treatment of acute fis-

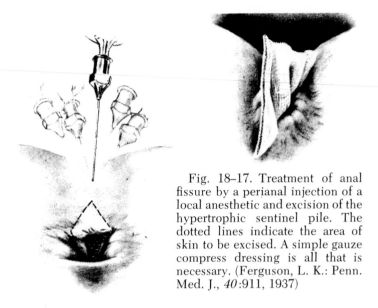

Fig. 18–17. Treatment of anal fissure by a perianal injection of a local anesthetic and excision of the hypertrophic sentinel pile. The dotted lines indicate the area of skin to be excised. A simple gauze compress dressing is all that is necessary. (Ferguson, L. K.: Penn. Med. J., *40*:911, 1937)

sure may be either conservative or operative. When the fissure is only a recent tear of the transitional epithelium at the anal orifice, stool softeners and hot applications or sitz baths may suffice to produce healing. Anesthetic ointments fail to add much to this regimen.

Stretching of the anal sphincter has proved to be a successful conservative treatment of acute anal fissure. Under adequate local anesthesia, the sphincter is gradually dilated, using at first two fingers, then three and four, introducing the fingers as a conical dilator into the anal canal. The index and ring fingers of each hand may be used to obtain further dilatation. This stretching produces a short-lived relaxation of the sphincter and a relief of anal spasm, allowing the acute ulcer to heal spontaneously.

When the fissure is really an anal ulcer with a flat grayish pink base, sharply demarcated by edema of the surrounding rim of transitional epithelium, conservative treatment should be abandoned. After infiltration under and around the ulcer with a local anesthetic, the base of the ulcer should be incised. The incision should be deep enough to divide a few fibers of the external sphincter and should

be continued for about ½ inch in a radial direction from the anal orifice. Often the edematous skin edge is cut away with curved scissors. A small gauze compress tucked into the wound is used as a dressing. The postoperative care is described below.

When the fissure is chronic, with a well-marked sentinel pile and a polypoid hypertrophied papilla at its upper margin, a more extensive procedure is necessary in order to effect a cure. In such cases, it is necessary to inject a local anesthetic in a wedge-shaped area around the sentinel pile and underneath the fissure. A wedge-shaped excision (Fig. 18-17) of skin extending from ½ to ¾ inch from the anal orifice is carried toward the anal canal, the sentinel pile and the fissure being removed. The dense fibrosis (pecten band) underlying the fissure should be divided with a light stroke of the knife and, with it, a few of the superficial fibers of the external sphincter muscle. When there is a hypertrophic papilla at the upper margin, this should be removed after ligation with a simple suture of fine catgut. After introducing a small piece of Gelfoam into the wound, the wound is packed with gauze, and a T-binder dressing is applied. The of the external sphincter muscle. When there is a hypertrophic papilla at the upper margin, this should be removed after ligation with a simple suture of fine catgut. After introducing a small piece of Gelfoam into the wound, the wound is packed with gauze, and a T-binder dressing is applied. The dressing is permitted to remain in place for about 24 hours, when it can be removed by the patient. As a rule, the patient is asked to take a sitz bath with the compress and the dressing in the wound; after the sitz bath the gauze is moist enough to permit its removal without much discomfort. Simple superficial dressings are all that are required, the area being kept clean by the use of sitz baths 2 or 3 times a day.

Practically all fissures can be taken care of in ambulatory patients. Only 7 of 125 patients with fissure in ano were admitted to the hospital.

POLYPS OF THE ANAL CANAL

Etiology. A polyp of the anal canal usually develops from a hypertrophied papilla. The papilla, as a result of repeated trauma in the anal canal, becomes enlarged and edematous, and, eventually, a fibrous nodule covered by squamous epithelium forms. Not infrequently, the inflammatory reaction extending from an anal ulcer may be the etiologic factor in the primary enlargement of the papilla. This accounts for the frequent finding of anal polyps at the cephalic end of chronic anal fissures.

These pedunculated hypertrophied anal papillae are covered with squamous or transitional epithelium, are pale pink, and never become malignant. They are not to be confused with adenomatous rectal polyps, which are also often pedunculated. The latter are red and velvety, bleed easily, and may be precancerous lesions.

Symptoms. The symptoms produced by anal polyps are easily understood. The usual complaint is anal pain and discomfort, especially at the time of bowel movements. As the polyps enlarge and the pedicle becomes longer, they frequently prolapse through the anal ring (Fig. 18-7), and many of them may remain outside the anal canal most of the time. Occasionally, ulceration of the polyp may take place and cause bleeding.

Treatment. The treatment is excision of the polyp. This operation may be performed under local infiltration and block anesthesia. A generous area at its base should be removed with the polyp. Hemostasis may be obtained by interrupted sutures of fine catgut. The postoperative care is the same as for other anal operations.

HEMORRHOIDS

Definition. Hemorrhoids is the name given to protruding masses of tissue in the anal canal and at the anal orifice. They are spoken of as external when they lie distal to the pectinate line and are covered with the modified skin tissue of ectodermal origin. They are called internal when they lie above the pectinate line and are covered by mucous membrane of endodermal origin. The combination of these two types, i.e., when the hemorrhoidal mass extends throughout the length of the anal canal, is spoken of as a mixed hemorrhoid.

Anatomy and Etiology. Under normal conditions there are two venous plexuses at the anal orifice and in the anal canal. These lie in the subcutaneous and the submucosal tissues and are loosely supported by the overlying tissues. The upper plexus lies above the pectinate line and drains into the middle and the superior hemorrhoidal veins. The lower plexus lies distal to the pectinate line and drains into the inferior hemorrhoidal vein. The two plexuses are united by numerous anastomotic branches, so that it is not unusual to find that both are involved in the same pathologic process. A distention of these venous plexuses may be caused by an increase of intra-abdominal pressure or a local obstruction of the venous return.

Most commonly, the cause of hemorrhoids is straining at stool, due to either

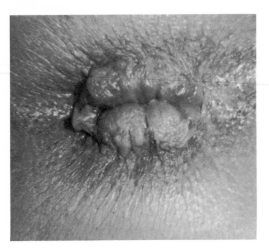

Fig. 18–18. External hemorrhoids. Note skin hypertrophy.

constipation or diarrhea; less commonly, other types of straining, associated with physical exertion, may be etiologic factors. The venous stasis produced by pregnancy and, especially, by childbirth is not infrequently the cause of hemorrhoids in women. Many female patients will date the onset of their hemorrhoidal symptoms from the birth of their first or second child. Another common cause of venous stasis is the partial obstruction of the venous return by the infiltration of carcinoma in the pelvic rectum; because of this frequent association, hemorrhoidal bleeding should be treated only after a thorough visual examination of the lower bowel with the proctoscope. Another factor, somewhat difficult to explain, but nonetheless easily recognized clinically, is relaxation of the external sphincter. With a lack of sphincter tone there is a thinning out of the anal canal in the act of defecation. This is associated with an eversion of the mucosa of the upper part of the anal canal.

External Hemorrhoids

Etiology. Dilatation of the external hemorrhoidal plexus is accompanied by stretching and hypertrophy of the skin tissue at the anal orifice. When venous stasis is produced by straining, the plexus becomes distended, and the overlying skin is stretched into round purplish masses at the anal orifice (Fig. 18-18). These are best demonstrated by doing the examination with the patient in the squatting position or lying on his side. They are most frequently noted by the patient as masses at the anal orifice following bowel movements. The distention of the plexus usually disappears soon after the straining that produced it has stopped, so that on observing the relaxed patient one notes only deep folds and plications indicative of hypertrophy of the skin at the anal orifice.

Symptoms. The only symptoms produced by external hemorrhoids are the feeling of enlarged masses at the anus after straining and, occasionally, itching due to the skin hypertrophy. These symptoms in themselves rarely demand treatment. Very frequently, however, the veins of the external hemorrhoidal plexus become thrombosed, the cause of which is probably local trauma, with or without an associated infection. The appearance of thrombosis in the external hemorrhoid adds the symptom of pain.

The severity of the pain in the thrombosed external hemorrhoid varies according to the severity of the inflammation accompanying the thrombosis. In a large majority of cases, only one or two small venous radicals become thrombosed. These appear as firm, rounded, purplish masses at the anal orifice (Fig. 18-19). They are tender on pressure and therefore give pain when traumatized by bowel movements, sitting on hard surfaces, or standing for long periods. If untreated, the smaller thrombi may undergo organization, and the hemorrhoidal mass will remain as a tab of skin overlying an area of fibrosis. Larger thrombosed masses may slowly progress to an ulceration of the skin overlying the thrombosed vein. A new symptom then develops, namely, bleeding in small amounts and not necessarily associated with bowel movements. The blood is dark and necessitates a protective dressing. Eventually, the clot will be discharged through the ulcer, and

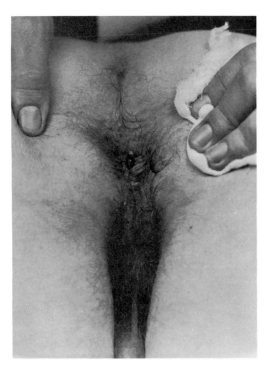

Fig. 18–19. Thrombosed external hemorrhoid seen as a mass at the anal orifice.

healing will take place by granulation. In other cases of thrombosis of the external hemorrhoidal veins, the inflammatory symptoms are much more marked. The overlying tissues become markedly edematous, and pain is a much more troublesome symptom. In such cases, it is often impossible to palpate a single large area of thrombosis; instead, multiple small thrombosed points, scattered throughout the area of diffuse edema, are apparent.

Treatment of External Hemorrhoids. Uncomplicated external hemorrhoids rarely demand treatment unless itching becomes a prominent symptom, in which case the hemorrhoidal mass, with the overlying skin, may easily be excised under local anesthesia. The excision should be performed by the use of elliptical incisions placed radially from the anal orifice. No sutures are necessary; bleeding may easily be controlled by simple pressure with a T-binder dressing.

Treatment of Thrombosed External Hemorrhoids. When thrombosis occurs in the external hemorrhoidal plexus, the patient usually seeks the help of a physician because of the pain experienced. Almost immediate relief can be given in those cases in which the thrombosis is confined to one or more well-defined masses without marked edema. In such cases, the pain seems to be due to tension in the area of thrombosis, and relief is obtained by incision and evacuation of the clot or by excision of the thrombosed segment of the vein. With the patient lying on his side, with the thrombosed area down, or in position on the proctoscope table, the area about the thrombosed vein and the overlying skin is infiltrated with a local anesthetic (Fig. 18-20). With tension on the skin away from the anal orifice, an elliptical incision is made around the thrombosed vein. The flap of skin is then picked up with forceps to expose the underlying thrombosed vein, which can often be excised with the skin. With Allis forceps placed on each lip of the incision, any other thrombosed veins in the area are sought and incised or are excised intact. A small square of Gelfoam is placed in the wound. The corner of a small square gauze compress, 3 x 3 inches, is then inserted with the forceps into the anal orifice and placed to lie in the wound. This takes care of hemostasis, and no further dressing is required. The gauze is left in place for a few hours. The patient is told to expect a slight amount of pain when the effect of the anesthetic disappears; this may easily be relieved by a potent oral analgesic. He is instructed to keep the area clean with soap and warm water after bowel movements and is warned that for a day or two there may be a slight amount of bleeding, which will necessitate the wearing of a pad or the continued use of small gauze squares held in the anus. After 3 or 4 days no dressing is necessary.

This method of unroofing a thrombosed hemorrhoid by the use of an elliptical incision gives better results than the simple single incision and evacuation of the clot. The lips of the latter type of wound

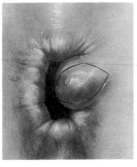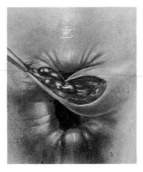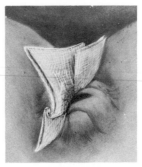

Fig. 18–20. Excision of a thrombosed external hemorrhoid. The area under and round the thrombosed mass is infiltrated with 1 percent procaine hydrochloride containing epinephrine. An elliptical incision is made over the thrombosed mass and the point of the ellipse is picked up in a hemostat or Allis forceps. The incision is then carried downward to remove the thrombosed vein with the overlying skin. A gauze compress is inserted into the anal canal to lie in the wound. No further dressing is necessary. (Ferguson, L. K.: Penn. Med. J., *40*:909)

often fall together, and infection in the small hematoma which frequently develops is associated with the prolongation of pain or discomfort. In addition, healing usually results in the formation of a large skin tab, which may be the source of considerable discomfort and itching.

The treatment of the thrombosed external hemorrhoid associated with marked edema is a much less simple matter. Occasionally, conservative treatment with the application of hot moist dressings will produce a gradual decrease in the inflammatory symptoms, so that the above procedure of unroofing the hemorrhoid may be performed. More often, however, the thrombosis is not confined to a few large segments of veins but is diffuse. In such cases, it is necessary to excise the inflammatory mass. This type of thrombosed hemorrhoid is frequently associated with thrombosis of the internal hemorrhoidal plexus and is perhaps treated more satisfactorily in the hospital. Occasionally, however, it may be possible to excise the hemorrhoidal masses under local anesthesia in an ambulatory patient.

Internal Hemorrhoids

Etiology and Symptoms. Dilatation of the upper hemorrhoidal plexus is as-

sociated almost invariably with a looseness and a laxness of the mucous membrane just above the pectinate line. It is a question not yet settled whether the dilatation of the hemorrhoidal vessels causes a stretching and a looseness of the overlying mucous membrane or whether the hypertrophy and the loose attachment of the mucous membrane offer such poor support for the underlying venous plexus as to permit it to become dilated. In any event, due to straining at stool, there is a distention of the hemorrhoidal mass, which bulges into the lumen of the anal canal. The passage of a hardened stool mass or the frequent straining in diarrhea traumatizes the protruding mucous membrane and causes it to bleed, and, frequently, the loose mucosa is dragged downward with the passage of the stool, so that it prolapses through the external sphincter. In extreme cases, the mucosa of the entire upper portion of the anal canal may be everted as a crimson rosette outside the anal sphincter. This is especially likely to occur when the external sphincter is relaxed and the anal canal becomes a ring during the act of defecation. In cases of internal hemorrhoids, the bleeding is not from the hemorrhoidal veins but from the capillaries and the arterioles of the traumatized mucous membrane which

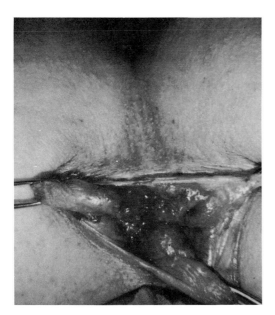

Fig. 18–21. Mixed hemorrhoids. Note the external element in what is a predominantly internal hemorrhoidal mass.

overlies them. The bleeding is bright red in color and may frequently appear in spurts. It may continue as long as the prolapse exists and even after the mucous membrane is replaced inside the anal canal, so that clots of blood are frequently found lying in the ampulla of the rectum in cases of well-developed internal hemorrhoids. In many patients, the prolapse appears not only at the time of bowel movements but also when the patient has been on his feet for a time, or when he is exercising, or when he is merely walking about. This troublesome symptom is most often noted in those in whom the external sphincter is relaxed. The symptoms of internal hemorrhoids, therefore, are bleeding and prolapse.

Thrombrosis of internal hemorrhoids occurs less frequently than does thrombosis of external hemorrhoids. When thrombosis of internal hemorrhoids is seen, the hemorrhoids are usually of the mixed type and are not the simple internal variety. However, thrombosis does occur in internal hemorrhoids; usually it is due to trauma, with or without infection.

These hemorrhoids are palpated as masses bulging from the wall of the upper anal canal. As a rule, they are not as hard and firm as most thrombosed external hemorrhoids. They are rarely as tender, and the inflammatory reaction subsides if the bowel is put at rest by the use of a liquid diet for 3 or 4 days.

Diagnosis. The diagnosis of internal hemorrhoids may often be suspected if a careful history is taken. However, other lesions which produce bleeding from the rectum must be kept constantly in mind. Even the finding of internal hemorrhoids should not deter the physician from making a careful examination of the entire lower bowel; other lesions, such as rectal polyp and carcinoma, may cause bleeding from the rectum. It follows, therefore, that a diagnosis cannot always be made at the patient's first visit unless the bowel is sufficiently clean to permit such an examination to be done. Internal hemorrhoids may be suspected on digital palpation, but one can be certain of their presence only on visual examination, which does not necessarily have to be done with instruments. If the patient has large hemorrhoids associated with a relaxed external sphincter, by pulling the buttocks apart as the patient strains, one can often see the mucous-membrane-covered hemorrhoidal masses presenting at, or prolapsing through the anal orifice.

Most often internal hemorrhoids present as three masses: on the right side, one posteriorly, at the 2 o'clock position, and one anteriorly, at the 5 o'clock position; on the left side, one laterally, at the 9 o'clock position (Fig. 18-21). These sites correspond to the positions of the venous radicals that drain upward from the rectum.

More definite knowledge can be obtained by examination with a lighted anoscope. With this instrument in place, the hemorrhoidal masses present into the scope and become more apparent as the patient strains. Often, as the hemorrhoidal mass is distended, bleeding appears from the part of the hemorrhoid nearest the pectinate line, frequently in spurts from a superficially placed arterial vessel.

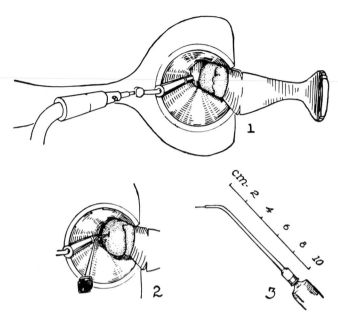

Fig. 18–22. (1) The internal hemorrhoidal mass appears in the lateral window of the Brinkerhoff anoscope as the patient strains. (2) The mass is injected at its midpoint, as near the upper edge as possible. The Frankfeldt hemorrhoidal needle may be used; the author prefers Vail's tonsil needle with the injecting tip filed down to a length of $1/2$ in ch. (3) Satisfactory type of needle.

Treatment of Internal Hemorrhoids.

When bleeding from internal hemorrhoids occurs only occasionally and is associated with periods of constipation or diarrhea, the hemorrhoidal masses are usually found to be so very small that ordinarily they give no symptoms. In such cases, it seems logical to treat the underlying cause, namely, the constipation or the diarrhea; often, regulation of the patient's bowel habits will entirely relieve the local disturbance. As an associated therapy, various sorts of astringents and sedatives made into suppositories or ointments may be applied.

When the bleeding appears at frequent intervals in spite of well-regulated bowel habits, some more active form of therapy must be employed. In such cases, excellent results may be obtained by the injection of some irritating solution into the hemorrhoidal mass. The injection is not made directly into the hemorrhoidal vein but into the area of the dilated hemorrhoidal plexus. The purpose of the solution is to set up an inflammatory reaction that will produce thrombosis and secondary fibrosis, so as to shrink up the hemorrhoidal mass and unite it more firmly to the underlying wall of the anal canal and the lower rectum.

Technique of Injection.

Injection is performed more conveniently with the patient on the proctoscopic table, although the knee-chest or the lateral position may be used. An anoscope is inserted to expose the hemorrhoidal mass. Either an end-opening or a lateral-opening scope may be used; we have found the Brinkerhoff type to be the most satisfactory. Internal hemorrhoids are usually found at three chief locations: to the right of the midline posteriorly, to the right of the midline anteriorly, and in the middle of the left lateral anal wall. As the patient strains, these hemorrhoidal projections can easily be seen through the scope as distended masses covered with bright red mucous membrane. The injection is best made with a hemorrhoidal needle, a long needle bent so that the syringe is out of the field of vision, which permits a view of the hemorrhoid during the injection. The needle is pressed into the center of the hemorrhoidal mass (Fig. 18-22), and the injection is made between the mucosa and the submucosa, and between the submucosa and the muscularis. No attempt is made to inject any certain vessel; the injection is a perivenous rather than an intravenous one.

Any one of several solutions may be

used; those used in the sclerosing of varicose veins may be employed. Sodium morrhuate, 5 percent solution, or any of the other oily solutions, such as monoethanolamine morrhuate and sodium psylliate (Sylnasol), may be used in amounts of from 0.5 to 1.0 ml. One or several hemorrhoids may be injected at a time, depending upon the size and the distribution of the hemorrhoidal masses. If a good reaction is obtained from the first injection, the mucous membrane will feel tough and leathery, and it may be wise to delay further injection until the reaction has subsided. Usually, from 1 to 4 injections are necessary to treat a single hemorrhoid, and they are given at intervals of from 5 to 7 days.

The injection treatment of hemorrhoids is one that can easily be carried out in the ambulatory patient; there is no particular pain incidental to the insertion of the needle into the insensitive mucous membrane. A very slight feeling of discomfort may be experienced at the time of the injection. Following injection, a sense of fullness may be felt in the lower rectum, but acute pain rarely occurs. Bleeding may continue for several days after injection, and the patient should be warned of this possibility. If pain occurs during or following an injection, the needle has been inserted too close to the mucocutaneous line.

By the injection treatment, practically all bleeding internal hemorrhoids without prolapse and some bleeding hemorrhoids with very minor degrees of prolapse may be treated successfully. One cannot promise that there will be no recurrence following this therapy, but the patient can be assured of relief from his bleeding, and, with normal attention to his bowel habits, the probability of recurrence is slight.

The injection treatment of internal hemorrhoids is contraindicated when the hemorrhoids prolapse, when there are other anal lesions which demand surgery, such as fissure or fistula, or when there is infection. External hemorrhoids are never treated by injection.

Hemorrhoidectomy. Internal hemor-

rhoids that prolapse are best treated by excision of the hemorrhoidal mass. When several large masses are present, hospital admission is preferable, but, in many cases with a single prolapsing mass, hemorrhoidectomy may be performed under local anesthesia in the ambulatory patient. In such cases, the entire circumference of the anal region does not have to be infiltrated to produce anesthesia sufficient for excision of the hemorrhoid. Usually, the infiltration is confined to the skin area and the underlying tissues in the region of the hemorrhoid. With the patient either on the proctoscopic table or in the lateral position, the anesthetic is injected and the hemorrhoid is brought into view with Allis forceps. A suture is then placed around the base of the hemorrhoid, fine chromic or plain catgut being used; this is tied, and the ends are left long for use as a tractor (Fig. 18-23). With traction on the ligature, on an Allis forceps over the middle of the hemorrhoid, and on the skin surface, the entire amount of hypertrophic tissue may easily be demonstrated. This is excised with scissors or a scalpel, the mucous membrane being united by interrupted sutures of fine catgut. By this method any bleeding is controlled. The ends of the sutures are left long and are grasped in a hemostat, so that by traction upon them the entire wound can be seen throughout the operation. After the excision has reached the mucocutaneous junction, a wedge-shaped area of skin and subcutaneous tissue is excised; this extends the incision to about $^{3}/_{4}$ inch lateral to the anal margin. No sutures are inserted into the skin. The ends of the sutures are left fairly long (about 1 inch). After covering the wound with a piece of Gelfoam, a simple pressure dressing of gauze is inserted into the wound, and a T-binder is applied. This operation requires an assistant; hence it is probably best performed in an outpatient department, rather than in the office. If a local anesthetic containing adrenalin is used, there is almost no bleeding.

These patients may be permitted to go home after such an operation; they are given potent analgesic tablets and are

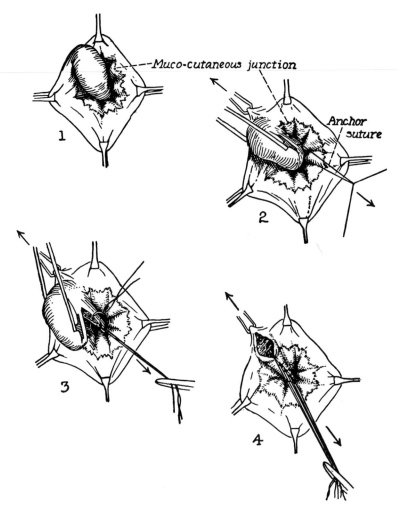

Fig. 18–23. Hemorrhoidectomy. (1) Hemorrhoid exposed. (2) Suture ligature placed. (3) Excision started, the second suture having been placed. (4) Suturing almost complete.

instructed to take one every 3 hours as needed for pain. The dressings may be removed and replaced as necessary, and, after the first 24 hours, hot sitz baths should be taken 3 or 4 times a day. Usually, a liquid diet is suggested for at least 2 days. As a rule, the wounds heal very kindly. The frequent postoperative complication of urinary retention is almost never seen in the ambulatory patient.

Management of the Patient After Hemorrhoidectomy

The patient who has had a hemorrhoidectomy should be examined a week after discharge from the hospital, and every 5 to 10 days thereafter until healing is complete. A digital examination is made to evaluate the state of healing. If this is done carefully and with gentleness,

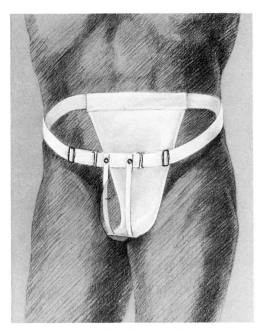

Fig. 18–24. Shield type of protective dressing for the postoperative care of anal and perineal wounds. The shield is made of cotton fabric protected by a rubberized backing and is fitted with adjustable elastic waistband and snap-on perineal straps. (Fuller Pharmaceutical Co.)

very little pain should be produced. In many cases there may be a heaping up of granulation tissue at the site of the excision. This should be reduced with scissors or with a silver nitrate stick. Occasionally the lips of the hemorrhoidectomy wound become edematous and painful. In such cases relief may be given by excising the edematous tags under local anesthesia.

Taking a hot sitz bath after each bowel movement and at least 3 or 4 times daily is the best method of keeping the area clean and of relieving the discomfort that comes from anal spasm. These baths should be continued as long as there is an open wound. At times, there is some excoriation and irritation of the perianal skin. This may be relieved by protecting the skin with zinc oxide ointment. The best dressing is the easily available sanitary napkin (Kotex), worn with an elastic belt.

There are also commercially available special protective dressings made especially for the postoperative care of anal and perineal wounds (Fig. 18-24).

Regulation of the bowels should aim for one formed stool daily. If the patient has a normal daily movement, no drugs need be given. If it is thought that some cathartic is necessary, one of the hydrophilic preparations, such as Hydrocil or Metamucil, may be used. In about 2 weeks, the patient should be able to return to work and have bowel movements without discomfort.

RELIEF OF PAIN AFTER ANAL OPERATIONS

Various methods have been suggested for the relief of pain after anal operations. These apply to ambulatory patients following the excision of thrombosed external hemorrhoids, fissure operations, hemorrhoidectomies, and even incision and drainage of acute inflammatory lesions such as perirectal abscess. Topical applications of ointments containing local anesthetics, such as Xylocaine and Nupercaine, have been used with rather mediocre results. They are better than plain gauze, but they do not give the relief of pain that might be expected in cutaneous wounds.

Postoperative pain due to adherent clotted dressings may be largely avoided by inserting soft packs of Gelfoam into the wound before the gauze dressing is applied. This not only results in a less painful wound but is also hemostatic; Gelfoam should therefore be used generously after all anal operations.

After considerable experience with various methods of relieving pain following anal operations, the author has reached some definite conclusions. Pain is due to traumatic irritation at the operative site. This irritation may be held to a minimum if approximation of mucosal or skin edges can be at least partially effected. The traumatic irritation of the wound site causes a secondary spasm of the anal sphincter; this is most marked at the time of bowel movement. The sphincter spasm grasps and squeezes the traumatic wound and so prolongs the pain after bowel movement. Applications of moist heat (hot compresses or hot sitz baths) are the most effective way to relax anal spasm and relieve anal pain. They should be used after each bowel movement and at least 4 times daily.

There is a general idea that the softer the stool, the less pain the patient will experience after anal operations. This is true up to a point. Even in the absence of an operative wound, the passage of a hard dry stool, produces discomfort. On the other hand, more trauma and a worse inflammatory reaction in the operative wound are caused by soiling from frequent loose or watery stools than are caused by a firm formed stool. One formed stool per day should be the aim. Usually, a cathartic is not advisable, but the hydrophilic stool softeners are useful.

The long-acting, oil-soluble anesthetics might seem to be ideal for use after anal operations. After considerable experience with them, however, the author has given them up completely. They are not necessary if the plan of postoperative care suggested above is followed, and, even with the most careful technique, there is danger of necrosis and slough, which are much more difficult to endure and treat than is the pain from an anal operation.

DISEASES OF THE RECTUM

All patients with anal, rectal, and bowel symptoms deserve an examination of the lower bowel with the proctosigmoidoscope. There are many types of instruments (of metal, nonconducting material, etc.) available with lights at the distal end of the scope and at the handle end of the scope. Fiber-optic sigmoidoscopes are also satisfactory. The scope should be provided with an airtight window and a bulb-type insufflator for distending the bowel during the examination.

A tube for suction, about 4 inches longer than the scope, is useful to remove liquid bowel contents. The cheapest and best suction tube is made of copper tubing about 1 cm. in diameter, bent proximally at a right angle, so that suction can be carried out under direct vision, with the hand holding the suction out of the line of vision. Suction is also useful to remove smoke produced with electrodesiccation. Suction can be attached to many electrodesiccating electrodes.

The author has found it best to do the planned procedure (e.g., biopsy, snaring off a polyp, electrodesiccation) the first time the lesion is seen through the scope. If the scope is advanced with the idea of coming back to the lesion as the scope is removed, many small lesions may be hard to find again or may be missed completely.

In making an endoscopic examination of the bowel, the scope should be advanced only when a lumen is seen. By manipulating the scope and inflating the bowel under direct vision, the lumen can usually be seen. A proctoscopic examination should be a painless procedure. If pain is produced, it usually indicates that the bowel is fixed in a position which will not allow it to be straightened out on the scope, and the examination should be discontinued.

The position on the table for the proctoscopic examination may not be comfortable, but it should be tolerable, for the patient. Tables adjusted so that the patient's weight is borne on his forearms and elbows are best. To allow the abdominal contents to drop away from the pelvis, the abdomen should not rest on the table.

Cleansing tissue or unsterile gauze may be used for cleansing and retraction of the buttocks. Wipes for this purpose are available (Chux, Johnson & Johnson).

POLYPS OF THE PELVIC RECTUM

Polyps of the pelvic rectum are not uncommon. Most frequently, they are nodules half the size of a pea; they arise from the mucosal surface of the bowel. They give no symptoms, but their prophylactic removal is recommended because they may become larger and may undergo carcinomatous change.

Treatment. Their removal with basket-type biopsy forceps or with a coagulating electrode is a simple matter. The tissue thus obtained should be sent for histologic examination. Hemostasis may be obtained by pressure with a swab soaked in epinephrine or by electrocoagulation.

PEDUNCULATED POLYPS OF THE RECTUM

Pedunculated rectal polyps may vary from masses the size of marbles to those so large as to encroach materially upon the lumen of the rectum. They may have broad or narrow peduncles attached to the rectal wall at a relatively broad base. They are often palpable on digital examination.

Symptoms. Pedunculated polyps practically always give symptoms. They are subjected to the trauma of peristalsis and of the passage of the fecal mass over them. Patients complain of a dragging sensation in the rectum at the time of bowel movements, and, if the polyp is large, there is the constant sensation of incomplete evacuation. Occasionally, polyps in the lower rectum may prolapse through the anus. The presenting symptom is frequently bleeding with the bowel movement. The cause of the bleeding is easily discovered on proctoscopic examination. The repeated trauma to the polyp causes an ulceration of its surface, from which bleeding occurs with each movement as the stool mass moves over the surface. The bleeding may be sufficient to cause clots to form in the rectum.

Treatment. To relieve the bleeding and the dragging sensation in the rectum, removal of the polyp is advisable. It is thought that the small polyps (less than 1 cm. in diameter) are true adenomas and rarely have malignant potential. Large polypoid growths, however, may be small early carcinomas. It is important, therefore, that all of these growths be subjected to pathologic examination. In some cases a biopsy is taken before excision; in

others, the polyp itself is removed and is used as the specimen.

The polyp is seen through the proctoscope, and with a snare attached to an electrocoagulating current, it may be removed at its base without bleeding (Figs. 18-25 and 18-26), or it may be destroyed by electrodesiccation at one or two sittings. No anesthesia is required. By this method the author has removed not only rectal but also sigmoidal polyps from ambulatory patients without complication.

Usually no specific aftercare is required. A low residue diet is prescribed for about 10 days or 2 weeks to reduce the trauma which may occur from a large hard stool mass. Stool softeners are given for the same reason. The ulceration resulting from the removal of the polyp heals in about 2 weeks, leaving a small scar. This area should be observed at frequent follow-up visits for a period of a year because of the danger of carcinoma in these lesions.

THE DIAGNOSIS AND BIOPSY OF RECTAL CARCINOMA

Patients who come into an office or outpatient clinic complaining of a change in bowel habits, the passage of blood in the stools, crampy abdominal pains relieved by the passage of gas, extremely foul-smelling stools, passage of ribbon-like stools, and the feeling of fullness in the rectum should be suspected to have a rectal carcinoma.

This diagnosis can be made in most cases by an examination performed on an ambulatory patient. With the patient in the knee-chest or proctoscopic position, a digital examination will disclose a soft fungating mass, a deep ulcer crater with heaped up edges, or a hard constriction of the rectal lumen. The diagnosis can be made on proctoscopic examination, which allows one to see the lesion that has produced the findings of the digital palpation. To confirm the diagnosis, a specimen is removed for pathologic examination.

The biopsy can be obtained with a

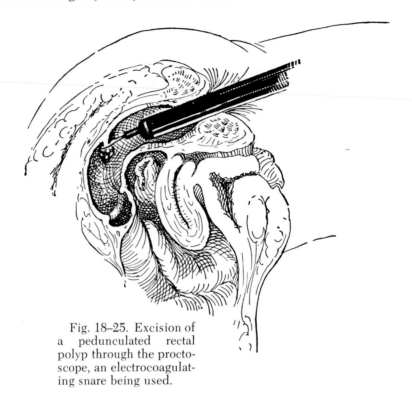

Fig. 18–25. Excision of a pedunculated rectal polyp through the proctoscope, an electrocoagulating snare being used.

long-handled biopsy forceps (Fig. 18-27), which is introduced through the proctoscope. With the lesion under direct vision, a piece of the edge of the tumor is snipped off and is preserved in a bottle of formalin for sending to the laboratory. To control the bleeding that usually occurs, electrodesiccation may be used. The long-handled electrode with a suction attachment for smoke removal is excellent for this purpose (Fig. 18-28).

OFFICE AND OUTPATIENT CARE AFTER RECTAL OPERATIONS PERFORMED IN THE HOSPITAL

Most patients on whom anal and rectal operations have been performed are discharged from the hospital before their wounds are healed, and they require further care in an office or outpatient clinic. The aftercare of patients who have had the common anal operations has been described above.

CARE FOLLOWING ABDOMINOPERINEAL RESECTION OF THE RECTUM FOR CARCINOMA

In many of these patients the perineal wound is almost healed by the time they are discharged from the hospital; in others, the wound may be widely open, with considerable discharge. In the latter group the drainage comes from gradual liquefaction of sloughing tissue in the pelvis. The pelvic wound will gradually heal by granulation. The healing process can be hastened and the drainage greatly decreased by mechanically removing as much as possible of the sloughing tissue from the perineal and pelvic wound. This is best done by irrigating the wound with saline solution, using a rubber catheter to lead the fluid from a reservoir or using a bulb syringe. After as much as possible of the slough and purulent material has been removed by irrigation, those pieces of sloughing tissue that float in the flow of the irrigating solution may be removed with scissors and forceps. Antiseptic so-

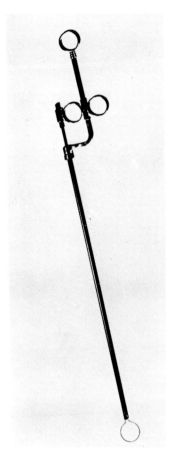

Fig. 18–26. Snare for the endoscopic removal of rectal and sigmoidal polyps by electrodesiccation. (Coles Electronic Corp.)

lutions are of no value in this process. After the slough has been cleared from the wound, simple perineal dressings are all that are necessary (Fig. 18-24). Excoriation due to irritation from the wound discharge can be prevented by applications of zinc oxide ointment.

Care Following Abdominoperineal Resection for Ulcerative Colitis

In the immediate postoperative period, the care of the perineal wound is the same after operations for ulcerative colitis as it is after operations for rectal carcinoma. However, after the slough has disap-peared from the wound, there is frequent-ly an overgrowth of granulation tissue from the chronically infected perirectal tissue. This produces a continuous thick purulent discharge, which continues in spite of all of the ordinary measures used to combat it.

The only effective treatment that has been found to date is the use of nitrogen mustard (Mustargen) locally. The nitrogen mustard is placed in solution by adding 10 ml. of sterile saline or water to the bottle. With the patient in the inverted (proctoscopic) position, the area about the wound is protected with a generous layer of petroleum jelly. The perineal wound is then packed loosely with plain gauze packing (1 inch) soaked in the Mustargen solution, or the solution is introduced into the wound with a cotton swab soaked in the solution. Care must be taken not to produce bleeding. After the application of Mustargen, any excess of the solution must be sponged away because the solution in contact with the skin produces a marked burn and blistering. The wound is protected with an absorbent dressing. Two or three applications of nitrogen mustard may be necessary before the chronically infected granulation tissue in the perineal wound is destroyed.

PILONIDAL CYSTS AND SINUSES

(Sacrococcygeal Cysts and Sinuses)

Etiology. Cysts and sinuses which develop in the sacrococcygeal area are common lesions that frequently require surgery. The origin of these cysts has not been well established, despite much embryologic and pathologic research. However, the evidence is that the lesion is primarily a typical foreign body (hair) granuloma.

Clinical Manifestations. Whatever the true etiology of these cysts and sinuses, the clinical symptoms are constant. In almost all cases, there are from one to several tiny openings in the midline of the intergluteal cleft over the lower portion of the sacrum. Hairs often protrude

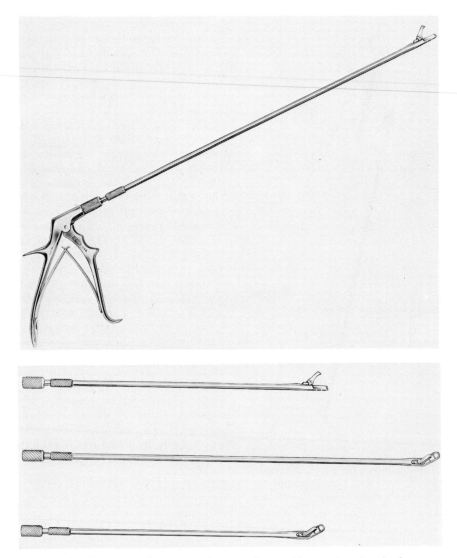

Fig. 18–27. Biopsy forceps with interchangeable cutting heads for use through the proctoscope to obtain specimens of rectal and sigmoidal lesions. (Welch Allyn)

from these openings, and there is frequently a discharge sufficient to keep the skin moist and, sometimes, macerated. Less commonly, there are no openings on the skin but simply a mass in the midline over the lower sacrum. As a rule, the sinuses are not noted by the patient until early adult life, and the first symptoms are the presence of moisture, maceration, itching, and, sometimes, burning in the region of the sinuses.

The usual reason for treatment of a pilonidal cyst is secondary infection. Most often, this follows mild and repeated trauma, such as sitting on hard surfaces. The infection may be relatively mild and may subside spontaneously by the drainage of pus from the tract for a few days. Often, secondary fistulous openings appear, usually at one or the other side of the midline. These secondary fistulas may be numerous and may be

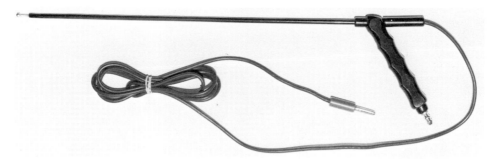

Fig. 18–28. Ball type of electrode with suction attachment for electrodesiccation of rectal lesions through the proctosigmoidoscope. This instrument is often used to destroy small polyps and to control bleeding after biopsy of rectal lesions (carcinomas). (Coles Electronic Corp.)

some distance away from the original cyst opening (Fig. 18-29).

When infection produces an abscess, a tender, red swelling appears in the midline over the lower sacrum. The patient complains of marked pain and tenderness, and, on examination, the abscess is easily demonstrated. Frequently pus appears at the sinus openings or following the removal of hairs which protrude from one of the sinus tracts.

Treatment. The treatment of pilonidal sinuses must be divided into treatment of the acutely infected pilonidal cyst or sinus and the treatment of a quiescent sinus or cyst.

Incision and Drainage. When an acute infection appears in a pilonidal cyst, it is unwise to attempt to do anything more than drain the purulent material and permit the acute inflammation to subside. It is inadvisable to attempt any radical extirpation of the cyst or the sinus at this time because of the marked cellulitis, edema, and inflammation of the surrounding tissues and because of the large area of tissue which must be excised and which cannot be closed by suture.

The treatment of an acute inflammation, therefore, consists of drainage of the purulent material and the application of hot moist dressings. In a few cases, drainage may be accomplished by simple dilatation of one of the sinus openings. Frequently, however, it is wise to incise the cyst. This can be accomplished under

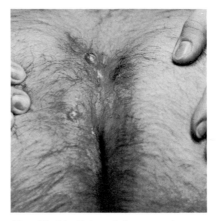

Fig. 18–29. Pilonidal cyst with secondary sinus opening.

local infiltration anesthesia in the ambulatory patient. The anesthetic solution is injected intradermally in the line of the proposed incision. If a suction apparatus is available, the pus in the abscess cavity may be aspirated without discomfort to the patient. All hairs in the abscess cavity should be carefully removed before gauze packing is inserted. Antibiotic therapy appears to aid in controlling the infection, although the inflammatory process will subside promptly without it if adequate drainage is provided.

The usual treatment with hot wet dressings, with removal of the packing in from 2 to 3 days, permits subsidence of the infection and of the inflammatory reac-

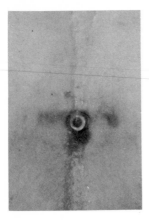
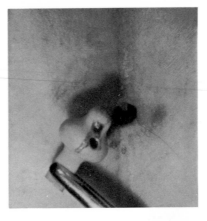

Fig. 18–30. (*Left*) Pezzer catheter in place after incision and drainage of acute pilonidal cyst. (*Right*) Pezzer catheter removed after 3 weeks.

tion. After removal of the packing at the first dressing, the wound is searched for hair collections or deep pockets. The hairs are removed with forceps. The lips of the wound are kept apart with gauze until the wound cavity begins to fill with granulation tissue. The wounds are allowed to heal and no further surgery is attempted in such cases for a period of from 2 to 3 months at least.

An alternative method of treatment of the acute pilonidal abscess is incision and drainage and insertion of a small Pezzer catheter to assure complete drainage (Fig. 18-30). This can be left in place for 3 or 4 weeks until the acute inflammation has subsided and definitive excisional therapy can be carried out. This is usually done in the hospital under general or subarachnoid block anesthesia. In selected cases, however, it can be done on ambulatory patients.

In a very few cases, recurrence will not take place following simple incision. This is especially true if the incision has been wide and adequate drainage has been obtained. More commonly, however, recurrence can be expected unless excision of the sinus tract is performed.

Peterson and Ames believe that recurrence can be prevented and permanent healing achieved, even in acute cases, by suturing the cyst wall to the skin. After wide incision of the abscess, they excise a wedge-shaped section of tissue between the skin and the cyst wall and unite these two structures with a running suture of wire or silk. This is a slight modification

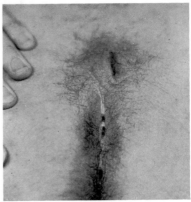

Fig. 18–31. Pilonidal cyst following incision and drainage of an abscess. The incision is seen above the midline sinus opening. The inflammatory reaction has subsided, and the cyst now is ready for excision.

of the marsupialization procedure long practiced by Buie.

Excision and Primary Suture. In the pilonidal sinus that has healed following incision for acute infection (Fig. 18-31) or in the chronic draining pilonidal sinus without marked inflammatory reaction, excision of the tract and primary suture of the wound is the method of treatment which has given the best result in the hands of the author.

The technique of the operation is simple. Procaine-epinephrine is injected around and under the sinus tract and cyst. The incision is then begun in the midline over the sinus tract and continued down-

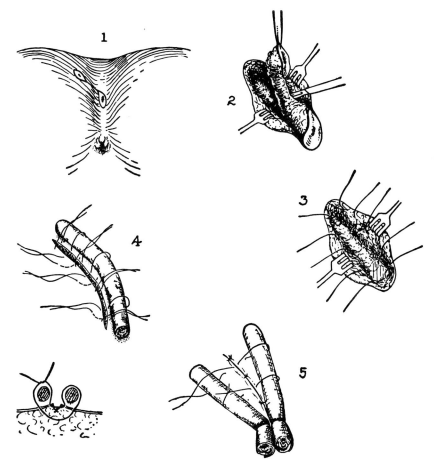

Fig. 18–32. Technique of excision of a pilonidal cyst. The patient is placed on the abdomen with a pillow under the hips. The area round the cyst tract is infiltrated with procaine solution. (1) Line of incision to include any accessory openings and midline opening. (2) The cyst and the sinus are excised as a narrow tract with a scalpel. It is important to keep the edges of the wound on tension with sharp rake retractors. (3) The dead space is obliterated with buried sutures of fine silk or catgut, all of which are placed before any are tied. (4 and 5) Method of wound closure with mattress sutures tied over gauze rolls and interrupted sutures between the mattress sutures. All the skin sutures are of steel wire.

ward to surround the sinus opening. Using sharp rakes as retractors, the incision is deepened to isolate the sinus opening entirely. An Allis forceps is then applied to close the sinus orifice and to serve as a tractor on the tissue to be removed. With the tissue constantly on tension, the dissection is then carried upward, the sinus and the cyst being isolated. The line of separation from the fascia overlying the sacrum is easily recognized, but the

lateral separation must be made with the scalpel. When there are secondary sinus openings, these are dissected out before the main cyst is attacked.

After removal of the cyst and the sinus, a clean wound remains, with normal fatty tissue on the sides and sacral fascia in the base. Closure is effected with two layers of sutures. The first layer is of fine alloy steel wire or fine silk; 4 or 5 interrupted sutures are placed so as to include the fatty tissue on each side of the wound and the sacral fascia at its base. These sutures are all inserted before any are tied, because the partial closure of the wound obtained by tying them as they are inserted makes it difficult and even impossible to insert accurately the last two sutures. This layer of sutures obliterates dead space in the base of the wound. The skin edges are approximated and dead space is further obliterated by the use of mattress sutures of alloy steel wire tied over gauze rolls (Fig. 18-32). Often these wire mattress sutures are placed first, so that the deep portion of each suture includes all the layers of the wound, including the sacral fascia. The superficial portions of the mattress sutures are not placed until the buried fine wire sutures have been introduced and tied. Usually, several interrupted sutures of fine wire are used to aid in the approximation of the skin edges. A pyramidal pressure dressing of gauze is applied and held in place with firm adhesive strips.

When primary closure cannot be effected without too much tension, the skin edge is sewn to the sacral fascia or to the base of the cyst, as recommended by Buie.

Our experience has shown that primary union is dependent on the obliteration of dead space and the prevention of serum collections, and to this end, pressure on the wound is further obtained by placing the patient on his back on a litter or an operating table for an hour after operation.

This method of therapy—excision under local anesthesia of pilonidal cysts and sinuses in the quiescent stage—has produced a cure in 92 percent of our patients, with few recurrences. The healing period, averaging 17.4 days in 37 patients, has been a factor in support of this treatment.

Most of the patients with pilonidal cyst are of the fat, hairy type. The hairs on each side of the gluteal cleft often grow downward and act as a bristle brush on the fresh scar tissue of the healed pilonidal wound. If this healed scar is not protected, it is often traumatized by the hairs on each side of the wound, and a new ulceration appears. To avoid this complication, it is necessary to keep the hairs away from the healed wound. The author has tried many ways to do this. Repeated shaving around the wound should be carried out. In some cases epilation doses of x-rays have been necessary to control hair growth.

BIBLIOGRAPHY

Fistula in Ano

Dunphy, J. E., and Pikula, J.: Surgery for fistula in ano. Surg. Clin. N. Am., *35*:1469, 1955.

Nesselrod, J. P.: Pathogenesis of common anorectal infections. Am. J. Surg., *88*:815, 1954.

Rosser, C.: Comments on the treatment of lesions resulting from anal infections. Am. J. Surg., *88*:181, 1954.

Turell, R.: Anal fistula: background and surgical treatment. New York J. Med., *58*:1473, 1958.

Fissure in Ano

Brossy, J. J.: Anatomy and surgery of anal fissure with special reference to internal sphincterotomy. Ann. Surg. *144*:991, 1956.

Bengt, F., and Rietz, K. A.: Treatment of fissure in ano. Acta Chir. Scand. *128*:312, 1964.

Swinton, N. W.: Anal fissure. Surg. Clin. N. Am., *22*:811, 1942.

Turell, R.: The surgical treatment of chronic anal fissure. Surg., Gynec. Obstet., *86*:434, 1948.

Watts, J. McK., Bennett, R. C., and Galigher, J. G.: Stretching of anal sphincters in treatment of fissure in ano. Brit. Med. J., *2*:342, 1964.

Pruritus Ani

Alexander, R. M., and Manheim, S. D.: The effect of hydrocortisone acetate ointment on pruritus ani (preliminary and short report). J. Invest. Derm., *21*:223, 1953.

Becker, G. L.: Recent advances in the local treatment of perianal skin lesions. Am. J. Surg., *88*:289, 1954.

Buie, L. A.: Anal pruritus. J. Iowa Med. Soc., *29*:185, 1939.

Hayden, E. P.: The Rectum and Colon. Philadelphia, Lea & Febiger, 1939.

Kile, R.: The use of hydrocortisone-neomycin ointment. Ohio Med. J., *49*:1047, 1953.

Sarner, J. B.: Etiology, diagnosis, and therapy of pruritus ani. Clin. Med., *70*:75, July, 1963.

Shapiro, A. L., and Rothman, S.: Pruritus ani: a clinical study. Gastroenterology, *5*:155, 1945.

Condyloma Acuminatum

Culp, O. S., and Kaplan, I. W.: Condyloma acuminatum: 200 cases treated with podophyllin. Ann. Surg., *120*:251, 1944.

Kaplan, I. W.: Condylomata acuminata. New Orleans Med. Surg., *94*:388, 1942. Abstr. Digest Treat., *6*:42, 1942.

Microenema

Lieberman, W.: Rapid patient preparation for sigmoidoscopy by microenema. Am. J. Proctol., *15*:136, 1964.

Hemorrhoids

Barron, J., and Fallis, L. S.: Nonoperative treatment of internal hemorrhoids. Canad. Med. J., *90*:910, 1964.

Bartlet, W.: Technic for hemorrhoidectomy. Arch. Surg., *78*:916, 1959.

Kratzer, G. L.: Improved technic in hemorrhoidectomy. Dis. Colon Rectum, *7*:177, 1964.

Polyps of the Rectum and Colon

Colcok, B. P.: Relation of polyps to carcinoma of the colon and rectum. Current Surgical Management, II, pp. 45-53. Philadelphia, W. B. Saunders, 1960.

Spratt, J. S., Jr., and Ackerman, L. V.: Treatment of polyps of the colon as benign lesions. Current Surgical Management, II, pp. 37-41. Philadelphia, W. B. Saunders, 1960.

Spratt, J. S., Ackerman, L. V., and Moyer, C. A.: Relationship of polyps of the colon to conic cancer. Ann. Surg., *148*:682, 1958.

Pilonidal Disease

Abramson, D. J.: A simple marsupialization technic for treatment of pilonidal sinus: long-term follow-up. Ann. Surg., *151*:261, 1960.

Block, R. I.: Early treatment of pilonidal abscess. Mod. Med. P., 97, March, 1964.

Buie, L. A.: Jeep disease (pilonidal disease of mechanized warfare), Southern J. Med., *37*:103, 1944.

Cherry, J. K.: Primary closure of pilonidal sinus. Surg., Gynec. Obstet., *126*:1263, 1968.

Culp, C. E.: Pilonidal disease and its treatment. Surg. Clin. N. Am., *47*:1007, 1967.

Currie, A. R., Gibson, T., and Goodsall, A. L.: Interdigital sinuses of barbers' hands. Brit. J. Surg. *41*:278, 1953.

Downing, J. G.: Barbers' pilonidal sinus. JAMA, *148*:1501, 1952.

Fox, S. L.: The origin of pilonidal sinus, with an analysis of its comparative anatomy and histogenesis. Surg., Gynec. Obstet., *60*:137, 1935.

Gage, M.: Pilonidal sinus: an explanation of its embryologic development. Arch. Surg., *31*:175, 1935.

Granet, E., and Ferguson, L. K.: Pilonidal disease: management of cysts, sinuses, and abscesses in naval personnel. Am. J. Surg., *70*:139, 1945.

Hardaway, R. M.: Pilonidal cyst—neither pilonidal nor cyst. Arch. Surg., *76*:142, 1958.

Heifetz, C. J.: Pilonidal disease: a study of fifty consecutive cases treated successfully by excision and primary closure. Am. J. Surg., *96*:405, 1958.

Hirshowitz, B., Mahler, D., and Kaufmann-Friedman, K.: Treatment of pilonidal sinus. Surg., Gynec. Obstet., *131*:119, 1970.

Jacobson, P.: Pilonidal disease: management without excision. GP, *19*:84, 1959.

King, E.S.J.: The nature of pilonidal sinus. Aust. New Zeal. J. Surg., *16*:182, 1947.

Kluge, D. N.: Hospital versus outpatient treatment of pilonidal sinus. Surgery, *57*:244, 1965.

McCaughan, J. S.: The results of the surgical treatment of pilonidal cysts. Surg., Gynec., Obstet., *121*:316, 1965.

Maurice, B. A., and Greenwood, R. K.: A conservative treatment of pilonidal sinus. Brit. J. Surg., *51*:510, 1964.

Notaras, M. J.: A review of three popular methods of treatment of postanal (pilonidal) sinus disease. Brit. J. Surg., *12*:886, 1970.

Patey, D. H., and Scarff, R. W.: Pilonidal sinus in a barber's hand with observations on postanal pilonidal sinus. Lancet, *2*:13, 1948.

Peterson, P., and Ames, R. H.: Pilonidal sinuses and cysts. Am. J. Surg., *65*:384, 1944.

Peterson, P., and Ames, R. H.: Pilonidal sinuses and cysts. Am. J. Surg., *65*:384, 1944.

Pulaski, E. J., Scavone, E., Brune, W. H., and Christopher, W. N.: The factor of infection in pilonidal (sacrococcygeal) disease. Ann. Surg., *144*:170, 1956.

Pyrtek, L. J., and Bartus, S. A.: Excision of pilonidal cyst with simplified partial wound closure. Surg., Gynec. Obstet., *118*:605, 1964.

Raffman, R. A.: A re-evaluation of the pathogenesis of pilonidal sinus. Ann. Surg., *150*:895, 1959.

Rickles, J. A.: The office treatment of pilonidal sinus. J. Int. Coll. Surg., *36*:61, 1961.

Stephens, F. O., and Sloane, D. R.: Conservative management of pilonidal sinus. Surg., Gynec. Obstet., *129*:786, 1969.

Thomas, D.: Pilonidal sinus: a review of the literature and a report of 100 cases. Med. J. Aust., *2*:184, 1968.

Turner, F. P., and O'Neil, J. W.: Treatment of pilonidal sinus by primary closure. Arch. Surg., *78*:398, 1959.

Warren, J. C.: Abscess, containing hairs on the nates. Am. J. Med. Sci., *28*:113, 1854.

19
Back

Hugo V. Rizzoli, M.D.

EXAMINATION OF THE BACK

In order to treat patients with low back lesions satisfactorily, the physician must attempt to make an accurate diagnosis. Though the etiology of the back problem may remain obscure in some patients, the evaluation of each patient requires a careful history, physical examination, and radiological study. Obviously, a careful history will allow the examining physician to determine whether the onset was insidious or sudden, whether or not it was related to an incident of trauma, whether or not there is a history of previous attacks, joint disease, malignancy, or tuberculosis or other infections. In addition, the history may give some indication of the patient's degree of emotional stability.

The physical examination includes a methodical evaluation of musculoskeletal and neurological functions. When possible the patient should be examined in the standing, sitting, and recumbent positions.

Musculoskeletal Examination. This examination includes evaluation of the following:

1. Posture and gait.
2. Lumbar lordotic curve. There is usually straightening or reversal of the normal lumbar curve with acute and chronic lesions of the lumbar spine.

3. Curvature of the spine. Scoliosis and kyphosis should be noted. With acute lumbar disc lesions there is often a sciatic scoliosis or a pelvic tilt. The listing of the spine is always away from the affected side, and the pelvis is almost always higher on the ipsilateral side.

4. Muscle spasm. Spasm of the erector spinal paravertebral muscles is commonly present during an acute back attack. Spasm of these muscles is often visible and always palpable and may be more marked on one side.

5. Mobility of the spine. Especially with acute lesions, flexion, extension, lateral flexion, and rotation are apt to be limited. The degree of restriction of motion is often related to the severity of the pathological process.

6. Local tenderness. Tenderness to palpation on percussion of the spinous process suggests involvement of the vertebra by an inflammatory, traumatic, or metastatic process, although in the sensitive and emotionally upset patient this may have no real significance. With disc protrusion, however, the tenderness is usually approximately 2 inches lateral to the spinous process at the level of disc protrusion. In addition, there is often tenderness over the sciatic notch on the affected side.

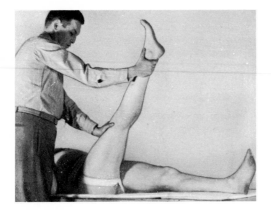

Fig. 19–1. The straight-leg-raising test. This maneuver stretches the sciatic nerve and yields pain if one of its lower roots is compressed. Pain may be experienced in the back and/or leg.

7. Straight-leg-raising test. This test is usually positive in patients with nerve root irritation and/or compression. The test is performed with the patient supine and with the legs extended. The leg to be examined is elevated by the examiner so that it is passively flexed at the hip with the knee extended (Fig. 19-1). Normally the leg can be elevated to 80 degrees or 90 degrees above the horizontal, depending upon the degree of hamstring tightness. This results in stretching of the sciatic nerve and its component roots. This maneuver is painless unless one of the roots is being compressed. When this is the case, the degree to which the leg can be raised is reduced, and the examiner experiences a feeling of resistance as he raises the leg. Coincident with this, the patient complains of pain in the back or pain radiating into the ipsilateral leg or both. The *contralateral straight-leg-raising test* is said to be positive when elevation of the normal leg is limited and results in pain in the opposite leg. This usually suggests a marked degree of nerve root compression, and when it is present, the chances are greater that the patient will not respond to conservative measures.

8. The femoral stretch test. This test is performed for evaluation of nerve root irritation at higher levels, e.g., involvement of the L_4 root at the level of the L_3-L_4 disc and the L_3 root at the L_2-L_3 disc. This test is performed with the patient prone. The examiner passively extends the leg at the hip with the knee flexed or extended (Fig. 19-2). The test is positive when the degree of extension is limited and is accompanied by pain in the anterior aspect of the ipsilateral thigh.

9. The fabere test. Because hip disease may result in pain referred to the thigh, it is important to rule out hip disease. The fabere test is always positive when there is significant pathological change in the hip. The test is performed with the patient lying supine. The examiner begins the test with the hip flexed at 90 degrees and the knee flexed to 90 degrees. The leg is then passively externally rotated and extended at the hip. The test is positive if there is limitation and pain in the hip when the examination is performed. The word "fabere" indicates the movements performed at the hip: *f*lexion, *ab*duction, *e*xternal *r*otation, and *e*xtension.

10. The jugular compression test. This test is best performed with the patient supine. Both internal jugular veins are compressed by the examiner for a few seconds. The accompanying rise in intracranial venous pressure is transmitted to the lumbar subarachnoid space and results in some stretching of the lumbar roots in their extrathecal course. When this is done to patients who have a significant degree of nerve root compression, the pain is increased, and this increment of pain subsides when jugular compression is discontinued.

Neurological Examination. With lesions of the lumbar spine resulting in nerve root compression, the resulting

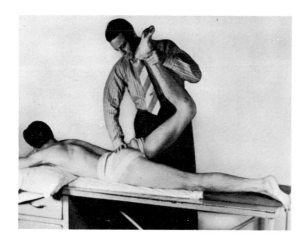

Fig. 19–2. Femoral stretch test. This maneuver yields pain in the anterior aspect of the ipsilateral thigh when the L_3 or L_4 nerve root is compressed.

neurological deficit in the motor sphere, if present, is of the lower motor neuron type. Therefore, motor weakness, atrophy, and decreased deep tendon reflexes may be present in the distribution of the involved nerve. Subjective sensory phenomena (tingling, numbness, and pain) and objective sensory impairment may also occur in the appropriate dermatome.

1. Motor function. Motor function is tested with the patient in the recumbent, sitting, and standing positions. Atrophy of the muscles of the calf, thigh, and buttock, if present, is usually visible. The degree of atrophy can be documented by appropriate measurements of calf and thigh circumferences. The calf circumference is best measured at the level of greatest circumference, and this measurement is compared with the measurement from the contralateral leg. The thigh circumference is measured at various distances above the upper edge of the patella and compared with similar measurements of the other leg. In evaluating the resulting measurements, the examiner should ask if the patient is right- or left-"legged." Gross degrees of motor weakness will be apparent from observation of the patient's gait. The ability to dorsiflex or plantar flex the ankle and toes can be evaluated quickly by having the patient walk on his heels and then on his toes. In addition, careful evaluation of individual muscles must be performed. With the patient supine, the patient is asked to flex

each hip against the examiner's resistance. Extension, abduction, and adduction of the hip are also tested against the examiner's resistance. The hamstring and quadriceps muscles are examined by having the patient flex the lower leg at the knee and then extend the lower leg at the knee against the examiner's resistance. Both plantar flexion and dorsiflexion of the ankle can also be tested with the patient supine. The patient performs these actions against resistance. It is extremely important to test extension of the big toe against the examiner's resistance for evidence of extensor hallucis longus weakness, since this is frequently present with disc lesions at the L_4-L_5 level (L_5 root) even though there is no evidence of weakness in dorsiflexion of the foot.

2. Sensory function. Sensory testing with pin or pinwheel is often helpful. Sensory loss may be present in the appropriate dermatome, that is, in the skin distribution of the irritated nerve root. Certainly sensory deficits occur more frequently than do motor defects.

3. Reflexes. The deep tendon reflexes may be tested with the patient supine or sitting. The Achilles tendon reflex is frequently depressed or absent with S_1 root lesions. The patellar reflex may be diminished or absent with L_3 or L_4 root involvement.

X-ray Examination. Adequate radiological examination of the lumbar spine is essential in all patients complaining of

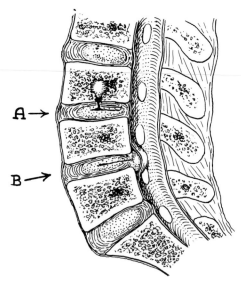

Fig. 19–3. Herniation of the nucleus pulposus. (A) Extrusion of the nucleus pulposus into a vertebral body (the Schmorl type), usually of little clinical importance. (B) Posterior herniation of the nucleus pulposus causing pressure on a nerve root.

low back and/or sciatic pain. Routinely, anteroposterior, lateral, and oblique views of the lumbosacral spine should be obtained. Often this study should include radiographic examination of the hips.

RUPTURED INTERVERTEBRAL DISC

This clinical entity is certainly the most common cause of low back pain with or without sciatica.

History. The patient's description of the onset, the cause, and the nature of his symptoms is often typical enough to enable the examiner to make a tentative diagnosis on the basis of the history alone. Though lumbar intervertebral disc lesions often produce a characteristic clinical syndrome, there does tend to be significant variation from patient to patient and from time to time in the same patient. The patient often gives a history of recurrent low back pain in the past and often, but not always, relates the attacks to a minor degree of trauma, such as

bending over to lift something heavy, as well as to more trivial episodes, such as bending over to dry his feet after a shower, bending over to brush his teeth, or coughing or sneezing. The traumatic incident may well occur several hours, or even days, before the onset of pain (Fig. 19-3).

Usually the first symptom of ruptured lumbar disc is low back pain, later followed by sciatic pain (Fig. 19-4). The severity varies from patient to patient, and the attack may be extremely acute, severe, and sudden in onset. When this is the case, the patient usually has marked spasm of the paravertebral muscles and is virtually immobilized in a rigid state. Later, unilateral sciatic pain may occur (Fig. 19-5). In some instances there may be dull, chronic low back pain of insidious onset, later followed by acute back and/or sciatic pain. Less frequently, the onset of symptoms may be heralded by unilateral sciatic pain without low back pain. Occasionally there is the simultaneous onset of low back pain and sciatic pain. Characteristically, coughing, sneezing, and movement intensify the pain. Patients with sciatic pain often describe areas of localized numbness and paresthesias. These symptoms may have localizing significance in that they may help to identify the involved nerve root (Fig. 19-6). A history of bowel or bladder dysfunction may be given; if such dysfunction present, it may indicate massive nuclear extrusion, which demands prompt surgical attention.

Examination. During an acute attack, patients with ruptured intervertebral discs will usually show spasm of the paravertebral muscles and a decrease of the normal lumbar lordosis, and, often, a tilt of the lumbar spine away from the affected leg. Movements of the lumbar spine are often limited. The straight-leg-raising test usually demonstrates limitation of motion; when there is a marked degree of nuclear extrusion with marked nerve root compression, the straight-leg-raising test is strongly positive and the contralateral straight-leg-raising test may be positive. When the lesion is at the

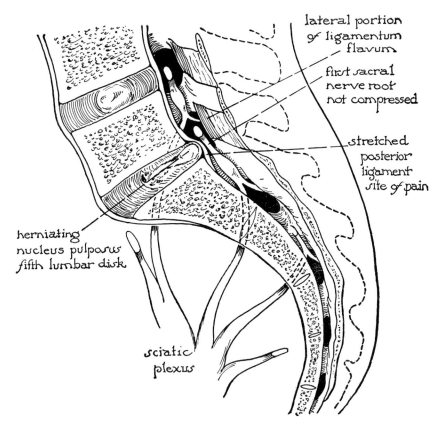

lateral portion
of ligamentum
flavum

first sacral
nerve root
not compressed

stretched
posterior
ligament
site of pain

herniating
nucleus pulposus
fifth lumbar disk

sciatic
plexus

Fig. 19–4. Posterior herniation of the nucleus pulposus of the fifth lumbar disc giving rise to low back pain without nerve root irritation. (Keegan, J. J.: JAMA., *126*:868, 1944)

L_3-L_4 level, the straight-leg-raising test may be negative and the femoral stretch test may be positive.

The neurological examination may be normal or it may show various degrees of neurological deficit, depending upon the degree of nerve root compression. Ninety-five percent of lumbar disc protrusions occur at either the L_4-L_5 or at the L_5-S_1 level. Most of the remaining lumbar disc protrusions occur at the L_3-L_4 interspace. With lesions at the L_5-S_1 level, the S_1 nerve root is usually compressed. When sensory loss is present, it occurs in the S_1 root distribution, namely, the lateral aspect of the leg and foot, including the lateral three toes. If weakness is present, it involves plantar flexion of the foot and toes. The Achilles tendon reflex may be depressed or absent. With lesions at the L_4-L_5 interspace, the L_5 root is compressed, and the sensory loss involves the lateral aspect of the calf and the dorsum of the foot, including the great toe. Weakness, when present, is noted on dorsiflexion of the great toe and, occasionally, of the foot. This can be quickly tested by having the patient walk on his heels. Usually there is no abnormality of the reflexes. With protrusion at the L_3-L_4 level, the L_4 root is compressed and leg pain is usually on the anterior aspect of the thigh. When present, the sensory loss is over the anteriomedial aspect of the lower thigh and proximal portion of the lower leg. Weakness and atrophy of the quadriceps muscles may be apparent. The weakness can be demonstrated by having

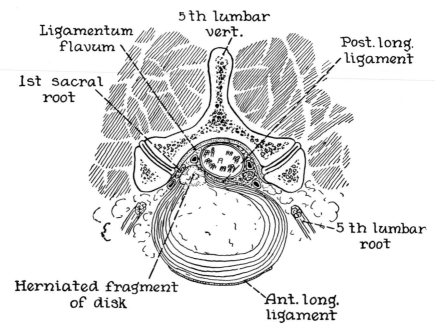

Fig. 19–5. Cross section through the lumbar intervertebral disk, showing posterior herniation of the nucleus pulposus with compression of root of first sacral nerve.

the patient extend the lower leg at the knee against the examiner's resistance. The patellar reflex may be diminished or absent.

Radiological examination should be done to help rule out other pathology. The x-ray films will usually show straightening of the normal lumbar curve because of the spasm present. Narrowing of the disc interspace at one or more levels may be demonstrated; however, the site of such narrowing may or may not be significant, since the disc protrusion responsible for the attack may be at an interspace which is normal by x-ray examination.

Treatment. Most attacks of low back pain can be treated conservatively if no profound neurological deficit exists, even though the attack may be discogenic in origin. When the attack is acute, rest on a firm bed, with the knees flexed, should be prescribed, and the patient is advised to use moist heat. Rest in bed from one to three weeks is often necessary. If the patient is treated at home and does not

improve after a week or two with rest in bed and the use of moist heat, a period of hospitalization for continued rest in bed, traction, hot packs, and observation may be indicated. When the patient is hospitalized, semi-Fowler's position is often the most comfortable for the patient. Although it may be difficult to defend the use of pelvic traction on a scientific basis, many clinicians feel that it is helpful.

Depending on the severity of pain, analgesic drugs, including narcotics, may be necessary. Muscle relaxants, such as Valium, Robaxin, and meprobamate, are also useful. Brief periods on anti-inflammatory medications, such as Butazolidin, alka, Tandearil, or Indocin, may be very helpful. Dramatic relief following the use of Butazolidin alka, 100 mg. four times a day after meals for four days, is often noted. The anti-inflammatory drugs are usually not used when there is a known history of peptic ulcer. These drugs should be used cautiously if there is a history of hiatal hernia.

When the patient is to be treated on an

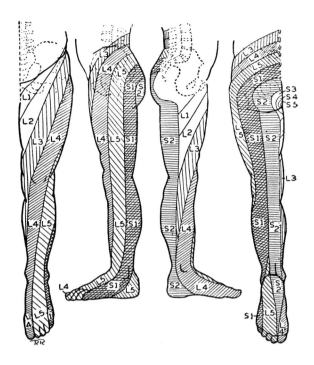

Fig. 19–6. Composite dermatome chart of the lower extremity. (Keegan, J. J.: Arch. Neurol, & Psychiat., *50*-:81, 1943)

ambulatory basis because symptoms are not acute enough to require complete bed rest or when he is allowed to become ambulatory following a period of rest in bed, a lumbosacral corset should be prescribed for several weeks (Fig. 19-7). When symptoms subside or disappear, the patient should be gradually weaned away from the corset.

When the spasm, the pain, and most of the limitation of motion have disappeared, the patient should be taught the postural back exercises. He should do exercises for many months after his pain has completely disappeared. Regular swimming should be encouraged when this is feasible.

Many patients with acute attacks of back pain have obtained relief through manipulation of the back. This may be done by an osteopath, an orthopedic surgeon, or another properly trained physician. Although this treatment was discussed in earlier editions of this book, it has been omitted here since this form of therapy is best administered only by those well experienced in its use. In patients with severe acute attacks of back pain, manipulation may not be advisable,

since it may result in the extrusion of a nuclear fragment.

When conservative measures fail and significant pain and disability persist, or if on the initial examination significant neurological deficit is present, operative intervention should be considered. The patient should then be referred to a neurosurgeon or an orthopedic surgeon who is experienced in this type of surgery. In most cases a myelogram will be done to verify the level of the lesion, to rule out neoplasms, and to help determine the advisability of surgery.

ACUTE BACK STRAIN

Although this diagnosis is frequently made, it is probable that in many of the cases so diagnosed there is some degree of discogenic disease. Undoubtedly, muscle and ligamentous strain do occur in the low back following sudden jerking movements, sudden lifting, and straining in an awkward position, as well as with falls, but it seems likely that in addition to strain there is some degree of disc injury. This diagnosis should be reserved for those patients who do not have radicular

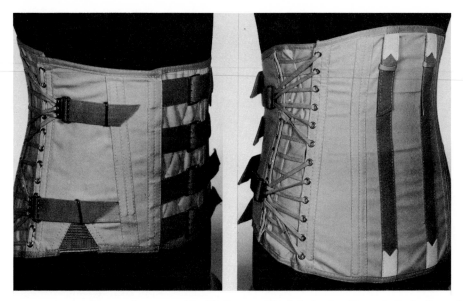

Fig. 19–7. Lumbosacral corset. (*Left*) Front. (*Right*) Back. (R and G Orthopedic Supplies, Washington, D. C.)

pain and in whom there is no evidence of nerve root compression or irritation. Even though many patients who are given this diagnosis subsequently show evidence of a ruptured disc, this diagnosis should be retained to imply that, even if some discogenic disease is present, the examination does not give any indication of nerve root irritation.

Treatment. Treatment is directed at relieving the pain and muscle spasm, and it is essentially as outlined above for the conservative treatment of ruptured intervertebral disc lesions. When well-localized tender areas can be found, each of these is injected with 5 to 10 ml. of a 1 percent procaine solution. In mild cases, the patient may immediately begin moderate activity, avoiding overexertion. When necessary, additional injections are given at intervals of 1 or 2 days. The addition of 25 mg. of hydrocortisone to each 5 or 10 ml. injection of procaine may increase and prolong the effect. The other local anesthetics and more potent steroids may be used in smaller doses. Lidocaine (Xylocaine), 1 percent, is supplied already mixed with dexamethasone (4 mg. per ml.). Two to 3 ml. of the mixture are used in each tender area.

RHEUMATOID STATES

Patients with known rheumatoid disease commonly have back pain. With active rheumatoid disease, other joints are commonly involved. Sedimentation rates are elevated and tests for rheumatoid disease are positive. Radiographs of the back may reveal nothing except straightening of the lumbar curve due to muscle spasm.

Commonly, acute and/or chronic back pain may be the result of an inflammatory lesion, often diagnosed as myositis or fibrositis. These patients frequently have negative tests for rheumatoid activity. They often give a history of other joint problems in the past, including episodes of bursitis. Often these patients have underlying discogenic disease and they may be more prone to have flare-ups due to inflammatory reaction. Apparently, patients with rheumatoid tendency tend to have their flare-ups of this reaction in areas of previous injury. Characteristically, these patients complain of stiffness after being in one position for a long time and are usually stiff in the morning when they first get out of bed. They often complain primarily of back pain and stiffness

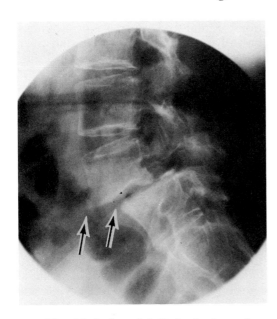

Fig. 19–8. Spondylolisthesis. Lateral view of the lumbosacral spine of a 45-year-old female with complaint of low back pain. There is marked forward displacement of the L₅ vertebra over the S₁ vertebra (arrows). (R and G Orthopedic Supplies, Washington, D.C.)

of the back, and, on examination, there is usually some degree of back limitation, with a relatively normal straight-leg-raising test. There is usually no neurological deficit. In the more chronic cases, the patient's complaints of disability are more striking than are the abnormalities on examination.

In the more acute cases, rest in bed, moist heat, analgesics, muscle relaxants, and, especially, anti-inflammatory drugs, such as Butazolidin alka or Tandearil, 100 mg. four times a day after meals for four days, are usually efficacious. In the less acute attacks, a lumbosacral corset and, later, the postural back exercises may be helpful.

OSTEOARTHRITIS

Arthritic changes in the lumbar spine are often associated with pain, limitation of motion, and paravertebral muscle spasm. Sciatic radicular pain may be present if there is any nerve root irritation or compression by a spur. Symptoms tend to be less acute than they are with typical ruptured disc lesions. The pain tends to be worse when the patient gets up in the morning and improves after the patient has limbered up. These patients have got relief from use of moist heat, analgesics, anti-inflammatory drugs, and postural back exercises.

CONGENITAL ABNORMALITIES OF THE LUMBAR SPINE

Congenital abnormalities of the lumbar spine may result in mechanical dysfunction in the low back, which often leads to disc disease and pain. However, even before disc degeneration occurs these conditions may be responsible for local back pain and, at times, leg pain.

Spondylolysis and Spondylolisthesis. Spondylolysis is a relatively common defect that is either congenital or of developmental origin. It is readily seen on radiographs, especially on the oblique views, which show a defect in the pars interarticularis, usually at either the L₄ or L₅ vertebra. This defect is more significant when it is bilateral, for then the entire posterior arch of the vertebra is attached to the vertebral body by fibrous union, and this makes the locking mechanism of the facets ineffective and often results in various degrees of anterior displacement of the body of the involved vertebra.

Spondylolisthesis is often associated with chronic back pain, aggravated by exertion. Occasionally the patient will have an acute exacerbation, with unilateral sciatic pain. Disc extrusion may develop at the level of the defect or at other levels. Of course, the diagnosis is readily made by x-ray examination; the lateral view will clearly show the anterior displacement of the body of the affected vertebra (Fig. 19-8). On physical examination this lesion may be suspected on palpation of the spinous processes, for the neural arch is usually displaced posteriorly, thus causing the spinous process at the level of the spondylolisthesis to be more prominent.

Acute episodes are treated as are ruptured discs. For more chronic pain, the flexion back exercises and a lumbosacral corset are frequently helpful. When surgery is indicated, ruptured disc must be ruled out. Surgery usually involves removal of the posterior arch to decompress the nerve roots and often, especially in the younger age groups, fusion is recommended.

Exaggerated Lumbosacral Angle. Many patients with chronic low back pain have marked increase of the lumbar lordotic curve due to increased lumbosacral angle, as measured anteriorly. This results in mechanical instability and in chronic low back pain which is aggravated by activity, prolonged walking, and standing. Examination is usually negative except for the exaggerated lumbar lordosis, which is readily verified by radiographic examination. The postural back exercises and the use of a lumbosacral corset for strenuous activity are helpful.

CHRONIC BACKACHE OF UTERINE, PROSTATIC, RECTAL, OR PELVIC MUSCLE ORIGIN

Lesions of the uterus and the adnexa, such as malposition, inflammation, and tumors, may cause dull, aching discomfort in the lower back. Examination of the back shows little to account for the pain, but a checkup on the history may reveal exacerbations associated with menstruation or leukorrhea, and vaginal examination may disclose significant lesions.

Prostatic inflammation or congestion sometimes causes pain in the region of the lumbosacral joint and the sacrum. The pain is apt to be dull and aching and radiating. Examination of the back shows little, but rectal examination may show a distended and tender prostate. Satisfactory relief of the back pain often follows suitable treatment of the prostatic condition.

Rectal lesions, such as cryptitis and fissure in ano, that cause sphincter spasm may also produce pain over the sacrum. The patient is often aware of the associa-tion. Digital and proctoscopic examination of the rectum is in order, and treatment of the anal or the rectal lesion should precede measures for the relief of the back pain.

Spasm of the perineal muscles may cause pain over the coccyx and the upper buttock with radiation down the thigh.

FRACTURES OF THE TRANSVERSE PROCESSES OF THE LUMBAR VERTEBRAE

The transverse processes in the lumbar region may be fractured by indirect violence due to muscular action, such as a sudden jerking movement of the back or a fall that causes extreme twisting or lateral bending of the back. Direct violence, such as a kick or a blow, may also be a cause. The quadratus lumborum muscle is attached to the transverse processes and is torn when the fracture occurs.

Diagnosis. The history of acute violence followed by severe pain on one side of the lower back, intense muscular spasm and tenderness on one side of the lumbar region, and severe pain on lateral bending to the opposite side will indicate the diagnosis. There is often pain on flexion of the thigh of the affected side, especially when resistance is offered. Roentgen examination confirms the diagnosis (Figs. 19-9 and 19-10).

Treatment. Although these injuries are usually treated by rest in bed, patients often make a more rapid and satisfactory recovery on ambulatory treatment. Using the roentgen films and local tenderness as a guide, from 10 to 20 ml. of a 1 percent procaine solution is injected into and around the site of fracture. This gives striking relief of pain and ease of motion. A firm crisscross adhesive back strapping from mid-buttocks to mid-thorax (Fig. 19-11) supplies adequate support and immobilization. Some discomfort often persists for several days, and the procaine injections may be repeated 2 or 3 times at invervals of from 1 to 3 days. Medication as for acute back strain should be given during the first few days.

When only one or two processes are

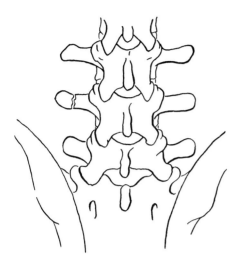

Fig. 19–9. Fracture of left transverse process, fourth lumbar vertebra. (Ferguson, L. K., and Erb, W. H.: Ann. Surg., *114*:304, 1941)

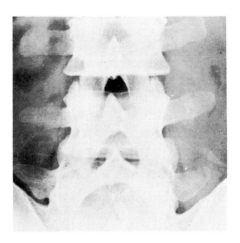

Fig. 19–10. Same case as Figure 19–9. 18 days after fracture, showing early callus formation. (Ferguson, L. K., and Erb, W. H.: Ann. Surg., *114*:304, 1941)

involved, this simple method produces excellent results without residual symptoms. When several processes are involved, the soft-tissue damage may be extensive. In addition to the procaine injections, the treatment program may include a few days' rest in bed and longer use of the strapping, or perhaps the application of a light plaster cast from the mid-buttock to the mid-thorax region for 3 or 4 weeks.

LESIONS OF THE COCCYX

Etiology. Pain in the region of the coccyx most often arises as a result of trauma. Because of the fact that the tubera ischii are separated somewhat more in females than in males, the coccyx is less protected and more often traumatized in females. The trauma producing this local injury may be a fall on the back; more often some projecting object is struck in the fall, as, for instance, a stair or a child's block; or it may be the result of a kick. In such instances, the coccyx is driven forward and, if the force is sufficient, dislocation or fracture may result. Another perhaps less frequent cause of pain in this region is injury to a fixed coccyx by internal forces, especially the pressure of the child's head on the coccyx during childbirth.

DISLOCATIONS AND FRACTURES

Diagnosis. Injuries of the coccyx, either dislocation or fracture, cause acute pain that is noted especially on sitting, on rising from the sitting position, and on walking. It is less noticeable when the patient is lying down.

On examination, there is tenderness over the area of the coccyx, especially on pressure. If the finger is so inserted into the anal canal that the coccyx can be grasped between the thumb and the forefinger, there is marked tenderness when the coccyx is pressed between the fingers and when it is moved.

Treatment. In cases of dislocation, the displacement may be palpated in this manner, and a reduction may be effected by gentle manipulation, often with complete and almost immediate relief of pain. In cases of fracture, however, little can be done in the way of a reduction, and there is no known method of fixation.

The accepted treatment in cases of injury to the coccyx is rest in bed with applications of heat. Sometimes 3 or 4 weeks of this therapy is necessary before pain is

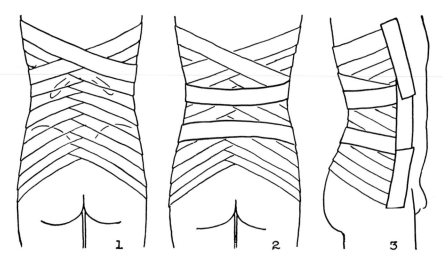

Fig. 19–11. Adhesive strapping for immobilization of a fracture of a transverse process. (1) A layer of crisscross adhesive is started at midbuttock level and ended at the middle of the thorax. (2) It is reinforced by transverse strips. (3) The free ends are fastened down by longitudinal strips.

completely relieved. As a rule, however, pain disappears before this if acute trauma is its sole cause. The pain of localized injuries of this area can often be greatly relieved by the injection of small amounts (2-5 ml.) of 1 percent procaine or lidocaine. Injection of procaine and hydrocortisone can be repeated as necessary. Ambulation can be started early if the injury has caused no displacement of the coccyx.

In some cases of fracture with fragmentation, persistent pain makes the removal of the coccyx necessary. This may be accomplished through a midline incision, the sacrococcygeal ligaments being divided and the coccyx being removed by rotating it downward and away from the rectum. The operation may be performed under local anesthesia and the wound closed with interrupted sutures or packed with gauze and allowed to heal by granulation. This procedure may occasionally be performed in the office, but for most patients hospitalization is preferable.

COCCYGODYNIA

Symptoms. Coccygodynia is a term applied to a throbbing, aching, or stabbing pain occurring in the region of the coccyx. It occurs spontaneously but is aggravated by any movement (such as walking, sitting down, getting up from a chair, or defecation) that brings into action the muscles attached to the coccyx.

Etiology. Although the initiating cause of coccygodynia may be trauma, the duration of the pain suggests that its persistence must be due to some other cause; perhaps a secondary trauma, such as that due to the involvement of some of the muscles or nerve fibers in scar-tissue formation, causes a persistent neuralgia in the region of the coccyx.

Diagnosis. The patient gives a history of definite pain in the coccygeal region, made worse by sitting on soft, upholstered chairs. Such discomfort is experienced that the patient is unable to sit for any length of time. He twists and squirms, sitting first on one tuber ischii and then on the other. To obtain relief, the patient frequently places his feet underneath his chair and sits forward, holding himself upon the tuber ischii and the thighs.

On examination, there is usually tenderness on pressure over the coccyx or, especially, along its edges. On rectal examination, no particular pain is caused by movement of the coccyx, but pain is caused by pressure of the index finger along the muscles attached to it. The roentgen examination fails to throw any light upon the cause of the symptoms.

Treatment. It is often difficult to relieve coccygodynia. In many cases, the marked pain caused by pressure along the edge of the coccyx with the finger in the rectum suggests spasm of the muscles attached to the coccyx, and relief has been obtained by daily massage of these muscles with long, sweeping strokes of the finger per rectum. Local applications of heat, in the form of sitz baths, hot compresses, and even diathermy, are of doubtful value. Certainly they do not give an immediate relief of symptoms.

We have had good results in some of these patients by injecting the tender areas at the sides or tip of the coccyx with local anesthetic solution (1 percent procaine, lidocaine, etc). If pain persists, the addition of steroids may be helpful.

Removal of the coccyx in these cases of coccygodynia should be reserved until all conservative measures have failed, since this surgery is frequently unsuccessful.

BIBLIOGRAPHY

Armstrong, J. R.: Lumbar Disc Lesions. Baltimore, Williams & Wilkins, 1965.

Bate, J. T.: A functional lumbosacral back support. J. Bone Joint Surg., *45-A*:1698, 1963.

Bradford, F. K., and Spurling, R. G.: The Intervertebral Disc. ed. 2. Springfield, Ill., Charles C. Thomas, 1945.

DePalma, A. F., and Rothman, R. H.: The Intervertebral Disc. Philadelphia, W. B. Saunders, 1970.

Ferguson, L. K., and Erb, W. H.: Procaine injection and early mobilization in the treatment of non-weight-bearing fractures. Ann. Surg., *114*:293, 1941.

Gurdgian, C. S., and Thomas, L. M.: Neckache and Backache. Springfield, Ill., Charles C. Thomas, 1970.

Keegan, J. J.: Diagnosis of herniation of lumbar intervertebral disks by neurologic signs. JAMA, *126*:868, 1944.

Steindler, A.: Differential diagnosis of pain low in the back. JAMA, *110*:106, 1938.

Steindler, A.: The interpretation of sciatic radiation and the syndrome of low back pain. J. Bone Joint Surg., *22*:28, 1940.

Watson-Jones, R.: Fractures and Joint Injuries. ed. 4. Baltimore, Williams & Wilkins, 1952.

Woodhead, B. H., and Fowler, J. R.: The dynamic treatment of low back strain syndrome. Canad. Med. Assoc. J., *90*:1152, 1964.

20

Genitourinary System

Richard G. Middleton, M.D. *and Douglas S. Dahl,* M.D.

URINARY INFECTIONS

General Considerations. An individual
with a normal urinary tract rarely develops a serious urinary infection. Even
though urine is a fairly good culture medium for a number of bacteria, those
organisms which gain entrance into the
urinary tract usually do not multiply sufficiently to produce symptoms and recognizable infection. Natural protective
mechanisms include continuous dilution
of bacteria by urine formation, intermittent complete emptying of the lower urinary tract by voiding, and the antibacterial effects of the healthy transitional
epithelum. However, many congenital
and acquired abnormalities of the urinary
tract result in obstruction of urinary flow,
residual urine, the presence of foreign
material, and the disruption of the normal
mucosa. In these situations the urinary
system is altered; bacteria can flourish
and produce clinical infection.

The derangement of the urinary tract
should be regarded as the basic cause of
the infection; bacteria are nearly always
opportunistic invaders of the altered urinary tract. Most urinary infections are
"nonspecific." There are, however, certain "specific" infections in which the
organism is sufficiently aggressive to invade the normal urinary system. Gonor-

rhea, renal tuberculosis, and some fungal
urinary infections are examples of specific urinary infection.

Acute Cystitis in Women is the most
common urinary infection encountered in
clinical medicine. When the woman is in
the early months of marriage this infection has often been called "honeymoon
cystitis." Although the patient is acutely
uncomfortable and may be very anxious,
cystitis is not a serious illness and is easy
to recognize and treat. Symptoms include
burning, urinary frequency, urgency,
lower abdominal cramps, and grossly
bloody urine at times. Pain in the flank
and fever are *not* a part of ordinary acute
cystitis.

On bimanual pelvic examination the
bladder is extremely tender. A catheterized urine specimen will contain in-
numerable white cells, many bacteria,
and often red cells. Cystoscopy should
generally be avoided in acute cystitis (the
bladder mucosa is fire red and edematous). Usually urine culture reveals a high
colony count of a gram-negative organism, most commonly *E. coli.*

Treatment with sulfonamides, nitrofurantoin, nalidixic acid, tetracycline
or ampicillin will ease the symptoms
promptly, and the infection is cleared in
several days. Sulfonamides are generally
effective and are recommended because

they are inexpensive and cause few side effects. Therapy for 5 to 7 days is sufficient, and therapeutic failure is uncommon. Flank pain, fever, or persistence of the infection for more than 5 to 7 days are indications for urologic investigation. However, urologic investigation in the woman with typical and periodic episodes of acute cystitis rarely reveals an anatomical abnormality of the urinary system.

A recurrence of symptoms in a woman who has received antibacterial treatment for acute cystitis can nearly always be proved to be a new infection with a different bacterial organism. Pyridium and other azo-dyes are thought to soothe the irritated bladder a little bit, but they are of dubious value in the management of acute cystitis.

Traditionally physicians have employed many schemes in the hope of preventing periodic acute cystitis in women. Regular urethral dilatation, urethrotomy, various bladder irrigations, and a variety of operations upon the distal urethra have all been advocated and frequently performed. There is little scientific basis to relate acute cystitis in women to an abnormality of the urethra. Exceptions to this would be the patient with a urethral diverticulum or chronic infection in periurethral glands.

Urinary Infection in Children. The great majority of children never have a single urinary infection. The child with a urinary infection will usually develop further episodes of infection after the initial one is treated with an antibiotic. A child with repeated urinary infections is extremely likely to have a congenital abnormality of the urinary tract. It is reasonable to perform an intravenous pyelogram and cystogram on any child who has had even one urinary infection. Waiting for the second or third infection before carrying out investigation of the urinary tract increases the yield of abnormal findings but unnecessarily delays the detection of serious urinary tract abnormalities at times. Certainly, complete and prompt urologic investigation is vital in any child

who has a *febrile* urinary infection, any infant with a urinary infection, and any boy upon the detection of any type of urinary infection.

MALE GENITAL INFECTIONS

Gonorrhea. Acute gonococcal anterior urethritis is extremely common and has reached epidemic proportions in many areas. Dysuria and profuse purulent urethral discharge begin within 7 days after coitus with an infected partner. The urethral discharge is thick and creamy and has a yellowish green tint. The diagnosis can be presumed upon inspection of the typical urethral discharge, but the demonstration of intracellular and extracellular gram-negative diplococci is necessary for definitive diagnosis. Specific culture media are available for gonococci but are rarely necessary to establish the diagnosis in men. Vaginal cultures for gonococci are valuable in women, in whom the infection may be insidious and asymptomatic.

Aqueous procaine penicillin G remains the preferred drug for treatment of gonorrhea. Its effectiveness has been somewhat diminished by the emergence of strains partially resistant to penicillin. Since resistance is relative and not absolute, the recommended dose of penicillin has increased somewhat in recent years. Probenecid enhances therapy by elevating and prolonging the blood levels of penicillin. The treatment recommended by the Public Health Service is 1.0 g. of probenecid given orally 30 minutes prior to the injection of 4.8 million units of aqueous procaine penicillin G, given in two intramuscular injections. An alternative treatment is the simultaneous oral administration of 3.5 g. of ampicillin and 1.0 g. of probenecid. When penicillin is ineffective or cannot be used because of allergy, alternative treatments include tetracycline hydrochloride, 1.5 g. initially followed by 0.5 g. 4 times a day for a total dose of 9 grams; or Vibramycin, 200 mg. orally followed by 100 mg. a day for 4 days.

Sexual intercourse should be completely proscribed until the infection has resolved. Any individual with whom the patient has had intimate contact should be examined and treated. With adequate antibiotic treatment, the urethral discharge and dysuria disappear completely over a period of 2 to 4 days. Without treatment, the discharge will continue for months and possibly several years. Untreated gonorrhea can result in gonorrheal prostatitis, epididymitis, late urethral stricture, and gonorrheal arthritis from hematogenous spread of this organism. Occasionally after adequate treatment of gonorrhea, a watery, scanty discharge will linger for several weeks or longer. Cultures of this nonspecific discharge are almost invariably sterile. Gonorrhea is occasionally seen in the rectum and in the mouth in homosexuals or those involved in other unusual sexual practices.

Nonspecific Urethritis. This is milder than gonorrhea and is not caused by the gonococcus. In the majority of instances, even though there is pyuria and a urethral discharge, cultures reveal no growth. Symptoms are burning on urination, frequency, urgency, and a watery, mucoid discharge. These may occur spontaneously or may follow sexual contact, although this is not necessarily a venereal infection. Microscopic examination of the urethral discharge reveals many white blood cells and usually no organisms. The majority of the white cells will be seen in the first portion of a three-glass test. Without the three-glass test this condition may be indistinguishable from chronic prostatitis.

Rational treatment is elusive since one rarely is able to identify an etiological agent. Sulfonamides, nitrofurantoin, and tetracycline are frequently given empirically. Nonspecific urethritis seems to resolve over a period of 2 to 3 weeks, whether or not the patient receives antibacterial treatment.

Acute Prostatitis. Acute bacterial prostatitis may occur abruptly in a patient without prior urinary disease, probably as a result of hematogenous spread. More often it occurs in a patient with pre-existing urinary infection. The patient with an indwelling Foley catheter, vesical calculi, urethral stricture, or residual bladder urine is a frequent victim of acute prostatitis. Generalized symptoms—myalgia, chills, fever, and anorexia—are accompanied by marked dysuria, frequency, perineal pain, and a weak urinary stream or even acute urinary retention.

The prostate is swollen, tense, and tender and may be very warm to palpation. Massage of the acutely inflamed prostate is risky, should be avoided, and is not necessary to make the diagnosis. The urine is loaded with white cells and bacteria, and urine cultures are usually positive.

Broad-spectrum antibiotics should be given until culture data are available; then specific antibacterial treatment can be employed. Narcotics may be necessary for pain. Aspirin is useful for the accompanying fever. Sitz baths may be soothing. Hospitalization is advised if the patient has high fever and is toxemic, or if he develops acute urinary retention. Acute epididymitis is common following acute prostatitis. If symptoms and fever persist despite antibiotic treatment, the possibility of a prostatic abscess should be considered. When febrile prostatitis occurs in a patient requiring long-term catheter drainage, he should be treated by suprapubic cystostomy and removal of the urethral catheter. Cystostomy diverts the urine from the deep urethra and allows removal of the irritating foreign body from the urethra.

Chronic Prostatitis. This is a common condition in men of all ages, although it does not occur before puberty. Symptoms are mild burning, frequency, and urgency, often in association with aching in the groins, scrotum, perineum, suprapubic and sacral areas. There may be slight watery urethral discharge, often noted only in the morning upon arising. Some patients describe a decrease in libido and a perineal ache after ejaculation. A bloody or brownish discoloration of the semen is also indicative of chronic prostatitis.

It is important on physical examination to exclude other diseases of the inguinal area, genitalia, and prostate. Hernia, hydrocele, epididymal cyst, and varicocele may give similar symptoms, as may prostatic cancer. In chronic prostatitis, the prostate is often soft and boggy, and areas of softness and of fibrosis may be palpable in the same prostate. A three-glass test will reveal few white cells in the first glass, but many white cells are seen in the prostatic fluid or in the voided urine after vigorous prostatic massage. Prostatic fluid expressed by prostatic massage will generally contain more than 8 to 10 white cells per high-power field.

The urologic literature is full of speculations, opinions, and "old wives tales" relating this condition to various sexual practices, diet, activity, local or distant infection, and trauma to the perineum. It is difficult to incriminate these factors scientifically, and almost always the urine and prostatic fluid are sterile on culture. Chronic prostatitis often seems to be a noninfectious swelling or congestion of the prostate.

Massage of the prostate yields fluid for microscopic examination and also seems to be therapeutic. Systematic stripping of the prostate from base to apex by the gloved finger in the rectum relieves the symptoms and promotes resolution of the chronic prostatitis. Many patients benefit from one or two subsequent massages of the prostate at intervals of 1 to 2 weeks. Too frequent massage of the prostate and an indefinite course of prostatic massage are of doubtful value. Antibiotics are frequently given in spite of negative cultures; they may seem to help at times, but their value is difficult to document in many cases. Traditionally the patient with chronic prostatitis is advised to alter the frequency of sexual intercourse (either increase or decrease the frequency) and avoid alcohol and spicy foods. The value of this advice is dubious.

HEMATURIA

No more than one to two red cells per high power field are ever seen in a normal urinary sediment. More than two red cells per high power field in a centrifuged urinary specimen should be regarded as microscopic hematuria. Many more red cells are required to color the urine pink or red. The presence of a reddish colored urine without red cells in the urinary sediment suggests hemoglobinuria or the ingestion of beets or azo-dyes.

There are scores of causes of hematuria, such as tumors of the kidney, ureter, bladder, prostate, and urethra; calculi at all levels in the urinary tract; prostatic hypertrophy; strictures; and urinary infections (Fig. 20-1). Red blood cells are found in the urine in various types of glomerulitis (glomerulonephritis, lupus nephritis, diabetic nephrosclerosis, etc.), but protein and casts, including red blood cell casts, will also be present. Hematuria occurs with various types of urinary tract infection; however, in infection the red blood cells will be accompanied by white cells and bacteria.

A lesion of the kidney or ureter is suggested by hematuria associated with flank pain. Dysuria with hematuria, especially terminal hematuria, suggests a source of bleeding in the bladder, prostate, or urethra. Many common benign conditions produce hematuria, but one must suspect a malignant neoplasm in the urinary tract in any patient with hematuria, gross or microscopic. Virtually every patient who experiences hematuria should be evaluated urologically by intravenous pyelography and cystoscopy. In the presence of gross hematuria, prompt cystoscopy during the period of active bleeding is often helpful in identifying the source of the bleeding. One can often identify blood efflux from the ureteral orifice at cystoscopy in instances of upper urinary tract bleeding. It is a common clinical mistake to assume that hematuria results from prostatic hypertrophy or an infection somewhere in the urinary system when an insidious neoplasm is the actual cause of the bleeding.

ACUTE URINARY RETENTION

Abrupt inability to void is painful. The patient experiences steadily increasing lower abdominal pain and progressive

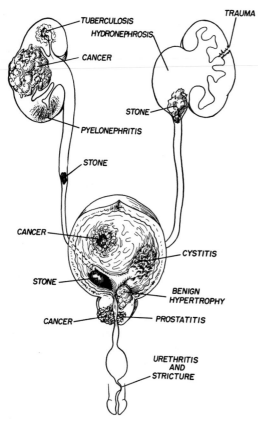

TRAUMA

TUBERCULOSIS
HYDRONEPHROSIS

CANCER

STONE

PYELONEPHRITIS

STONE

CANCER

CYSTITIS

STONE

BENIGN
HYPERTROPHY

CANCER

PROSTATITIS

URETHRITIS
AND
STRICTURE

Fig. 20–1. These are common causes of hematuria. There are other causes. Hematuria is a sign of serious disease until proved otherwise. (Marshall, V. F.: Textbook of Urology. New York, Hoeber-Harper, 1964)

bladder distension with the passage of time. The elderly man with acute urinary retention is often in great agony; drainage of his distended bladder with a catheter is a simple humanitarian act greatly welcomed by the miserable patient. The typical patient is a man over the age of sixty who previously has had increasing symptoms of prostatism. Usually urinary retention is acute, but occasionally a man may have been in retention for days, weeks, or even months, with marked frequency or continuous overflow urinary dribbling and a distended bladder. Rarely, a patient with "silent prostatism" has a distended bladder and a markedly elevated residual urine and yet is unaware that his voiding pattern has changed significantly. While

some urologists advocate the gradual withdrawal of urine from the distended bladder, it is safe and often easier to evacuate the bladder at once and completely with a catheter.

Generally, urinary retention in the elderly man is caused by either benign prostatic hypertrophy or prostatic cancer. Acute retention in women is the result of neurologic disease, pelvic tumor, drug abuse, or is a psychologic phenomenon—often associated with unusual emotional stress.

Urinary retention in the elderly man is a prime indication for prostatic surgery, and requires prompt admission to the hospital for preoperative evaluation and prostatic surgery. If one simply evacuates the bladder and sends the patient on his way, the chances are great that he will return within a few hours, again in urinary retention. In managing the woman in acute urinary retention, the following are important: evacuation of the bladder, bimanual pelvic examination, cessation of all anticholinergic and sedative drugs, and reassurance. Recurrence of retention in women is rare in the absence of a neurologic disease or mechanical obstruction.

URETHRAL CATHETERIZATION

Types of Catheters (Fig. 20-2).

1. Straight, soft rubber or plastic catheter (Nelaton): This is the catheter most commonly used for a simple catheterization in a male or female patient. Number 16 or 18 French is appropriate and convenient for the adult patient of either sex.

2. Coudé-tip catheter. This is more rigid than the ordinary soft rubber catheter and is named for the fixed, upturned (Coudé) tip of about 15 degrees. The single eye of this catheter is set back from the upturned tip. This catheter is extremely useful in the patient with prostatic enlargement and will often pass readily into the bladder when a soft rubber or plastic straight catheter buckles in the prostatic urethra. The slight angulation of the tip can often make a difficult catheterization in an elderly male patient a simple maneuver.

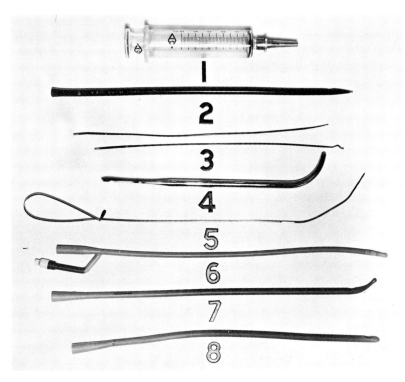

Fig. 20–2. Common urologic instruments. Calibration of these instruments is on the French scale and is expressed in units. Each French unit equals $1/_3$ mm. For example, a #24 F. instrument has a diameter of 8 mm. 1. Toomey syringe. 2. Woven follower. 3. Woven filiforms. 4. Van Buren sound. 5. Catheter guide (Mandrin). 6. Foley catheter. 7. Olive-tip catheter with Coude curve. 8. Straight, or Robinson, catheter.

3. Metal catheter. This is a hollow metal tube, fashioned in the shape of a urethral sound, that provides maximum stiffness and can be used in catheterizing the man with prostatic hypertrophy. This catheter can cause great damage if not used carefully and properly, and should be used only by an experienced physician when rubber catheters have failed.

4. Filiform and woven catheter follower. A straight or corkscrew-shaped urethral filiform is used for probing a urethra that has a stricture or is tortuous. Once the tract into the bladder has been negotiated, the woven following catheter is screwed firmly onto the filiform tip and is passed into the bladder.

5. Foley catheter. This is a catheter with an inflatable bag near the tip. The inflated bag secures the catheter within the bladder.

Technique of Catheterization Urethral catheterization requires proper positioning of the patient, cleansing of the urethral meatus, and the use of sterile instruments. The catheter should be passed gently and with due consideration of the anatomy of the urethra. A male patient can be catheterized in the supine or the lithotomy position. A female patient can be catheterized satisfactorily only in the lithotomy position. In the male, the foreskin must be retracted and the glans cleansed with an antiseptic solution. In the female, the labia must be held widely apart to expose the urethral meatus for proper cleansing and for insertion of the catheter. Negotiating the female urethra is rarely difficult, but the male urethra regularly presents two problems: the angulation in the bulbous urethra and the negotiation of the prostatic urethra and bladder neck. If a straight soft rubber catheter will not pass through either of these problem areas, a coudé catheter should be tried next. A filiform and following catheter is the next resort, and rarely should one resort to a metal catheter. The catheter should be lubricated generously with a sterile water-soluble lubricant, and its passage should be gentle.

DISEASES OF THE FEMALE URETHRA

The Urethral Syndrome of adult women is the combination of dysuria, suprapubic discomfort, frequency of urination, and a sensation of incomplete voiding attributed to nonspecific urethral inflammation. The symptoms mimic cystitis; yet urinary infection is absent. Fatigue, anxiety, and neurotic tendencies accentuate the symptoms. Although rarely required, cystoscopic examination reveals inflammation of the urethra and a normal bladder mucosa. A presumptive diagnosis can be established from the history and the negative urinalysis. Various therapeutic plans have been advocated for the urethral syndrome; however, simple periodic outpatient urethral dilatation has been effective. Xylocaine or cocaine is applied topically to the urethra with a cotton swab, following which the urethra is dilated to 30 to 40 French with steel sounds. A sulfonamide or nitrofurantoin may be prescribed for several days following each treatment. The dilatations are repeated as necessary to control the symptoms. Mild sedatives, urinary antispasmodics, and optimistic reassurance are valuable adjuncts to treatment.

Urethral Caruncle. Caruncles are polypoid, vascular, red lesions which protrude from the posterior urethral meatus. Benign but often tender, they may cause dysuria, postmicturation bleeding, and pain on sexual intercourse. Symptomatic lesions are treated by excision or fulguration after the application of 10 percent cocaine to the distal urethra. A simple method of removal is as follows: the lesion is stretched taut, the base is clamped with a hemostat, the lesion is excised, and the base is fulgurated before removing the clamp.

Mucosa Prolapse. Mild degrees of prolapse of the urethral mucosa are common and do not require treatment. Extensive full-circle prolapse occurring in prepubertal girls and elderly women appears as a dramatic, violaceous, boggy, bleeding mass which obscures the meatus and is often mistaken for a neoplasm. The lesion is easily cured by applying a strangulating ligature over an inlying catheter. After 10 percent cocaine has been applied to the lesion, a number 20 French Foley catheter is inserted through the urethra and the balloon is inflated. The prolapsed mucosa is drawn taut, and a 2-0 silk ligature is passed around the lesion and tied tightly over the catheter. After several days the necrotic lesion sloughs and the catheter can be removed.

DISEASES OF THE PENIS AND MALE URETHRA

Phimosis. The normal prepuce is supple and can be retracted easily to expose the entire glans penis. When constriction or thickening of the leading edge of the prepuce prevents complete retraction, the condition is termed phimosis. Unless the prepuce can be retracted easily, inflammation of the glans, or balanitis, is inevitable. Acute suppurative balanitis with phimosis causes a bulbous inflammation of the distal penis, at times associated with fever, lymphadenopathy, and even urinary retention. An immediate dorsal slit allows drainage of pus, free voiding, and resolution of the infection (Fig. 20-3). When the inflammation has subsided, circumcision is advised. Paraphimosis results when the retracted prepuce becomes fixed proximal to the glans. With time, lymphatic and venous obstruction cause progressive swelling of the glans, resulting in ischemic necrosis in neglected cases. Manual reduction is possible early in the disease, but if reduction cannot be accomplished it is imperative that the constricting band be incised to permit

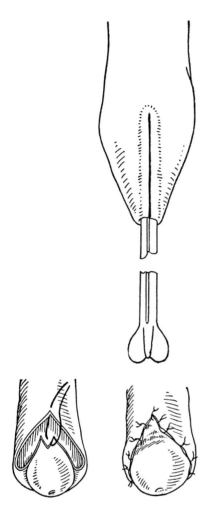

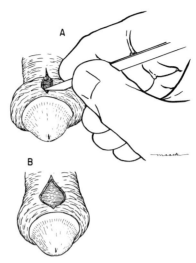

Fig. 20–4. Dorsal slit for relief of paraphimosis.

Fig. 20–3. (*Top*) A grooved director is inserted under the prepuce to the corona; then the prepuce is divided along the director with a pair of pointed scissors. (*Bottom*) Edges of dorsal slit united with interrupted sutures of fine chromic catgut.

reduction of the prepuce (Fig. 20-4). The area of constriction is recognizable as a blanched fibrotic ring. A local anesthetic is so instilled that a small wheal forms and the area is incised vertically, allowing the prepuce to slide forward. Circumcision is performed electively.

Urethral Strictures. Strictures of the male urethra cause decreased force, narrowing, splitting, and spraying of the urinary stream. Strictures often perpetu-

ate nonspecific urethritis. In the past, most strictures were due to gonorrhea; currently, the common etiologic factors are inlying catheters, urethral instrumentation, and trauma.

A stricture is present when a lubricated number 16 French catheter is arrested in the urethra. Definitive diagnosis requires a retrograde urethrogram, and urethral endoscopy is helpful. When the location, length, and caliber of a stricture are defined, proper treatment can be planned. Periodic urethral dilatation is acceptable treatment for many patients; however, urethroplasty is recommended for complicated strictures, those which require frequent dilatation, and strictures in young men. A patient who has experienced many dilatations can offer valid advice about the best instruments for his own case.

The following outlines the technique of urethral dilatation: the urethra is filled with 8 to 12 cc. of 4 percent Xylocaine, which is then retained in the urethra for 2 to 3 minutes by pinching the meatus. A well-lubricated number 18 Van Buren sound is passed according to the diagrams (Fig. 20-5 and 20-6). If the sound meets resistance and is gripped by the stricture, forceful passage is dangerous, and filiforms and following sounds or catheters

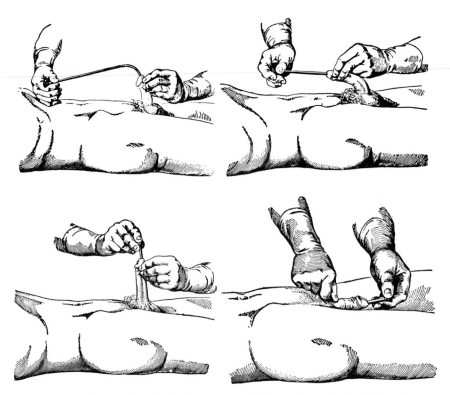

Fig. 20–5. (*Top, left*) While the penis is held steady with the left hand, the tip of the sound is inserted into the meatus with the right hand. (*Top, right*) The sound is advanced into the urethra as the penis is drawn up over the instrument. (*Bottom, left*) Resistance is encountered by the sound at the bulbomembranous junction. (*Bottom, right*) The handle of the sound is depressed slowly by the left hand. In this way, the tip of the sound follows easily the curve of the posterior urethra. The right hand makes pressure downward over the root of the penis to relax the suspensory ligament.

should be substituted. The urethra is filled with a sterile, water-soluble lubricant instilled with a catheter-tipped syringe. Then a spiral-tipped filiform is introduced and advanced; if it reaches the bladder, a number 16 French follower is screwed on and passed into the bladder. If the first filiform fails to reach the bladder, it is left in the urethra and a second, third, and fourth are inserted and manipulated to and fro until one slips past the obstruction and enters the bladder (Fig. 20-7). Progressive dilatation with larger caliber instruments is then possible by attaching them to the guiding filiform. As a rule, a 2 to 4 French enlargement of the urethral caliber at each dilatation is suf-ficient. Excessively vigorous dilatation aggravates the stricture and risks hemorrhage.

Short strictures of the urethral meatus result from urethral instrumentation, meatal ulceration, and balanitis xerotica obliterans. The last is related to lichen sclerosus et atrophicus and produces atrophy and fibrosis of the glans and prepuce, with obliteration of the urethral meatus. Regardless of the etiology, meatal stenosis is treated by meatotomy. A local anesthetic is infiltrated at the ventral lip of the meatus, and this area is crushed with a hemostat. In the crushed area, a sharp cut with a scissors is nearly bloodless. Then the mucosa is sutured to the skin with

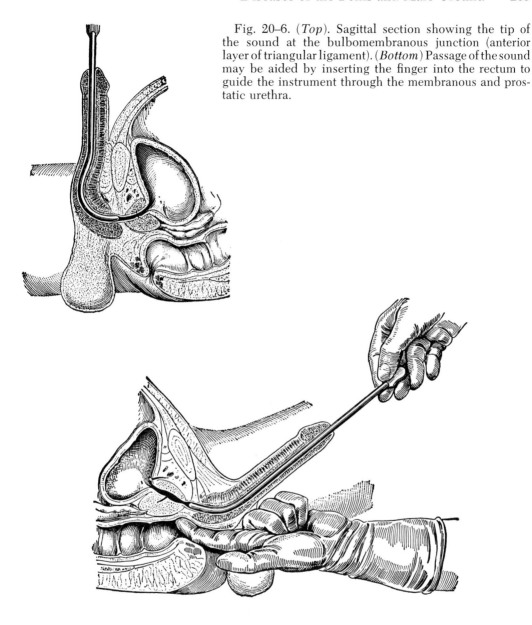

Fig. 20–6. (*Top*). Sagittal section showing the tip of the sound at the bulbomembranous junction (anterior layer of triangular ligament). (*Bottom*) Passage of the sound may be aided by inserting the finger into the rectum to guide the instrument through the membranous and prostatic urethra.

interrupted 4-0 chromic catgut sutures (Fig. 20-8).

Condylomata Acuminata. These lesions can arise in the urethra and cause persistent urethral discharge or hematuria. Rarely solitary, condylomata on the glans and prepuce provide a clue to intraurethral lesions. Lesions visible at the meatus can be excised or fulgurated. Deep lesions require endoscopic fulgura-

tion. Podophyllin should not be instilled into the urethra, but it is effective when applied to surface condylomata.

Urethral Foreign Bodies. Patients who have placed foreign bodies into the urethra for autoeroticism or to support a flaccid penis during coitus present with bleeding, urethral pain, discharge, and, possibly, urinary retention. Plain x-ray films and contrast urethrograms are use-

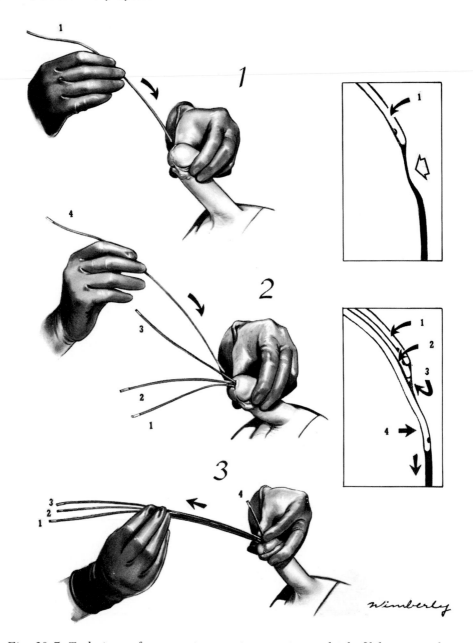

Fig. 20–7. Technique of overcoming a stricture using multiple filiforms attaching a follower.

ful to define the location of the foreign object. Pencils and swizzle sticks can be palpated and milked out of the proximal urethra after filling the urethra with lubricating jelly. Objects in the deep urethra and bladder demand hospitalization for surgical removal, via cystotomy or urethrotomy.

CIRCUMCISION

Circumcision of the ambulatory man can be performed painlessly by employing regional block anesthesia (see Fig. 20-9). Premedication with Valium, 10 mg. by mouth, or Seconal, 100 mg., plus Demerol, 75 mg., is usually helpful. The

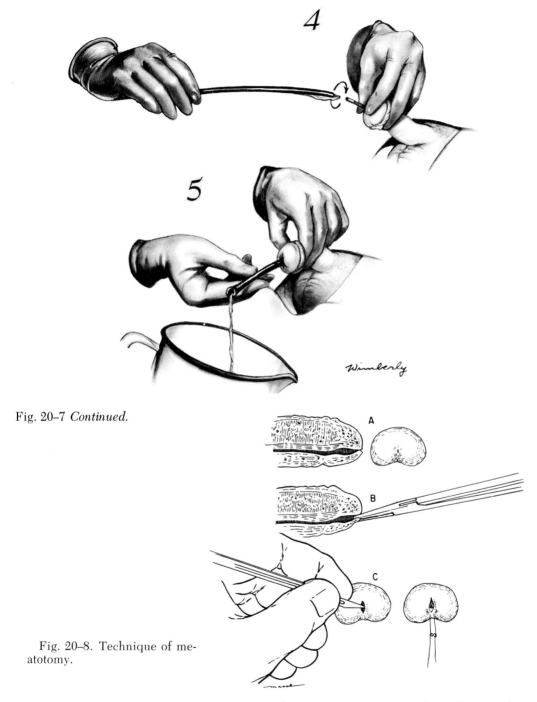

Fig. 20–7 *Continued.*

Fig. 20–8. Technique of meatotomy.

patient is instructed to shave the hair at the base of his penis and thoroughly wash his genitalia at home before the procedure.

Following skin preparation with Beta-dine, Ioprep, or a similar solution, the penis is draped with sterile towels or an eye drape. The base of the penis is injected with 1 or 2 percent Xylocaine in four separate spots, as follows: a small

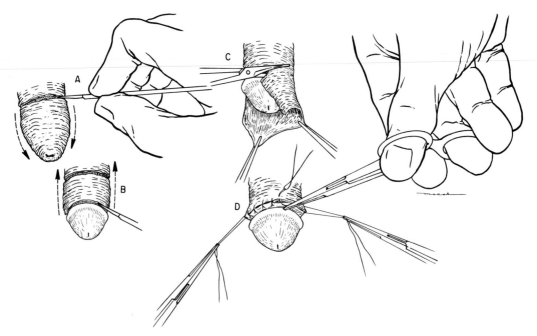

Fig. 20–9. Technique of circumcision.

wheal of anesthesia is produced by subcutaneous injection at the 10 o'clock, 2 o'clock, 4 o'clock, and 8 o'clock positions. A 23-gauge needle is used. The needle is then passed through the wheal and through the fascia of the penis, slowly injecting as the needle is advanced. Approximately 2 ml. is injected in each site. The prepuce will become insensitive shortly.

The tip of the prepuce is placed on slight tension, and a short transverse cut is placed at the level of the coronal sulcus. The penis is held upright, and short marking incisions are made on the ventral and lateral aspects of the skin of the penile shaft. An exact circumferential incision is made by connecting the marking cuts. The prepuce is then retracted to expose the glans. If the prepuce cannot be retracted because of phimosis, the edge of the prepuce is incised by making a dorsal slit to permit full retraction. A transverse incision is started in the precoronal skin and is extended circumferentially, perpendicular to the shaft. The incision must divide a full thickness of skin; this allows the edges of the incision to retract slightly. The free edge is lifted with forceps and is undermined with a dissecting scissors. Hemostats are placed on a free edge and lifted, to permit further dissection. When the subcutaneous dissection has tunneled beneath the preputial skin to the first incision, a long hemostat is placed through the tunnel, and the blades are spread. A sharp cut is made in the groove of the open blades, and the free cut edges are clamped with hemostats. Dissection is continued in the loose subcutaneous tissue until the preputial skin is completely excised and discarded. Several veins are cut and must be clamped and ligated with fine plain gut. After the surgeon is certain that all bleeding points have been ligated, he can proceed. Four-o chromic sutures are placed at the 12 o'clock, 3 o'clock, 6 o'clock, and 9 o'clock positions, uniting the skin of the penile shaft with the precoronal skin. The sutures are grasped with hemostats, providing traction which aids in further suturing. A suture is then placed in the center of one quadrant of the wound, and then in the center of 1/8 of the wound, and so forth; thus asymmetrical closure, which can result in torsion of the penis is avoided. Throughout the operation, care is exercised to avoid roughly grasping the skin with tissue forceps. Careless handling results in postoperative pain and edema. After all of the sutures have been placed, the incised area is covered with a 1-inch strip of Telfa and wrapped snugly with 1-inch Kling. The dressing is removed in 48 hours, and the patient is allowed to bathe. Virile young patients are provided with a bottle of ethyl chloride spray, which when applied to the erect penis promptly produces detumescence.

DISEASES OF THE SCROTUM AND SCROTAL CONTENTS

The Acute Scrotum. The triad of abrupt pain, swelling, and redness of the scrotum indicates either torsion of the testis or acute epididymitis. Differentiating between the two diseases is critical because torsion demands prompt surgical exploration to restore the testicular circulation, whereas epididymitis is treated by nonsurgical means. Epididymitis is rare before puberty; in the mature male, however, epididymitis is more common than torsion. The acute scrotum in prepubertal males is usually due to torsion. Pyuria, when present, suggests epididymitis because of the frequent association of the latter with urinary infection. Although the patient's symptoms and the appearance of his scrotum may be similar in both diseases, a large tender epididymis is usually palpable in the early stages of epididymitis. In acute testicular torsion, one cannot differentiate among the structures in the scrotal mass. Often the twisted testis lies high in the scrotum; in contrast, acute epididymitis produces a mass involving the dependent scrotum. When the diagnosis of epididymitis is certain, the patient is treated with rest in bed, elevation of the scrotum, cold compresses, and necessary analgesics. Either ampicillin, 500 mg. 4 times a day, or tetracycline, 250 mg. 4 times a day, is administered in conjunction with the anti-inflammatory agent oxyphenyl butazone, 100 mg. 4 times a day. Treatment is continued until swelling and tenderness are markedly decreased and the patient can walk without pain. The patient must be examined repeatedly until there is complete resolution of the inflammation and a normal testis can be distinguished from the epididymis. When pyuria is present, urine culture is obtained and antibacterial treatment is based on the results of the sensitivity studies. Rarely, the acute scrotal syndrome is the result of insect bite, cellulitis, or a viral orchitis. Viral orchitis does not occur before puberty, and in the adult male it is usually part of the generalized viral illness. Mumps orchitis is usually associated with mumps parotitis. Viral orchitis is treated by rest in bed, analgesics, scrotal elevation, and anti-inflammatory agents. It is essential that scrotal exploration be performed whenever the diagnosis of the acute scrotum is in doubt. None of the lesions which mimic testicular torsion are harmed by scrotal exploration.

Solid Lesions of the Scrotal Contents. An exact diagnosis of a solid scrotal mass should be made by the first physician consulted. Solid masses can be differentiated from cystic lesions by transillumination. The use of a fiberoptic light source in a dark room provides a high degree of accuracy. A nontransilluminating, solid mass of the testis must be considered a cancer and the patient hospitalized for inguinal orchiectomy. A "watch and wait" attitude toward testicular masses often robs the patient of his best chance for a cure.

Cystic Lesions of the Scrotum. Cystic lesions of the scrotum include spermatocele (epididymal cyst), hydrocele of the cord, hydrocele of the testis, and communicating hydrocele, in which the processus vaginalis is patent from the peritoneal cavity to the testicle. Since all cystic lesions transmit light, transillumination is the first step in diagnosis. In the common hydrocele of the testis, a spherical mass obliterates all details of the testis and epididymis. In contradistinction, a spermatocele arises from the head of the epididymis and thus can be palpated distinctly above the testis. Often a spermatocele is considered a supernumerary testis by the layman.

Surgical repair of hydroceles is only required when they produce significant symptoms. Tapping a hydrocele is a temporary treatment which has little therapeutic value and carries a significant risk of infection. When a hydrocele prevents urethral instrumentation or obscures a testicular lesion, percutaneous aspiration is performed with a 14-gauge intravenous catheter or a trocar needle.

Acute Pheblitis of the Spermatic Cord. Varicocele, or varices of the pampiniform plexus, occurs in 10 to 20 percent of men and is confined to the left hemiscrotum. The varicocele becomes tense when the patient stands, and it feels like a "bag of worms." Occasionally, trauma or infection result in acute pheblitis of the varicocele. This painful lesion is identified by the presence of tender, indurated varices. General treatment consists of rest in bed, scrotal elevation, the application of warm compresses, and, possibly, antibiotic therapy.

Acute Dermatitis of the Scrotum. The scrotum can be involved by many generalized dermatological diseases which require the specialized care of a dermatologist; however, acute dermatitis, regardless of the underlying cause, can be treated effectively by the primary physician. Red, painful, weeping dermatitis is common on the crural areas and the scrotum. Obesity, diabetes, hot weather, and poor hygiene are predisposing factors. Chronic tinea cruris may have acute flare-ups when irritated with friction, heat, and sweat. Regardless of etiology, immediate palliative treatment consists of wet dressings soaked in Burow's solution (available in packets, as Domeboro powder). Mix one packet in one pint of cool water. A piece of folded soft cotton sheeting is soaked in the solution, applied sopping wet, and changed frequently. Severe discomfort and anxiety should be treated with sedatives and analgesics. After the acute phase has subsided, treatment is continued with a water-soluble steroid plus iodochlorohydroxyquin cream (Vi-oform-hydrocortisone ointment, 1 percent Domeform-HC ointment, etc.).

VASECTOMY

The Operation. Interruption of the vas deferens is performed to prevent recurrent epididymitis and for voluntary male sterilization. When epididymitis is the result of chronic prostatitis, vasectomy may prevent recurrence. In cases of chronic epididymitis with persistent epididymal thickening, epididymectomy is a more reliable operation.

The indications for voluntary sterilization encompass a myriad of ethical, moral, religious, and intellectual considerations. Sound judgement is required in patient selection. Detailed preoperative interviews, consultations with the entire family, consultation with other physicians, and psychiatric evaluation should all be used freely to avoid error. Explicit, detailed, written consent should be obtained from the patient, and preferably also from his wife. Sample consent forms are available from several sources.

Vasectomy is easily performed in the outpatient operating room. The patient is required to shave his scrotum at home before the operation. Sedation with 5 to 10 mg. of Valium by mouth one half hour before the procedure is helpful. With the patient supine, the scrotal skin is prepared with Betadine, pHisoHex, or other nonastringent solutions. The field is draped with a three-towel triangular drape. The vas is grasped near the neck of the scrotum and is rolled between the thumb and forefinger, isolating it from other cord structures and fixing it directly beneath the skin. The scrotal skin and the tissues around the vas are infiltrated with 1 or 2 percent Xylocaine, using a small needle. An incision 1 cm. long is made directly over the vas (Fig. 20-10). Spreading the incision with a small hemostat permits visualization of the vas deferens. An Allis clamp is gently closed about the vas, which is then lifted through the skin incision. Longitudinal, shallow cuts directly over the vas free it from its fascial

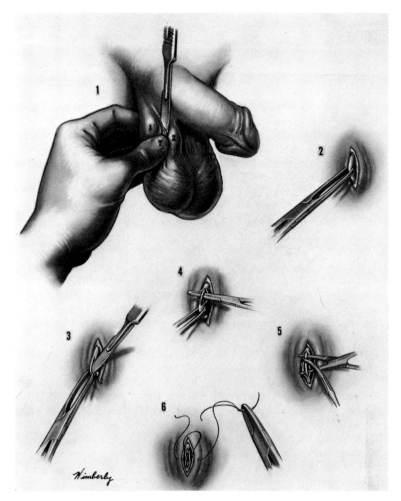

Fig. 20–10. Steps in the technique of vasectomy. See text.

envelope. The naked vas is further isolated by passing a hemostat beneath it. It is helpful to infiltrate the spermatic cord before proceeding with this step. The vas is stripped for 2 to 3 cm., and each end is crushed with a hemostat. A segment 1 to 3 cm. long is removed, the crushed ends are ligated with 2-0 chromic gut and are allowed to fall back into the wound. The ends may be doubled back upon themselves and religated. The skin is closed with a single mattress suture of 2-0 chromic gut. Sterile gauze is placed within a scrotal suspensory and allowed to remain in place for 48 hours.

Postoperative Care. The patient is urged to return home immediately and to lie in bed for 6 to 8 hours with an ice bag on his scrotum. Full activity is resumed in 24 hours. The scrotal suspensory can be discarded and bathing resumed after 48 hours. When vasectomy is done for sterilization, the patient must continue his usual birth control methods until his ejaculate contains no more sperm by microscopic examination. A clean-catch ejaculate is submitted for microscopic study after the 10th ejaculation. Should any sperm remain, every 5th ejaculate is analyzed until no sperm are seen. Although sperm should be absent after 10 ejaculations, certain patients show an occasional immobile spermatozoan up to 30 ejaculations.

Complications. Scrotal hematoma is an infrequent but distressing complication. A hematoma larger than a golf ball is best treated by incision and evacuation of the clotted blood. Aspiration has proved futile. Exploration can be performed in an outpatient operating room. The scrotum is thoroughly prepared with soap and an antiseptic solution. Sterile conditions are necessary. The scrotum is infiltrated with Xylocaine along a 6-cm. line over the hematoma. The skin is incised and the edematous connective tissue is spread bluntly; usually, this reveals a mass of "current jelly" clots. Rarely, an active bleeding point can be identified and ligated. Penrose drains are placed in the wound, each end of the drain emerging at one of the extremities of the incision. The skin is closed with 2-0 chromic sutures. Antibiotics and a scrotal suspensory are prescribed. Usually the drains can be removed in 3 to 5 days. Smaller scrotal hematomas are managed with analgesics, local heat, and scrotal support.

Acute funiculitis and epididymitis have been observed weeks or months following vasectomy. The patient complains of unilateral or bilateral pain in the groin. A tender mass extends either proximally or distally from the point of ligature of the vas. Often the inflammation is due to a spermatic granuloma. Patients may have pyuria or pus in the prostatic fluid. However, often no genitourinary infection is demonstrable. Empirically, broad-spectrum antibiotics, either tetracycline or ampicillin, and oxyphenyl butazone are prescribed. The patient is instructed to apply a heating pad to the groin and to avoid vigorous activity until the inflammation has subsided.

REPLACEMENT OF THE NEPHROSTOMY TUBE

Changing a nephrostomy tube is easy if the tube has been in place at least six weeks following the original surgery and if the tract into the renal pelvis is straight. The new tube should be ready for prompt insertion after removal of the old tube. A Malecot catheter must be inserted with a stylet, whereas a Foley catheter can usually be passed directly into the tract without a stylet. At times the catheter will not pass easily into the renal pelvis and may be impeded at the point where the tract penetrates the renal parenchyma. Forcing the tube often results in the creation of a false passage and makes further attempts at inserting the catheter unsuccessful. Difficulty replacing the tube is common if the previous tube has been out of the tract for several hours or longer. If difficulty is encountered, a smaller caliber coudé catheter is often successful. If the position of the tube is uncertain, injection of dye through the tube will identify the location of the catheter. Surgical placement is occasionally necessary if the catheter cannot be replaced.

21
Female Reproductive Tract

Morton A. Stenchever, M.D.

THE GYNECOLOGIC EXAMINATION

The gynecologic examination begins with a complete history. This includes a description by the patient of her gynecologic symptoms and further questioning by the physician with respect to such things as age at menarche, interval of menstrual cycle, and duration of flow.

Examination includes a complete physical examination, but emphasis is placed on the breasts, abdomen, and pelvic organs.

Examination of the pelvis is carried out in the same fashion as are all other physical examinations. It begins with inspection. This includes an observation of the hair pattern, of the presence of any skin diseases, alopecia, discoloration, or lesions, and observation of redness, edema, or discharge coming from the vagina. The introitus is inspected for symmetry and for signs of parity. Scarring and signs of old obstetrical damage are noted. The size and shape of the clitoris is important if endocrinologic disease is considered. The urethral meatus is observed for evidence of pathology. The condition of the hymen is noted. Should the individual be presenting herself for premarital exam and the hymen be imperforate, the physician may recommend stretching maneuvers or surgical excision. The rectum is inspected for signs of external hemorrhoids and other pathology.

Next, the speculum examination is carried out. In order to carry out a complete and adequate pelvic examination, attention must be given to the needs of the patient with respect to comfort and modesty. She should be placed on a comfortable table, well draped, and the stirrups properly adjusted. A female chaperone should be in the room, even if the physician doing the examination is herself a female. Instruments to be used should be well lubricated and warm. Movements in the examination should be made gently and without any sudden maneuvers. Where pain is anticipated, the patient is warned and, if necessary, an analgesic or local anesthetic is used.

Speculum examination is carried out using the appropriate-sized Grave's (duckbill) speculum. In the case of a virginal individual, a narrow, but nonetheless long, speculum should be used. A typical example of this is the Pederson speculum. The speculum is inserted with the transverse axis of the speculum in the anteroposterior axis of the introitus. After passing through the introitus, it is rotated with downward pressure, since upward pressure would cause pain against the rigid pubic symphysis. The speculum is then opened and adjusted and the vagina is visualized. Observations are made on the condition of the mucous membrane, the presence of discharge, or the presence of lesions. Discharges that are present may be cultured or smeared or placed into saline wet mounts or potassium hydroxide wet mounts. Cultures and smears are helpful when gonorrhea is suspected. Saline wet mounts will make it possible to visualize trichomonads, and potassium hydroxide will make it possible to visualize mycelia if monilia infections are present. Inspection is then made of the cervix for such things as erosions, eversions, polyps, and other lesions. The cervix is also observed for signs of parity and for obstetrical damage. At this point the Papanicolaou smear is taken. Although there are many ways of taking a good Papanicolaou smear, an example of one which is useful is to scrape the endocervical canal, using a cotton-tipped applicator or a wooden spatula, and to smear the material obtained on a slide. The material then found in the posterior cul-de-sac of the vagina is picked up with either a cotton-tipped applicator or a spatula and is smeared on a slide. The slides should be fixed immediately, as air-drying will injure cells and make diagnosis difficult. A worthwhile variant of this means of obtaining a Papanicolaou smear is to aspirate mucus from the endocervical canal, using a glass aspirator, and to crush the material between two slides. The squamocolumnar junction is then scraped and smeared. Obvious lesions of the cervix may be biopsied using a Gaylord biopsy curette. Bleeding is usually not a great problem, but where continuous oozing is noted, silver nitrate cautery may be carried out.

A bimanual examination should now be carried out.

AMBULATORY PROCEDURES

Vulva

A variety of surgical procedures may be carried out on an ambulatory basis on the vulva.

Incision of Hymen. Although a physician may feel that some young patients who are relatively unsophisticated would do better being admitted to the hospital than they would having their hymens incised on an ambulatory basis, occasional hymenotomy may be carried out using preoperative analgesia and infiltration of the hymen with 1 percent procaine or lidocaine. Incisions are made using a scalpel at 2, 4, 8, and 10 o'clock. When hemostasis is a problem, fine catgut sutures may be placed. A small gauze sponge impregnated with Vaseline jelly may be left in the introitus for a few hours, and postoperative care consisting of keeping the area clean and sitz baths two to three times a day may be prescribed.

Incision and Drainage of Bartholin's Gland Abscess. When a patient presents with a Bartholin's gland abscess, she is generally in great pain. A small amount of 1 percent procaine or lidocaine may be injected in the skin above the abscess in the area where it is pointing. This is generally near the mucocutaneous junction. An incision of one-half to three-quarters of an inch is made with a scalpel, and a specimen of pus is immediately cultured. The gland should be inspected internally, using a Kelly clamp or the finger to insure that the abscess is monolocular. Loculations should be broken up, and solid portions which might signify a solid carcinoma of Bartholin's gland should be sought. A ½-inch iodoform drain is placed in the abscess and sitz baths are prescribed. Healing is generally rapid, but a Bartholin's gland cyst may be present following the healing.

Marsupialization of a Bartholin's Gland Cyst. When a Bartholin's gland cyst is present, either after an acute episode of bartholinitis or as an incidental finding, marsupialization may be done on an ambulatory basis. The skin above the cyst in the area of the mucocutaneous junction of the introitus is infiltrated with 1 percent procaine or lidocaine. An incision is made at the junction and an elliptically shaped piece of cyst wall and skin above is removed using iris scissors. It should measure approximately one inch in length and ½ to ¾ of an inch in width,

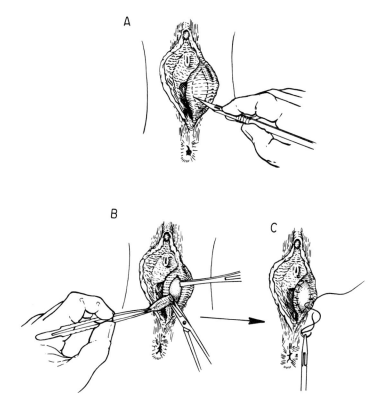

Fig. 21-1. Marsupialization of Bartholins' gland cyst. (*A*) Dotted line depicts incision line. (*B*) Full thickness of cyst wall is removed, and (*C*) cyst lining is sutured to skin edges.

depending upon the size of the cyst. The skin is then sutured to the cyst wall with a row of interrupted fine catgut sutures, and sitz baths are prescribed. Resolution of the cyst is usually complete within a few weeks. Again, inspection of the interior of the gland is important to rule out solid portions which may be carcinoma (Fig. 21-1, *A, B,* and *C*).

Biopsy of Leukoplakic Areas. Frequently, women who are postmenopausal develop leukoplakic plaques on the skin of the vulva. These may be precancerous lesions. They are observed to be thickened, white areas, frequently on a reddened base. They are frequently multiple and are found in any of the regions of the vulva. Because of their potential for malignant change, biopsies are frequently carried out. These may be done by infiltrating the region with 1 percent procaine or lidocaine and removing small areas of tissue for biopsy with a scalpel. Adjacent normal skin should also be included in

the biopsy. When necessary, sutures of fine catgut may be placed. Postoperative care consists in keeping the region clean.

Biopsy of Vulvar Masses. When masses are seen on the vulva, they should be biopsied. Delay in treatment of carcinoma of the vulva is frequently due to denial by the patient, but all too often, to neglect by the physician. When the lesion is small, an excisional biopsy may be done, again using local infiltration and fine sutures where necessary. When a lesion is large, the corner of the lesion should be removed, including some area of adjacent normal skin.

Treatment of Condylomata Acuminata (Venereal Warts). In general, venereal warts are bothersome but are self-limiting; they are caused by a virus. The problem is that they may resemble carcinoma of the vulva or vice versa. They are easily treated by applying a solution of 25 percent podophyllin in benzoin to the lesion. After three hours, the area is washed with soap solution. The lesion should disappear within one to two weeks, although it may require a few treatments. The lesions are frequently multiple and may occur in the vagina as well as on the vulva. If the lesion does not disappear rapidly with podophyllin treatment, excisional biopsy should be carried out to rule out carcinoma.

VAGINA

Vaginal Cysts. Cystic lesions are frequently seen in the vagina and, in general, are of two types. The first is an inclusion cyst formed within a region of the vagina by production of some caseous material secondary to old laceration or episiotomy. When these are small they need not be removed, but if they are large and bothersome they may be removed using local anesthesia. The other type of vaginal cyst is the cyst found in the lateral vaginal wall; this is filled with clear fluid and is known as a Gartner's duct cyst, or a remnant of the wolffian duct. If small, they may be left alone, but if noted to be large or growing, they may be excised. Frequently, because of their size and the difficulty in treating them on an ambulatory basis, the patient should be admitted to the hospital and excision carried out under general anesthesia.

Biopsy of Lesions of the Vagina. Solid lesions of the vagina should be biopsied. Frequently this can be carried out with a Gaylord punch-biopsy instrument without any anesthesia. When the lesion is extensive, when the procedure is expected to be accompanied by significant bleeding, or when the lesion is in a difficult place to reach in an ambulatory situation, the patient should be admitted to the hospital for proper management.

CERVIX

Treatment of Erosion of the Cervix. Erosion of the cervix is a condition in which columnar epithelium migrates down onto the portio vaginalis and appears as a beefy, mucousy membrane. This may occur congenitally when the squamocolumnar junction is located on the portio vaginalis or following such circumstances as pregnancy, abortion, or the use of birth-control pills. The region is frequently prone to infection, and this condition may be treated with electrocautery, in which case the electrocautery instrument is allowed to make furrows in a cartwheel fashion all around the external os. Healing is generally rapid, and postoperative care consists of the use of antibiotic or sulfonamide suppositories for about six days to keep the region clean. Since the cervix has no pain fibers that respond to heat or incision, no anesthesia is necessary. Occasionally the squamous epithelium will attempt to reestablish itself in the region of the erosion and in so covering the columnar epithelium cause inclusion cysts. These cysts may be seen on many cervices and are known as nabothian cysts. They, too, may be managed by electrocautery (Fig. 21-2, *A* and *B*).

An *eversion* of the cervix is somewhat different and represents the healing of an obstetrically lacerated cervix in such a fashion that the external os is turned out, exposing portions of the endocervical canal. Although this resembles an erosion, it is not such a condition and no treatment is necessary. Occasionally, when the eversion is extensive and chronic infection is bothersome to the patient, reconstructive surgery on the cervix may be necessary. However, this is more extensive and requires hospitalization.

Excision or Evulsion of Cervical Polyps. Endocervical polyps will frequently present themselves at the external os. They are usually on pedicles and may be removed by grasping the pedicle with a Kelly clamp and twisting, thus evulsing the polyp. Bleeding is usually minimal and no other care is necessary. Occasionally the polyp originates from a wide base. This type of polyp is frequently seen at the squamocolumnar junction. Excision is of necessity by use of a scalpel, and electrocautery of the bed is frequently necessary. One should constantly be aware of the fact that a chancre may appear on the cervix and resemble a poly-

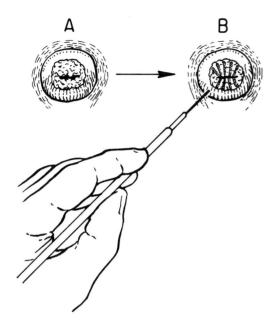

Fig. 21–2. Electrocautery of cervical erosion. (*A*) Erosion before cautery. (*B*) Erosion after cautery.

poid structure. When such is suspected, a dark field preparation should be made for detection of the spirochetes.

Biopsy of the Cervix. If a lesion that appears to be a neoplasm is seen on the cervix, a punch biopsy may be taken, using the Gaylord punch-biopsy curette. A visible lesion of the cervix limited to the cervix would be a Stage I carcinoma. A visible lesion that has extended to the upper vagina or into the parametrium would be a Stage II. A lesion that has extended to the lateral pelvic wall or to the lower one-third of the vagina but has no distant metastases is a Stage III carcinoma of the cervix. A carcinoma of the cervix with distant metastases is a Stage IV. All visible lesions may be safely punch-biopsied for diagnosis. When a Papanicolaou smear is read as suspicious or positive but no lesion is present on the cervix, a proper work-up requires admission of the patient to the hospital, the staining of the cervix with Lugol's solution to differentiate areas of the cervix where cell activity is such that glycogen storage of the cells is poor, and then a cone biopsy of the cervix carried out to include all areas of the cervix which do not take up the stain. In addition, curet-

tage of the endocervix not included in the cone and of the endometrium must be carried out. It is inappropriate to punch-biopsy a cervix which has no obvious lesion when a positive or suspicious Papanicolaou smear is found. Punch biopsy will only give a diagnosis on the area biopsied and will not define the extent of the disease in areas that are not biopsied. A microscopic tumor of the cervix or a tumor of the endocervical canal is not visible but may be nonetheless invasive and dangerous. Some authors feel that multiple punch biopsies are as good as a conization. However, I feel that the only sure way of diagnosing the complete extent of a tumor is by conization.

UTERUS

Endometrial Biopsy. Diagnostic procedures concerning the uterus that may be carried out on an ambulatory basis are essentially those related to infertility and those related to the diagnosis of cancer. In diagnosing the cause of infertility, it may be appropriate to carry out an endometrial biopsy to detect evidence of ovulation and to date the endometrium properly. In this respect, an endometrial biopsy is carried out, using one of a variety of biopsy instruments, some time after the 23rd day of the menstrual cycle. Many people, fearing that a pregnancy would be interrupted, wait until the first day of menstruation to carry out such a biopsy. However, it has been shown that if the biopsy is taken along the lateral wall of the uterus, a pregnancy would probably not be interrupted, as most ova implant on the anterior or posterior wall.

To carry out an endometrial biopsy, the cervix is grasped with a single-toothed tenaculum and a biopsy curette is gently placed into the endometrial cavity, applied to one of the lateral walls, and then removed with steady outward pressure. A small piece of tissue is thus obtained and may be sent to the laboratory fixed in formalin. In the case of postmenopausal bleeding, endometrial biopsies are occasionally used to detect cancer. This is a poor test and should not be carried out. When a postmenopausal bleeder is found, dilatation and curettage is mandatory.

Endometrial Washings. Recently a variety of instruments to obtain cells from the endometrium for the detection of tumors have been developed. The latest of these is the Gravalee jet washer, which combines the washing of the endometrium with a negative pressure system to produce a cell block for study. Although in the best of hands this may improve the possible diagnostic ability of the physician to as much as 95 percent, in the case of a postmenopausal bleeder or someone with whom there is a strong suspicion of serious pathology, dilatation and curettage should be carried out.

Dilatation and Curettage. Diagnostic dilatation and curettage may be carried out under local anesthesia on an ambulatory basis. A paracervical block is carried out by infiltrating the paracervical region with approximately 5 cc. of 1 percent lidocaine or mepivacaine bilaterally. The endometrial cavity is then sounded with a uterine sound and the cervix dilated with progressive Hegar-type dilators. For most diagnostic curettages, dilatation to approximately a number 8 to

10 French is sufficient. The endocervical canal is then systematically curetted with a small sharp curette, and any curettings obtained are sent to the laboratory in a separate container. The purpose of this is that if there is an endometrial tumor, one wishes to know whether it has extended to the cervix, as treatment would be different. Then, systematic curettage of the endometrial cavity is carried out, using a small or medium-sized sharp curette. The technique suggested is that of placing the curette into the cavity at 12 o'clock until it just reaches the end of the endometrial cavity and then removing, with an upward, firm motion, a portion of the endometrium. The curette is then reinserted at 12 o'clock and moved to the 1 o'clock position. Each movement of the curette is carried out by replacing it at the 12 o'clock position and then turning it to the proper position in the cavity. If the uterus is retroflexed, the curette is placed at 6 o'clock instead of at 12 o'clock. In other words, the axis of the uterine cavity is always followed. The cavity should never be curetted in a hurky-jerky or back-and-forth fashion, as perforation may take place. Attention is always given to irregularities in the uterus, such as submucous fibroids or the presence of septa within the uterus. Septa occur in about 5 percent of all uteruses. Following the curettage, an exploration with a polyp forceps for endometrial polyps is carried out.

TUBES AND OVARIES

It is possible to perform laparoscopy or culdoscopy for diagnostic inspection of the tubes and ovaries on an ambulatory basis. Local anesthesia is used. Through the laparoscope or culdoscope, it is possible to biopsy the ovary, ligate the fallopian tubes, or lyse adhesions. However, skill in laparoscopy or culdoscopy depends on experience. In most cases, referral to an individual with such experience is necessary, and many individuals with such skill require that the patient be admitted to the hospital for adequate anesthesia of a general or regional nature.

PREGNANCY

Two procedures may be carried out on the pregnant uterus on an ambulatory basis. One is dilatation and curettage for incomplete abortion and the second is dilatation and curettage for therapeutic abortion. The former is generally associated with a dilated or partially dilated cervix. After an analgesic is given, a paracervical block may be carried out as previously described and the uterus emptied either by the use of a suction curette or with the ring forceps and a standard medium-sized sharp curette. Care must be taken to avoid perforation of the uterus. To avoid this, an oxytocic agent, such as 0.2 mg. Ergotrate maleate or 10 I. U. Pitocin or Syntocinon, may be injected intramuscularly or intravenously to help the uterus contract. In addition, all mechanical maneuvers should be carried out with great care and gentleness.

Dilatation and curettage for therapeutic abortion may be carried out with relative safety until about 10 to 12 weeks' gestation. Thereafter, other means of emptying the uterus, such as intra-amniotic infusion of hypertonic saline or glucose or of a prostaglandin, or hysterotomy, should be considered. When dilatation and curettage is planned, paracervical block anesthesia is used. An option which may be exercised is to insert a laminaria tent into the cervix 8 to 12 hours prior to the procedure. These tents produced from the seaweed plant *Laminaria digitatum* are available commercially and are hydrophilic, causing a slow steady swelling, with dilation, of the cervix. Dilation may be then completed easily under paracervical block anesthesia with Hegar-type dilators. Curettage may be then carried out with either the suction curette or with ovum forceps and a medium-sized sharp curette. Again, gentleness and the use of an oxytocic are extremely important.

When a patient aborts or is aborted, attention should be paid to her hematocrit and to blood loss. If heavy bleeding is anticipated or encountered, blood should be crossmatched and available. Blood typing should be carried out on each patient, as an Rh-negative patient should be given RhoGam (anti-D human gamma globulin) within 72 hours of abortion to avoid isoimmunization. Postoperatively, the patient should be observed for bleeding and signs of infection.

22

Thorax, Clavicle, Scapula, and Chest Wall

Mark W. Wolcott, M.D.

CONTUSIONS OF THE CHEST WALL

Etiology. In these days, when numerous types of accidents occur, injuries to the chest wall are not infrequent. In automobile accidents, a person may be struck by the steering wheel or thrown against the dashboard, or bruises may be obtained through various other mechanisms.

Examination for Fracture. In this area, contusions must always be suspected of overlying a fracture of the ribs. It is not possible to make a diagnosis of fracture without a roentgenogram, but one can obtain a fairly certain clinical impression by moving the involved part of the chest cage without pressing upon the injured area. For instance, if the injury is along the side of the chest, with the hands anterior and posterior, the ribs may be sprung by pressing the hands toward each other. This gives excruciating pain at the site of a fracture, whereas in the case of a simple contusion, if pain is elicited, it is not nearly so marked.

Symptoms. Contusions of the chest differ little in their pathology from those elsewhere in the body, but, because they overlie an area which is constantly in motion with each respiration, they are associated with prolonged periods of disability and accompanying discomfort.

Treatment. Immobilization of the area by adhesive strapping which extends beyond the midline, front and back, or, better, which encircles the entire chest at the site of the injury, will prevent movement of the chest under the area of contusion and so lessen discomfort. Immediate strapping is the most effective method of treatment, and the strapping may be applied even though a fracture is suspected. The application of cold during the first 24 hours, and later, of heat, over the adhesive strapping is of value. The acute soreness of the contusion usually is relieved in from 5 to 7 days of strapping, but there may be residual soreness for a considerably longer period. This may be controlled effectively by the injection of an anesthetic into the area of the contusion.

WOUNDS OF THE CHEST

Wounds of the chest are dangerous because they may be associated with wounds of the thoracic viscera, the most commonly associated injuries being pneumothorax, damage to an intercostal vessel, or damage to the lung, the great

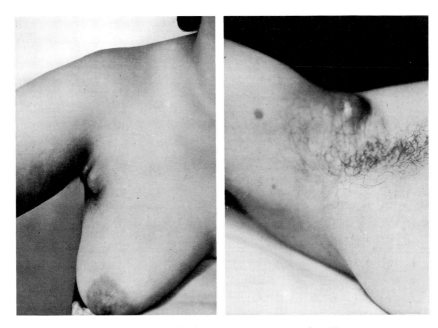

Fig. 22–1. Hidradenitis suppurativa of axilla.

vessels, or the heart. The type of wounding agent is of great importance and should be ascertained as quickly as possible. A very careful examination must be made of every thoracic wound. If there is any suspicion of an underlying visceral injury, hospital admission is necessary.

Treatment. The care of superficial wounds of the chest does not differ from that of wounds elsewhere in the body. After the wound has been cleansed, if it is not more than 6 hours since the injury was received, primary suture may be attempted. Immobilization is best effected by adhesive strapping which encircles the chest at the site of the wound. A bandage of elastic gauze is particularly helpful, since it molds and clings to the thoracic cage but does not constrict unduly. A penetrating wound should make one suspect internal injury following trauma and is an indication for prompt hospitalization.

HIDRADENITIS SUPPURATIVA

This disease, which may occur wherever apocrine sweat glands are found, appears most commonly in the axilla (Fig. 22-1). It may occur, however, in the inguinal and gluteal cleft areas.

It is characterized by the formation of painful erythematous swellings ("blind boils"). These are really small abscesses which eventually rupture, forming chronic drainage tracts. The process repeats itself, with the result that extensive fibrosis may scar the axilla. Treatment consists of careful frequent cleansings of the axilla with an antibacterial soap or detergent and the use of appropriate antibiotics systemically. Sensitivity tests should be carried out as soon as possible because the infecting organisms may be resistant to the usual antibiotic therapy. Fluctuant "blind boils" should be incised under local anesthesia and the abscess cavity packed lightly with gauze.

The use of corticosteroids has given some promise in the treatment of hidradenitis suppurativa. Hydrocortisone, in doses of 60 to 80 mg. per day, or prednisolone or another adrenal steroid in comparable dosage, is given for 7 to 14 days; then the dosage is gradually reduced until the drug is stopped in 2 to 3 weeks.

Occasionally it will be necessary to admit the patient to the hospital to carry out radical excision of the involved area and subsequent skin grafting.

FRACTURES OF THE RIBS

Etiology. The ribs may be fractured as a result of violent sneezing or coughing, but more frequently they are fractured by the transmitted force of a blow on the front of the chest. Much more commonly, the force is direct and is due to, for example, a fall against a table or the side of the bathtub, an automobile accident, or the impact of a fist. The fracture may be single or multiple and incomplete, complete, or comminuted. Slight overriding sometimes accompanies complete fracture, but most often there is no displacement.

Some irritation or injury of the subjacent pleura always accompanies fracture of the ribs. When the violence is great, the pleura and the lung may be perforated, and paradoxical motion, subcutaneous emphysema, hemothorax, penumothorax, or pulmonary hemorrhage may follow rapidly. Empyema or atelectasis of the lung may occur later. Careful search for such complications must be made when the patient is first seen. Such complications often require a chest roentgenogram for diagnosis. When they are present, hospitalization for observation and treatment is necessary. External or internal fixation may be necessary in some cases, especially when paradoxical motion exists.

Diagnosis. A history of injury and the characteristic aspect of the patient usually suggest the diagnosis at a glance. The patient tends to immobilize the affected rib by speaking deliberately, by hunching himself to the affected side, and by compressing the affected area with his hands. Breathing may be labored; it is always shallow. Agonizing spasms of pain accompany coughing or sneezing.

After direct violence, localized swelling and skin injury may indicate the site of fracture; the patient can localize it accurately. On palpation, well-defined areas of tenderness, and possibly also irregularity of contour and crepitus, may be found. To differentiate incomplete fracture from simple contusion of the chest wall, compression of the chest with one hand on the back and the other on the sternum may be useful. When a fracture is present, distinct pain should be elicited at the site of fracture. Routine roentgen examination of the chest frequently fails to demonstrate fractures about the anterior and the posterior axillary lines; therefore, oblique views may be necessary. In the presence of a typical clinical picture, a negative roentgenogram must be regarded simply as failure to demonstrate the fracture rather than as assurance of its absence.

Roentgen examination is advisable after every chest injury that produces signs of fracture. Medicolegal reasons necessitate x-ray examination in most situations where trauma has been sustained by the thorax.

Treatment. No reduction is attempted. The patient with an uncomplicated fracture of the ribs primarily requires relief of pain. This may be obtained by strapping the chest and administering liberal doses of codeine and acetylsalicylic acid during the first few days. When pain is severe or when there are multiple fractures, rest in bed must be insisted upon for a period of 1 to 3 weeks or more. Injection of 10 to 20 ml. of a 1 percent procaine solution directly into the fracture site and/or into the intercostal nerves along the lower borders of the fractured and the adjacent ribs often gives prolonged relief of pain. This may be repeated several times if necessary.

The ordinary semicircular strapping of the chest is inefficient at its best; it loosens rapidly, and the tension on the skin frequently causes blebs. Complete circular strapping, with the tension so adjusted that the strapping is just tight enough to immobilize the ribs but not tight enough to choke the patient, gives greater relief and less trouble. The circular adhesive may be reinforced by vertical straps (Fig. 22-2), that cross the shoulder from back to front. Giving the skin a good alcohol rub and covering hairy areas with gauze help to avoid pustular dermatitis

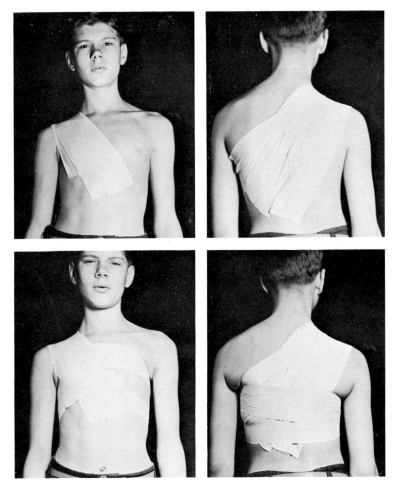

Fig. 22–2. Strapping for pain over the costochondral junctions of the right second and third ribs following an injury. The right upper chest is compressed and immobilized by the vertical and the horizontal straps. The same type of strapping is used for fractures of the lower ribs.

due to the adhesive. Tincture of benzoin may often be used to protect the skin. After measuring the circumference of the chest below the fracture level, tear off three or more straps of adhesive, each slightly longer than the circumference and from 2 to 3 inches wide. With the arms elevated, the patient takes a deep breath and exhales fully; then, starting in the anterior midline well below the level of the fracture, the strap is carried around the unaffected side to the back and forward over the affected side, the starting point finally being overlapped. The next strap is applied higher, half of the width of the first strap being overlapped. This is continued until the highest strap is 2 or 3 ribs above the fracture site. When the upper ribs are fractured, 2 additional straps are placed across the shoulder. In women with pendulous breasts, it may be impossible to strap the chest over the fracture. In this event, 1 or 2 bands of adhesive may encircle the lower chest with moderate tension; this limits the respiratory excursion and gives considerable relief from pain. An elastic adhesive bandage also may be used.

The strapping becomes loose in from 2 to 4 days in many patients. If it has been tolerated well, it need not be removed, and a tight second layer may be applied directly over it. This may be repeated as often as necessary. Very often, the strapping produces a mild dermatitis with itching or pustules. When this happens, the strapping is removed gently and a nonadhesive elastic bandage from 4 to 6 inches wide is applied instead. Alcohol rubs 3 times daily will be helpful, and in 3 or 4 days the strapping may be reapplied after covering the most irritated areas with gauze. The immobilization of the chest is continued until pain on breathing and local tenderness disappear. This may take from 3 to 8 weeks. In the author's experience, less than half of the patients can tolerate strapping for more than a day or two. In such people, repeated infiltration of a local anesthetic into the intercostal nerves above and below, and into the intercostal nerve supplying the rib fractured, is quite successful. This may be repeated daily. Great care must be taken not to produce a pneumothorax.

Fractures of the ribs in elderly fat women may be one of the most exasperating lesions to treat. Because of the resulting skin lesions and abdominal distress, strapping may cause greater discomfort than does the fracture. Rest in bed, sedatives, and mild laxatives constitute the mainstay of treatment in these patients.

COSTOCHONDRAL SEPARATION; FRACTURE OF THE COSTAL CARTILAGES

Occasionally, as a result of direct trauma, a fracture may occur at the costochondral junction; this has been called costochondral separation. Fractures through the costal cartilage also may occur; they are more apt to involve the lower ribs at the costal margins.

Diagnosis. The clinical picture is that of fracture of a rib close to the sternum or at the costal margin. The patient often experiences a snapping sensation on deep inspiration. A roentgenogram usually is negative, since cartilage is radiolucent.

Treatment. These lesions are treated in the same manner as are fractures of the ribs (Fig. 22-2), either by strapping or by local injection of an anesthetic agent. Pain may persist for several months, since cartilage heals very slowly. It is generally impractical to maintain adhesive strapping for more than a week. The patient must be warned to avoid injury to the site until healing occurs; otherwise a prolonged period of disability may occur.

In old cases of costal cartilage fracture, suture may be performed under local anesthesia, after first freshening the fracture ends of the injury. Repair should be done with stainless-steel wire.

FRACTURES OF THE STERNUM

Etiology. Fractures of the sternum have been more common in recent years because of the frequency of automobile collisions. In such accidents, the driver is thrown forward against the steering wheel; at high speed, the impact may be so great that, not only is the sternum fractured, but there also may be multiple fractures of the ribs, injury to the thoracic viscera, and fractures of the spine, the jaw, and the skull. A fracture of the sternum may then be the least of the injuries, and, if it exists without displacement of the fragments, it is easily overlooked. Fractures of the sternum may be caused also by a fall on the head or the shoulders. This fracture is rare in persons under 20 years of age, which is the age at which the upper segments of the bone fuse.

The site of the fracture tends to be at or near the junction between the manubrium and the body. Usually this is the most prominent and narrow part of the bone. Backward displacement of the upper fragment on the lower may take place, and overriding may occur.

Diagnosis. When fracture of the sternum occurs without displacement, the site of the pain and tenderness and the associated severe pain on breathing and coughing suggest the diagnosis immediately. The patient tends to hunch

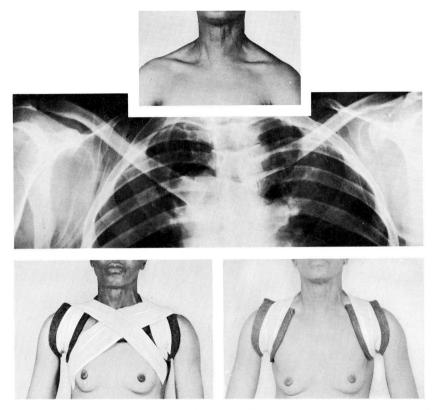

Fig. 22–3. Sternoclavicular dislocation. There is an upward dislocation of the sternal end of the right clavicle. The dressing is applied as shown in the pictures at the bottom.

himself, and his breathing is shallow in an effort to ease the pain. Lateral roentgen films usually demonstrate the fracture well, but oblique views may be necessary. When displacement of the fragments occurs, the severity of the pain, the associated dyspnea, and the palpable deformity should make the diagnosis easy.

Treatment. Careful observation of the patient and a careful search for associated injuries at a minimum require an electrocardiogram and appropriate roentgenograms of the chest. Since there is usually minimal motion at the fracture site, no treatment other than relief of pain by giving codeine is required. Patients with displaced fractures may require hospitalization and operation, with wiring of the fragments.

Prognosis. The prognosis in uncomplicated cases is good, even though there may be residual deformity.

STERNOCLAVICULAR DISLOCATION

Anatomy and Etiology. Dislocation at the sternoclavicular joint is relatively uncommon. The joint lies obliquely, facing upward and outward. A fibrocartilage lies between the clavicle and the sternum, and it is bound strongly to both bones. In addition, dislocation is resisted by the sternoclavicular, the interclavicular, and the rhomboid ligaments, which tear when dislocation occurs. The rhomboid ligament may remain intact in forward dislocations. A thurst inward on the shoulder may force the inner end of the clavicle upward or forward on the sternum, as well as medially. The very rare backward, or retrosternal, dislocation may occur as a result of direct violence.

Diagnosis. The diagnosis of forward-upward dislocation may be made on inspection and palpation (Fig. 22-3). because the dislocated end of the clavicle is prominent both to the eye and to the finger. Localized tenderness at the sternoclavicular joint may be quite acute. Roentgen examination is advisable for verification and for exclusion of associated fractures. Sternoclavicular dislocation may be partial or complete. The partial type can usually be reduced and maintained in position after reduction, whereas the complete type may be irreducible or impossible to maintain in the reduced position.

Treatment. Reduction of the forward-upward displacement is not difficult unless an infolding of the torn ligaments occurs. Anesthesia may not be necessary, but, when it is, infiltration of 10 to 15 ml. of 2 percent procaine hydrochloride solution about the joint will give complete freedom from pain. The maneuvers are the same as those for reduction of a fractured clavicle. The patient lies on a table with a sandbag between the scapulae. While an assistant holds the opposite shoulder to the table, with one hand the surgeon presses the shoulder of the injured side toward the table and cephalad, and with the other hand he forces the inner end of the clavicle downward and caudad. Maintenance of reduction always has been difficult. A felt pad about 3 inches square and 1 inch thick can be made to press on the dislocated end of the clavicle by 2- or 3-inch adhesive cross straps applied with considerable tension after the patient enhales forcibly (Fig. 22-3). When any tendency to recur is present, a clavicular T splint or a posterior figure-of-eight bandage also is applied to hold the shoulders backward and outward; otherwise, a sling for the arm on the affected side is enough. Very gentle use of both arms may be encouraged from the beginning. The adhesive strapping and the splint must be inspected every second day for 2 or 3 weeks. From 5 to 6 weeks' immobilization is advisable; a shorter period may result in recurrence of the dislocation. Usually, however, good function may be expected, even with a persistent partial dislocation.

The retrosternal type of dislocation may be manipulated as described above, except that the inner end of the clavicle should be pulled forward.

If a dislocation is irreducible or if it is impossible to maintain reduction, operative correction should be considered. This is especially true in women in whom a deformity is of cosmetic consideration.

Prognosis. After partial dislocation, no permanent effect other than slight thickening about the joint may be expected. After complete dislocation, failure to maintain a good reduction may require operation, the result of which is usually good.

Spontaneous subluxation of the sternoclavicular joint occurs occasionally. It has been ascribed to joint relaxation and degenerative changes that occur with advancing age. It is usually asymptomatic and very slowly progressive or stationary. Usually no treatment is necessary.

FRACTURES OF THE CLAVICLE

Anatomy and Etiology. The clavicle functions as a rigid prop or pivot for the shoulder girdle, maintaining the shoulder joint at a fixed distance from the sternum. It is the only bony connection between the upper extremity and the trunk.

The clavicle is one of the bones most often fractured. In every fall on the outstretched hand or arm and in every fall on the point of the shoulder, the shoulder is thrust toward the chest. The clavicle receives this thrust and usually breaks at its weakest point, the junction of its two curves, between the middle and the outer thirds. Occasionally, this fracture is found in a newborn infant. Fractures also may occur by direct violence when the bone is struck directly on its anterior or superior surface.

Displacements. The fracture line is

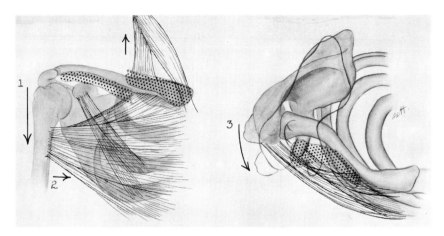

Fig. 22–4. Fracture of the clavicle as seen from in front and from above. The medial fragment is pulled upward slightly by the sternocleidomastoid muscle. The lateral fragment moves with the shoulder (1) downward, due to the weight of the arm and the shoulder, (2) inward, due to the tension of the pectoralis muscles, and (3) forward, due to the added action of the serrarus magnus and to the shape of the chest.

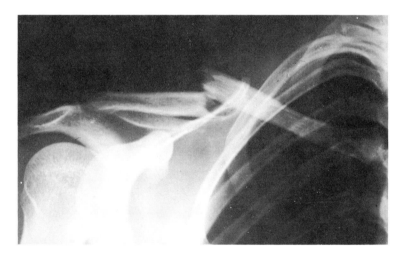

Fig. 22–5. Typical fracture of the clavicle. The inner fragment is elevated, and the outer fragment is displaced downward and inward.

usually oblique, but it may be transverse or comminuted. When the fracture is complete and the fragments separate, a characteristic displacement follows (Figs. 22-4 and 22-5). The medial fragment is drawn slightly upward by the sternocleidomastoid muscle. The outer fragment moves downward, inward, and forward, due to the weight of the shoulder and the arm and to the tension of the muscles that attach the scapula and the humerus to the chest. These muscles are mainly the pectoralis major and minor, the serratus magnus, and the latissimus dorsi.

In children, the fracture frequently is of the greenstick type, with a relatively slight displacement consisting mainly of increased angulation.

Diagnosis. When the fracture is complete, the patient may have a characteris-

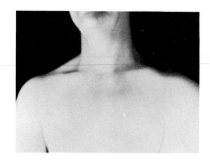

Fig. 22–6. Fracture of the left clavicle. The characteristic deformity is visible.

tic posture; the head is carried forward and to the injured side to relieve the tension on the inner fragment. The arm on the affected side is cradled in the opposite hand to relieve the tension on the outer fragment caused by the weight of the arm. Inspection may reveal a typical deformity (Fig. 22-6). Palpation and comparison with the unaffected side disclose thickening, angulation or sharp edges associated with localized acute tenderness, and crepitus. Motion of the arm causes pain at the fracture site. Practically always, an accurate diagnosis can be made in a moment or two, except when there is an unusual amount of swelling.

When the fracture is incomplete, the diagnosis may be made from the history, the slight swelling, and the localized acute tenderness, which are accompanied by some pain on motion and limitation of elevation of the arm. The actual disability of the arm on the affected side may be very slight. Not infrequently, a child is brought in by a parent because of a "lump near the shoulder" that proves to be a fracture of the clavicle of 1 or 2 weeks' duration with excessive callus formation resulting from lack of immobilization.

Roentgen examination serves to show the exact type of fracture and, in complete fractures, the degree of displacement; and to verify the diagnosis when the fracture is incomplete. Roentgenograms may be necessary to differentiate the rare fractures very close to either the sternal or the acromial end from sternoclavicular or acromioclavicular separations.

Treatment of Incomplete and Green-stick Fractures. Many methods for treating of the clavicle have been described. Their value varies according to the type of fracture and the age and the sex of the patient. Practically always, these fractures unite with good subsequent function, so that the problem is one of selecting the form of treatment best suited to the particular case.

Incomplete and greenstick fractures require very little treatment. A posterior figure-of-eight dressing provides adequate immobilization. The materials required are an elastic bandage, such as Kling or a similar loose-weave material, 2, 3, or 4 inches wide, depending on the size of the patient; 3 felt or cotton pads, 1 inch thick and 6 x 8 inches wide for adults (smaller for children); and 3 safety pins. Felt pads should be wrapped in gauze.

The patient elevates the uninjured arm, and an assistant elevates the other. A strip of bandage is laid across the chest in front of the shoulders, and one pad is placed just in front of and below each shoulder joint, and one, over the scapulae. The posterior figure-of-eight is then applied with moderate tension and pinned in the back. The ends of the bandage previously laid across the chest are pulled together, and each side is pinned to an anterior turn of the figure-of-eight bandage (Fig. 22-7). A similar dressing may be made with a plaster bandage. Felt pads are placed in each axilla and on the back, and the wet plaster bandage is used to make a posterior figure-of-eight. No anterior band is used. Beneath the axilla, the plaster is molded into a narrow thick band, so that the arm may be brought to the side without too much discomfort (Fig. 22-8).

In the first few days, the patient may complain of axillary discomfort, and so instructions are given to rest the arm in the horizontal position if necessary. We encourage the use of both arms freely within the limit of pain. The bandage dressing usually needs to be adjusted and tightened every 3 or 4 days. The skin of the axilla and over the shoulder should be watched carefully, and at every opportunity it should be washed thoroughly,

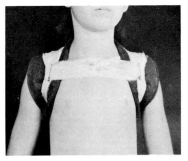 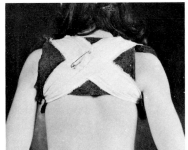

Fig. 22–7. Anterior and posterior views of figure-of-eight dressing. Double-thickness felt is used for the axillary pads; the 2 loops are prevented from slipping by the strip of bandage which is pinned on each side. Three thicknesses of felt are applied over the back. The

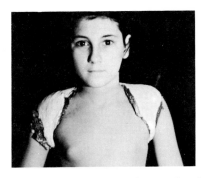

Fig. 22–8. Posterior figure-of-eight plaster dressing for fracture of the clavicle. The plaster was applied after the anterior aspects of the shoulder, the axilla, and the back had been protected by felt.

rubbed with alcohol, and powdered. Cotton may be inserted under the felt pads to prevent chafing. Callus forms rapidly and becomes palpable in 2 to 3 weeks, but the dressing is maintained until union is solid, usually 4 weeks. The plaster dressing seldom requires replacement.

Reduction of Complete Fractures with Displacement. In reducing fractures of the clavicle, difficulty is seldom encountered in aligning the fragments. Maintenance of reduction is the problem, and, of the 200 and more methods devised so far, none is entirely satisfactory.

Infiltration of 10 to 15 ml. of 2 percent procaine hydrochloride solution into the hematoma about the fracture produces

excellent anesthesia in 10 minutes. Frequently, no anesthetic is necessary if the maneuvers are carried out gently. The displacement of the medial fragment is rarely marked, and in any event it can be controlled but poorly. The displacement of the outer fragment can be corrected easily by bringing the shoulder up, out, and back. One of two methods may be used. In the first, the patient sits on a stool. The assistant stands behind him, puts his knee between the scapulae, and draws both shoulders upward and backward forcibly. The surgeon stands facing the patient and manipulates the fragments into alignment, the assistant maintaining the traction until the splint has been applied.

A wood or an aluminum clavicular T splint may be used (Fig. 22-9). The crosspiece must be the full width of the shoulders, and the vertical piece must be

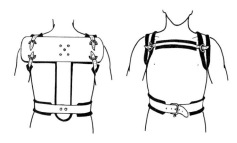

Fig. 22–9. T splint for fracture of the clavicle.

long enough to reach from the base of the neck to the sacrum. The anterior surfaces of both are covered with felt, and the felt axillary pads must be at least 1 inch thick. The vertical piece is bent to conform to the shape of the back in the upright position, and the low webbing strap is fastened about the trunk below the iliac crests. While both shoulders are held upward and backward, they are strapped to the crosspiece. An anterior transverse strap holds the 2 shoulder straps in position. These splints must be inspected frequently, and the skin, especially of the axilla, must be watched carefully.

A satisfactory dressing for fractures that are stable after reduction is a snugly fitted posterior figure-of-eight plaster dressing. The patient is instructed to relieve axillary discomfort by elevating the arms and to continue active use of both arms within pain limits. There is often considerable discomfort during the first 48 hours after reduction; this may be relieved by taking codeine or morphine tablets by mouth.

The fracture is usually stable in 4 weeks, and active use is begun. After removal of the cast or other cumbersome dressing, usually in 4 weeks, a strap type of splint (Fig. 22-10) can be useful for support; occasionally it makes a good initial dressing.

For fractures that cannot be readily maintained, operative fixation, using a stainless steel wire, is recommended. Usually, this will require general anesthesia and, therefore, either hospitalization or the use of an inpatient/outpatient surgiclinic facility.

Prognosis. When the fracture is incomplete or when a complete fracture can be reduced and maintained in good position, the functional result will be excellent. There will be visible thickening at the fracture site, which will decrease after a lapse of time. When a satisfactory position of the fragments cannot be maintained, the functional result is usually good, but the visible deformity may be considerable. (In very rare instances, nonunion, accompanied by persistent pain and symptoms of pressure on the brachial plexus, may require operation.)

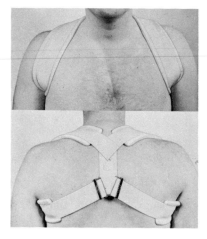

Fig. 22–10. McLeod strap type of splint—a variation of the figure-of-eight dressing, particularly useful when the fracture is in good position and also as a supporting dressing after the removal of other, less comfortable, types of immobilization. (Zimmer, Warsaw, Indiana)

ACROMIOCLAVICULAR DISLOCATION

Etiology. Acromioclavicular dislocation occurs comparatively often. It is a very common injury in contact sports, especially football. A blow on the top of the shoulder that forces the acromion downward and inward may shear through the acromioclavicular ligaments and cause subluxation. Greater violence results in torn coracoclavicular (conoid and trapezoid) ligaments and complete dislocation (Fig. 22-11).

Diagnosis. Immediately after the injury, the patient complains of inability to use the arm and the shoulder. Later, there are swelling and pain at the tip of the shoulder, increased by elevation of the arm. The displacement is characteristic, the outer end of the clavicle becoming much more prominent; it is movable on the acromion, especially when the dislocation is complete (Fig. 22-12). Palpation reveals the deformity, even in the presence of considerable swelling. Determining the exact point of wincing tenderness and comparison with the opposite side help to differentiate this lesion from frac-

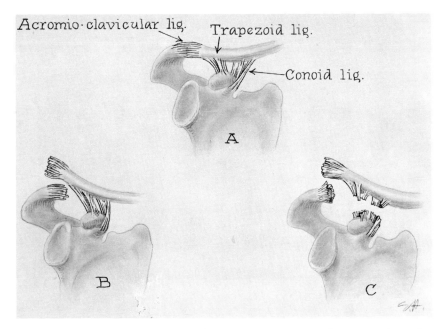

Fig. 22–11. Acromioclavicular dislocation. (*A*) Normal acromioclavicular attachments. (*B*) Incomplete type of dislocation, in which the conoid and the trapezoid ligaments suffer little injury. (*C*) Complete dislocation, in which all ligaments are torn.

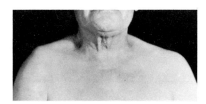

Fig. 22–12. Complete dislocation of the right acromioclavicular joint.

ture of the outer end of the clavicle. Since a fracture may complicate this dislocation, roentgen examination always is in order.

The subluxations offer some difficulty in diagnosis, and even the roentgenologist may have his troubles. Examination of films of both shoulders and determination of the comparative mobility of both acromioclavicular joints under the fluoroscope are of value in doubtful cases.

Treatment. The downward pull of the weight of the arm and the shoulder tends to maintain the displacement. Reduction can be effected by outward and backward traction on the shoulder, accompanied by downward pressure on the prominent end of the clavicle, but the displacement tends to recur almost instantaneously. Reduction must be maintained while the retentive dressing is applied, and the adhesive straps of the dressing must be made tight every 2 or 3 days.

For a temporary dressing, a thick (2-inch) pad is tied in the axilla, and a felt pad about 3 inches square and 1 inch thick is placed over the acromial end of the clavicle; a similar pad is held against the undersurface of the flexed forearm just below the point of the elbow. A 2-inch adhesive strap is started on the midline of the back below the scapula and is carried upward and outward over the clavicular felt pad, then down the anterior surface of the arm, over the lower felt pad, and up the opposite surface of the arm, until it crosses the clavicular felt pad again and continues across the front of the chest to a little beyond the midline. A 3-inch muslin bandage is used to make a wrist sling, the forearm remaining at a

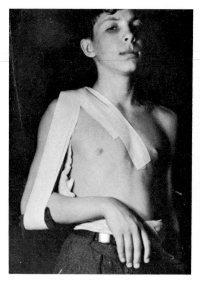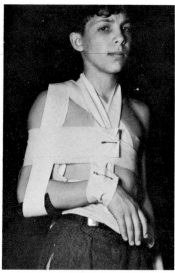

Fig. 22–13. Dressing for acromioclavicular subluxation.

right angle to the arm (Fig. 22-13). A snug Kling-type bandage swathe then is tied about the chest and the arm. The axillary pad acts as a fulcrum, and the shoulder moves outward, lessening the tendency to recurrence of the displacement.

Good union of the ligaments occurs in 4 to 6 weeks in subluxations and in about 8 weeks in complete dislocations. Every 3 to 5 days the swathe must be removed and the adhesive loop tightened by placing a new loop on top of the old. Otherwise, the dressing becomes loose, and the displacement recurs. A piece of the adhesive in front of and behind the arm may be removed and replaced by rubber tubing, thus providing constant elastic pressure.

Dislocations irreducible because of infolded ligaments, failure to maintain reduction, and longstanding dislocations of 1 to 2 months or more may necessitate operative correction. Operation should be advocated as the primary procedure when severe injuries occur in patients who do heavy manual work.

Prognosis. Incomplete dislocations heal rapidly and leave no effects. Complete dislocations may require open reduction, the result of which is usually good. The chief difficulty with this injury is that the patient begins to use the arm before healing is complete. This is seen

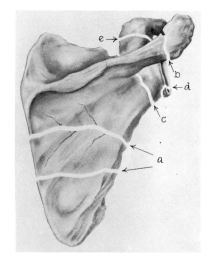

Fig. 22–14. Fractures of the scapula: (*a*) body, (*b*) acromion, (*c*) neck, (*d*) glenoid, and (*e*) coracoid.

most often in football, where the players are reinjured each Saturday. A partial dislocation may become complete if adequate healing is not permitted to occur.

FRACTURES OF THE SCAPULA

Fractures of the scapula may be classified according to the part of the bone

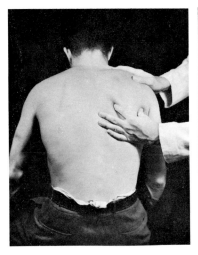 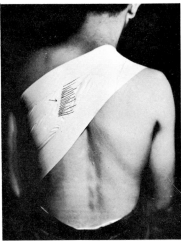

Fig. 22–15. (*Left*) Examination for fracture of the body of the scapula. The acromion is pressed down with one hand, and the other hand grasps and moves the angle of the scapula to determine mobility and crepitus. (*Right*) Adhesive strapping for a fracture of the body of the scapula. The straps begin in the anterior axillary line on the injured side. They are pulled tight over the scapula and pass over the opposite shoulder to beyond the clavicle. A sling is to be added.

This patient had an injury to the rhomboideus muscle at its insertion into the vertebral border of the scapula. The arrow points to the tender area. The muscle is relaxed when the scapula is taken toward the spine.

involved: body, acromion, neck, glenoid, and coracoid (Fig. 22-14).

FRACTURE OF THE BODY OF THE SCAPULA

This fracture, which occurs only rarely, is caused as a rule by direct violence. The body is a flat plate of bone covered on both sides by thick muscular masses; hence, separation of the fragments is seldom of any importance. Body fractures may be single or comminuted.

Diagnosis. A history of direct trauma followed by pain over the bone on moving the shoulder and localized tenderness and swelling usually indicate a fracture. If the acromion is pressed down with one hand and the angle is pushed medially by the other, localized pain, crepitus, and mobility of fragments may be disclosed (Fig. 22-15, *left*).

Treatment. When the fracture is a simple fissure, an adhesive strapping (Fig. 22-15, *right*) and a triangular sling im-

mobilize it adequately. After 3 or 4 days, mild heat and gentle massage are started. In 2 or 3 weeks, healing is sufficient to permit full use.

When the fractures are more extensive, the accompanying pain and swelling are considerable, and rest in bed, application of ice bags, and sedatives may be needed for from 24 to 48 hours. As soon as the patient is up, an axillary pad, sling and swathe dressing is applied. At the end of 1 week, baking, massage and gentle exercises are begun and continued until the shoulder is free of pain and has a full range of motion. After the second or the third week, a triangular sling may be adequate, and daily active use of the part may be permitted. Full active use is resumed at the end of 4 or 5 weeks.

FRACTURE OF THE ACROMION

Diagnosis. This fracture results from a blow on the top of the shoulder. The tension of the deltoid and the weight of the arm then tend to carry the outer portion of the acromion downward. The diagnosis may be made from the history, the local swelling and tenderness, and the irregularity of contour.

Treatment. If pain is severe, rest in bed with the arm abducted is helpful for 2 to 3 days. In the ambulatory patient, an adhesive loop dressing such as that used for acromioclavicular separation (Fig. 22-12) is applied. It presses the flexed forearm upward, makes counterpressure on top of the shoulder medial to the fracture site, and tends to bring the other fragment into line. A wrist sling and a swathe complete the dressing. The immobilization is continued for from 4 to 6 weeks. Active exercise of the hand and baking and massage of the arm and the shoulder are started after 3 or 4 days. After the dressings are discarded, exercises are begun, and baking and massage are continued until the patient can move the arm through the full range of motion without pain, usually about 7 or 8 weeks from the time of injury.

When there has been no displacement of the outer fragment, a sling and swathe dressing is adequate, and shoulder motion may be started after 2 or 3 weeks.

FRACTURE OF THE NECK OF THE SCAPULA

Fracture of the scapular neck may follow falls on the hand or the arm. When the fracture is complete, the weight of the arm pulls the glenoid downward, and the space between the acromion and the head of the humerus becomes wider (Fig. 22-16.)

Diagnosis. After a violent injury to the shoulder, the diagnosis may be suspected when pain and swelling are marked, but there is no definite fracture or dislocation of the humerus. Widening of the acromiohumeral space and palpable irregularity of the axillary border of the scapula may be present. When the displacement is not enough to interfere materially with the mechanics of the shoulder joint, ambulatory treatment is satisfactory.

Treatment. During the acute post-

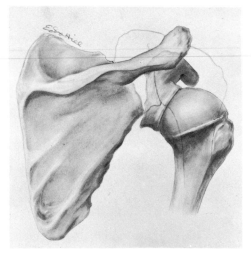

Fig. 22–16. Fracture of the neck of the scapula. The articular fragment is pulled down by the weight of the arm.

traumatic phase, rest in bed, ice bags locally, and sedatives are indicated. After 2 or 3 days, an adhesive loop dressing similar to that described for acromioclavicular separation is applied. This forces the head of the humerus and the glenoid upward. A wrist sling and a swathe complete the dressing. Physiotherapy is instituted as for fractures of the acromion. When very marked displacement of the head threatens to interfere seriously with shoulder function, reduction may perhaps be effected by traction on the abducted arm, accompanied by upward pressure on the distal fragment of the scapula in the axilla. If the malposition is persistent, consultation with an orthopedist is advisable.

FRACTURE THROUGH THE GLENOID

Occasionally, this accompanies dislocation at the shoulder, and, unless very great comminution or displacement is present, it requires no special treatment beyond that for the dislocation.

FRACTURE OF THE CORACOID

This fracture is very rare. A pressure pad is strapped over the coracoid, and an axillary pad, sling and swathe dressing is applied. Immobilization is continued for from 3 to 5 weeks.

PROGNOSIS OF FRACTURES OF THE SCAPULA

Fractures of the body of the scapula rarely leave any permanent disability. Fractures of the acromion, the neck, the glenoid, and the coracoid practically always unite and cause little trouble. Rare and atypical cases of body or glenoid fracture may require operation.

BIBLIOGRAPHY

Bonnin, J. G.: Spontaneous subluxation of the sternoclavicular joint. Brit. Med. J., *2*:274, 1960.

Coleman, F. P., and Coleman, C. L.: Fracture of ribs—a logical treatment. Surg., Gynec. Obstet., *90*:129, 1950.

Danto, J. L.: Preliminary studies of the effect of hydrocortisone on hidradenitis suppurativa. J. Invest. Derm., *31*:295, 1958.

Geckeler, E. O.: Fractures of the clavicle in adults. Am. J. Surg., *81*:333, 1951.

Horn, J. S.: The traumatic anatomy and treatment of acute acromioclavicular dislocation. J. Bone Joint Surg., *36B*: 194, 1954.

Howard, F. M., and Shafer, S. J.: Injuries to the clavicle with neurovascular complications. J. Bone Joint Surg., *47A*:1335, 1965.

Hurley, H. J., and Shelley, W. B.: Disorders of the apocrine sweat glands: diagnosis and treatment. American Practioner, *11*:101, 1960.

Murray, G.: A method of fixation for fracture of the clavicle. J. Bone Joint Surg., *22*:616, 1940.

Neviaser, J. S.: The treatment of fractures of the clavicle. Surg. Clin. N. Am., *43*:1555, 1963.

Panel-Instructional Course, Lecture of the American Academy of Orthopedic Surgeons: Treatment of complete acromioclavicular dislocations. J. Bone Joint Surg., *44A*:1008, 1962.

Quigley, T. B.: Injuries to the acromioclavicular and sternoclavicular joints sustained in athletics. Surg. Clin. N. Am. *43*:1551, 1963.

Sage, F. P., and Salvatore, J. E.: Injuries of the acromioclavicular joint: a study of results in 96 patients. Southern Med. J., *56*:486, 1963.

Shelley, W. B., and Cahn, M.: The pathogenesis of hidradenitis suppurativa in man. Arch. Derm. Syph., *72*:562, 1955.

Stein, A. J., Jr.: Retrosternal dislocation of the clavicle. J. Bone Joint Surg., *39A*:656, 1957.

23

Upper Limb

Part I—Soft Tissues

Mark W. Wolcott, M.D.

BENIGN TUMORS

The forearm and, especially, the upper arm are not unusual sites of benign tumors. These vary from simple skin blemishes, such as pigmented moles, which usually are hairy and often occur round the forearm and the elbow, to large lipomas and fibromas (Fig. 23-1).

Treatment. Most of these tumors may be removed easily under local anesthesia through an elliptical incision. Primary suture of the wound and a pressure bandage of elastic adhesive are sufficient to give an excellent result. As a rule, splinting is not necessary following these operations because adequate pressure and immobilization can be obtained by means of the bandage.

In the removal of larger skin defects, such as scars or tattoo marks, the method employed by Davis is of value. In such cases, instead of removing the entire lesion in one step, an elliptical excision is made from the center of the lesion, and the skin edges are approximated. After healing and stretching of the approximated skin has occurred, a second similar operation is performed, the scar previously made and and another elliptical portion of the remaining blemish being

excised. Two or three operations are necessary for complete removal of the lesion. In the end, a single linear scar is left, and a considerable area of the skin may be removed without the necessity of grafting. However, it is quite possible in many such cases to excise the entire skin area and apply a primary skin graft. This operation may be performed easily under local anesthesia in the ambulatory patient.

LESIONS OF THE OLECRANON BURSA

OLECRANON BURSITIS (MINER'S ELBOW)

Etiology. The olecranon bursa overlies the olecranon and is one of the subcutaneous bursae most frequently involved. It develops between the skin and the bony prominence of the olecranon in response to friction. If friction and trauma continue for a long time, a chronic inflammatory change takes place in the bursa, with the result that it becomes thickened and rubbery. Trauma may result in a secretion of fluid in the bursa, with the formation of a tense swelling under the skin over the point of the elbow. If acute trauma has occurred, there

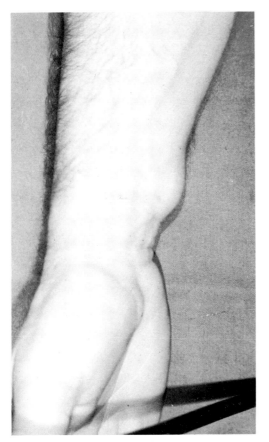

Fig. 23–1. Neurofibroma of forearm, removed under local anesthesia in ambulatory patient.

is definite tenderness and the swelling may be painful, whereas usually in the chronic cases it is painless.

Treatment. In younger persons, it is often possible to aspirate the bursa and apply a firm elastic pressure dressing and an elbow splint. Usually, a rubber sponge applied with a firm bandage is adequate. In such cases, formation of the effusion may not recur, but if it does, it will recur in slight amounts only.

In older individuals, when the bursa has definitely thickened, the swelling usually is not painful, and on palpation small hard movable bodies within the bursa may be noted. These often are mistaken for chips of bone, especially if there is a history of previous injury, but really they are fibrous villi or bands that extend across the bursa. Pressure upon these fibrous projections gives acute pain.

In chronic olecranon bursitis, subcutaneous incision of the bursal walls under local anesthesia has proven to be very successful. If one cuts the fibrous supports, thus separating the roof from the floor, the bursa is obliterated completely, and it disappears (Fig. 23-2). This is an ambulatory procedure.

In some cases of olecranon bursitis of the chronic type, excision of the bursa is carried out. The operation may be performed easily under local anesthesia. The patient lies on the table with the arm across the chest. An elliptical incision is so made that the scar will not lie over the tip of the elbow. The bursa is found to be a tense structure that is separated easily from the overlying skin but is densely adherent to the fibrous tissue over the olecranon. When the bursa is opened, a yellowish fluid escapes, and usually the fibrous villi and the bands that extend into the lumen of the bursal cavity may be seen. Care must be taken to obtain good hemostasis, after which the skin flap is sutured in place, and a pressure dressing is applied. When hemostasis is not absolute, it is wise to insert a small rubber tissue drain for 24 hours. Usually, an internal right-angled splint is used for 2 or 3 days. Skin sutures are removed at the end of a week or 10 days, at which time normal function is resumed almost at once.

The treatment of chronic olecranon bursitis by the injection of sclerosing solutions has not proven to be too successful in our hands. Other bursae, such as the prepatellar, frequently respond very well to injection, but usually the olecranon bursa continues to secret fluid, and the swelling does not subside.

SUPPURATIVE OLECRANON BURSITIS

Occasionally, the olecranon bursa becomes the site of a secondary infection following a furunculosis over the tip of the elbow. In such cases, the bursa becomes distended and tender.

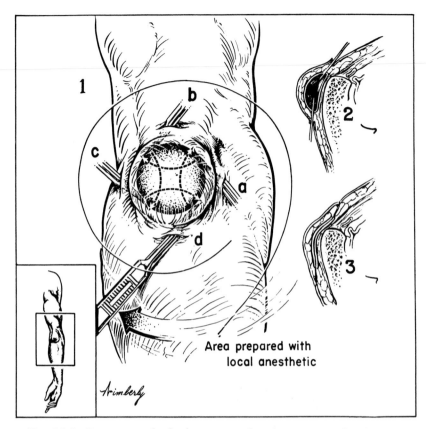

Fig. 23–2. Burgess method of treatment for chronic superficial bursitis. After infiltration round and at the edge of the bursa, a pointed knife is inserted at each of 4 puncture sites and swept round in an arc to separate the roof from the floor of the bursa. Very slight bleeding can be controlled by a pressure dressing. The bursa becomes obliterated by the formation of a scar as the roof and the floor of the bursa grow together.

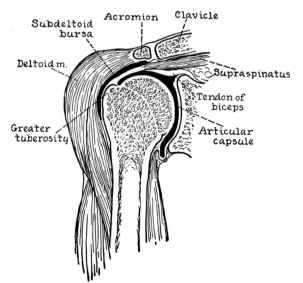

Fig. 23–3. Diagrammatic longitudinal section of the shoulder area, showing the relation of the subacromial bursa to the deltoid muscle, the greater tuberosity, the supraspinatus tendon, and the acromion.

Treatment. Conservative therapy, consisting of antibiotics, hot wet dressings, and splinting, may be tried; however, as a rule, incision and drainage of the bursa are necessary. Following simple incision, the bursa usually becomes obliterated, and the wound heals. There may be a few cases in which healing will be incomplete because of the large amount of chronic fibrous tissue in the bursa wall. At the base of the wound, there is a chronic granulating area that refuses to heal, and excision of this area is necessary to obtain rapid healing.

LESIONS OF THE SUBACROMIAL, OR SUBDELTOID, BURSA

As the arm is elevated, the greater tuberosity of the humerus slides beneath the acromion. This requires a smoothly functioning subacromial bursa (Fig. 23-3). Any lesion of the structures that form the floor or the roof of the bursa may cause a disturbance of motion associated with pain. These lesions fall into two main groups: those that are traumatic and post-traumatic and those that are nontraumatic and degenerative.

TRAUMATIC AND POST-TRAUMATIC LESIONS

Acute Traumatic Subacromial Bursitis

Etiology. Whenever a thrust is made by the hand or the forearm, the force is transmitted to the area of the subacromial bursa. The coraco-acromial arch prevents upward dislocation of the head of the humerus, so that a fall on the hand or the forearm may cause contusion of the bursal surfaces with slight, or even severe, bursitis. Injury to the bursa occurs also in all dislocations at the shoulder and in fractures of the upper humerus. This fact is often overlooked in dealing with the more evident bony lesions, but it is a factor in the disability produced by these injuries. In young individuals, the bursitis results in little or no final disability,

but in the elderly, if the bursal lesion is neglected, it may cause persistent trouble.

Acute traumatic bursitis with severe pain also may follow a fall in which the point of the shoulder impinges forcibly on a hard object, or it may be secondary to a tear of the supraspinatus tendor or a fracture of the greater tuberosity, both of which underlie the floor of the bursa.

Diagnosis. The patient complains of severe shoulder pain and declines to move the arm, holding it rigidly at the side. Even passive motion causes severe pain. The arm may be elevated passively through 30° to 60°, but close inspection reveals this motion to occur by rotation of the scapula on the chest rather than at the scapulohumeral joint. Reflex muscle spasm in acute bursitis may be so great that abduction is almost impossible, simulating partial or complete tear of the supraspinatus tendon. Palpable swelling and fluctuation may be present, but always there is acute diffuse tenderness just below, and anterior to, the acromion.

The diagnosis of simple acute traumatic subacromial bursitis may be made only when dislocations and fractures of the head of the humerus and tears of the short rotator tendons have been excluded, since injuries to these structures may be manifested by an acute bursitis if by no other signs. Therefore, x-ray examination is usually necessary.

Treatment. Injury to the bursal surfaces is important because of its sequelae. If the arm is held at the side for a sufficient length of time, dense adhesions form between the opposed surfaces and limit humeroscapular motion. In addition, muscle atrophy occurs rapidly with disuse. During the first 24 to 48 hours after injury, treatment is aimed at relieving the pain and at obtaining rapid subsidence of the acute reaction to trauma. If fluctuation is present, the bursa is aspirated, and from 5 to 10 ml. of 1 percent procaine is injected, often with 25-50 mg. of hydrocortisone. Immediate relief of pain and spasm follows, and the diagnosis of laceration of the rotator cuff tendons may be made if elevation of the arm cannot be initiated or is very weak. The shoulder is immobilized in partial abduction; a thick

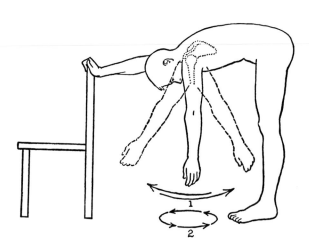

Fig. 23–4. Relaxed circumduction exercises for shoulder lesions (after Codman). The patient bends forward, grasping a chair with the hand of the sound arm; the painful arm falls forward of its own weight to become perpendicular to the floor. In this position, the patient is asked to swing the arm forward and backward gently, raising it as far as possible up toward the head. In addition, circular motions should be performed, carrying the arm in an arc forward and backward. Often it is advisable to have the patient hold something in his hand during this exercise. The old-fashioned flatiron is a good substitute for a dumbbell for this purpose.

axillary pad is used to obtain abduction, and a sling and a swathe are applied to relieve the tension of the shoulder muscles. If adhesions form, these will separate when the arm is brought to the side later. Ice bags are advised during the first 24 to 48 hours, and sedatives are given if necessary.

After 3 to 5 days, when the acute symptoms have subsided, relaxed circumduction exercises (Fig. 23-4) are begun to avoid adhesions and stiffness. They should be performed for from 2 to 5 minutes, 4 times daily. Heat and gentle massage twice daily are helpful at this time. Recovery often is complete in from 7 to 14 days.

Post-traumatic Adhesions in the Subacromial Bursa

Etiology. It has been indicated that this condition may follow simple acute bursitis as well as the acute bursitis associated with dislocations, fractures, and tendon injuries. It is due to neglect of early motion of the shoulder.

In addition, any injury to the shoulder, even without bursal injury, that causes pain on motion and keeps the arm at the side without exercise for a few weeks may be complicated by bursal adhesions. This is particularly likely to occur in elderly patients who have had prior attritional changes, that is, a fraying out of the rotator cuff and the biceps tendons.

Diagnosis. After a few weeks, the clinical picture of bursitis with adhesions may be superimposed on the picture of the acute lesions described above. It is obvious that accurate diagnosis becomes extremely difficult. The well-advanced clinical picture of post-traumatic bursitis with adhesions is typical. The pain of injury subsides after a week or two and is replaced by ill-defined pain over the shoulder that radiates to the insertion of the deltoid, to the elbow, or to the wrist and the fingers and becomes progressively more severe.

Usually, examination discloses atrophy of the supraspinatus, the deltoid, and the arm muscles, often associated with vasospastic phenomena, such as coldness and stiffness of the hand and a glossy, atrophic skin. The bursal area is quite tender. Active elevation of the arm is limited strikingly and is painful. If the scapula is prevented from rotating, the patient may be able to abduct the arm only from 10° to 30°. This is the characteristic physical sign of this condition. Internal and external rotation also become restricted greatly.

Treatment. Treatment is directed toward separating the adhesions and re-

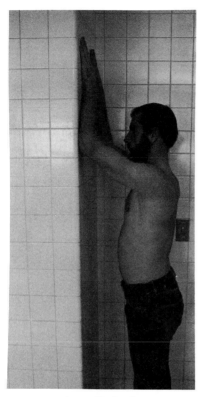

Fig. 23–5. Wall-climbing exercise. Note position of forearms close to body and position of body 4 to 6 inches from the wall. One "crawls up the wall" with his fingers to the highest point he can reach. The arms are not allowed to drop; instead, the patient "crawls back down" once he has "climbed up."

storing normal motion. Until this is accomplished, no permanent relief of pain is to be expected.

When the symptoms are mild and motion is restricted only moderately, relaxed circumduction (Fig. 23-4) and wall-climbing exercises (Fig. 23-5) are prescribed for 10 minutes, 3 to 5 times daily. The patient is advised to use the arm as much as possible and to sleep with the arm above the head. Adequate doses of salicylates and barbiturates should be given at first.

If improvement is not marked and continuous with this form of conservative therapy, cortisone may be given. Usually, 3 oral doses of 25 mg. each are given daily for a week. As a rule, decreased pain and increased motion in the shoulder become apparent in from 2 to 3 days. Depending on the improvement noted, cortisone may be continued in the above dosage or reduced to 50 mg. daily in 3 to 4 divided doses. Exercises and salicylates should be continued. Cortisone is gradually reduced and stopped when the pain has disappeared and shoulder motion has returned to normal. Cortisone should not be continued past 3 to 4 weeks, whether the problem subsides or not.

Local injections of hydrocortisone acetate also have been used in the treatment of the post-traumatic form of bursitis. The results are less dramatic than those obtained in acute bursitis. Usually, from 25 to 50 mg. of hydrocortisone is injected after the area has been infiltrated with 1 percent procaine. The injection may be repeated in from 3 to 5 days.

NONTRAUMATIC AND DEGENERATIVE LESIONS

Calcareous Tendinitis of the Rotator Cuff Muscles

Calcareous deposits form frequently in the supraspinatus tendon close to the greater tuberosity. Less frequently, such deposits may be found in the subscapularis and the infraspinatus tendons.

Etiology. The cause of this condition is not known, but it appears to be due to some local disturbance, possibly of the blood supply, rather than to any toxic or infectious cause. There may be some relationship between this condition and the calcification seen in ischemic or necrotic areas. Injection studies of the vascular supply of the rotator cuff of the shoulder fail to confirm the theory of reduced blood supply as the cause of the calcification and degenerative lesions of the rotator cuff.

In the acute forms of the condition, the symptoms appear to be due to an increase in local tension about the area of calcification, possibly because of an inflammatory reaction excited by the calcareous material. Usually, the area of calcification is large and soft, and it lies well out over

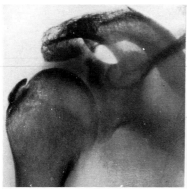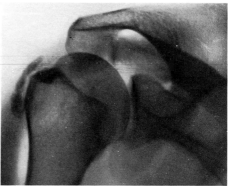

Fig. 23–6. Roentgenograms of two patients showing large deposits of calcareous material over the greater tuberosity. Both patients were operated upon under local anesthesia, and the calcareous deposits were drained by incision. (Ferguson, L. K.: Ann. Surg., *105*:243, 1937)

the greater tuberosity (Fig. 23-6). To relieve the tension relieves the symptoms.

In the milder forms, the symptoms are due to the mechanical effect of the calcareous material. When the calcification is present in the supraspinatus tendon and causes some roughening of the floor of the subacromial bursa, there is an irregularity in the rhythm of elevation accompanied by discomfort. When the deposit so lies in the substance of the tendon that it causes no roughening of the floor of the bursa, it may cause no symptoms whatever. Most often these deposits are chalky hard and are found to lie above the head of the humerus in the roentgen film.

Symptoms and Findings. The calcareous deposits may cause acute or mild symptoms, or they may not cause any symptoms whatever. Roentgen films taken with the arm in internal and external rotation help to locate the site and to determine the type of calcium deposit.

Acute Form. Following insignificant trauma or without obvious cause, the patient begins to have pain in the shoulder that is localized over the bulge of the deltoid and occasionally radiates down the arm. The pain grows worse rapidly, and in a few days it may be agonizing. Motion at the shoulder intensifies the pain, and this forces the patient to hold

the arm rigid at the side. On examination, there may be visible swelling over the subacromial bursa. Intense spasm of the muscles of the shoulder prevents passive motion, and the intense pain permits little or no active motion. On palpation, acute agonizing tenderness is found over the greater tuberosity when the calcification is in the supraspinatus tendon, or a little in front of or behind the tuberosity when the other tendons are involved. When the history of some injury has been given, it is important for the purpose of differential diagnosis to establish the violence and the character of the injury. In most cases, it will become apparent that the injury to which the condition is attributed has not been violent enough to cause laceration of the rotator cuff tendons or fracture of the greater tuberosity, the two conditions which may simulate acute calcareous tendinitis most closely.

Mild Form. The patient becomes aware of some vague discomfort in the shoulder that becomes more annoying after several weeks. Usually, the pain is localized over the deltoid, and it may radiate down the arm. It is apt to be brought on by full elevation of the arm. In these cases, the calcareous deposit lies just beneath the floor of the bursa and impinges against the edge of the acromion when the arm is abducted. As a rule, the symptoms do not

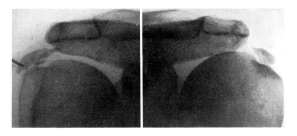

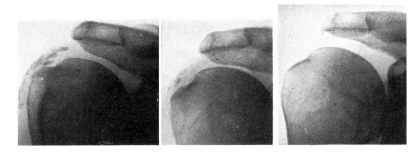

Fig. 23–7. (*A*) Roentgenogram of right shoulder with needle in center of the deposit before infiltration therapy. Note the presence of a deposit also over the left shoulder (*B*) Which was completely symptom free at that time. (*C*) Roentgenogram of right shoulder 5 days after infiltration therapy. Note fragmentation and spreading of the deposit over a much larger area and beginning of absorption. (*D*) Roentgenogram of right shoulder 4 months after infiltration therapy. Note practically complete disappearance of the deposit. (*E*) Roentgenogram of right shoulder 1 1/2 years after infiltration therapy. Note complete disappearance of the deposit on the right side. Roentgenogram of the left shoulder taken at the same time showed the same findings as in *B*. (Lapidus, P. W.: Surg., Gynec. Obstet., *76*:715, 1943)

vary much for the better or the worse if the patient is watched for a few weeks, although ultimately, if the arm is used constantly, the symptoms will disappear. Failure to use the arm may result in adhesions between the bursal surfaces; the result may be, in addition to mild calcareous tendinitis, distubances incidental to bursal adhesions.

In the uncomplicated form, on examination there usually is little visible or palpable change in the shoulder. A tender spot may be found proximal to the greater tuberosity. The patient can lift the arm through its full range of motion, but he has some difficulty in doing so and shows a disturbed rhythm of elevation accompanied by pain.

Asymptomatic Form. Occasionally, in a patient who has symptoms in one shoulder, roentgenograms are made of both shoulders for comparison, and calcareous deposits are seen in both, although only one is painful (Fig. 23-7). This brings out two points: first, that the simple presence of a calcareous deposit does not in itself cause symptoms and, second, that the symptoms are due either to inflammatory reaction about the deposit or to some mechanical interference with shoulder motion at the subacromial bursa.

Treatment. In the acute form, the symptoms are often so severe that relief is required urgently. Several methods of therapy may be used. If one believes that the acute pain is due to an inflammatory reaction around the calcium deposit in the supraspinatus tendon, it is logical to assume that relief of tissue tension will cause relief of pain. This may be accomplished by needling or incising the calcareous deposit. If needling is to be tried, a skin wheal is made with procaine over the point of maximum tenderness. The subcutaneous tissues are infiltrated, and a large-bore, 16-to gauge needle is directed into the calcified area. The area is infiltrated with from 5 to 10 ml. of 1 percent procaine solution. Without withdrawing the needle from the skin, several punctures of the calcified area are made, and each time, a small amount of procaine solution is injected. Even better than this is the introduction of a second needle into the calcified area. One percent procaine solution is injected through the first needle, and very often it can be seen running out of the second needle, carrying flakes of calcareous material with it. The calcareous material does not need to be removed completely. In most instances, it is sufficient to remove enough to relieve tension around the calcareous deposit and to allow the rest to disperse into the tissues, from which it is absorbed rapidly (Fig. 23-7, *E*). If the calcified area has been punctured and some of the calcareous material escapes into the bursa or is aspirated through the needle, almost immediate relief of pain is obtained. The residual soreness due to the trauma of the needling can be relieved by appropriate sedation for 1 or 2 days.

If the needle cannot be introduced into the calcareous area and if the symptoms are very severe, dramatic relief may be obtained by operation. Under local anesthesia, an incision is made downward from the anterior margin of the acromion for a distance of from 1 to 2 inches. The fibers of the deltoid are split, and the roof of the subacromial bursa is picked up with hemostats and incised. With the elbow flexed to a right angle, the arm is rotated very gently by an assistant, and the floor of the bursa is examined. A zone of hyperemia with a central yellowish area will come into view. Often this hyperemia is about 1 cm. in diameter. An incision is made into this area in the direction of the fibers of the supraspinatus tendon, and immediately a mass of pasty yellowish-white material is extruded. The symptoms usually are relieved immediately, and they may disappear entirely within 24 hours. No attempt is made to close the roof of the bursa. The deltoid fibers are approximated with 2 or 3 sutures of plain catgut, and the skin is closed with sutures or clips. If discomfort is considerable and there is a disinclination to use the arm, a thick axillary pad should be applied to maintain a slight degree of abduction. Active motion should be started as soon as it can be tolerated by the patient. Relaxed circumduction exercises may be used initially.

In rare instances, the calcareous deposit may rupture spontaneously into the subdeltoid bursa (Fig. 23-8). When this occurs, almost immediate relief of pain and early resumption of normal function occur.

Roentgen therapy may be employed and gives the best results when the symptoms are severe. It may be used also in females who object to having scars about the shoulder and in patients who dread operation. In many instances, there will be considerable relief after 1 or 2 treatments. If there is no relief after treatments on 2 successive days, it is unlikely that further roentgen therapy will be beneficial, and this method of treatment should be abandoned and one of the other forms of treatment tried. It has been the author's experience that at times roentgen therapy gives surprising relief of pain in acute "bursitis" after a single treatment, but that less dramatic results are obtained in the subacute types of bursitis.

The most recent, and often successful, method of treatment of acute subdeltoid bursitis is the local injection of hydrocortisone. It is not known how this acts, but it is presumed to bring about a decrease in inflammation in the calcareous area. The injection of hydrocortisone gives the best results when there is a localized area of pain and tenderness. The injection is made into this area, but there is probably some "spreading" of the effect.

The injection may be carried out as an

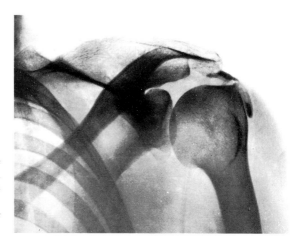

Fig. 23–8. Large area of calcification with spontaneous rupture into the bursa; the patient had spontaneous relief of the agonizing pain from which he had been suffering. —he calcified material that has escaped into the bursal sac may be seen outlining the lower portion of the sac over the greater tuberosity.

office procedure. A search with the examining finger easily identifies the most tender area, and the skin over this area is marked with a pencil. After the skin preparation with alcohol, the skin, the subcutaneous tissues, and the muscle are infiltrated with 1 percent procaine. Then, with a syringe and an 18-gauge needle, hydrocortisone, 0.5 to 1.0 ml. (12.5 to 25 mg.), is injected into the painful area. The needle should be advanced slowly until it impinges upon a firm structure (the supraspinatus tendon), then withdrawn slightly and the injection made.

The results of hydrocortisone injections in the acute type of bursitis have been dramatic. Usually, there is an increase in pain or soreness during the first 24 hours after injection, and, thereafter, complete relief of pain and resumption of normal function. The patient should be provided with sedation for use during the first day and night after the injection. If complete relief of pain has not been obtained, the injection may be repeated in amounts of up to 2 ml. in from 3 to 5 days.

In the mild form, in which symptoms consist mainly of some discomfort during shoulder motion, no radical form of treatment is indicated. Procaine injection is of benefit, but operation seldom gives any considerable relief. Roentgen therapy may be tried. Hydrocortisone injections give results that are less striking than those obtained when they are used for acute bursitis, but they may give partial relief of pain and discomfort. For the majority of cases, it is advisable to have the patient continue active use of the arm, to prescribe heat and massage at home, and to assure the patient that the symptoms will subside after a certain length of time.

In the asymptomatic form, no treatment is indicated.

Bursal Lesions Due to Wear

After many years of use, the shoulder may exhibit evidence of wear. The ordinarily smooth surface of the supraspinatus tendon shows fibrillations and possibly minute tears, and the floor of the subacromial bursa becomes roughened. The tendon of the long head of the biceps may undergo similar changes, which may be accompanied by mild symptoms. However, if active use of the arm continues, the patients rarely complain of more than occasional slight discomfort or stiffness. If the arm is immobilized for any reason, the roughened bursal surfaces may become adherent and produce pain on motion. Because of the pain, motion is limited, and the adhesions grow more dense; thus, lesions due to wear are especially important as etiologic factors in subacromial bursitis with adhesions.

Bony Excrescences, Villi, and Bands in the Bursa

Symptoms. Chronic bursitis also occurs without adhesions. There is a gradual onset of mild pain at the shoulder; this is brought on by motion and disappears when the arm is at rest. The total range of motion is impaired very little, if at all; motion at the shoulder, however, may exhibit a definite change in rhythm. Examination often discloses nothing but mild tenderness over the subacromial bursa. The patient may twist and turn his arm uncomfortably during the process of elevating it, although the total range of motion may be good.

Etiology. Roentgen examination of such shoulders may show no abnormalities, or a tiny bony excrescence may be visible at the lateral margin of the acromion or on the upper surface of the greater tuberosity. When such excrescences are present, the pain occurs usually when the greater tuberosity is about to slide beneath the acromion. When the roentgenogram is negative, the discomfort may be due to thickened folds of bursal lining or to the formation of villi in the bursa. These cause some mechanical irritation of the bursa and interfere to a variable extent with motion.

Treatment. If symptoms are mild and not progressive, no treatment other than gentle home physiotherapy is indicated. On the other hand, if symptoms are progressive and troublesome, it is advisable to perform an exploratory operation on the bursa and remove any bony excrescences, villi, and bands that may be present.

FROZEN SHOULDER

Frozen shoulder is a term loosely applied to shoulder conditions of uncertain etiology and characterized by pain, atrophy, and limited mobility, and patients often are given this diagnosis by exclusion. The condition is usually seen in the fourth to sixth decades of life, and often it is associated with radiation of pain to the arm and the fingers. Roentgen examination is negative except for evidence of bone atrophy in the upper humerus.

In many of these cases Neviaser found the condition to be an adhesive capsulitis between the head of the humerus and the capsule of the shoulder joint. Tenderness may be present over the bicipital groove, and this had led Lippmann and DePalma to believe that in many of these cases the condition is really due to a tenosynovitis of the tendon of the long head of the biceps. In other cases, myalgic trigger points may be found in the muscles of the shoulder girdle. Travell, Rinzler, and Herman found these areas most often in the serratus posterior superior and in the infraspinatus. They were identified by applying pressure to produce pain in the reference zones in the arm, the forearm, and the hand. These authors were able to relieve the pain and disability by injection of the trigger points with procaine solution.

In our experience, most patients have responded eventually to repeated procaine infiltration along the anterior part of the bursa and the bicipital groove and of any other tender spots that can be demonstrated. This must be coupled with persistent attention to the shoulder exercises by the patient. He should be assured that recovery will take place eventually if the prescribed exercises are carried out faithfully. These exercises are those prescribed for the patient with subdeltoid bursitis and consist of wall-climbing and rotary motion of the dependent arms. Low-intensity diathermy, hot towels, or infrared lamps are types of heat that are helpful. Light stroking massage helps to produce relaxation of tense muscles. Russek believes that muscle spasm is one of the primary factors in the pain mechanisms of the shoulder. If progress is slow, or if it ceases, manipulation under general anesthesia may be performed, followed by exercises and procaine injections as before. This condition often is a test of the patience of both physician and patient, but persistence in treatment usually will be rewarded by a full recovery.

If motion does not increase and pain is not reduced by a week's trial of physical therapy as described, cortisone may be added. Coventry usually gives 3 oral doses of 25 mg. of cortisone daily. This dosage is continued for a week, or even longer, up to 3 to 4 weeks. If the response is good, the dosage may be reduced to 50 mg. daily in divided doses and gradually reduced or discontinued as the improvement warrants. Coventry believes cortisone to be a most valuable adjunct to the treatment of frozen shoulder.

One should be aware of the complications that may follow cortisone therapy. Usually, prolonged administration of the drug is not recommended.

THORACIC OUTLET SYNDROME

A syndrome that until fairly recently was called scalenus anticus syndrome, cervical rib syndrome, hyperabduction syndrome, and several other terms, has now been clarified and is more properly called thoracic outlet syndrome. The problem in all shoulder girdle compression syndromes is compression of the brachial plexus and of the subclavian artery and vein, usually by the clavicle and the first rib.

Etiology. The first rib is unique in several ways. Its superior surface is nearly flat. The subclavian artery and vein and the inferior trunk of the brachial plexus cross this rib, separated by the anterior scalene muscle. The clavicle directly overlies the first rib. There are several forces tending to pinch the clavicle and first rib together. The scalenus anticus, the scalenus medius, and the levatores costarum muscles tend to lift the first rib toward the clavicle. Several congenital anomalies of the ribs tend to lead to development of the thoracic outlet syndrome. A cervical rib, which occurs in about 1 percent of the population and is bilateral in 80 percent of the cases, is the most common of these. When the first rib is abnormal and does not reach the sternum but rather fuses with the second rib, one is quite likely to develop a thoracic outlet syndrome.

Symptoms. The symptoms vary depending on the structure or structures compressed—vein, artery, or nerve. Compression of the nerve gives pain, numbness, tingling, and loss of strength in the fingers and hand. The ulnar distribution is by far the most common. The symptoms of arterial insufficiency are diffuse pain, numbness, pallor, coolness, and sensitivity to cold; these are all aggravated by elevation of the arm. Symptoms often occur when the patient sleeps, especially if he sleeps on his back or with his arm behind his head. Venous compression gives aching, swelling, and bluish discoloration of the upper extremity.

Contributory factors are often seen. The position of the shoulder girdle is relatively high in infants and children, and it gradually descends to the adult position. In females and in the aged, the descent is greatest, so that the shoulders droop considerably. An occupation factor sometimes is present. The patient works as a typist or as a housewife and has the pain while the arms are down at the sides; it subsides on rest and elevation of the arm.

About half of the patients give a history of injury, with pain beginning immediately or after a lapse of a few hours. The other half give no history of injury, the pain being mild at first and increasing gradually in severity. The location and the distribution of the pain vary. Most commonly, it is over the shoulder and the upper arm, with radiation to the neck or the scapula, or down the arm to the elbow, the wrist, or the fingers. In some instances, the pain may be mainly over the shoulder, the scapula, and the axilla; in others, it is most severe over the arm and the elbow and radiates down the ulnar side of the forearm and the hand. The character of the pain varies from case to case. It may be dull, aching, and twisting; sharp or burning; or combinations of these types. It often increases with work, such as typing or sweeping, and subsides when the arm is raised and rested. Very often, the pain is much worse at night.

Signs. These may be divided into vascular and neurologic and may be best elicited by 90° abduction and external rotation of the arm without shoulder elevation. In this position, the clavicle swings posteriorly from its fixed point of attachment at the sternoclavicular joint, creating a scissorlike entrapment of the plexus and the subclavian vessels against the first rib. The neurologic signs are reproduced by compression with the thumb in the supraclavicular fossa over the subclavian artery and the brachial plexus. Pinprick hyperesthesia in the hand, most commonly in the C_8-T_1, or ulnar, dermatome, weakness of the interosseous muscles of the hand supplied by this nerve, and, sometimes, weakness of the biceps and the triceps muscles are frequent neurologic signs. The ulnar distribution is so common since the ulnar nerve is formed from the C_8-T_1 cervical roots, which join to form the lowest cord of the brachial plexus; this lies on the first rib, where it may be readily compressed by the bony scissors formed by the clavicle and the rib.

Diagnosis. The diagnostic signs are: (1) pain in part or all of the brachial distribution; (2) absence of a local cause of pain, such as a muscular or a bursal lesion; (3) tenderness over the scalenus anticus muscle just behind the lateral edge of the sternocleidomastoid; (4) vascular disturbances; (5) muscle atrophy; and (6) temporary relief of pain by infiltrating the scalenus anticus muscle with 10 ml. of 1 percent procaine. This last is a most valuable and constant finding. The absence of signs 3, 4, and 5 does not exclude the diagnosis.

Recently Urschel has developed more objective tests for demonstrating the thoracic outlet syndrome; these are especially valuable for assessing the severity of the syndrome and, therefore, the type of treatment. They are based on measuring the velocity of nerve conduction over the ulnar nerve at three points on the arm. When conduction is only moderately prolonged, conservative management, by the use of exercises, often will suffice. When it is prolonged past 70 milliseconds, surgery with removal of the first rib is usually successful.

Usually, there is striking relief of pain, partial or complete, within 5 to 10 minutes if pain was present immediately prior to injection. Often this is accompanied by increased mobility of the arm and the shoulder. In many instances, a Horner's syndrome (drooping eyelid,

enophthalmos, constricted pupil, dilated subconjunctival vessels, and lacrimation) appears on the affected side, indicating anesthesia of the cervical sympathetic fibers. This lasts from 30 to 60 minutes.

It is important to exclude subacromial bursitis with adhesions and calcification in the supraspinatus tendon, since this may induce thoracic outlet syndrome that is relieved temporarily by injection. Cervical rib as a cause of thoracic outlet syndrome can be excluded only by roentgen examination, since it is also likely to be relieved temporarily by injection. Marked hypertrophic changes in the cervical vertebrae, with narrowing of the intervertebral foramina through which the cervical nerves make their exit, can cause typical pain in the brachial distribution. In this condition, injection gives no relief, and oblique views of the cervical spine show the narrowed foramina.

Treatment. In very mild forms of the thoracic outlet syndrome, benefit is obtained through rest, correction of faulty posture, and exercise of the muscles of the shoulder girdle. The diagnostic procaine injection often gives relief for many hours or days, and in these instances repeated procaine injections, from 10 to 20 ml. each, may be of great value.

In the past, division of the scalenus anticus muscle was considered all that was necessary for those cases not responding to exercise and posture correction. The results, however, were not predictable, and today most authorities favor removal of the first rib by an anterior approach, a transaxillary approach, or a posterior approach. If a cervical rib is present, the posterior approach is necessary. Hospitalization for a few days is necessary for any of these operations.

LESIONS OF THE MUSCLES AND THE TENDONS

Acute Traumatic Myositis And Tendinitis

Etiology. Acute traumatic myositis and tendinitis occur quite commonly about the shoulder as a result of falls or twisting injuries that suddenly overstretch one or more muscles. Direct violence also may cause traumatic myositis, in which case the lesion is essentially a contusion. The exact pathology present in a suddenly overstretched muscle is not always clear; there may be actual lacerations of some muscle or tendon fibers, but it is quite possible that these lesions are essentially functional and are analogous to sprains of ligaments.

Symptoms. Immediately after the injury or within a few hours of it, there is an onset of pain over the muscles involved. This pain may be mild or severe. The patient tends to carry his shoulder in a position that allows the affected muscle to be relaxed.

Diagnosis. The pain is well localized over the affected muscle, which is spastic and tender. There may be swelling of the muscle. Active motion is painful and restricted in the direction that stretches the muscle. Thus, involvement of the trapezius muscle will result in pain on raising the shoulder actively and on passive depression of the shoulder or on flexing the neck to the opposite side. Involvement of the rhomboid muscles, which attach the scapula to the spinous processes of the upper thoracic vertebrae, causes pain when the patient pulls his shoulders backward and "throws out" his chest; also when the arm is elevated actively. Involvement of the deltoid muscle also gives pain on elevation of the arm. In each instance, the localization of the pain and the tenderness indicates the particular muscle involved. The pectoralis major and the biceps and the triceps muscle bellies are seldom affected. The tendon of the biceps, however, is often the site of an acute traumatic tendinitis. In this condition, there are pain and tenderness well localized over the bicipital groove at the anterior aspect of the shoulder, and aggravation is likely when the patient attempts to flex the forearm against resistance while raising the arm.

We have seen instances in which there apparently had been an active traumatic myositis of the scalenus anticus muscle, as judged from localized tenderness over the muscle and from pain on stretching the muscle, which can be done by rotating the head to the same side and hyperextending the neck. In these cases, there may be pain over the side of the neck and the top of the shoulder that radiates to the insertion of the deltoid or down the arm. This pain indicates some irritation of the brachial plexus, which lies immediately beneath the muscle.

Treatment. The general principles governing the treatment of any traumatic lesions apply to myositis and tendinitis. Rest, immobilization, and application of cold during the first 24 to 48 hours after the injury usually are very helpful. The immobilization dressing must be made according to the needs of the patient. Usually, an adhesive strapping can be applied in such a manner that the origin and the insertion of the muscle involved can be drawn toward each other. This aids relaxation of the muscle, prevents it from being overstretched, and relieves the pain to a considerable extent.

When the acute symptoms subside, home physiotherapy in the form of an electric pad or a hot-water bottle applied to the painful area for from 15 to 20 minutes, 3 times daily, followed by gentle massage with a 10 percent methyl salicylate ointment is prescribed. Active use should be started as soon as the acute symptoms subside; otherwise, there are likely to be fibrosis and contracture of the involved muscles that result in loss of function.

We have had many satisfactory results from repeated infiltrations of such injured muscles with a 0.5 or 1.0 percent solution of a local anesthetic. The local anesthetic solution should contain no vasoconstrictor drug, and it should be given liberally, from 10 to 50 ml., as required. Active exercise of the part may start immediately. The infiltration may be repeated several times if necessary. Tendinitis of the long head of the biceps often responds very well to infiltration. The tissues above the bicipital groove should be well distended with solution.

RUPTURE OF THE SUPRASPINATUS TENDON

The supraspinatus muscle originates from the supraspinous fossa of the scapula and passes beneath the acromion to

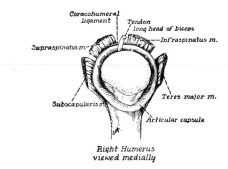

Fig. 23–9. Musculotendinous cuff about the neck of the humerus.

insert into the greater tuberosity of the humerus. Its function is to help initiate elevation of the arm and, with the other rotator cuff muscles, to hold the head of the humerus against the glenoid. The tendon of the supraspinatus fuses with the other tendons of the rotator cuff muscles (Fig. 23-9) to form a cuff that inserts into the sulcus at the outer margin of the articular surface of the humerus. This cuff forms part of the floor of the subacromial bursa. The rotator cuff muscles serve to hold the head of the humerus against the glenoid as well as to rotate the arm. The fused tendinous cuff may be torn as a complication of fractures and dislocations about the shoulder; rupture of the supraspinatus tendon occurs also as an isolated injury. It is caused by the same mechanism that produces avulsion fracture of the greater tuberosity of the humerus, that is, sudden adduction of the arm while it is being elevated, so that an abrupt and a violent increase of tension on the tendon occurs. The rupture may be partial or complete.

Partial Rupture

Diagnosis. An intact supraspinatus is necessary for powerful elevation of the arm. Partial rupture weakens the action of the muscles and makes elevation difficult. The immediate symptoms are mainly those of an acute traumatic subacromial bursitis, manifested by pain, tenderness, and swelling about the bursa. Muscle spasm is present, and this limits motion. In addition, there is likely to be a spot of acute tenderness just proximal to the greater tuberosity, weakness on attempting to raise the arm, and pain when the injured area passes beneath the acromion. A fracture must be excluded by roentgen examination. During the acute phase, it is not easy to determine whether difficulty in raising the arm is due to pain and muscle spasm or to actual injury to the rotator cuff tendons. When partial rupture is suspected, the bursa may be infiltrated with procaine solution to abolish pain and spasm. If definite weakness on elevation remains, the patient should be treated for partial rupture.

As an alternative diagnostic procedure, the patient may be treated for acute subacromial bursitis until the acute symptoms subside. This takes perhaps 3 or 4 days. Then the patient is re-examined, and if elevation is definitely weak and difficult, a diagnosis of partial rupture is made.

When a patient with partial rupture is seen long after the injury, adhesions in the subacromial bursa often complicate the clinical picture.

Treatment. In addition to the measures commonly used for acute tramatic bursitis, the arm should be immobilized in partial or full abduction for at least 2 or 3 weeks, depending on the estimated extent of the rupture. When weakness of elevation and irregularity of the rhythm of motion are very slight, immobilization should be in moderate abduction through an abduction cast or a splint (Figs. 23-24 and 23-26) for a short period. When these findings are quite marked, full abduction for a long period of immobilization is desirable. After the period of immobilization, home physiotherapy and massage are indicated. Relaxed circumduction exercises, as used in the management of subdeltoid bursitis, are of value in order to prevent bursal adhesions. If the symptoms persist after an adequate period of immobilization followed by exercises, the floor of the subacromial bursa should be explored through an incision as described in the operation for complete rupture of the tendon.

Complete Rupture

Diagnosis. If the patient is seen shortly after injury, the signs of acute sub-acromial bursitis may be present in addition to the inability to raise the arm from the side. This disability is often simulated by the pain and muscle spasm incidental to acute bursitis, and to rule out the latter a procaine infiltration of the bursa to abolish the pain may be given. If the patient still is unable to lift the arm from the side, the diagnosis of extensive rupture is certain. If the rupture is not extensive, the patient may be able to abduct the arm in one position of rotation but not in another; that is, he may be able to abduct in full internal rotation but not in external rotation.

When the patient is seen after the acute phase, other diagnostic signs are present. Although unable to lift the arm from the side, if it is passively elevated to the horizontal, the patient then can raise the arm to the vertical; this is due to the action of the deltoid. The patient can lower the arm slowly from the vertical position until it becomes horizontal. At this point, he loses control of the arm, because of the absence of supraspinatus action, and the arm falls to the side. The total range of motion is diminished little, if at all. When the tuberosity passes beneath the acromion, there is apt to be a jog or a bump, which may be palpable and visible and is accompanied by a soft, gristly crepitus. Palpation of the shoulder may disclose a tender spot over the greater tuberosity of the humerus. The tuberosity may feel unduly prominent, and there may be a sulcus proximal to it at the point of laceration of the tendon. In cases of long standing, marked atrophy of the spinatus muscles may be present.

Treatment. When a diagnosis of extensive rupture of the supraspinatus tendon is made, conservative treatment is not likely to be of value. However, since considerable improvement may follow subsidence of the acute symptoms in a week or two, and since repair may be difficult in the elderly patient due to extensive degenerative changes in the tendon, a definite decision often may be deferred for a short time.

Under local anesthesia, an anterior incision 5 to 7 cm. long is made downward from the tip of the acromion. The fibers of the deltoid are separated, and the roof of the bursa is exposed, grasped with hemostats, and incised. The crescentic tear in the tendon is visible in the floor of the bursa, and the torn edges are approximated with a synthetic suture if a sufficient distal stump of tendon is present; otherwise, the proximal portion must be sutured directly to the greater tuberosity. A sharp heavy-gauge needle is used to drill four canals through the tuberosity, into which the sutures are threaded. It may be necessary to bring the arm into some degree of abduction to secure approximation of the tendon to the tuberosity. The deltoid muscle is closed with plain catgut or silk sutures, and the skin is closed with sutures or clips.

The arm is immobilized at the side in moderate abduction by means of a thick axillary pad with a sling and a swathe dressing or an abduction splint. Passive exercises are started after 7 to 10 days, and active use is begun after 2 to 3 weeks, depending on the security with which the tear has been repaired. Without operation, prognosis for a good functional shoulder is very poor.

Calcareous Tendinitis at the Elbow

The etiology of this condition is not well understood. Probably, calcium deposition follows trauma with injury. It occurs at the lateral epicondyle of the humerus.

Diagnosis. There is a slow or a rapid onset of pain, which may be related to some mild trauma. The pain grows worse and may be disabling. In mild forms, the condition resembles tennis elbow. However, roentgenograms will show a typical area of calcareous deposit at the lateral epicondyle, and it is at this point that pain, acute tenderness, and, perhaps, swelling will be found.

Treatment. Conservative treatment by means of procaine infiltration and multiple punctures of the area with a large-bore needle is likely to be effective. Active motion should be started in a day or so. If these measures fail, evacuation of the deposit through a small incision will relieve the symptoms.

TENNIS ELBOW

Tennis elbow is the name given to a painful disability in the area of the lateral epicondyle of the humerus. In an effort to identify the syndrome with a pathologic process, the names of epicondylitis, radiohumeral bursitis, and radiohumeral synovitis are often used. In most cases, the causative factor is repeated violent contraction of the extensor-supinator muscles of the forearm, which have their origin from the lateral epicondyle of the humerus.

Etiology and Pathology. Most commonly, tennis elbow is seen on the side used most. It is common in those who practice sports and occupations requiring extension and supination of the forearm—tennis, fly-fishing, wringing clothes, etc. Some authors believe that these repeated strains at the origin of the common extensors from the epicondyle may result in an incomplete tear and a periostitis or an epicondylitis. It has been suggested that the symptoms are due to an imflammation in a bursa under the common extensor origin, but no bursa has been demonstrated in this area in the author's experience. Some believe that tennis elbow is due in some cases to a synovitis of the radiohumeral joint and that the pain is the result of the pinching of the synovium between the head of the radius and the capitellum when the arm is used with the elbow in extension and the hand is used to grasp objects.

Symptoms. The patient complains of pain and tenderness in the region of the lateral epicondyle. This pain is "accentuated" by grasping an object or by making a fist with elbow and the wrist extended and the forearm pronated. Pain or soreness often radiates over the extensor muscles of the forearm. A weakness in the grip and/or a pain when grasping appears, so that patients may drop inadvertently even such light objects as a cup; or there may be difficulty with the finer hand-and-finger movements, such as tying a tie or buttoning a shirt. Supination of the forearm with the hand in the grasping position, such as turning a door knob, causes acute pain.

Diagnosis. The gradual onset of pain associated with a specific activity requiring pronation-extension of the forearm is characteristic. Examination discloses a tender spot just below the lateral epicondyle or in the extensor group of muscles close to it. The elbow joint is normal, but there may be slight limitation of extension if the forearm is pronated. This condition may be tested. If the wrist and the fingers are flexed fully and the forearm is pronated, complete extension of the elbow is restricted and painful. Supination of the forearm against resistance produces marked pain in the area of the elbow.

Calcareous tendinitis at the lateral epicondyle may simulate tennis elbow, but the pain is likely to be quite severe, and roentgenograms will show the characteristic calcareous deposit.

Treatment. Rest and immobilization will relieve the pain, at least temporarily. The forearm is splinted with the wrist in dorsiflexion and is suspended in a sling. If pain recurs persistently, one of three methods of treatment may bring relief. The manipulative and the operative methods are effective probably because a partial rupture of tendon fibers is made complete, or because the tendinous insertion is lengthened, by stretching or by incision. Injection may be employed to produce a local inflammatory reaction at the site of the origin of the extensor group. As the inflammation subsides, the painful syndrome disappears gradually.

Manipulation. Mills advises manipulation, particularly in chronic cases exhibiting limitation of movement. With the patient under general anesthesia, he forces the elbow into full extension with the wrist and the fingers flexed and the forearm pronated. At the same time, firm pressure is made over the tender point, the thumb of the hand controlling the elbow. The elbow may straighten suddenly, with a click; or it may straighten gradually with continued effort. If the condition is not relieved completely, this procedure may be repeated after 4 days.

Hydrocortisone. In the hands of the author, injections of hydrocortisone, 25 mg. (1 ml.), at the most tender spot over the elbow have given almost immediate and complete relief of the symptoms of tennis elbow.

Operation. This may be advisable when other methods fail. Probably this was first performed to excise an inflamed radio-humeral bursa which was believed to be the cause of the pain; although no bursa was found, the symptoms were relieved. It appears that any operation in which the fibrous origin of the muscle is partly divided will relieve the pain.

Under local anesthesia, an incision is made over the lateral epicondyle and the tendinous origin of the supinator-extensor muscles is incised. Often this will expose an area of denuded bone or a ganglionlike area of degenerated fibrous tissue, which may be scraped away with the edge of the knife. However, the essential curative effect seems to come from incision.

BIBLIOGRAPHY

Shoulder Pain and Disability

Brewer, A. A., and Zink, O. C.: Radiation therapy of acute subdeltoid bursitis. JAMA, *122*:800, 1943.

Cerino, L. E., and Lipscomb, P. R.: The painful shoulder. Minnesota Med., *47*;365, 1964.

Cotton, R. E., and Rideout, D. F.: Tears of the humeral rotator cuff. J. Bone Joint Surg. *46B*:314, 1964.

Coventry, M. B.: The use of cortisone and hydrocortisone (compound F) in treatment of the painful shoulder. Proc. Mayo Clin., *29*:58, 1954.

———: Problem of the painful shoulder. JAMA, *151*:177, 1953.

DePalma, A. F.: Loss of scapulo-humeral motion (frozen shoulder). Ann. Surg., *135*:193, 1952.

Hollander, J. L.: Intra-articular hydrocortisone in the treatment of arthritis. Ann. Intern. Med., *39*:735, 1953.

Lippmann, R. K.: Frozen shoulder; periarthritis: bicipital tenosynovitis. Arch. Surg., *47*:283, 1943 (Abstr. in Surg., Gynec. Obstet., *78*:239, 1944).

McLaughlin, H. L.: Lesions of the musculotendinous cuff of the shoulder; differential diagnosis of rupture. JAMA, *128*:563, 1945.

Michelsen, J. J., and Mixter, W. J.: Pain and disability of the shoulder and arm due to herniation of the nucleus pulposis of cervical intervertebral discs. New Eng. J. Med., *231*:279, 1944.

Moseley, H. F., and Goldie, I.: The arterial pattern of the rotator cuff of the shoulder. J. Bone Joint Surg., *45B*:780, 1963.

Neviaser, J. S.: Adhesive capsulitis of the shoulder; study of pathological findings in periarthritis of shoulder. J. Bone Joint Surg., *27*:211, 1945.

Quigley, T. B.: Injection therapy of calcium deposits. Surg. Clin. N. Am., *43*:1495, 1963.

Russek, A. S.: Role of physical medicine in relief of certain pain mechanisms of shoulder. JAMA, *156*:1575, 1954.

Semmes, R. E., and Murphey, F.: Syndrome of unilateral rupture of sixth cervical intervertebral disc, with compression of seventh cervical nerve root; report of 4 cases with symptoms simulating coronary disease. JAMA, *121*:1209, 1943.

Travell, J., Rinzler, S., and Herman, M.: Pain and disability of the shoulder and arm. JAMA, *120*:317, 1942.

Tennis Elbow

Bailey, R. A. J., and Brock, B. H.: Hydrocortisone in tennis elbow: a controlled series. Proc. Roy. Soc. Med., *50*:389, 1957.

Lamphier, T. A., Pepi, J., Covino, J., Ostroger, J., Rosenthal, C. E., and Brusch, C.: Prednisolone (Meticortelone) in treatment of epicondylitis. Arch. Surg., *78*:492, 1959.

Michele, A. A., and Krueger, F. J.: Lateral epicondylitis of the elbow treated by fasciotomy. Surgery, *39*:277, 1956.

Mills, G. P.: Treatment of tennis elbow. Brit. Med. J., *2*:212, 1937.

Poretta, C. A., and Janes, J. M.: Epicondylitis of the humerus. Proc. Mayo Clin., *33*:303, 1958.

Slowick, F. A.: Sodium morrhuate in treatment of epicondylitis of humerus. New Eng. J. Med., *222*:1071, 1940.

Stein, I., Stein, R. O., and Beller, M. L.: Hydrocortisone in tennis elbow. Am. J. Surg., *86*:123, 1953.

Wall, J.: Tennis elbow. Indust. Med. Surg., *29*:173, 1960.

Thoracic Outlet Syndrome

Judovich, B., Bates, W., and Drayton, W., Jr.: Pain in the shoulder due to scalenus anticus syndrome. Am. J. Surg., *63*:377, 1944.

Nachlas, I. W.: Scalenus anticus syndrome or cervical foraminal compression. Southern Med. J., *35*:663, 1942.

Nelson, R. M., Davis, R. W.: Thoracic outlet compreesion syndrome. Ann. Thorac. Surg., *8*:437, 1969.

Reichert, F. L.: Compression of brachial plexus: the scalenus anticus syndrome. JAMA, *118*:294, 1942.

Spurling, R. G., and Grantham, E. G.: The painful arm and shoulder with especial reference to the problem of scalenus neurocirculatory compression. J. Missouri Med. Assoc. *38*:340, 1941 (Abstr. in Digest Treat., *5*:573, 1942).

Urschel, H. C., Razzuk, M. A., Wood, R. E., Parekh, M., and Paulson, D. L.: Objective diagnosis (ulnar nerve conduction velocity) and current therapy of the thoracic outlet syndrome. Ann. of Thorac. Surg., *12*:608, 1971.

23

Upper Limb
Part II—Fractures

Andrew C. Ruoff III, M.D.

MECHANISM OF THE SHOULDER

The upper limb is attached to the trunk by a mechanism of great flexibility. Normal arm elevation is a synchronization of many motions. Essentially, the humerus rotates upward on the scapula, and the scapula rotates on the chest wall, so that the glenoid fossa faces more and more upward as the arm is elevated. The humerus rotates on the scapula at the shoulder joint proper and at the subacromial bursa, where the greater tuberosity must slide beneath the acromion for full elevation. The scapula rotates on the chest wall and on the outer end of the clavicle. The inner end of the clavicle rotates on the sternum. Disturbances of shoulder function may occur at any of these points and may originate from fractures and dislocations or from lesions involving the shoulder joint, the subacromial bursa, the acromioclavicular or sternoclavicular articulation, or the muscles, tendons, and nerves concerned in shoulder motion.

Lesions involving the cervical spine may be responsible for shoulder pain, as may lesions of the thoracic and abdominal viscera. Compression of the neurovascular bundle at the thoracic outlet may also result in shoulder and arm pain.

The five major points at which shoulder motion occurs when the arm is elevated above the head are:

1. The scapulohumeral joint, which lies between the head of the humerus and the glenoid fossa of the scapula; this joint is surrounded by a loose capsule. The stability of the joint relies largely on muscular balance, since the capsule is a very loose structure and the joint configuration does not lend stability.

2. The greater tuberosity and the rotator cuff slide under the acromion as full abduction is attained. The subacromial bursa facilitates the gliding mechanism in this area.

3. The scapulothoracic plane of motion occurs between the serratus anterior and the chest wall. The scapula rotates when the arm is elevated, and the glenoid moves up. The scapula can also move forward and backward on the chest wall.

4. The acromial end of the clavicle moves upward and rotates at the acromioclavicula joint as the arm is elevated.

5. The sternoclavicular joint acts as a stabilizing pivot for the shoulder girdle. The clavicle rotates somewhat on its one axis, and the angle between its long axis and the sternum increases as the arm is elevated.

DIAGNOSIS OF LESIONS ABOUT THE SHOULDER

History. A detailed history is mandatory, and the main points to be considered are:

1. The nature and extent of antecedent violence, or the absence of violence.

2. The time of onset of symptoms and their progress.

3. The distribution of pain, and its persistence or degree of intermission, its re-

lation to use and movement, its character, its occurrence during sleep, and the amount of analgesia required for its relief.

4. The extent of disability, or its absence.

5. The occurrence of parethesias in the shoulder region or in the arm and hand.

6. The occurrence of vascular disturbance distal to the shoulder.

Examination. A thorough examination is essential for accuracy of diagnosis. It should be conducted with the patient stripped to the waist, sitting on a stool, and squarely facing a good light. Comparison with the nonaffected shoulder is most important.

In the case of dislocation of the humerus, fracture of the clavicle, or injury to the neck, inspection may disclose a characteristic posture. Swelling, discoloration, muscle spasm, muscle atrophy, and signs of circulatory disturbance should be noted.

When palpating the shoulder, the examiner must avoid causing any unnecessary pain. Starting at the sternoclavicular joint, the outlines of the clavicles, the acromioclavicular joints, the heads of the humeri, and the scapulae are compared. Deformity and tenderness should be noted. The muscles of the neck, the shoulders, and the scapular regions are explored by means of firm deep pressure for tenderness and spasm. The degree of disability and the range of motion of the shoulder must be determined by gentle examination limited by the presence of pain and resistance. The ability to elevate the arm actively and the range of passive motion are of particular interest and should be recorded. Limitation of rotation should be noted, as should be the points at which pain is produced by motion. Localized tenderness and pain on motion at any point usually indicate an underlying lesion, especially when the spontaneous pain of which the patient complains is in the same region.

Examination cannot be considered complete until the circulatory, sensory, and motor changes of the limb have been determined.

More than one injury may be found,

and muscular, joint, and bursal injuries should receive their share of attention. In the presence of obvious fractures and dislocations, soft tissue injuries that often lead to prolonged disability may easily be overlooked.

DISLOCATIONS OF THE HEAD OF THE HUMERUS

The head of the humerus is much larger than the glenoid fossa, and the capsule is loose about its entire circumference. The acromion and the coraco-acromial ligament prevent upward displacement of the head. Dislocation takes place through the lower and anterior portion of the capsule. As a rule this is resisted by the muscular attachments about the head of the humerus. When dislocations occur, extensive muscle and tendon injury may accompany them.

Types. There are several varieties of dislocation.

The common form is an anterior, or subcoracoid, dislocation. The head bursts through the anterio-inferior portion of the capsule and comes to rest beneath the coracoid process. Rarely, when violence is very great, the head may be carried farther in, to rest beneath the clavicle (subclavicular dislocation).

The second most common type is the subglenoid dislocation, in which the head lies directly beneath the glenoid and the arm is moderately fixed in full abduction (luxatio erecta).

Posterior dislocation is relatively rare and is often associated with neuromuscular or psychiatric abnormalities.

MECHANISM OF ANTERIOR DISLOCATION

When the arm is so rotated and elevated that some part of the humerus lies against the acromion, the normal limit of glenohumeral motion is reached. When the humerus is forced beyond this limit, the acromion becomes the fulcrum on which the head is levered away from the glenoid and tears through the anterio-inferior portion of the capsule. There may be an

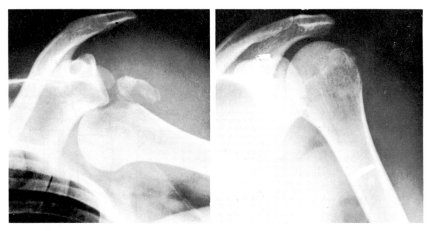

Fig. 23–10. (*Left*) Subglenoid dislocation complicated by fracture of the tuberosities. (*Right*) After reduction the tuberosities resumed their normal positions. If the tuberosities had retracted under the acromion (Fig. 23–27), and good position could not have been obtained, operation would have been indicated.

associated compression fracture of the head from forced contact of the head against the anterior or inferior glenoid margin (Hill-Sachs lesion). As the head leaves the glenoid fossa, the rotator cuff muscles may be torn or stretched, the greater tuberosity may be fractured (Fig. 23-10), or a portion of the glenoid may be broken off. The head assumes its final resting position when the arm falls to the side by its own weight.

DIAGNOSIS

Frequently the diagnosis can be made as the patient walks into the room. The elbow may be supported well away from the body. Comparison of the two shoulders will demonstrate a flattening in the region of the deltoid and the absence of the head of the humerus from its usual position beneath the acromion.

Measurement with the arm at the side may demonstrate increase in length from the acromion to the point of the elbow. The hand of the affected side cannot be brought to the opposite shoulder when the elbow is held against the chest wall.

After the diagnosis has been made, motor, sensory, and vascular changes in the limb indicative in injury to the neurovascular bundle must be sought and the presence or absence of these abnormalities noted. Although roentgen examination is not necessary for diagnosis, it is advisable in order to document the original injury and to recognize the prereduction presence of associated fractures of the tuberosities, the glenoid, or the humerus. Adequate films must include anteroposterior views of the shoulder and an axillary view, since no other view can accurately assess the relation of the head of the humerus to the glenoid. Posterior dislocations are frequently not diagnosed if an axillary view is omitted.

TREATMENT

Reduction should be carried out without delay. It can usually be accomplished in fresh dislocations within an hour, or sometimes longer, utilizing intravenous or intramuscular analgesics, such as morphine or meperidine, in the absence of contraindications. Intravenous analgesia has the advantages of prompt maximum relaxation and rapid vitiation of effect; the latter allows the patient to return home shortly after reduction without fear of lingering effect. In some muscular and tense patients, local anesthesia may be useful. If other methods fail, and in some apprehensive or difficult individuals, general anesthesia may be indicated.

When utilizing any method of reduction, traction should be applied steadily, with a *gradual* increase in pull. Sudden force or intermittent traction causes increased spasm and resistence and is self-defeating.

Local Anesthesia. After surgical preparation of the skin, a wheal is made one inch below and anterior to the acromion. A long needle is inserted into the joint space, and 10 ml. of 1 percent procaine hydrochloride solution is injected. An additional 10 ml. of solution is injected above the dislocated head. After 10 minutes, manipulation may be started.

Traction Method Without Anesthesia

Stimpson's method requires no anesthesia. After sedation with an analgesic given intramuscularly or intravenously, the patient is placed in a prone position on a high table or litter with a sandbag under the clavicle. In some cases, after a few minutes in this position, the weight of the arm will be enough to allow the head of the humerus to return to its normal position. Commonly, traction is necessary. Adhesive or sponge rubber friction strips and elastic bandage are applied to the forearm, and a weight carrier with 5 pounds is attached (Fig. 23-11). After a minute or two, another 5-pound weight is added. After 5 or 10 minutes, if reduction has not occurred, passive pendulum motion with rotation, gently applied, may aid reduction. Total traction time should not exceed 15 minutes. If reduction has not taken place, local or general anesthesia should be given and another method of reduction tried.

Parvin has described a similar method. The position of the patient is the same. Instead of applying traction by means of weights, the operator sits on a low footstool or on the floor and grasps the patient's wrist, making steady downward traction. If no reduction occurs after 5 to 6 minutes of sustained traction, reduction may be obtained by flexing the elbow 25° and slightly rotating the arm externally while the traction is continued.

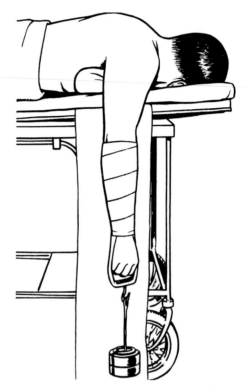

Fig. 23–11. Stimpson's method of reducing shoulder dislocation without anesthesia. (Tronzo, R. G.: JAMA, *184*:1043, 1963)

The Hippocratic Method

For reduction of an anterior dislocation, the Hippocratic method is often satisfactory. This makes use of manual traction and leverage of the humerus over a heel placed in the axilla. The patient lies flat on his back on the table, and the surgeon grasps the wrist of the affected side, placing his stockinged foot in the axilla so that it lies between the chest wall and the upper end of the humerus, and traction is made on the arm (Fig. 23-12). The arm is brought close to the side, so that the heel acts as a fulcrum, forcing the head of the humerus outward. If the head does not slip in, gentle external rotation of the arm may help.

A similar method is one in which the patient lies supine and an assistant holds a sheet around the thorax to give countertraction. Gentle, constant, and increasing

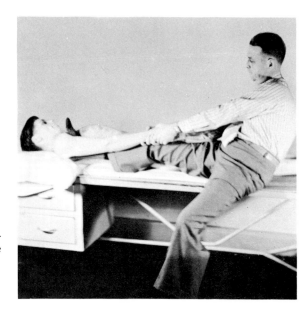

Fig. 23–12. Reduction of a dislocation of the head of the humerus by the
Hippocratic technique.

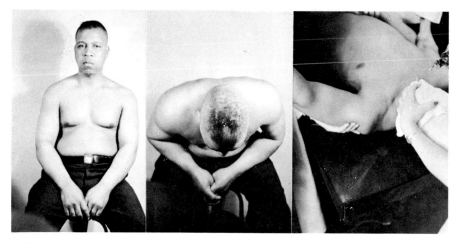

Fig. 23–13. Posterior dislocation of the left shoulder. (*Left*) The flattening
of the deltoid bulge; (*center*), the increased anteroposterior dimension of the
shoulder; and (*right*), reduction by traction and pressure.

traction is applied to the arm involved
with the elbow flexed at a right angle—the
forearm being held in a vertical position
and the arm moderately abducted. The
patient is asked to breathe deeply and
relax the shoulder muscles. While steady
traction is maintained, the flexed arm is
rotated gently toward the head, and reduction frequently occurs with ease.

A posterior dislocation can usually be
reduced by pressure from behind with
gentle traction and rotation of the arm
(Fig. 23-13).

POSTREDUCTION CARE

After reduction, the arm is held comfortably at the side, with an axillary pad to
prevent maceration. Position is maintained with a sling and a swathe (Fig.
23-14). A simple method of maintaining
satisfactory position is the utilization of a

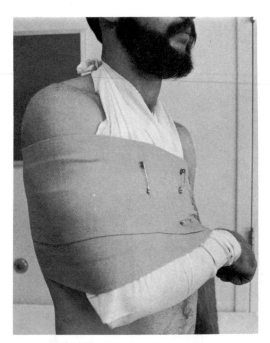

Fig. 23-14. Sling and swathe. This type of immobilization has many uses and is one of the most useful for immobilizing the shoulder and arm. The sling is applied first. A swathe of wide elastic bandage is then wrapped over the sling, and the safety pins go through both the elastic bandage and the sling. This dressing gives good support and prevents abduction and external rotation, while allowing some freedom of elbow motion and finger motion.

normal sling with a swathe of wide ACE bandange or Elastofoam over the sling. This swathe is pinned to both layers of the sling in several locations and comfortably prevents abduction and external rotation. This type of immobilization is not rigid and allows some elbow, hand, and wrist motion. Active use of the hand and wrist should be encouraged in the postreduction period.

If this is the first documented dislocation, the shoulder must be protected from abduction and external rotation for 6 weeks, although, after about 4 weeks, the sling and the swathe may often be discontinued during the day if the patient is cooperative. Recurrent dislocation is much more likely to occur if the first

dislocation is not protected until the motor power of the rotator cuff has returned to normal.

COMPLICATIONS

Fracture of the inferior lip of the glenoid is often present but requires no special treatment. Fracture of the greater tuberosity may be present. The fragments usually lie in good relation to each other after reduction and no special treatment is indicated; however, when the tuberosity has been retracted by the supraspinatus muscle, measures for approximation of the tuberosity to its bed must be taken. These are described under fractures of the greater tuberosity. The subacromial bursa often suffers extensive trauma, and this accounts for the prolonged disability that sometimes follows dislocation. When any evidence of injury to the brachial plexus or to the circumflex nerve (deltoid) is present, immobilization in abduction and slight external rotation may be indicated.

OLD DISLOCATIONS OF THE HEAD OF THE HUMERUS

One occasionally sees a patient who has long complained of pain and disability in the shoulder, and x-ray examination may show a dislocation which has been present for a long period of time. Often these patients have a surprisingly satisfactory range of motion and relatively little pain (Fig. 23-15). For the most part, no open operation is indicated in these cases. Surgery is occasionally indicated, but the results can be far from acceptable; therefore, clinical judgment is extremely important in this situation.

FRACTURES OF THE HEAD AND THE NECK OF THE HUMERUS

ANATOMY AND ETIOLOGY

The cylindrical humerus has a knoblike proximal end. The shaft is strong cortical bone, while the proximal end is spongy bone. The transition occurs at the surgical

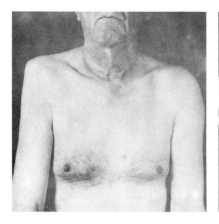 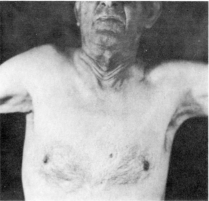

Fig. 23–15. (*Left*) An old subcoracoid dislocation of the humerus. (*Right*) Showing good range of motion obtained by exercise; no operation was performed.

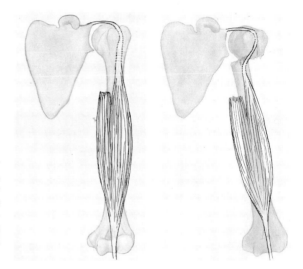

Fig. 23–16. (*Left*) Showing the tendon of the long head of the biceps, which is fastened securely in the bicipital groove. (*Right*) After fracture of the neck of the humerus, the fragments usually remain attached to the tendon. If the tendon is made taut, the fragments tend to fall into alignment.

neck, which also represents the line of division between the attachments of the rotator cuff muscles above and the powerful thoracic muscles, such as the pectoralis major and the latissimus dorsi, below.

Dense fibrous tissue bridges the groove between the two tuberosities, and, in the canal so formed, the tendon of the long head of the biceps passes upward to pierce the capsule, cross the joint space, and become attached to the posterosuperior margin of the glenoid (Fig. 23-16, *left*). The biceps tendon does not move during elevation; rather, the head and the

neck of the humerus move on it as on a guide wire.

After fracture, both fragments usually remain threaded on the biceps tendon (Fig. 23-16, *right*). Tear of the tendon is rarely a complication. Commonly, some untorn periosteum and rotator cuff tendon expansion also connect the fragments to each other. Falls on the hand and on the arm and, sometimes, direct violence cause these injuries. The fracture line is irregularly transverse, often with comminution or impaction (Fig. 23-17). The greater tuberosity often splits off as a separate fragment. The position of the arm and the

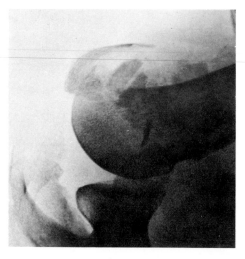 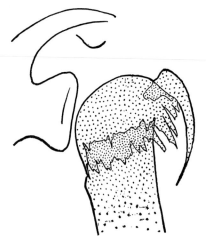

Fig. 23–17. (*Left*) Comminuted fracture of the neck of the humerus and the greater tuberosity in a 65-year-old woman. Reduction was not performed. The patient was treated with a sling and a swathe (Fig. 23–14) and relaxed circumduction exercises; an excellent result was obtained. (*Right*) Showing more clearly the position of the fragments in the same fracture.

direction of the fall often determine the displacement of the fragments. In only a few cases can the exact mechanics of displacement be determined.

Some shortening usually accompanies the fracture; this may be a few millimeters when position is good and as much as 3 or 4 cm. when the fragments overlap.

DIAGNOSIS

Pain at the shoulder after a fall or a blow, with swelling and tenderness localized over the head or the neck of the humerus and pain on elevation or rotation of the arm and on tapping the point of the flexed elbow, should alert the examiner to the possible presence of a fracture. On comparison with the uninjured side, deformity may be visible. The examiner may grasp the head of the humerus firmly with one hand and rotate the flexed forearm with the other (Fig. 23-18). If the head fails to rotate with the shaft, or if crepitus and increased pain are elicited, a definite diagnosis may be made. Ecchymosis along the medial side of the biceps muscle usually appears in from 24 to 48 hours.

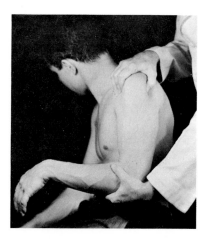

Fig. 23–18. Examination for fracture of the neck of the humerus. The examiner grasps the head of the bone firmly with one hand and rotates the flexed forearm with the other.

TREATMENT

Immediately after the examination, the arm should be immobilized with an axillary pad, sling, and swathe dressing (Fig. 23-14), and a roentgen examination should be made. The films should be read at once and the treatment delineated. This will vary with the amount of displace-

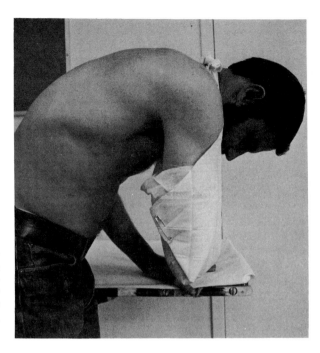

Fig. 23–19. Relaxed circumduction exercises. The patient bends forward, supporting himself with his good arm, and allows the injured arm to swing away from the body; with the help of gravity, the shoulder can then be moved in all directions.

ment of the fragments. In discussing treatment, it is convenient to classify these fractures into four groups:

Fractures Without Displacement or with Unimportant Displacement of Fragments

If no displacement of fragments has occurred, no reduction is required. In a young person, angulation of 15° to 25° and lateral displacement that is less than half the diameter of the shaft is unimportant; no disturbance of function and no deformity should result.

In older people, possibly an impaction with from 35° to 45° of angulation and less than two-thirds diameter of lateral displacement also may be considered to be unimportant, since little disturbance of function will result if treatment is carried out properly. The normal range of motion at the shoulder is so great that a loss of 30° of the full 180° is relatively unimportant. The risk of anesthesia and the trauma of reduction should be weighed against the expected benefits in these cases.

When no reduction is indicated, the initial dressing should remain undis-turbed. If the patient's general condition warrants, he may go home with instructions to apply an ice bag and to take a sedative as often as necessary. Acetylsalicylic acid, 60 mg., and phenobarbital, 30 mg., every 3 or 4 hours, or a suitable narcotic may be prescribed. The patient should be re-examined in 24 hours, with inspection of the dressing and of the limb; thereafter, twice weekly is usually sufficient. Full exercise of the hand and the wrist should start at once. After 2 weeks, a sling may be substituted for the sling and swathe, and daily relaxed circumduction exercises of the shoulder (Fig. 23-19) and guarded exercises of the elbow may be started. For at least a week after discontinuation of the use of the swathe during waking hours, the swathe may be useful at night to avoid unguarded abduction or external rotation while asleep.

In elderly patients, relaxed circumduction exercises and exercises of the elbow should be started as soon as acute pain and swelling subside, usually within 3 to 5 days. Neglect of early exercise and prolonged immobilization cause persistent pain, stiffness, and disability of the shoulder.

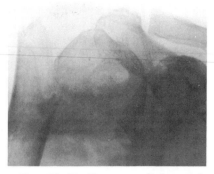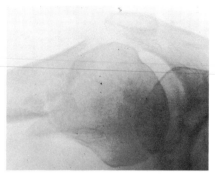

Fig. 23–20. Fracture of the neck of the humerus. The head lies in the abducted position. Alignment was obtained by bringing the arm into abduction and holding it there in an abduction cast.

The position of the fragments should be verified by taking roentgenograms at the end of the first week. Further roentgen examination is usually not needed until it is desirable to determine the amount of callus formation, unless there is a sudden increase of pain at the fracture site, which could denote displacement of the fragments.

After 4 to 5 weeks, callus can usually be palpated, and tenderness is absent if union has occurred. The extent of union should be verified by means of roentgenograms. At this time, full use may be resumed, with the exception of those duties requiring considerable exertion, such as pushing, pulling, and twisting, which should be deferred for another month.

If a program of exercise can be followed, little formal physiotherapy need be used. During the early period of immobilization, heat and gentle massage may be of some value. After relaxed circumduction exercises have been begun, the patient may use a hot-water bottle or an electric pad for 15 minutes, followed by massage with a mild counterirritant ointment for from 5 to 10 minutes. This can be repeated twice daily. Exercises and massage must be continued until a full range of motion is regained.

Transverse Fractures
with Displacement

In this group are placed those cases with more or less transverse fractures, with or without slight comminution, and with displacement beyond the limits described above. Overlapping may occur and may be associated with marked rotation of the head in relation to the shaft. In these cases, the head often lies in a position of abduction, external rotation, and forward flexion (Fig. 23-20). Invariably, the patient carries his forearm across his chest, and so brings the shaft into internal rotation. The proximal end of the shaft may lie anterior or posterior to the head. Roentgen examination in two planes is necessary, the regular anteroposterior view being supplemented by an axillary view taken with the roentgen plate above the shoulder and the beam directed proximally along the thoracic wall and aimed at the axilla. In low surgical-neck fractures in children, the proximal fragment may be abducted and flexed anteriorly without much external rotation, the proximal end of the shaft moving outward and the elbow inward. There are numerous other types of displacement, frequently with comminution.

Anesthesia. Local anesthesics or short-term inhalation anesthetics are extremely useful (Fig. 23-21). If local anesthesia is used, from 10 to 15 minutes should elapse after injection of the anesthetic before reduction is attempted.

Reduction. The usual methods of reduction are as follows:

With the patient sitting upright, supporting the injured arm across the body with the opposite hand, a folded face

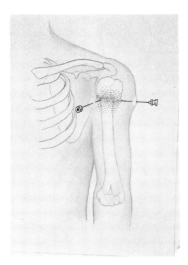

Fig. 23–21. Local anesthesia for reduction of a fracture of the neck of the humerus.

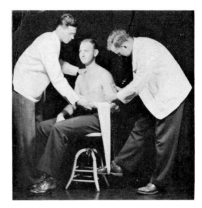

Fig. 23–22. Reduction of a fracture of the neck of the humerus with the patient sitting.

towel is placed over the forearm just below the elbow. A 4-inch or 6-inch heavy muslin bandage is looped over the towel and tied in a sling, so that its lower end hangs from 8 to 12 inches from the floor. An assistant grasps the wrist of the injured arm and, bringing the forearm to a right angle with the body in the sagittal plane (pointing forward), maintains right-angled flexion of the elbow. The surgeon then places one foot in the sling, grasps the upper arm with both hands below the line of fracture, and slowly and steadily increases the amount of pressure on his foot (Fig. 23-22). It is often an advantage to have the patient on a stool, in order to use the lower rung as a fulcrum for the toe of the foot applying the traction force. This not only steadies the foot, but increases the amount of force one can use. The two hands grasping the arm below the fracture site are used to force the upper end of the distal fragment laterally, anteriorly, or posteriorly, as required by the displacement. In those fractures with marked abduction of the upper fragment, it is well to have an assistant bear down upon the upper fragment while traction is being applied.

This method makes use of the taut tendon of the head of the biceps as a guide for both fragments. It requires less force than traction in abduction, in which the tension of the pectoralis major must be overcome.

When general anesthesia or the condition of the patient necessitates having the patient supine, a slightly different method is used (Fig. 23-23). For countertraction, a swathe or webbing strap 6 inches wide is passed around the patient's chest and fastened to the table or to an assistant on the uninjured side. The forearm is flexed to a right angle, and a folded towel is placed over it just below the elbow. A heavy muslin bandage is tied on over the towel and then passed around the waist or the shoulders of another assistant, who then holds the forearm at a right angle and produces traction by leaning backward. The pull should be very steady and increased slowly over a period of from 5 to 8 minutes. The axis of traction may be in line with the body or in from 30° to 45° of abduction, as seems best. The surgeon then manipulates the fragments into alignment by pressure, and the arm is taken slowly to the side.

If the fragments remain in good alignment, the arm is fixed to the side with an axillary pad, a sling, and a swathe (Fig. 23-14). Treatment is then continued as for a fracture in good position. For some patients, in whom shoulder stiffness is feared much more than elbow stiffness, the hanging cast makes a good dressing. The weight tends to maintain reduction, and the daily shoulder exercise prevents

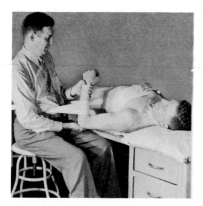

Fig. 23–23. Reduction of a fracture of the neck or the shaft of the humerus with the patient in the supine position. The assistant makes traction by leaning backward. The surgeon (not shown) uses both hands to adjust the position of the fragments.

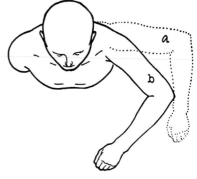

Fig. 23–25. The correct position for the abducted arm, as seen from above. (*a*) Incorrect position, in which the pectoral muscles are tense. (*b*) Correct position of muscle balance.

stiffness. The cast should be light enough to prevent distraction of the fragments.

In some instances, displacement recurs when the arm is taken to the side. If satisfactory position can be maintained only in abduction, the arm must be held in an abduction cast or splint (Fig. 23-24). The most favorable position is usually 30° to 60° of abduction but midway between the coronal and the sagittal planes and midway between external and internal rotation (Fig. 23-25).

Application of an Abduction Cast. After the skin has been washed with alcohol and powdered, a stockinet jacket is applied to the chest, and sheet wadding is wrapped around the body from the neck to below the iliac crests. Two plaster splints, 6 inches wide by 3 feet long and $1/8$ inch thick, are made and are laid on the arm from the hand to above the elbow, up

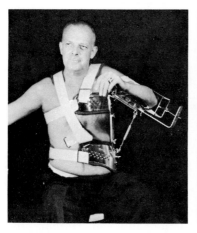

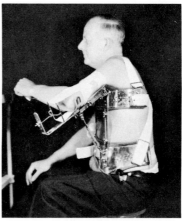

Fig. 23–24. (*Left*) Adjustable abduction splint arranged for continuous traction. Without the traction, the splint often is used for other lesions, such as rupture of the supraspinatus tendon. (*Right*) Abduction splint, lateral view. Note that the arm lies well forward of the lateral position. (Zimmer, Warsaw, Ind.)

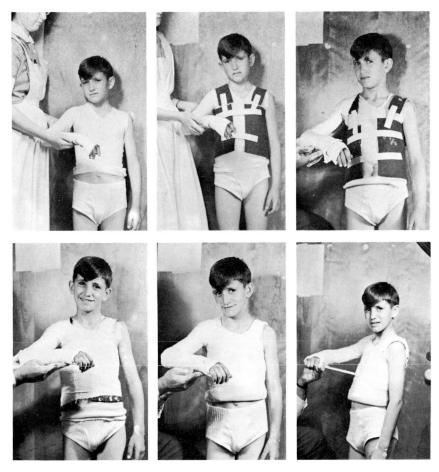

Fig. 23–26. Application of an abduction cast. (*Top, left*) A stockinet jacket and sleeve have been applied. (*Top, center*) Felt in position at the sides of the body and over the shoulders. (*Top, right*) The molded plaster splints have been applied from the knuckles to the back. (*Bottom, left*) Application of circular plaster. (*Bottom, center*) The stockinet has been turned back at the knuckles, the shoulders, and the abdomen, and held with a few extra turns of plaster bandage. (*Bottom, right*) A piece of board has been placed between the arm and the chest and fastened with turns of plaster to prevent the breaking of the cast at the shoulder.

the arm to the shoulder, and then across the back and the chest (Fig. 23-26). Six-inch plaster bandages are then wrapped about the forearm, the arm, and the chest until a cast of about 3/16-inch uniform thickness has been made. The free ends of the sheet wadding and the stockinet at the wrist, the opposite axilla, and the waistline then are turned over the edges of the plaster and are fastened with two additional turns of plaster bandage.

Since displacement of the fragments may occur during application of the cast, it is advisable to have an additional roentgen examination made as soon as the plaster has set.

Postreduction Care. The hand must be exercised from the beginning. After a week, the plaster may be removed from the dorsum of the forearm to permit active exercise of the forearm and the elbow. After 2 or 3 weeks, the cast may be bivalved to the shoulder to permit gentle exercise and massage of the shoulder. A

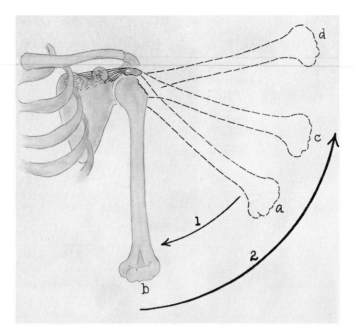

Fig. 23–27. When the supraspinatus is tense during abduction, sudden adduction (1) from the position at *a* results in avulsion of the greater tuberosity. The arm comes to the side, *b*. The tuberosity may be retracted as shown; when it is, the arm must be abducted (2) to the position shown in *c* or *d*.

roentgen examination should be made at the end of one week to verify maintenance of position. At the end of 4 to 6 weeks, the amount of callus formation is determined, both by palpation and by films; if it is adequate, the cast is removed entirely, and heat, massage, and active use are started. The physiotherapy must be continued until there is a full range of painless motion.

Extensively Comminuted Fractures

When extensive comminution and displacement are present, hospitalization or treatment by continuous traction is usually advisable. An exception to this may be the elderly patient in whom some loss of shoulder function is not of much practical importance. Many such patients can be treated satisfactorily by the hanging-cast method described below, provided exercise is started from the beginning and is performed faithfully.

Avulsion Fractures of the Greater Tuberosity

Avulsion fracture of the greater tuberosity is an uncommon injury, but it deserves extended description because of the disability that may follow. The greater tuberosity is the point of insertion of the supraspinatus muscle, the prime initiator of all abduction. The muscle works at great mechanical disadvantage, and the tuberosity is subjected to relatively great tension during elevation.

Etiology. Fracture of the tuberosity frequently complicates dislocation of the shoulder. The tuberosity, to which the taut supraspinatus tendon is attached, tears off or is pulled off. Usually it moves back into position when the dislocation is reduced. If the tuberosity remains retracted, there is probably an extensive rupture of the rotator cuff or of the retaining periosteum.

Avulsion fractures follow another type of violence, a fall against the side of the partly abducted arm (Fig. 23-27). The elbow is held away from the side to take the force of a fall against a wall or a floor. At impact, an abrupt tension is applied to the supraspinatus muscle, tendon and to the greater tuberosity. In older patients, the tendon, weakened by attritional changes or ischemia, tears either partly or completely. In younger people, the tuberosity often snaps off. The unopposed tension of the supraspinatus muscle permits retraction of the fragment toward the scapula. When the fracture is complete and the retaining periosteum is torn through, it may come to rest in the position that it normally would occupy only with full elevation of the arm. However, very often enough periosteum remains untorn to retain the fragment in relatively good position. Since the tuberosity forms part of the floor of the subacromial bursa, hemorrhage and exudation into the bursa may follow this injury.

Diagnosis. As may be expected, the clinical picture resembles that of acute traumatic subacromial bursitis and rupture of the supraspinatus tendon. Spasm of the shoulder muscles, severe pain on elevation of the arm, and tenderness over the bursa are present. Fracture may be suspected from the agonizing localized tenderness over the tuberosity and possibly by the presence of a slight notching at the site of the tuberosity when a large bone fragment has been detached and retracted. Roentgenograms must be obtained to determine the degree of displacement.

Treatment. When the fragment remains in good position, immobilization in slight abduction for from 4 to 6 weeks may be desirable. A thick triangular axillary pad, base down, and a sling and a swathe make a satisfactory dressing. Daily relaxed circumduction exercises, heat, and massage should be started after 1 or 2 weeks and continued regularly until full function returns. Failure to begin exercises early and to continue them regularly often results in a stiff, atrophic, and extremely painful shoulder.

When the tuberosity has been retracted substantially by the supraspinatus, open operation should be performed.

COMPLICATIONS OF FRACTURES OF THE HEAD AND THE NECK OF THE HUMERUS

Injury to the circumflex (axillary) nerve, as manifested by deltoid paralysis, may occur. The axillary blood vessels and the brachial plexus may be injured. Addition-al fractures or soft tissue injuries may be present.

Failure to reduce displacement, or rupture of the biceps tendon may make it necessary to operate.

FRACTURES OF THE SHAFT OF THE HUMERUS

Fractures of the shaft of the humerus may result from falls on the hand or the forearm; from direct violence, such as a blow with a club; or from muscular violence, such as occurs during wrestling or when throwing a ball. The fracture may be transverse, oblique, or comminuted. Complete displacement and overriding of the fragments are common. The biceps and the triceps go into spasm and increase the deformity.

DIAGNOSIS

Deformity makes the diagnosis easy. There may be shortening, angulation, thickening and irregularity of the shaft. Normally, the lateral epicondyle lies in the plane of the greater tuberosity. When this relationship changes, rotary displacement has occurred. Tenderness at the fracture site is usually acute and well localized. After a few hours, swelling and muscle spasm are present. Later, ecchymosis appears. Anteroposterior and lateral roentgenograms should be taken.

TREATMENT OF FRACTURES IN GOOD POSITION

If there is sufficient apposition for stability, slight degrees of angulation and rotary deformity may be corrected without anesthesia at the time of applying the immobilizing dressing. Incomplete fractures require only an axillary pad, sling, and swathe. Otherwise, a plaster sugarong splint or coaptation splints (Fig. 23-28) are applied. With the forearm at a right angle and the patient leaning forward with the humerus hanging away from the body, the splint is applied from the medial side of the axilla down the inner side of the arm, across the extensor

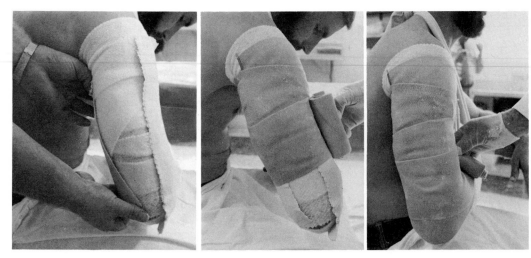

Fig. 23–28. (*Left*) With the patient bending forward and the arm hanging down toward the floor, anterior and posterior plaster splints are applied over sheet wadding. (*Center*) Elastic bandage molds the plaster splint to conform to the arm. (*Right*) The completed dressing.

surface of the forearm at the elbow, and up the outer side of the arm across the top of the shoulder. A gauze bandage or an elastic bandage may then be used to fasten the splint securely. The arm is then allowed to fall to the side when the patient resumes the erect position, and an axillary pad, sling, and swathe are applied. Another roentgen examination should be made in 1 week to make certain that the fragments have not slipped.

The patient must exercise his hand from the beginning. After 1 or 2 weeks, the swathe may be removed 2 or 3 times daily for relaxed circumduction exercises of the shoulder.

Transverse fractures of the shaft of the humerus unite slowly at best. Delayed union and nonunion in these cases are not rare. Eight weeks of uninterrupted immobilization appear to be a safe minimum. At the end of this period, the splints are removed, the part is examined for callus formation, and the findings are verified by films. If union is satisfactory, heat, massage, and graduated exercises are recommended and are continued until the maximum return of function is obtained. If after 8 weeks callus formation is meager and if the fracture still shows on the films, the use of an axillary pad, sling, and swathe should be continued. Hot soaks, massage, and motion of the elbow should be begun in addition to the relaxed circumduction exercises of the shoulder. Active use should not be started until there is reasonably solid union. In the presence of marked delay in union or frank nonunion, open reduction and bone graft, with some form of internal fixation, is often necessary.

TREATMENT OF TRANSVERSE FRACTURES IN POOR POSITION

Transverse and slightly oblique fractures of the shaft offer more difficulty in management when overriding of the fragments occurs.

When the level of the fracture lies above the insertion of the deltoid, this muscle, with the assistance of the biceps and the triceps, tends to bring the distal fragment proximally and laterally, while the proximal fragment is usually adducted by the pectoralis major and the latissimus dorsi (Fig. 23-29). When the level of the fracture lies below the insertion of the deltoid, the action of this muscle is counterbalanced more or less

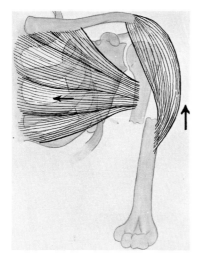

Fig. 23–29. Fracture of the shaft of the humerus between the pectoralis and the deltoid insertions. Shows muscle pull.

by the action of the adductors, and the displacement of the fragments is variable. Spasm of the biceps and of the triceps tends to produce and maintain overriding.

A simple rule for reduction is to bring the axis of the distal fragment, which can be controlled easily, into line with the axis of the proximal fragment. Sufficient traction overcomes the shortening, and gentle manipulation secures apposition. Occasionally, angulation may be increased to allow the edges of the fragments to come into apposition, and reduction may then be obtained by leverage.

Facilities for image intensification may be of real value. If not more than 24 or 36 hours have elapsed since the accident, local anesthesia is usually preferred. Brachial block anesthesia is also satisfactory, and it may be used even longer after the injury. Reduction may usually be accomplished more easily with the patient in the sitting position, rather than recumbent, and it is much simpler to apply the immobilizing dressing with the patient sitting.

Local anesthesia is induced by injecting a suitable anesthetic solution into the hematoma at the level of the fracture. Ten to 15 minutes should elapse before manipulations are begun. The patient is seated on a stool with suitable support, and reduction is accomplished. Using steady traction, the shortening is gradually overcome, and the fragments can then be moved into apposition. Traction must be slow and steady, and the manipulation must be gentle. If alignment seems satisfactory with the arm at the side, gentle traction is maintained while a plaster sugar-tong splint and an axillary pad, sling, and swathe dressing are applied, as previously described. If the distal fragment can be aligned with the proximal fragment only in a position of abduction, an abduction splint or cast should be used. The best position is usually with the arm in sufficient abduction and about midway between the coronal and the sagittal planes.

In some circumstances, general anesthesia may be preferred for reduction. Steadily increasing traction is applied to the flexed forearm until the shortening disappears. This may take from 5 to 15 minutes. The fragments are then manipulated into apposition, and their position is determined by roentgenography or by utilizing the image intensifier. When the position is felt to be satisfactory, the traction is decreased, but it is maintained until the immobilizing dressing is completed and the patient can sit up. The plaster of Paris sugar-tong splint and an axillary pad, sling, and swathe dressing are used unless a position of abduction is required.

For older patients, the hanging cast (Fig. 23-30) has some advantages. Although it does not immobilize the fracture site well, it produces relatively good constant traction, and it does permit relaxed circumduction exercises to be done from the onset of treatment. The usual late stiffness and pain at the shoulder may be prevented. There is also less restriction and compression of the thoracic cage. Treatment is continued as for fractures in good position.

If a good position of the fragments cannot be obtained or maintained, continuous traction must be instituted. Open reduction is occasionally advisable.

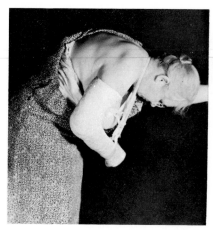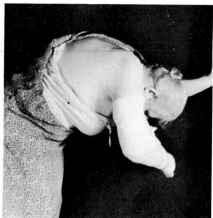

Fig. 23–30. Hanging cast. Relaxed circumduction exercises of the shoulder shown were begun 4 days after the injury.

TREATMENT OF OBLIQUE AND COMMINUTED FRACTURES

When shaft fractures are oblique or severely comminuted, the fragments often cannot be maintained in position by the methods of splinting described above. Continued suspension and traction are often necessary. The guiding principles are:

1. Sufficient traction to overcome shortening, and no more, should be applied. *Any* distraction of the fragments invites a delay in union, or nonunion.

2. The direction of traction must be such that the axes of the proximal and the distal fragments are in line.

3. The flexed forearm is brought to the position of rotation assumed by the uncontrolled proximal fragment, usually midway between external and internal rotation.

Continuous traction may be obtained with the patient either confined to bed or ambulatory. In the ambulatory patient, an abduction splint or a hanging cast must be used, and the traction must be obtained with the assistance of one of these devices.

Abduction Splint. The abduction splint (Fig. 23-24) should be applied with the arm in sufficient abduction for alignment of the fragments, i.e., about midway between internal and external rotation, and halfway between the coronal and the sagittal planes (Fig. 23-25). Strong traction should be made for approximately 24 hours, after which time a roentgen examination is made. If the position is satisfactory, the traction is gradually decreased during the next few days.

The Hanging Cast. Good position of the fragments often can be obtained by the use of the hanging cast. This method is particularly useful in elderly patients, in whom considerable angulation and shortening can be permitted. It allows immediate exercises and causes little restraint of the chest. Care must be taken to avoid distraction. A *light* cast is indicated, a plaster or wire loop being incorporated in the cast to support the sling in order to allow the cast to hang in an optimum position (Fig. 23-30).

A plaster sugar-tong splint is made and is applied from the axilla down the medial side of the arm, beneath the elbow, and up the outer side of the arm to the insertion of the deltoid. A second splint, 4 inches wide and from 24 'to 30 inches long, is applied from the knuckles along the extensor surface of the semipronated forearm, around the back of the elbow, and then along the flexor surface of the forearm to the flexion crease of the hand. Each sugar-tong splint should be made of one 4-inch-wide commercial plaster bandage. Two 3-inch bandages are then applied around the previously applied sugar-tong splints to complete the cast, a plaster or wire loop being incorporated in the cast just proximal to the wrist. If the above directions are followed, the cast will usually not be too heavy.

Next, a neck sling is passed through the loop and so fastened that the forearm lies horizontally, or slightly higher than the horizontal, to avoid pressure of the posterior portion of the cast against the humerus. The patient must allow the cast to hang freely and must not support the elbow with his knee when sitting or with pillows. He will be obliged to sleep in a semireclining position for 2 or 3 weeks.

On the day following reduction, the position of the fragments should be determined by roentgen examination. Traction may be increased, if necessary, by adding some weight at the elbow with more plaster. If the facture is angulated, a thick pad may be interposed between the cast and the chest to improve alignment. If it is seen in the anteroposterior views, angulation should be corrected by lengthening or shortening the sling. If overtraction is observed, a lighter cast should be used, and this can usually be obtained by cutting out a portion of the previously applied plaster.

The hand should be exercised from the beginning; relaxed circumduction exercises of the shoulder should be started immediately and continued hourly for a short period while awake. After removal of the cast, heat, massage, and active use will help to diminish stiffness at the elbow.

The position of the fragments must be determined approximately 1 week after reduction and subsequently in another week or 10 days. After 3 to 4 weeks, the tendency for the fragments to slip is reduced, and further roentgen examination may be postponed until clinical union is apparent. The cast should be removed when clinical and roentgen evidences of union are present, which usually takes from 5 to 8 weeks. A sling may be used for a short time, until the elbow can be extended. Physiotherapy is continued as outlined above.

COMPLICATIONS OF FRACTURES OF THE SHAFT OF THE HUMERUS

Interposed muscle may prevent reduction and make operation necessary. This complication should be suspected when crepitus is not felt readily on manipulation of the fragments.

Involvement of the radial (musculospiral) nerve may occur. This nerve lies in direct contact with the middle third of the shaft of the humerus as it winds round from behind. Involvement produces wrist drop and sensory loss over the radial distribution. If evidence of nerve injury presents itself at the original examination, contusion or laceration may have occurred. If this complication is present, immediate consultation should be obtained. Later involvement usually means constriction by scar or callus.

In the case of fractures of the lower third of the shaft, angulation is common. Ordinarily, the biceps aids the forearm supinators in opposing the strong pronators. When the humeral shaft loses its rigidity, the supinating effect of the biceps diminishes, and the pronators may act unopposed. If the forearm is supinated fully, rotation may occur at the fracture site, producing angulation of the fragments; the angle opens medially. The pronators relax in full pronation, overcoming this effect. Forced pronation must be avoided, or the opposite effect may be obtained (Fig. 23-31).

FRACTURES OF THE HUMERUS AT THE ELBOW

The strong cylindrical shaft of the humerus broadens, thins out, and bends forward as it approaches the elbow. The articular surfaces resist fracture, but the less dense, spongy bone immediately above is hollowed out for the coronoid

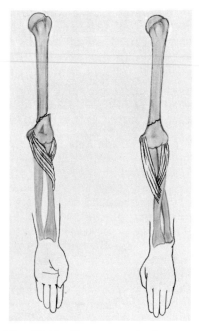

Fig. 23–31. Fracture at the lower end of the humerus. When the forearm is supinated, the fracture site becomes an accessory point of rotation. Pronation relaxes the pronators, and the angulation disappears.

process of the ulna anteriorly and for the olecranon posteriorly, and is vulnerable.

Epiphyseal Development
(Fig. 23-32)

The epiphyses at the lower end of the humerus vary considerably in time of appearance, contour, and time of fusion

with the shaft. Very often, in childhood the roentgenograms show irregularities that must not be interpreted as fractures except after comparison with the opposite normal side.

Anatomy

The brachial artery and the ulnar, the median, and the radial nerves may become involved in fractures at the elbow. The brachial artery lies at the medial border of the biceps muscle and tendon, and passes under an aponeurotic slip from the tendon, the bicipital fascia, just distal to the bend of the elbow (Fig. 23-33). It is accompanied by the median nerve. The radial nerve lies between the brachialis and the brachioradialis, anterior to the lateral condyle and the head of the radius. The ulnar nerve lies posteriorly, in a groove between the medial condyle and the olecranon.

Etiology and Displacement

In the adult, falls on the hand with the forearm extended may cause posterior dislocation at the elbow (Fig. 23-34, *B*). In children, supracondylar fracture of the humerus of the extension type occurs more often (Fig. 23-34, *C*). The line of fracture is more or less transverse in the anterior view, but frequently it is oblique when seen from the side. The lower fragment moves backward and upward as the expanded thin end of the shaft moves downward and forward into the ante-

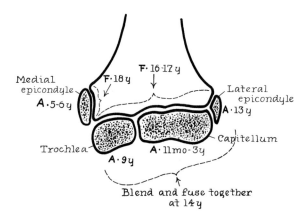

Fig. 23–32. Epiphyses at the lower end of the humerus. (*A*) The time of appearance of the centers of ossification. (*F*) The time of fusion of the epiphyses with the shaft. The trochlear, the capitellar, and the lateral epicondylar epiphyses fuse together at 14 years of age and unite with the shaft at from 16 to 17 years of age. The epiphysis of the medial epicondyle fuses with the shaft independly of the others.

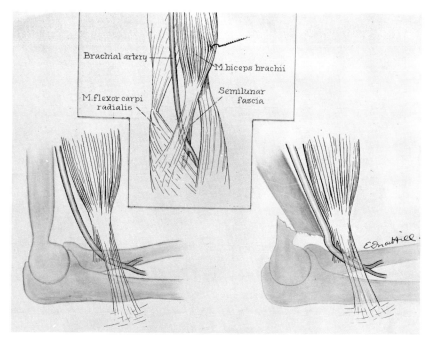

Brachial artery

M. biceps brachii

M. flexor carpi radialis

Semilunar fascia

Fig. 23–33. Showing the brachial artery passing beneath the semilunar (bicipital) fascia. The projecting sharp end of the upper fragment of the humerus may compress or sever the vessel.

cubital fossa, where it may tear or compress the brachial artery and the median nerve or the radial nerve. It may even protrude through the skin. Lateral and rotary displacement may also occur.

When the fracture follows a fall on the flexed elbow, the uncommon flexion type may occur (Fig. 23-34, *E*). The fracture line runs from behind upward and forward, and the distal fragment moves upward and forward.

Falls on the flat of the ulna may wedge the olecranon between the condyles, the result being either the T or the Y type of fracture (Fig. 23-34,*F*).

Falls which put the medial side of the elbow on tension or which make sudden tension on the flexor-pronator muscles may result in avulsion of the medial epicondyle. This type of violence may cause lateral dislocation at the elbow joint. The joint space widens from tension, and the epicondyle, drawn downward and medially by the pronators, may fall into the

joint and be caught when the abrupt tension stops.

Falls on the olecranon that thrust the olecranon to either side probably account for isolated single fractures of the trochlea or the capitellum.

DIAGNOSIS

Aside from avulsion of the medial epicondylar epiphysis, simple epiphyseal separation is rare.

When fracture or epiphyseal separation occurs without displacement, the signs are swelling, local tenderness, and pain on motion. In very young children, before ossification centers appear, the films may appear negative, even after extensive injuries, but the treatment should be instituted as for fracture, since roentgen signs of epiphyseal separation may not be apparent until later.

When displacement of the fragments has occurred, the diagnosis of fracture

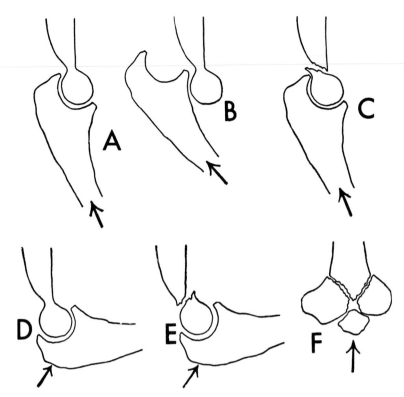

Fig. 23–34. The mechanism of fractures at the elbow. (*A*) The common type of thrust during falls with the elbow extended. (*B*) The posterior dislocation that tends to occur in adults. (*C*) The extension type of supracondylar fracture that tends to occur in children. (*D*) The direction of the thrust in falls on the point of the flexed elbow and (*E*) The flexion type of supracondylar fracture that results. (*F*) Falls on the olecranon tend to wedge it between the trochlea and the capitellum, and to fracture one or both.

may be made more readily. In addition to local tenderness and swelling, there may be visible (Fig. 23-35) or palpable deformity of the bones. To differentiate fracture from posterior dislocation at the elbow, the epicondyles and the tip of the olecranon are palpated and compared with the normal side. The tip of the olecranon is the apex of a triangle, of which a line between the epicondyles forms the base (Fig. 23-36). With the forearm flexed to a right angle, the triangle lies in the plane of the long axis of the humerus. With the forearm extended, the olecranon lies directly behind the line

between the epicondyles. This relationship is altered characteristically in dislocations of the elbow. In extension fractures, the lower end of the shaft may be palpable in the antecubital fossa; in flexion fractures, it appears over the olecranon, which has moved forward with the lower fragment. A difference in the contour of the epicondyles on comparison with the normal side suggests epicondylar or condylar fracture, as does any lateral mobility of the joint, which is normally almost rigid in this plane.

A history of dislocation in a child, with marked restriction of motion and pain

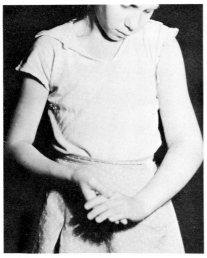
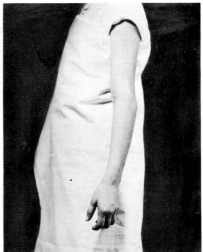

Fig. 23–35. (*Left*) Supracondylar fracture of the left humerus without displacement. Note the marked swelling. (*Right*) Deformity produced by a supracondylar fracture, extension type.

over the medial aspect of the elbow after reduction, requires accurate comparison of both medial epicondylar epiphyses and films of both elbows. The medial epicondyle may lie in the joint space.

A suspicion of any complication warrants hospitalization. An open fracture is an obvious and urgent complication; a diminished or absent radial pulse demands emergency care. Rapid swelling of the elbow and the forearm suggest extensive soft tissue damage and venous obstruction. A careful examination of motor power and sensory function must be made and recorded.

PRELIMINARY CONSIDERATIONS IN TREATMENT

The objectives of treatment are (1) the prevention of interference with circulation and of Volkmann's contracture; (2) the prevention of nerve injuries; (3) alignment of the fragments to prevent deformities and loss of function; and (4) prevention of myositis ossificans, extensive fibrosis, and persistent muscle spasm.

When the initial examination is completed, a snug bandage is applied about the elbow, and the joint is immobilized as it lies. The arm is elevated when the

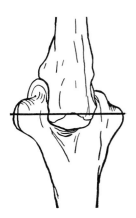
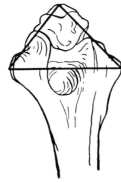

Fig. 23–36. Posterior aspect of the elbow. In extension, the tip of the olecranon is in line with the epicondyles. In flexion, the 3 points make a triangle.

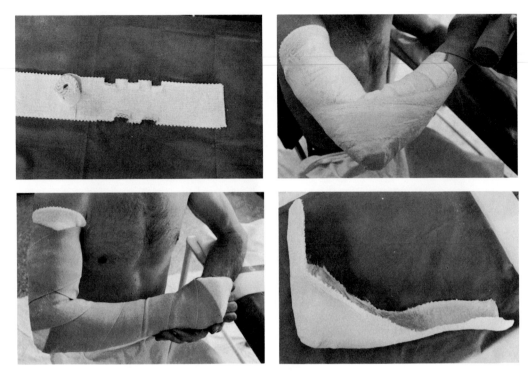

Fig. 23–37. Application of posterior molded splint for injuries about the elbow. This splint is one of the most useful devices available and has many applications. (*Top, Left*) Several thicknesses of plaster, long enough to extend from the upper arm to the edge of the metacarpals, are laid out on a table. The area which will be over the elbow is cut, as illustrated, to allow them to be smoothly interdigitated. The only other portion of plaster needed is a small roll of two-inch plaster bandage. (*Top, right*) Over a light layer of sheet wadding, the posterior splint is thoroughly moistened and smoothed out on a firm surface, after which it is applied to the arm over light padding. The splint should extend from the upper arm to the metacarpal heads. The circular bandage is then applied as shown in the illustration to reinforce the splint and obviate the need for a very heavy splint. The entire splint is then allowed to conform to the arm by light application of an elastic bandage. (*Bottom, left*) The completed posterior splint in place. This gives some lateral stability and does not give any compression in the antecubital area. It is important, as mentioned above, to carry the splint to the metacarpal heads since any shorter splint will allow the wrist to sag over the edge of the splint and will be quite uncomfortable. (*Bottom, right*) The completed splint after it has been removed.

patient is not walking, and the region of the elbow is surrounded with icebags. Protection is maintained until a decision is made concerning further treatment.

TREATMENT OF UNCOMPLICATED FRACTURES IN GOOD POSITION

When displacement of the fragments is absent or negligible and when no complications are present, treatment is simple. A posterior plaster splint may be applied from the hand to the axilla (Fig. 23-37). An elastic bandage helps to immobilize and aids in controlling swelling. Whether present or anticipated, swelling is controlled further by elevation of the limb to the shoulder level on pillows and application of ice bags for from 24 to 48 hours after injury. Full active use of the fingers and of the shoulder should begin immediately. The patient should return on

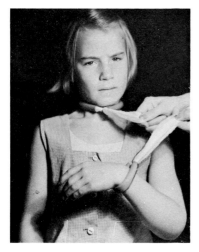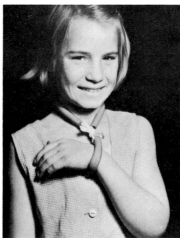

Fig. 23–38. Horse-collar dressing for elbow injuries. A piece of wide rubber tubing is cut to fit around the neck, and another is cut to fit the wrist. Bandage or tape is threaded through each piece of tubing and tied so as to hold the arm in acute flexion.

the following day to have the dressing inspected and to report the presence of any pain; thereafter, a weekly visit may suffice. At the end of 2 to 5 weeks, depending on the patient's age and the type of fracture, the splint is removed and active use is recommended. There should be no attempted passive stretching of the elbow. Active use should be the watchword. Adults may have a little swelling of the forearm for a few weeks, which, along with stiffness, may be diminished by daily hot soaks and gentle massage.

For younger children, the "horse-collar" dressing (Fig. 23-38), with the arm in the flexed position, may be used instead of the splint when there is little displacement and minimal swelling. A satisfactory dressing for the very young may be made as shown in Figure 23-39.

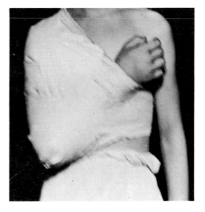

Fig. 23–39. A body-swathe type of dressing useful for undisplaced shoulder, humerus, and elbow fractures in small children. When covered with plaster, it makes a light and comfortable cast. A thin guaze pad is placed in the crease of the elbow, and a large pad is placed between the chest and the arm and forearm.

TREATMENT OF FRACTURES WITH DISPLACEMENT

The elbow functions as a hinge joint. The axis of the hinge, measured on the outer side, lies at an angle of about 80° with the long axis of the humerus. The forearm deviates laterally to allow a carrying angle. Displacement of the distal fragment medially diminishes or reverses the angle; displacement laterally increases it (Fig. 23-40).

Full flexion and extension depend on the thickness of the hinge. Unreduced forward or backward displacements heal with thickening, and motion is blocked (Fig. 23-41). Rotary displacement has this

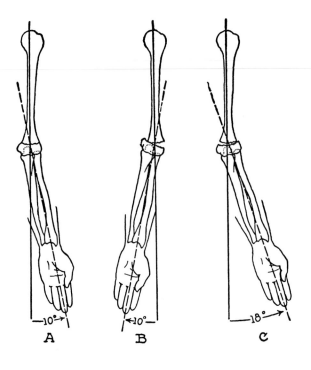

Fig. 23–40. The effect mediolateral displacement of the lower humeral fragment on the carrying angle. (*A*) Normal, (*B*) medial displacement, and (*C*) lateral displacement.

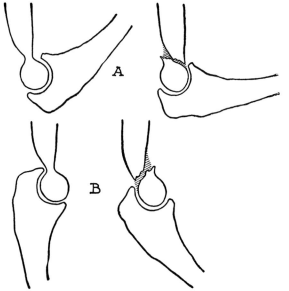

Fig. 23–41. Loss of mobility in supracondylar fractures. The effect of unreduced forward displacement of the shaft (*A*) is loss of flexion. The effect of unreduced backward displacement of the shaft (*B*) is loss of extension.

effect as well as that of changing the distal axis.

The ulna and the radius, in parallel motion, flex on the axis of the hinge. Fractures of the trochlea and the capitellum may change the mediolateral position of the ulna and the radius and may therefore affect the carrying angle; they may also change the anteroposterior position of these bones, so that they rotate on different axes, with limitation of motion (Fig. 23-42).

The brachial artery and the median nerve pass downward along the medial side of the biceps; then they pass through an almost rigid canal formed by the ulna,

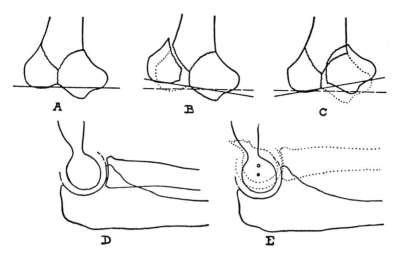

Fig. 23–42. The effect of displacement of the trochlea or the capitellum. (*A*) Normal contour of the articular surface. (*B*) Capitellar fracture; the forearm would shift to the outer side with an increase in the carrying angle, (*C*) Trochlear fracture; the carrying angle would be decreased or reversed. (*D*) Normally, the ulna and the radius flex on the same axis. (*E*) When the capitellum is displaced, the axis of flexion of the radius moves proximally; the two bones rotate on different axes, and motion becomes limited.

the radius, and the interosseous membrane below; the biceps tendon laterally; and the bicipital fascia medially. The distal end of the shaft may come down far enough to cause pressure on the artery (Fig. 23-43), or circulation may be obstructed when the tension in the antecubital space increases after extensive soft tissue injury.

Reduction

Displacement of the fragments threatens the blood supply, the nerve supply, the function and the appearance of the arm.

Manipulation and immobilization is the method of choice for:

1. Simple supracondylar and transcondylar fractures which are uncomplicated by excessive swelling and bleb formation, by actual or threatened interference with the blood supply, as determined from the radial pulse, or by obliquity of the fracture line.

2. Longitudinal fractures of the trochlea or the capitellum alone if there is some prospect of successful reduction.

3. Simple epicondylar fractures.

This group may be reduced and treated safely in ambulatory patients.

Hospitalization for continuous traction is the method of choice:

1. When there is actual or threatened interference with the blood supply.

2. When severe swelling and bleb formation are present. (The swelling may defeat attempts at reduction, and the trauma of reduction may increase the swelling further.)

3. For Y, T, and comminuted fractures with displacement and for other severe displacements.

4. For fractures of the trochlea or the capitellum which are unsuitable for manipulation because of swelling, nerve injury, or wide displacement.

Hospitalization for continuous traction becomes the method of choice:

1. When manipulation fails to effect reduction.

2. When the fragments cannot be held in place by splinting.

3. When excessive swelling or diminished radial pulse follows reduction and immobilization.

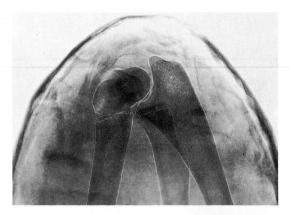

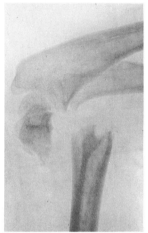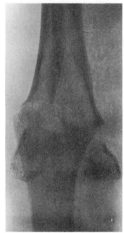

Fig. 23–43. Supracondylar fractures. (*Top*) Showing the marked displacement visible in the lateral view. (*Bottom*) Showing successful reduction. Less flexion is usually desirable.

Hospitalization and open reduction are urgent:

1. For open fractures.

2. When the radial pulse does not return after 30 to 45 minutes in traction.

3. When excessive swelling, uncontrolled by continuous elevation, threatens the venous return.

Open reduction is indicated:

1. For certain Y, T, tochlear, capitellar, and epicondylar fractures that are otherwise irreducible.

2. For irreducible supracondylar fractures.

Reduction of displacement is best done without delay, even in the presence of considerable swelling. Alignment of the fragments increases the soft-tissue space and helps to reduce swelling by reducing the pressure on veins and lymphatics.

Anesthesia. For children, general anesthesia is preferred. Good relaxation makes it easier to align the fragments and causes less soft-tissue trauma. For adults, local infiltration of the hemotoma or brachial plexus block anesthesia may be used. The latter is preferred by many.

The position of the fragments should be recorded on roentgen films immediately after application of the immobilizing dressing.

Manipulation of Supracondylar Fractures, Extension Type

The patient lies supine, with a wide strap about the upper chest fastened to the table or to an assistant for countertraction. For a fracture of the right arm, the surgeon clasps the patient's hand in a normal grip and makes steadily increasing traction on the semipronated hand for 4 or 5 minutes while the left hand palpates the fragments. Slight hyperextension may be needed to release impaction. When the shortening has been overcome, the mediolateral alignment is adjusted, and the left hand is placed on the arm with the fingers anteriorly on the shaft and the thumb posteriorly on the lower fragment. The thumb makes strong pressure to engage the fragments and the semipronated forearm is brought into moderately acute flexion. While gentle thumb pressure is maintained, gentle motion of the elbow tests the stability and the alignment. Reduction should be checked by roentgen examination and repeated if necessary. Failure to obtain or maintain reduction indicates obliquity of the plane of the fracture, and suspension and continuous traction must be instituted.

For more muscular patients, more effective traction may be produced with the pronated forearm flexed to a right angle. After shortening has been overcome by 5 to 8 minutes of traction, any mediolateral displacement is corrected by direct pressure. The surgeon then places the palm of one hand beneath the olecranon posteriorly and the other hand over the arm anteriorly and reduces the posterior displacement by direct pressure.

Immobilization. Most often, a position of moderate flexion (beyond a right angle) maintains the position of the fragments. The elbow should never be flexed to a point where the radial pulse is diminished. While the surgeon holds the arm, the posterior splint is applied over suitable padding; the elbow portion of the splint is reinforced by a plaster bandage, as illustrated in Figure 23-37, and the plaster is molded to the arm with an elastic bandage. The arm is supported by a wrist sling. The patient is then treated as for a fracture in good position.

When the reduction of a simple posterior displacement is stable and is maintained easily by simple flexion, the use of horse-collar dressing (Fig. 23-38) to keep the limb in acute flexion may be satisfac-

tory. A posterior molded plaster may be used if additional security is required. A powdered cotton or sheet-wadding pad may be placed in the crease of the elbow to avoid maceration of the skin. The untorn periosteum and the tense triceps tend to splint most of these fractures satisfactorily with the elbow flexed.

Traction and Suspension. It should be emphasized that there are those who strongly advocate traction and suspension for all supracondylar fractures with complete or marked displacement or comminution. Skin traction (Dunlop) or skeletal traction may be used. This, of course, requires hospitalization.

Manipulation of Transcondylar Fractures

When the fracture level lies low, so that the lower end of the proximal fragment is in the very thin portion of the humerus, traction and suspension rather than manipulation must be considered. Accurate reduction is very difficult, and residual displacement means trouble later.

Manipulation of Supracondylar Fractures, Flexion Type

In these cases, the lower fragment is displaced forward. Reduction may be effected by traction on the flexed semipronated forearm. When shortening has been overcome, and lateral displacement corrected, the surgeon presses the shaft forward and the articular fragment backward, and attempts to engage the fragments. When this can be accomplished, the traction is continued, and a posterior plaster splint is applied.

Good results may be obtained in these cases by reduction and immobilization in the fully extended position. Traction is made on the fully extended arm, lateral displacement is corrected, and the fragments are engaged by cross pressure. A plaster molded splint may be applied in full extension. The arm is elevated until swelling subsides and is then carried at the side. Active use of the shoulder and the fingers is encouraged.

Manipulation of Fractures of the Trochlea Alone

This is an adult type of fracture resulting from a fall on the proximal ulna. The trochlear fragment and the ulna move proximally (Fig. 23-42, C). The pull of the flexor-pronator muscles attached to the epicondyle also rotates the fragment. There is loss of the carrying angle. Reduction is attempted by traction in hyperextension with abduction of the forearm on the humerus, followed by pressure on the fragment and flexion of the forearm.

If reduction can be accomplished, a plaster splint, 4 or 6 inches wide, is applied from the axilla down the medial side of the arm, beneath the elbow, and up the lateral side of the arm to the deltoid. It is molded snugly to the lateral contours of the distal humerus. A second splint is applied from the axillary fold, down the arm, over the point of the elbow and down the ulnar side of the forearm to the knuckles. A snug elastic bandage must be applied from the knuckles to the deltoid.

More often than not, this fracture requires open reduction for accurate maintenance of position.

Manipulation of Fractures of the Capitellum Alone (Fig. 23-42, B)

Two types of fracture occur here. In one type, the fracture line passes lateral to the trochlear notch. In the second type, the fracture line goes through the trochlear notch or medial to it. Lateral displacement of the ulna accompanies the second type. This second type requires open reduction. Closed reduction may be tried in the first type if there is no dislocation of the ulna and if there is no significant displacement of the lateral fragment. Very accurate reduction is desirable. If this is not obtained, open reduction is indicated.

Reduction is attempted by traction in hyperextension with adduction of the forearm on the humerus, followed by

pressure on the fragment and flexion of the forearm in supination. The arm is splinted as for a fracture of the trochlear side.

Manipulation of Fractures of the Medial Epicondyle

Avulsion of the medial epicondylar epiphysis may be a complication of lateral dislocation of the elbow, especially in childhood. Isolated fracture of the epicondyle also occurs from direct violence. The amount of displacement varies. Pronation of the forearm and direct pressure may reduce the displacement. When the epicondyle is caught in the joint space, the forearm is supinated and the elbow, the wrist, and the fingers are extended. The forearm then is abducted in order to increase the gap between the trochlea and the ulna; this may allow the epicondyle a free route of exit from the joint, as it is pulled by the tension of the flexor-pronator muscles that originate from it. Some surgeons prefer to operate immediately when the fragment is in the joint space, or when ulnar nerve injury is present, without attempting closed reduction.

Manipulation of Fractures of the Capitellar Epiphysis (Fig. 23-44)

This fracture probably occurs when a posterolateral dislocation carries the fragment posteriorly. Clinically, no dislocation appears to be present because the dislocated joint surfaces fall forward to approximately the normal position, and the fragment lies anterior to the humerus. Closed reduction may be obtained by redislocating the elbow posterolaterally, reducing the fragment, and then reducing the dislocation. If this is possible, quite often the fragment is held accurately in place. Care must be taken to move the radius and the ulna medially to obtain accurate position. Even a slight displacement of the capiteller epiphysis can result

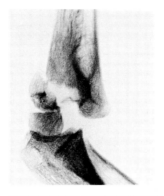
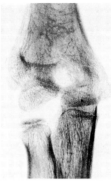
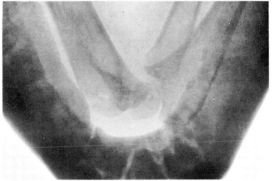

Fig. 23-44. (*Top*) Intercondylar fracture, with the capitellar portion broken off and displaced posteriorly. (*Bottom*) Showing the fracture reduced and fixed by a posterior plaster splint in acute flexion.

in deformity. Open reduction without delay is indicated if accurate replacement is not obtained.

Manipulation of Fractures of the Lateral Epicondyle

This rare fracture follows direct violence or avulsion of the radial collateral ligament. Considerable displacement rarely occurs, but when it does occur, it may be corrected by direct pressure with the forearm fully flexed and fully supinated. Immobilization in full supination is continued for 3 or 4 weeks. Open reduction is occasionally necessary.

TREATMENT OF EPIPHYSEAL SEPARATIONS AT THE LOWER END OF THE HUMERUS

Simple epiphyseal separation without diaphyseal fracture is not common. When

it does occur, it is treated in the same way as is an uncomplicated supracondylar fracture, (p. 38).

EARLY CHOICE OF TREATMENT FOR FRACTURES OF THE HUMERUS AT THE ELBOW

Although many fractures in the region of the elbow can be reduced and treated safely in ambulatory patients, there are many others that, by reason of comminution, displacement, or complications, such as nerve or vascular injuries or swelling, cannot be treated satisfactorily without hospitalization and traction. It is essential to recognize these latter fractures at an early stage of treatment and not to attempt prolonged or repeated reductions by manipulation. Traction and suspension are the safest methods of handling some of the more severe and complicated injuries.

TREATMENT AFTER REDUCTION

After immobilization, the part must be elevated, with the hand higher than the rest of the arm, and kept at rest until the swelling subsides. The patient should be examined within 6 or 8 hours after reduction to note any difficulty in circulation. The dressings should be loosened without hesitation if the edema of the hand increases, if the hand becomes cold or cyanotic, or if the patient complains of pain in the forearm or parethesias in the hand. If no improvement occurs in 10 or 15 minutes, the immobilizing dressing should be removed and the patient should be hospitalized.

Exercise of the hand must begin at once. Roentgenograms are required immediately after application of the immobilizing dressing and again 1 week later. If the position changes during this period, it can often be corrected. Additional films are made from time to time as indicated.

As the swelling subsides, the immobilizing dressing may become loose and should be snugged as necessary.

After removal of the immobilizing dressing in 2 to 4 weeks, active use is continued. No physiotherapy need be used, or at the most a daily warm bath and gentle massage. Any attempt to increase the range of motion by manipulation or passive force is contraindicated. Active use will more rapidly increase the range of motion of an injured elbow than any other modality. The prognosis in uncomplicated fractures treated by closed reduction is usually good.

POSTERIOR DISLOCATION AT THE ELBOW

Etiology and Anatomy. The capsule of the elbow joint is loose and thin anteriorly and posteriorly; laterally, the capsule is reinforced by lateral ligaments. The ulnar articulation is the strong point; there is a close fit of the coronoid process and the olecranon on the trochlear hinge, and the wide flange of the trochlea on the medial side bears against the transversely convex olecranon. When the normal range of extension is exceeded, the capsule tears, and posterior dislocation tends to occur. During a fall that hyperextends or abducts the forearm, the forward thrust of the humerus completes the dislocation.

The radius is bound to the ulna by the strong orbicular ligament and the interosseous membrane; the two bones usually dislocate as a unit.

The coronoid process, the head of the radius, and the lateral ligaments resist dislocation. Most of the posterior dislocations are complicated by fracture of the coronoid process, the head of the radius, or the epicondyles, which are torn away when the lateral ligaments do not give. The brachialis muscle and the triceps may also be injured.

Diagnosis. The patient may hold his arm extended or partly flexed. The anteroposterior diameter of the elbow is increased greatly, the antecubital space bulges, and, seen from the front, the forearm looks short. Swelling increases rapidly, but rarely to the point that the epicondyles and the olecranon cannot be defined and compared. With the forearm flexed, the olecranon lies far behind its normal situation, and the forearm appears shortened when compared with the opposite side. The normal relationship of olecranon to epicondyles is maintained in supracondylar fractures. Motion of the joint is much less than normal and very painful when dislocation is present. Roentgen examination should precede reductions; complicating fractures are the rule rather than the exception (Fig. 23-45).

Treatment. Parvin has described a method of reducing uncomplicated dislocations without anesthesia. The patient lies prone on a high table with the affected limb hanging over the side. In really apprehensive patients a suitable dose of narcotic may be given. After a few minutes, gentle downward traction is applied at the wrist.

All the time necessary is taken. After 1 to 2 minutes of traction, the olecranon will be felt to ride distally over the humerus. At this point, the operator, while

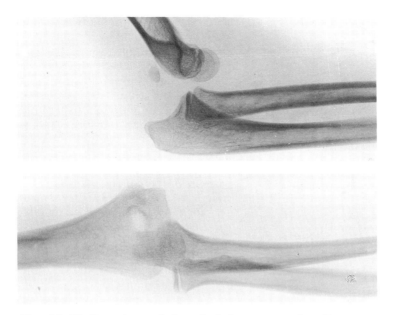

Fig. 23–45. Posterior and lateral dislocation at the elbow in a 7-year-old child. (*Top*) Posterior dislocation and separation of the medial epicondylar epiphysis with backward displacement. (*Bottom*) Lateral dislocation. The medial epicondylar epiphysis is seen faintly behind the medial condyle.

maintaining traction at the wrist with one hand, gently lifts the humerus laterally to flex the elbow about 20°, often completing the reduction (Fig. 23-46). Reduction in this fashion is so gentle that frequently, on lifting the humerus, the elbow is found to·be reduced, and one is not certain when reduction actually occurred.

Lavine has described another simple method. He places padding over the back of the chair on which the patient sits and then hangs the arm over the back of the chair (Fig. 23-47). The patient is assured that there will be little or no discomfort, and he is allowed to rest until the arm relaxes. The surgeon places one hand over the upper arm and pulls down on the patient's hand with the other. Lavine states that usually the dislocation reduces with ease. No anesthetic is required. Post-reduction treatment is given as described below. Reduction with the elbow in flexion may result in less soft tissue damage than does reduction in full extension.

Anesthesia. General anesthesia is preferred when anesthesia is needed. When

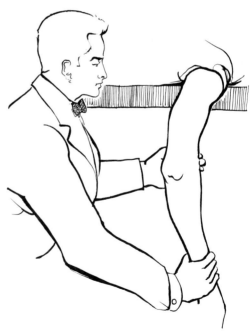

Fig. 23–46. Reduction of dislocation of elbow with dependent traction. Humerus is lifted laterally with traction maintained on wrist. (Parvin, R. W.: Arch. Surg., 75:972, 1957)

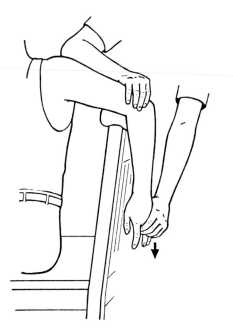

Fig. 23–47. Reduction of posterior dislocation of the elbow. After allowing the forearm to hang until relaxed, the surgeon makes traction as indicated. (Lavine, L. S.: J. Bone Joint Surg., *35A-*:786, 1953)

general anesthesia is contraindicated, brachial plexus block or local infiltration may be used. A suitable time must be allowed to elapse after the injection of the local anesthetic before manipulation is attempted.

Manipulation. The patient is placed on the table as for reduction of a fracture of a humerus. After any lateral subluxation has been reduced, traction is made on the forearm in partial flexion to bring the coronoid process of the ulna below the trochlear portion of the humerus. After a few minutes, the shaft of the humerus is pressed toward the table and additional upward traction is made on the hand. With a gentle rocking motion, the bones disengage, the forearm comes forward, and a distinct snap indicates that reduction has occurred. Flexion, extension, and rotation are carried out so that any obstruction to movement may be identified. A padded posterior molded splint should be applied and supported with an elastic bandage (Fig. 23-37).

Elevation and ice bags for the next 2 or 3 days tend to decrease swelling and pain. Full active use of the shoulder and the fingers is recommended from the beginning. Immobilization for from 2 to 3 weeks is usually satisfactory.

Following removal of the immobilizing dressing, hot soaks and gentle massage may be useful. Passive motion and stretching of the joint are prohibited. In the absence of complicating fractures, the prognosis is excellent if active use is started early and continued regularly.

Complications. Extensive injury to the soft tissues, and especially to the brachialis muscle, often occurs. Aside from the stiffness, the most troublesome complication may be ossification in the brachialis muscle or elsewhere about the joint.

Fractures of the head of the radius, the apex of the coronoid process, or the medial epicondyle may accompany dislocations. The medial epicondyle may remain in the joint space after reduction of the dislocation. It may be brought out by the method described on page 61. Fractures of the condyles, the capitellum, and the bones elsewhere in the forearm may occur.

When fractures are present, the dislocation is reduced in the usual way, and the fracture then is manipulated in whatever manner is necessary. The elbow is immobilized in the position that best maintains reduction of the fracture. Unreduced fractures are treated as described under the individual fractures, the reduced dislocation requiring no special additional treatment.

SUBLUXATION OF THE HEAD OF THE RADIUS: "PULLED ELBOW"

Peculiar to young children, usually under 8 years of age, is the injury called "pulled elbow." This is a subluxation of the head of the radius following a sudden pull on a child's extended arm, perhaps to keep him from falling or to lift him up over a curb. Usually the child cries out, dangles the arm at the side, and refuses to move it. He resists examination. A typical history, tenderness over the radial head,

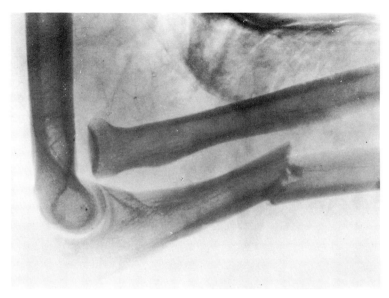

Fig. 23–48. Fracture of the ulna and anterior dislocation of the head of the radius.

and restriction of rotation make the diagnosis. There is no gross abnormality in the appearance of the limb, and roentgen examination is usually normal.

Treatment. The subluxation can usually be reduced without difficulty and without anesthesia. The forearm is flexed slightly and rotated gently while making pressure over the radial head and putting some pressure on the elbow to increase the lateral joint space. Quite often there is a palpable click, followed by a quick change in the condition of the youngster and his renewed ability to actively move the limb. Some people believe that no immobilization is necessary; others advise the use of a sling for a few days or a plaster posterior splint for no more than a week.

DISLOCATION OF THE RADIUS AT THE ELBOW WITH FRACTURE OF THE ULNA

(The Monteggia Fracture-Dislocation)

When the proximal ulna is fractured and displaced, there must be an associated displacement of the radius, either a fracture or a dislocation, proximally or distally. The most frequent type of displacement is a dislocation of the head of the radius (Fig. 23-48).

Diagnosis. Any fracture of the shaft or the proximal portion of the ulna may be complicated by dislocation of the head of the radius. Roentgen films of a fracture of the ulna or the radius must always include the entire bones and the adjacent joints, since deformity of one bone must always be associated with some displacement of the other.

Treatment. Closed reduction should be attempted using local, regional, or general anesthesia. The displacement of the ulnar fragments must be corrected first. Simple traction and extension may be attempted, or traction may be applied with the elbow flexed. As the shortening is corrected, the displacement of the head of the radius may correct itself, or it may be aided by direct pressure over the head of the radius. Failure to obtain satisfactory reduction of both the ulna and the head of the radius may necessitate hospitalization for open reduction. If closed reduction is successful, subsequent treatment is similar to that for fracture of the ulna (p. 67). Repeat roentgenograms can be taken after

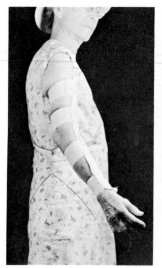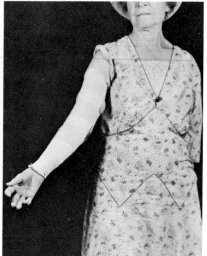

Fig. 23–49. Fracture of the olecranon with displacement. An anterior plaster splint is fastened with 2-inch adhesive; a firm flannel bandage completes the dressing.

a few days to ascertain that the head of the radius remains satisfactorily reduced.

FRACTURES
OF THE OLECRANON

Anatomy and Etiology. The proximal ulna is composed of spongy bone, and it is weak in the hollow of the sigmoid fossa. Falls on the forearm and elbow may cause fractures through the fossa. When the fracture is complete and the periosteum and the aponeurosis of the triceps are torn, the triceps draws the olecranon into extension and proximally. Hematoma and torn aponeurosis may occupy the space between the fragments, but the separation may be slight because of the large fibrous expansion of the triceps, which may maintain the fragments in satisfactory apposition.

The epiphysis for the olecranon usually appears between the eighth and the eleventh years and fuses with the shaft between the seventeenth and the nineteenth years. Epiphyseal separation occurs very rarely, and the epiphyseal line should not be mistaken for a fracture.

Diagnosis. Discoloration, swelling, and tenderness over the olecranon may be present after an injury, even if no separation of the fragments occurs. There is

pain on attempted motion of the elbow, especially when the patient attempts to extend the arm against resistance, and there may inability to fully extend the elbow. Palpation of the subcutaneous border of the ulna will usually disclose acute tenderness and irregularity or notching when displacement has occurred. When the fragments are widely separated, the deformity is both palpable and visible.

Acute traumatic olecranon bursitis may simulate fracture without displacement. In this situation, however, the swelling is usually limited to the bursa, and the tenderness is not localized sharply. Patients who have had previous attacks of bursitis will often have hard villi in the bursal floor; these are acutely tender after a hard blow and make the subcutaneous border of the ulna feel irregular. In these cases, active extension of the elbow against resistance does not usually cause pain. Preliminary examination should always include a search for additional fractures of the limb.

Treatment. If no separation of the fragments is palpable, an anterior molded splint (Fig. 23-49) is applied and roentgenograms are taken. If these show no separation of the fragments, elevation and ice bags are applied for from 24 to 48 hours.

Active use of the hand and shoulder is encouraged. The splint may be removed after 4 weeks, and hot soaks and massage are instituted to avoid stiffness.

When separation of the fragments is found at the preliminary examination, the arm should be splinted from the palm to the axilla in a little less than full extension (Fig. 23-50). Roentgenograms can then be made, and if the fragments remain separated appreciably with the arm extended, open reduction is indicated.

If the fragments are in good contact with the arm extended, either the splint is not disturbed or a plaster splint is applied from the palm to the axilla, with the elbow flexed about 10° (Fig. 23-49). A pressure dressing is applied, and elevation and ice bags are advised until the post-traumatic reaction subsides. Active use should be begun without delay. After 4 to 5 weeks, the splint is removed and the roentgenograms again are made. If definite union is present, an elastic bandage is applied about the extended elbow and active, but limited, flexion is allowed. Hot soaks and massage should be prescribed twice daily for stiffness. If there is only meager evidence of union, the splint should be reapplied for an additional 2 or 3 weeks. Treatment is then continued as described above.

Some olecranon fractures are so comminuted that even at operation it may be impossible to reconstruct the bone in good position. Excision of the fragments and repair of the triceps insertion will usually allow good elbow function.

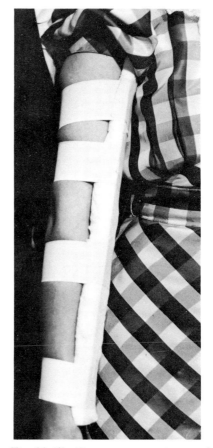

Fig. 23–50. Temporary anterior wooden splint for fracture of the olecranon when the fragments are displaced.

FRACTURES OF THE HEAD AND THE NECK OF THE RADIUS

ANATOMY

The head of the radius glides over the capitellum when the forearm is flexed and rotates on the capitellum and the lesser sigmoid fossa of the ulna during pronation and supination. The orbicular ligament holds the head against the fossa of the ulna in rotation and makes the radius follow the ulna in flexion and extension. The lateral, thickened portion of the joint capsule also adds to the stability of the articulation. When the orbicular ligament and the lateral ligament tear, dislocation of the proximal end of the radius occurs.

The epiphysis for the head appears between the fifth and the seventh years and fuses with the shaft between the seventeenth and the twentieth years.

ETIOLOGY

During a fall on the pronated hand, the head of the radius may be thrust against the capitellum with force sufficient to split the head or impact it on the neck. Falls on the elbow frequently cause fractures of the head and neck, as do blows on the outer side of the forearm below the elbow.

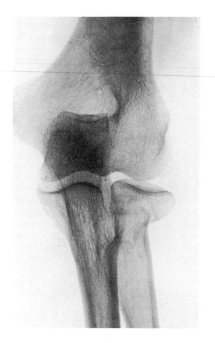

Fig. 23–51. Fracture of the head of the radius with negligible displacement.

DISPLACEMENTS

Splitting or comminution of the head is the common form of fracture (Fig. 23-51). The orbicular ligament may retain the fragments in good position, or they may be displaced from beneath the ligament anteriorly, near the muscle mass laterally, or into the joint space proximally. The entire head may be broken off and displaced from beneath the orbicular ligament. This is the common type of displacement after separation of the proximal epiphysis of the radius.

After fracture of the neck, the fragments may be angulated with the angle open medially and posteriorly due to the pull of the biceps. With comminution of the neck, the head tends to move distally and rotates.

DIAGNOSIS

After severe elbow injuries, the roentgenologist must show the head and the neck of the radius clearly. Some fractures are identified only after repeated roentgenograms in oblique views.

The clinical diagnosis of fractures of the head or the neck of the radius is based on pain at the site of the fracture, swelling over the anterolateral aspect of the elbow joint, and painful and limited rotation and flexion of the forearm. There is localized tenderness, which is accentuated by rotation with the thumb pressing on the head of the radius. In occasional cases, on palpating the lateral aspect of the forearm just distal to the lateral epicondyle, it will be noted that the head does not rotate with the shaft, that crepitus is present, or that there is some deformity when compared with the opposite side.

In many cases, fractures cannot be identified or excluded except by means of roentgenograms. Even when a definite diagnosis is made on the basis of physical signs, roentgenograms are still urgently needed to determine the degree of displacement.

TREATMENT

Immediately after examination, a snug elastic bandage is applied about the flexed elbow, and a sling is applied. As an alternative, the flexed elbow is covered with cotton or sheet wadding, which is bound firmly with a bandage, and a sling is applied. Roentgen examination should be done.

Treatment of Separation of the Upper Epiphysis of the Radius. This usually occurs between 7 and 15 years of age. In smaller children, the ossified center of the epiphysis represents only a small part of the large cartilaginous head. Even when clinical signs are definite, repeated oblique views of the elbow may be necessary to demonstrate a displacement of the head in small children.

When displacement is slight or absent, the separation is treated as is a fracture in good position (Fig. 23-52). When there is marked tilting of the head, manipulation should be attempted to improve position. With the patient under general anesthesia, the elbow is extended and the forearm is adducted by making lateral pressure on the medial side of the joint. The forearm is so rotated that the most prominent part of the head lies laterally. Strong digital

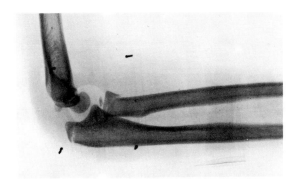

Fig. 23–52. Fracture of the neck of the radius in a 4-year-old child. The center of ossification is very small. The olecranon shows a fracture without displacement. The forearm was immobilized by means of an internal right-angled splint for 25 days; a perfect result was obtained.

pressure is then made on the head to replace it. A plaster splint is applied with the elbow at a right angle, and the forearm in neutral position.

When the head has slipped beneath the orbicular ligament into the joint space or toward the muscle mass, and if attempts at closed reduction fail, early open reduction must be performed. In a child, the head of the radius should *never* be excised.

Choice of Treatment for Fractures. The disc-shaped head of the radius fits snugly beneath the orbicular ligament and rotates smoothly. Fracture of the head tends to destroy a portion of this articular surface and leaves it roughened. When comminution and displacement are slight, simple treatment produces good results. When the destruction of the head is more extensive, the ultimate result of conservative treatment will be a thickened irregular head, with considerable impairment of elbow function and pain. In these cases, the best results are obtained by removal of the head of the radius. Operation should be performed during the first week to 10 days or delayed until after the acute results of trauma have subsided.

Fractures Amenable to Simple Treatment. Certain fractures will heal with little distortion of the articular surfaces and with little change in the size of the head. These are: (1) incomplete fractures of the head; (2) simple splitting of the head without displacement; (3) chip fractures without displacement or with displacement of the chip into the muscle mass laterally, the chip being disregarded unless it produces symptoms later; (4) fractures involving less than one-fourth

or one-third of the articular surface and in good position; (5) impacted fractures of the head with slight displacement; and (6) fractures of the neck with no displacement or moderate displacement that does not limit motion. These fractures should be immobilized in a posterior molded splint, with the elbow at a right angle and the forearm in neutral position, for 10 to 14 days; then active motion is started with the partial protection of a sling for a short period. Active use is then encouraged.

Displaced fractures of the neck of the radius may be reducible. With the elbow extended and the forearm supinated and an assistant exerting strong proximal traction on the arm, lateral pressure should be made over the medial humeral condyle until the carrying angle is reversed, the lateral joint space thus being opened. Direct pressure, anteriorly or posteriorly, should be made on the proximal fragment to replace it.

Fractures Treated Best by Operation (Fig. 23-53). These are fractures with (1) extensive comminution of the head and neck; (2) displacement of the head or more than one-third of the head from beneath the orbicular ligament; (3) impaction of the head or angulation at the neck causing marked distortion of the ulnar or the capitellar articulation; or (4) the presence of loose fragments in the joint space. In fractures of this type, early open reduction and excision of the head of the radius is the treatment of choice except in children.

PROGNOSIS

The results of treatment of simple frac-

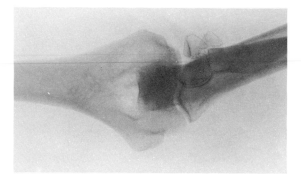

Fig. 23–53. Comminuted fracture of the head of the radius. There is likely to be limitation of motion after any method of treatment in this type of fracture. If the fragments are removed, the prognosis is improved.

tures are usually good, although slight limitation of motion may persist. Following resection of the head of the radius, there is usually little residual disability, although there may be slight limitation of motion and some discomfort on heavy activity.

FRACTURES OF THE SHAFT OF THE ULNA

Anatomy and Etiology. The ulna is thick at its proximal end and tapers off toward the distal end. The sharp posterior border is subcutaneous and readily palpable.

Fractures occur most often in the middle and distal thirds of the bone. Direct violence received in fending off a blow or when holding the elbow out of an automobile is the common cause. Open fractures are common. The fracture line may be transverse, oblique, or comminuted. Fractures of the proximal third with overlapping are always accompanied by displacement of the radius, due either to fracture or to dislocation of the head (Monteggia fracture) (Fig. 23-48). The ulnar fragments form an angle open posteriorly, the proximal fragment being flexed; they also move toward the radius. In fractures of the middle or the distal third, the pronator quadratus tends to pull the distal fragment toward the radius, but overlapping rarely occurs unless there is an associated fracture or dislocation of the radius. As stated above, any displaced fracture of the ulna must be accompanied by displacement of the radius, and roentgenograms must always include the entire forearm to identify the proximal and distal abnormalities.

Treatment. A well-padded internal right-angled splint from palm to axilla, covered by a snug bandage and a triangular sling, provides a good preliminary dressing. An air splint it also frequently useful. The splint should be broad enough to prevent direct pressure on the ulna, thus avoiding angulation of the fragments. Immediate roentgen examination is required.

If the fragments are in good position, a long arm cast with light padding should be applied from the proximal humerus to the knuckles, with the elbow at a right angle and the forearm in neutral position. When used as an initial dressing, the cast should always be split to the skin along the ulnar border to allow for early relief of swelling, and the hand should be carried with the fingers elevated until the swelling subsides. Early use of a sling can be pernicious in that it allows maintenance of a dependent position, and it should be discouraged for the first few days. Preferably, the injured arm should be carried with the opposite hand under the elbow and with the fingers elevated for the first few days. The cast should always support the fifth metacarpal and should always stop at the proximal palmar crease to allow full finger flexion. Active use of the arm should be begun promptly. Another roentgen examination should be obtained in a week to 10 days. Usually 5 weeks of immobilization is satisfactory. After this time, the limb is examined for union and the condition is verified by films. If union is incomplete, another cast is applied.

If the fragments are not in good position, reduction must be performed without delay. The patient is prepared as for reduction of a fracture of both bones of the forearm. General, regional, or local anesthesia may be used. Powerful, steady traction is applied to the hand for about 10 minutes to secure alignment of the fragments. Pressure then is made on the head of the radius to reduce the dislocation. While traction is continued, anterior and posterior molded splints are applied over suitable light padding, from the knuckles to the axilla, with the elbow flexed 80° to 90° and with the forearm in mid-rotation. These are secured with elastic bandages. The position of the fragments is verified by obtaining films as soon as the plaster is fixed. After 3 or 4 days, new films should be obtained. If the position is still satisfactory, the immobilizing dressing may be converted into a cast and treatment continued as for fractures in good position.

For fractures low in the shaft, reduction may be achieved by having an assistant hold the forearm in supination and the elbow in flexion while the surgeon makes direct pressure with his thumbs and forces both fragments posteriorly until he has converted the deformity into a posterior bowing. Then he presses between the radius and the ulna and forces the two bones apart to restore the normal interosseous space; the posterior bowing is corrected by direct pressure. If the radius is not fractured or dislocated, it may help if traction is made on the forearm with the hand forced to the radial side while the surgeon reduces the posterior bowing.

Failure to secure reduction necessitates operation. An open fracture always requires immediate operation.

FRACTURES OF THE SHAFT OF THE RADIUS

Anatomy and Etiology. The proximal radius is slender and cylindrical as compared with the large distal end. The proximal four-fifths is composed of dense, strong bone, while the distal portion is composed of spongy bone. The bone curves outward distal to the bicipital tuberosity, and the interosseous space is widest at about the junction of the middle and distal thirds. The proximal third is well covered by muscle; the distal portion is covered by tendons and is more easily palpable. This distal portion is slightly concave on the flexor side.

The radius is the more movable bone of the forearm and receives the pull of the pronators and the supinators. After fracture, muscle pull largely determines displacement, and muscle tension, lengthwise and spirally, contributes to overlapping and to angulation of the fragments toward the interosseous space. Fracture of the lower portion usually occurs by indirect violence, such as falls on the hand. Fracture of the proximal portion frequently results from the direct violence of a blow or from compression.

Displacements. The most powerful muscle attached to the proximal portion of the radius is the biceps, which acts at the bicipital tuberosity. It flexes and supinates the forearm. Normally, the supinator action of the biceps is opposed by the pronator quadratus. The pronator teres attaches to the radius about one-third of the way down the shaft, and the pronator quadratus attaches distally. Therefore, fracture of the proximal third of the bone (Fig. 23-54) permits the biceps to flex and supinate the proximal fragment, while the pronator teres and pronator quadratus pronate the distal fragment.

Fractures of the middle third do not exhibit this type of displacement. Both the biceps and the pronator teres are attached to the proximal fragment, and they tend to balance each other, so that the proximal fragment tends to lie in midposition, while the distal fragment tends to lie in pronation. Encroachment on the interosseous space may be the principal displacement.

In the distal third of the bone, the cross pull is less active, and displacement is often due to the original violence. The pronator quadratus pulls the distal fragment toward the ulnar and flexor side, and the tension of the extensors of the thumb,

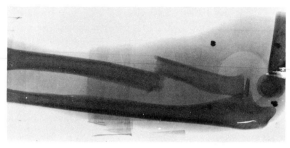

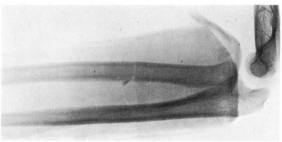

Fig. 23–54. (*Top*) Fracture of the shaft of the radius at the junction of the middle and the upper thirds. The proximal fragment is held flexed by the biceps. The distal fragment has moved toward the ulna, and the interosseous space has decreased. (*Bottom*) After reduction.

which are wrapped around the radius in pronation, also forces the fragment in the same direction. The distal fragment always rotates with the hand.

Diagnosis. Fractures without displacement exhibit only localized tenderness in addition to swelling and pain. Crepitus and pain on rotation may or may not be present.

Fractures without displacement in the distal portion are identified readily by inability to supinate, and perhaps by an unusual prominence of the distal end of the ulna resulting from subluxation. It is more difficult to identify fractures without displacement in the proximal third because of the large surrounding muscle mass.

Treatment. Fractures of the radius in good position are treated in the same manner as are those of the ulna (p.   ). Pressure on the subcutaneous border of the bone must be avoided, lest the fragments be pushed toward the interosseous space. Pressure of the fingers on the wet plaster directly between the bones helps to hold them apart. Fractures in the proximal third that appear at all unstable require immobilization in a fully supinated position as a rule. Fractures with displacement require reduction without delay unless the fracture line is oblique or

comminuted, in which case hospitalization is preferable. With the patient under suitable anesthesia (i.e., general, intravenous perfusion, local, or brachial block), strong, steady traction is made on the flexed and supinated forearm by way of the thumb and index finger, so that the hand is forced towards the ulnar side. After shortening has been overcome, direct pressure on the distal fragment may secure alignment. Always bring the distal fragment into line with the proximal. Fractures in the proximal third are usually best immobilized in supination; those in the middle or the distal third may be fixed in midposition or even in some pronation. Prereduction x-ray films, taken with the roentgen plate, parallel to the arm, the humeral condyles against the plate, the olecranon about one-third of the way down the plate, and the x-ray tube directed toward the elbow joint at about 20° from the horizontal, can be used to determine the amount of rotation of the proximal radius. The forearm should be immobilized with the distal fragment in this predetermined degree of rotation, using the view of the bicipital tuberosity as a guide to rotation of the proximal fragment.

Simple angulation may be corrected by firm pressure in the interosseous space to

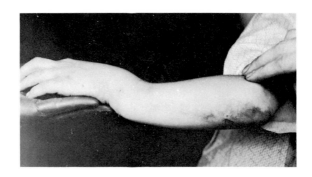

Fig. 23–55. Fracture of both bones of the forearm with considerable angulation. The point of the angle is toward the flexor side.

overcome the narrowing, combined with direct pressure at the fracture site. It is helpful if an assistant makes traction on the forearm as described above, so that the surgeon may use both hands in manipulation. Extreme caution must be exercised to avoid causing an overlap.

Closed reduction of fractures of the distal third of the radius is always unsatisfactory; these fractures require open reduction.

If subluxation has occurred at the inferior radio-ulnar joint, it is advisable to press the bones together in the dressing at this point to avoid later difficulty.

FRACTURES OF THE SHAFTS OF BOTH BONES OF THE FOREARM

ANATOMY AND ETIOLOGY

The main anatomic points have been covered. These fractures result from both falls and direct violence.

DISPLACEMENTS

Direct violence usually breaks both bones at the same level. Indirect violence due to a fall on the hand usually breaks the radius at a higher level than that of the break of the ulna. The radius takes the thrust and breaks; then the thrust is transmitted to the ulna by the fibers of the interosseous membrane, which attach at a lower level on the latter bone.

The bones are concave on the flexor and the interosseous surfaces. The interosseous space always is narrowed by the action of the pronators and by the extensors of the thumb, which draw the frag-

ments together. The distal end of the radius tends to move proximally, and the head of the ulna becomes more prominent. When the proximal third of the radius is fractured, the displacement is similar to that of a fracture of the radius alone; the proximal fragment lies in supination; the lower, in pronation. When the fracture is through the middle or the distal third, the proximal fragment tends to lie closer to the midposition, and the distal fragments tend to be pronated. Overlapping is common, the distal fragments usually lying posteriorly. Greenstick fractures are common in children, the displacement here being mainly angulation, usually with the angle open toward the posterior surface.

DIAGNOSIS

The common types of overlapping and greenstick fractures usually are recognized at a glance (Fig. 23-55). Careful examination for multiple fractures must be made. Fractures in good position may be identified by localized swelling, by the sharply localized acute tenderness, and by some palpable irregularity of contour. Crepitus and mobility should be sought with caution, if at all, to avoid further displacement of the fracture. Roentgen examination is necessary in all cases for accurate determination of the position of the fragments.

EMERGENCY CARE

After the initial examination has been completed, the forearm is immobilized from the knuckles to the axilla on a heavily padded internal right-angled splint, the dorsum of the forearm being protected by an additional padded splint extending from the knuckles to the elbow. A firm bandage and a triangular sling complete the dressing. Plaster splints or air splints may also be used. The patient is instructed to keep the arm elevated, with the hand higher than the rest of the arm, and to apply cold in the form of ice bags. Films are made immediately, so that reduction may be performed without delay.

TREATMENT

Treatment of Fractures in Good Position

Fractures are in good position if the interosseous space is not narrowed, if no considerable angulation is present, and if, for each bone, the fragments are in stable apposition for from one-third to one-half of the diameter at the fracture site.

When little or no displacement of the fragments has occurred, the forearm is flexed to a right angle and is rotated to the appropriate degree of rotation. A plaster splint or cast is applied from the knuckles to the axilla and is compressed smoothly over the interosseous space to maintain separation of the fragments. The patient is instructed to keep the arm elevated, with the fingers higher than the elbow. Initially, the use of a sling is often pernicious, since the patient often thinks this is an important part of the treatment. It should be stressed to the patient that the hand should be elevated whenever possible to allow drainage from the fingers toward the heart. The fingers and the shoulder should be exercised from the beginning. If a circular cast is used, it should always be split along the ulnar border to allow prompt relief of abnormal pressure, and the circulation should be watched carefully. Active use of the fingers and the shoulder should be started from the very beginning. Films are made after 1 week and are repeated as necessary. In children, from 4 to 6 weeks of immobilization usually is adequate. In adults, the cast is removed after 6 weeks, and the extent of union is estimated by palpation and roentgenography. If union is reasonably solid, no dressing is applied. If little callus has formed, a cast is reapplied for an additional period. Union tends to be slow in most of these fractures. Patients who use the hand constantly during the period of immobilization usually have little difficulty with stiffness of the wrist or elbow, and soaks and gentle massage twice daily rapidly overcome what disability there is.

Treatment of Fractures With Angulation Only

In children, the bones often break incompletely, and bend, producing a greenstick type of fracture (Fig. 23-56). After the films have been inspected, reduction is performed. An assistant makes traction on the patient's hand with the forearm flexed to a right angle, and countertraction is maintained either with a flannel sling or by another assistant. The surgeon grasps the forearm above and below the fracture site, his thumbs pressing into the interosseous space and his fingers flat on the opposite surface. A common error is to grasp the bones so as to press them toward each other; the interosseous space thus is narrowed, and it is very difficult to overcome this later. Angulation should be overcome sharply, and the bones should be permitted to spring back to normal position. The normal concavity of the flexor side must be borne in mind. A plaster cast should be applied from the knuckles to the axilla (Fig. 23-57) and molded with firm pressure over the interosseous space. If circular plaster is used, it should be immediately split to the skin along the ulnar border to allow relief if swelling should occur subsequently. The patient is then treated as for a fracture in good position.

Treatment of Fractures With Displacement

Open fractures require immediate operation.

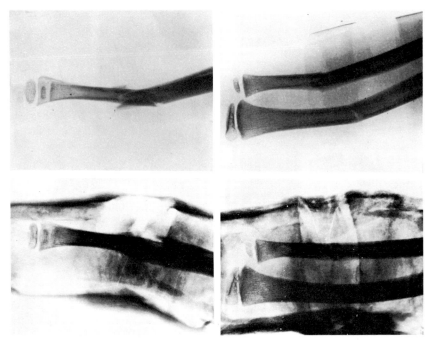

Fig. 23–56. (*Top*) Greenstick fracture of both bones of the forearm. (*Bottom*) After reduction. Same patient as in Figure 23–57.

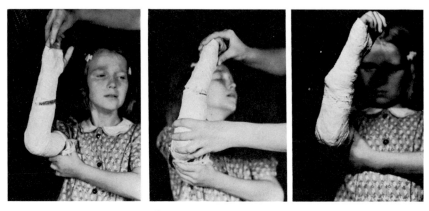

Fig. 23–57. Correction of angulation of a greenstick fracture. The point of the angle was toward the flexor surface. The cast was cut on the dorsal surface, and a wedge was removed on the flexor surface. The angulation then was corrected, and the correction was maintained with circular plaster. (See Fig. 23–56)

In the case of closed fractures, the films must be inspected for obliquity or comminution of the fracture. When these conditions occur, reduction must be supplemented by internal fixation to maintain position. In the presence of considerable soft tissue injury with much swelling, reduction is likely to be extremely difficult and hospitalization is indicated.

Reduction must be performed as promptly as possible. Adequate facilities for anesthesia, expert roentgen control,

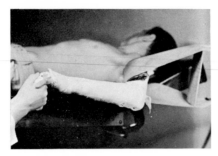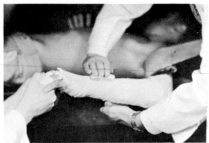

Fig. 23–58. (*Left*) Setup for reduction of fractures in the forearm. A wide strap is placed about the upper arm; it is padded anteriorly with 2 or 3 thicknesses of felt. Plaster splints are applied and fastened with gauze bandage after reduction. (*Right*) Application of Pressure to maintain the interosseous space. The surgeon has reversed the position of his right arm for the photograph. With his foot on a stool, his knee is used to brace his left hand. Circular plaster then is applied, and the procedure is repeated until the plaster is hard.

good assistance, and a means of preparing and applying plaster rapidly are basic necessities. It is extremely difficult to reduce these fractures and to maintain them in position, and, unless the practitioner has both the facilities and the experience, expert help should be obtained, or the patient should be transferred to the hospital.

In children, slight overlapping of the fragments, if alignment is good is usually compatible with a good result.

For reduction, we use a modification of Böhler's method (Fig. 23-58), employing general, regional, or local anesthesia. The roentgen films are hung within sight of the surgeon. With the patient in the supine position on the table, the injured arm over the side, the forearm is flexed to 90°, and a piece of felt is placed in front of the arm just above the elbow. A wide strap is passed over this and is fastened to a fixed object beyond the head of the table. An assistant then seats himself and makes steady traction on the thumb with one hand and somewhat less traction on the second, third, and fourth fingers with the other. For fractures in the proximal third, the hand is held in moderate supination; for those in the middle or lower third, it is held in appropriate rotation. After 5 to 10 minutes, the overlapping and the subluxation at the distal

radio-ulnar joint are usually overcome. The assistant continues the traction, and the surgeon presses on the interosseous space, with his thumbs on the flexor surface and his fingers on the extensor surface, to force the bones apart into normal relationship. End-to-end apposition of the radial and ulnar fragments then easily may be adjusted.

When reduction is complete, and while traction is continued, a molded, lightly padded, plaster splint is applied to the extensor surface, from the knuckles, over the point of the elbow, and up to the axilla, and is fastened with an elastic bandage. Another splint is applied to the flexor surface, from the flexion crease of the palm to the elbow. As soon as the plaster is hard, the strap, but not the felt, is removed from above the elbow and traction is continued, holding the hand elevated, while the original elastic bandages are removed and the circular cast is completed. The position of the fragments is determined by a film. If the position of the fragments is unsatisfactory, the cast is removed and a new reduction is attempted. The patient is then put to bed with his hand elevated. If swelling occurs, the plaster cast may be split, usually along the ulnar border. It is good practice whenever using a circular cast on an upper limb to split the cast to the skin along the ulnar border and to hold the integrity of the cast with a few strips of $1/2$-inch circular adhesive. If swelling becomes a problem, it is a simple matter to release the adhesive and to spread the cast through the previously made split without losing the molding benefits of the cast. As swelling subsides, adhesive may again be used to snug the cast satisfactorily.

When the fracture lines are oblique or comminuted, or when marked dislocation of the distal radio-ulnar joint has occurred, the position of the fragments may often be maintained by transfixing the ulna above, and the radius and ulna below, with pins or wires, these subsequently being incorporated into the cast. This should usually be done in the hospital. Failure to reduce these fractures or to maintain reduction usually requires subsequent surgical intervention.

The aftercare of these patients is described under the treatment of fractures in good position. The cast should remain in place for about 6 weeks for fractures of the middle third, and for from 5 to 6 weeks for fractures of the distal or proximal third. A roentgenographic examination should always be made after the first week. Films are made immediately after removal of the cast; a second cast may be applied for an additional 4 weeks or more if union is not firm.

DORSIFLEXION FRACTURE OF THE LOWER END OF THE RADIUS (COLLES' FRACTURE) WITH OR WITHOUT FRACTURE OF THE ULNAR STYLOID

ANATOMY

The radius acts as the proximal continuation of the hand, and takes the thrust in falls on the hand. The lower end is spongy bone, dense cortex appearing about 1 to 2 cm. from the distal end; the level 1 to 2 cm. from the articular surface is the common site of fracture. The tip of the radial styloid normally lies about 1 cm. distal to the tip of the ulnar styloid, and its articular surface lies not at right angles to the long axis but inclined about 25° toward the ulnar side. In the lateral view, the articular surface faces toward the palm rather than straight ahead (Fig. 23-59). The angle with the long axis is about 15° beyond the right angle.

In girls, the epiphysis for the lower end of the radius appears in the sixth to the tenth month of age; in boys, it appears between the twelfth month and the third year. The epiphysis fuses with the shaft between the twenty-first and the twenty-fifth years. The epiphysis for the distal end of the ulna appears in the sixth year and fuses with the shaft between the twentieth and the twenty-fourth years. There may be a separate epiphysis for the ulnar styloid.

DISPLACEMENT

During a fall forward on the palm of the hand, the body continues to go forward after the palm becomes fixed against the ground, the wrist being forced beyond the normal bony limit of dorsiflexion.

The protruding dorsal outer margin receives the impact, and following fracture the distal fragment thereby is driven proximally and toward the dorsum as well as toward the radial side (Fig. 23-60). As the distal fragment moves toward the radial side, the tense triangular ligament frequently pulls off the ulnar styloid. Considerable bone compression with loss of bone substance often occurs. This compression of the cancellous bone accounts for the ease with which deformity recurs after good reduction.

The fractures vary greatly in displacement. In children, there may be only very slight buckling of the bone or slight dorsal displacement of the distal epiphysis of the radius. There may be marked impaction on the dorsal side or complete overlapping without impaction. Comminution with extension of the fracture lines into the wrist joint and the radioulnar joint occurs frequently. Slight subluxation at the radio-ulnar joint is common; the ulnar styloid becomes more prominent and the hand deviates toward the radial side.

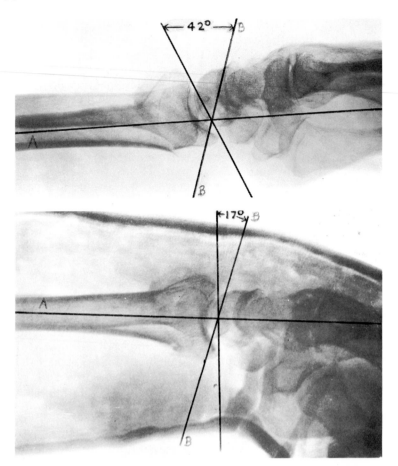

Fig. 23–59. Lateral view of dorsiflexion fracture. (*Top*) Rotation (42°) and impaction on the dorsal surface are shown. (*Bottom*) Reduction was incomplete; the articular surface still lies rotated 17° backward. Note lines *A*, bisecting the lower end of the radius lengthwise, and *B-B*, the normal position of the articular surface.

DIAGNOSIS

When dorsal displacement has occurred, the wrist exhibits a typical dinner-fork deformity (Fig. 23-61). Swelling may obscure this. When compared with the normal side, the site of fracture shows thickening, irregularity of contour, and acute tenderness, and the radial styloid lies close to the level of the ulnar styloid. There is pain on full flexion of the hand. Tenderness over the ulnar styloid usually indicates a fracture at that point. There may be additional fractures or dislocations of the carpal bones.

TREATMENT

After the examination has been completed, a suitable splint is applied to the dorsal surface from the knuckles to the elbow with the hand in the midpositions of rotation and flexion. Films are made, the angulation of the articular surface is determined, and reduction is performed, when necessary, without undue delay.

Treatment of Fractures in Good Position

If no displacement has occurred, or if the articular surface still inclines toward

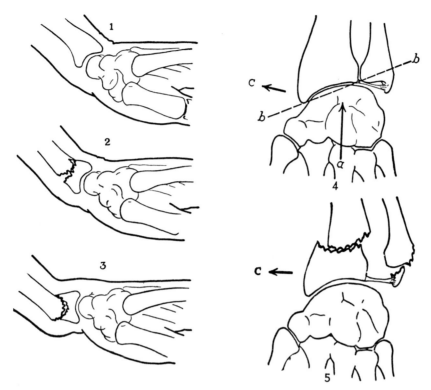

Fig. 23–60. Mechanism of dorsiflexion suprastyloid fracture. (1) the patient falls forward on the dorsiflexed hand. (2) The radius breaks in its weak, spongy portion proximal to the articular surface. (3) The hand is fixed on the ground. If the force is great, the shaft of the radius is driven downward and into the distal fragment, producing the typical deformity. (4) Seen from in front, the plane of the articular surface (b) lies at an oblique angle to the long axis of the bone. When the hand is thrust proximally in direction (a) against the oblique surface, there is a component of the resulting force in direction (c) which carries the distal fragment toward the radial side (5). The ulnar styloid is torn away if the triangular ligament does not rupture. The radio-ulnar joint may be completely disrupted.

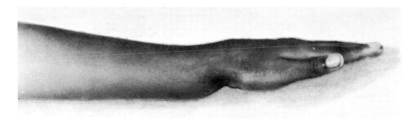

Fig. 23–61. Typical deformity seen in a dorsiflexion suprastyloid fracture of the lower end of the radius.

the palm and there is no appreciable outward displacement, the original splint may be left undisturbed for 3 to 4 days, during which time the patient should keep the arm elevated and exercise the fingers fully. The splint is then removed and is replaced by a circular cast. Normal use of the whole arm and hand must be resumed immediately. Special care should be taken to exercise the fingers through their full range of motion, to pronate and supinate as fully as possible, and to move the shoulder and the elbow through its full range of motion at least 3 times daily. Elderly patients frequently sustain mild injuries about the elbow and shoulder, and if they are supplied with a sling without instructions to exercise, severe disability may follow.

The cast may be removed in about 4 to 6 weeks, and at this time the wrist will usually be found to move freely. After a week or two of hot soaks and energetic use, the range of motion often returns to normal. Early removal of the cast to give physiotherapy is not advised. The best form of therapy is active use, and this is performed most safely while the fracture is protected by the cast.

Treatment of Fractures with Displacement

The displacement of the fragments may be estimated accurately from the films. The anteroposterior view shows the shift of the distal fragment to the radial side, the amount of shortening of the bone, and the disturbance of the lower radio-ulnar joint. Fracture of the ulnar styloid may also be present. The lateral view shows the rotation of the articular surface toward the dorsum and the degree of impaction of the fragment. Impaction of spongy bone means crushing and loss of structure. After reduction, an actual gap may be visible at the dorsum, or the radius may remain shortened due to loss of substance after crushing.

When crushing of bone and comminution have occurred, the fracture may be unstable and reduction may be difficult to maintain. Often the stability of the reduction may be improved by immobilizing the elbow as well as the wrist. When bony damage is very extensive, hospitalization for wire transfixion and casting may be advisable as the initial step in treatment.

Reduction. Reduction should be performed without undue delay, but it should not be attempted without ade-

quate anesthesia and assistance. Local anesthesia is usually satisfactory early and when the fragments are loose, i.e., when the anesthetic can reach the bone ends by diffusion through the hematoma. Ordinarily, 10 to 15 ml. of a 1 percent solution of a local anesthetic is injected at the dorsal site of the fracture, and about 3 ml., at the ulnar styloid. The addition of 1 cc. of hyaluronidase (Wydase) may facilitate diffusion of the anesthetic solution and be of assistance in reducing postoperative swelling. When there is impaction, somewhat less solution is necessary, since there is not usually as large an area available for diffusion.

Short-acting general or regional anesthesia is sometimes preferable.

The patient lies on the table with the arm arranged as shown in Figure 23-62. About 10 minutes after the local anesthetic has been injected, an assistant makes traction on the thumb with one hand and on the 2nd, 3rd, and 4th fingers with the other, pulling the hand into pronation, flexion, and ulnar deviation. After 3 to 4 minutes of traction, the surgeon disengages any impaction by direct pressure on the distal fragment. He completes the reduction by grasping the forearm with his two thumbs on the dorsum, one above and one below the fracture site, and his fingers on the flexor side, and then pressing the distal fragment toward the flexor side (Fig. 23-63).

When reduction is complete, a plaster cast is applied over light sheet wadding and is molded to maintain reduction with the wrist in some flexion and ulnar deviation. When the plaster becomes firm, the cast should always be split to the skin along the ulnar border to allow for easy relief if swelling occurs. The cast should be molded firmly in the palm and about the distal radius; it should extend across the knuckles posteriorly and to the proximal flexion crease in the palm anteriorly and should be relieved around the base of the thumb. Traction is discontinued as soon as the plaster has set, and a film is made. It is preferable to approximate the normal as closely as possible. If residual displacement is seen, the plaster should

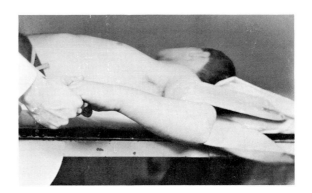

Fig. 23–62. Arrangement for reduction of a fracture of the lower end of the radius.

be removed and reduction repeated immediately. In certain extensively comminuted fractures, closed reduction and fixation may not be sufficient. Satisfactory position may occasionally be maintained by external skeletal fixation with a pin through the radius and another through the second metacarpal; these pins are then incorporated in a plaster cast.

If satisfactory position has been maintained, the patient should be instructed to keep the hand elevated to allow dependent drainage from the fingers, and flexion and extension of the fingers should be started immediately. Particularly when the forearm is short and fat, the cast should also include the elbow, but this is not always necessary. As stated previously, a sling is not supplied immediately, since this tends to encourage most patients to maintain the hand in a dependent position.

In the presence of swelling, ice bags are usually helpful for a short period of time. The patient is advised to report immediately if the hand becomes cold, blue,

or numb or develops a "pins and needles" feeling. If any circulatory disturbance is manifested, the pressure may be relieved by judicious spreading of the cast along the previously split ulnar border. The circulation of the part should be examined the day following application of the cast, and the cast should be tightened or loosened as necessary. If a short arm cast is used, it should be trimmed at the elbow to allow easy flexion of the elbow. Treatment is continued as for a fracture in good position. Roentgen films should be made again in one week. If the fragments have moved appreciably, which is quite rare, the displacement may still be corrected at this time. Additional films are made as indicated.

The cast is usually removed in 4 to 6 weeks, and the fracture is examined for callus formation; the findings are checked by films. In extensively comminuted fractures, the cast should remain in place for 8 to 12 weeks. The wrist usually moves through half of its normal range of motion immediately if the fingers have been ex-

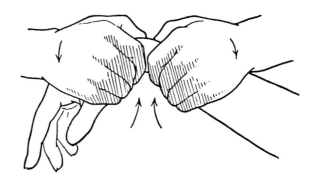

Fig. 23–63. Method of reducing a dorsiflexion suprastyloid fracture. If the fragments are impacted, this motion may be reversed at first to disengage the fragments.

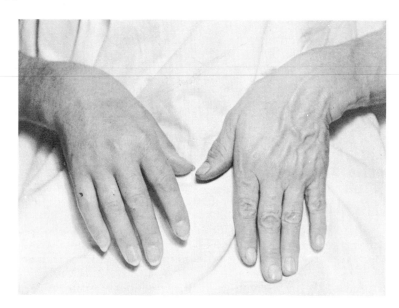

Fig. 23–64. Hands of a 55-year-old woman who sustained a fracture of the lower end of the right radius 10 weeks before this photograph was taken. Because the fracture was unreduced and poorly immobilized, the right hand became extremely painful, stiff, and duskier and warmer than the left. Duskiness, swelling, and loss of the normal skin wrinkles can be seen.

ercised adequately; and with daily, hot soaks, massage, and active use, full function frequently is recovered in as short a time as 2 to 3 weeks. Elderly patients with extensively comminuted fractures tend to have late bone resorption and recurrence of the deformity, so that immobilization of the fracture site with the hand molded toward the ulnar side must be maintained until the films show adequate callus formation.

COMPLICATIONS

Residual disability is common. Swelling and stiffness of the fingers and the hand occur often in patients who seek treatment late and in those who do not exercise adequately. An occasional occurrence in the older age group is persistent, painful swelling in the hand, associated with limitation of motion of the fingers and increased local temperature (Fig. 23-64). It occurs perhaps even more frequently with the palmar-flexion type of fracture of the lower end of the radius. When the condition has been present for a

considerable length of time, definite demineralization of the bones of the hand and the wrist (Sudek's atrophy) may be seen on roentgenograms. This is a complex sympathetic neurovascular disturbance, best described as a reflex vascular dystrophy. Extensive soft-tissue injuries, severe comminution of the bony fragments, failure to obtain good reduction, poor immobilization of the fragments, lack of immediate measures to control swelling (pressure dressings, elevation), excessive immobilization of fingers from the beginning, may all be contributing factors. Damage to, or persistent irritation of, the sensory nerve fibers probably also contributes to the problem. Exercises and occupational therapy should be prescribed.

In about half the cases exhibiting fractures of the ulnar styloid, no bony union occurs between the fragments, but symptoms from this are quite unusual, and it requires no specific treatment.

Mild pain often persists at the wrist when the fracture line has extended into the articular surface.

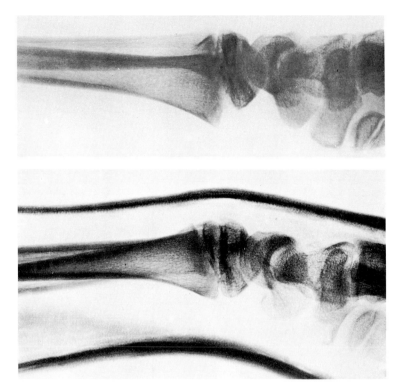

Fig. 23–65. (*Top*) Epiphyseal separation of the lower end of the radius with dorsal displacement of the distal fragment. (*Bottom*) After reduction.

Secondary to irregular healing of the distal radius, the extensor pollicis longus tendon occasionally ruptures late. Irritation of the median nerve as it passes through the carpal tunnel sometimes occurs and requires surgical relief.

EPIPHYSEAL SEPARATION AT THE LOWER END OF THE RADIUS

In children, the lower radial epiphysis may separate after a fall on the palm of the dorsiflexed hand (Fig. 23-65). Fracture of the ulnar styloid or separation of the lower ulnar epiphysis usually accompanies displacement of the radial epiphysis.

Epiphyseal separations really are dorsiflexion fractues with the following characteristics:

(1) Separation without displacement often may not be identified or excluded by the original roentgenogram unless diaphyseal fracture has occurred.

(2) When displacement occurs, a mushy crepitus may be elicted.

(3) Great force may be necessary to effect reduction.

(4) Residual displacements usually are overcome by later bone growth.

(5) Fractures extending through the epiphysis may be followed by disturbance of bone growth.

The treatment is similar to that for dorsiflexion fracture, but postreduction immobilization is usually not necessary for as long a period of time.

SMITH'S FRACTURES, OR REVERSED COLLES' FRACTURE

Etiology. Fracture of the radius 1 to 2 cm. above the wrist joint with palmar displacement of the distal fragment (Smith's fracture) has been attributed to a

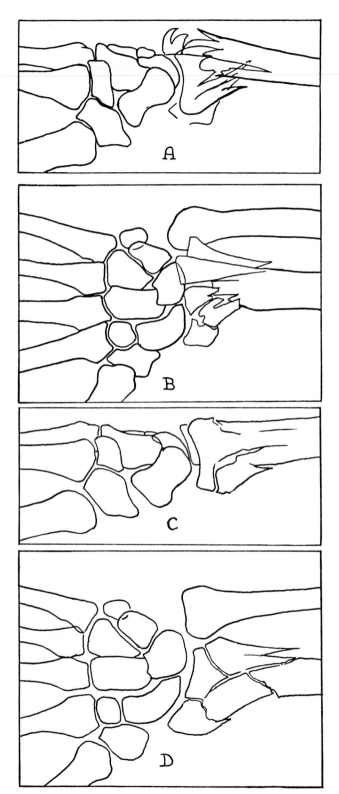

Fig. 23–66. (*A* and *B*) Comminuted suprastyloid fracture, flexion type, before reduction. (*C* and *D*) Comminuted suprastyloid fracture flexion type, after reduction.

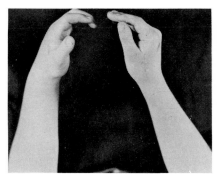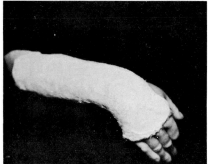

Fig. 23–67. (*Left*) Suprastyloid fracture, palmar flexion type, of the left arm. Note the swelling and the displacement of the hand toward the palmar side. (*Right*) Unpadded cast from the knuckles to the elbow, with the hand in extreme ulnar deviation; used to maintain the length of the radius after communution of the bone. This was necessary in the case shown on the left.

fall on the dorsum of the palmar-flexed hand. More likely, this fracture results from a fall on the dorsal or palmar side of the hand when the hand is tensed toward pronation.

The position of the hand and the tension of the extensor tendons force the distal fragment toward the flexor side (Fig. 23-66). The fragment also moves to the radial side, and the triangular ligament may be torn, or the ulnar styloid may be fractured. The fracture line is frequently oblique, running, from behind, upward and forward, and there may be extensive comminution.

Diagnosis. The hand is displaced toward the flexor and the radial sides (Fig. 23-67). This is visible unless the swelling is very great. Palpation discloses the changed relationship of the ulnar and the radial styloids, and the typical displacement of the distal fragment. Films show the radial displacement and the rotation of the articular surface toward the flexor side.

Treatment. If little or no displacement has occurred, the treatment follows that for dorsiflexion fracture, except that the wrist is immobilized in the functional position.

When there is considerable displacement, reduction is difficult, due to the obliqobiliquity and comminution of the fracture line. The method and the maneuvers of reduction follow those for reduction of a dorsiflexion fraction, except that the surgeon's thumbs are placed on the flexor side and the distal fragment is pressed toward the dorsum. Powerful traction toward the ulnar side and toward the dorsum is helpful. Full supination of the hand may aid reduction.

Stability of the fragments is obtained best by accurate molding of the plaster about the lower end of the radius and in the sapace between the thumb and the index finger, moderate *dorsiflexion* and ulnar deviation of the hand being maintained. The hand should be put in a full cast, applied with the elbow at a right angle.

Reduction must be followed by repeated roentgenograms for the first few weeks. Failure to obtain adequate reduction or to maintain position may require operation and skeletal fixation. The complications are similar to those occurring after dorsiflexion fracture.

BIBLIOGRAPHY
Dislocation of the Shoulder

Baker, D. M., and Leach, R. E.: Fracture dislocation of the shoulder—report of three unusual cases with rotator cuff avulsion. J. Trauma, 5:659, 1965.

Bush, L. F.: Dislocations of the shoulder. Am. J. Surg, *67*:520, 1945.

d'Aubigné, R. M.: Nerve injuries in fractures and dislocations of the shoulder. Surg. Clin. N. Am. *43*:1685, 1963.

McLaughlin, H. L.: Dislocation of the shoulder with tuberosity fracture. Surg. Clin. N. Am. *43*:1615, 1963.

Milch, H.: Pulsion-traction in the reduction of dislocations or fracture dislocations of the humerus. Bull. Hosp. Joint Dis., *24*:147, 1963.

Parvin, R. W.: Closed reduction of common shoulder and elbow dislocations without anesthesia. Arch. Surg., *75*:972, 1957.

Shaftan, G. W., and Herbsman, H.: Intravenous methocarbamol in reduction of shoulder dislocations. JAMA, *188*:69, 1964.

Smith, W. S., and Klug, T. J.: Anterior dislocation of the shoulder—a simple and effective method of reduction. JAMA, *163*:182, 1957.

Tronzo, R. G.: Reduction of dislocated shoulders using methocarbamol. JAMA, *184*:1044, 1963.

Fractures of the Humerus

Aitken, A. P.: Fractures of the proximal humeral epiphysis. Surg. Clin. N. Am., *43*:1573, 1963.

Bickel, W. E., and Perry, R.E.: Comminuted fractures of the distal humerus. JAMA, *184*:553, 1963.

Böhler, L.: Conservative treatment of fresh closed fractures of the humerus. J. Trauma, *5*:464, 1965.

Drapanas, T.: Initial treatment of fractures of the surgical neck of the humerus. Geriatrics, *18*:538, 1963.

Dunlop, J.: Transcondylar fractures of the humerus in childhood (suspension and traction). J. Bone Joint Surg., *21*:59, 1939.

El-Sharkawi, A. H., and Fattah, H. A.: Treatment of displaced supracondylar fractures of the humerus in full extension and supination. J. Bone Joint Surg., *47B*:273, 1965.

Hammond, G.: The management of supracondylar fractures of the humerus in children. Surg. Clin. N. Am., *32*:747, 1952.

Holstein, A., and Lewis, G. B.: Fractures of the humerus with radial nerve paralysis. J. Bone Joint Surg., *45-A*:1382, 1963.

Howard N. J., and Eloesser, L.: Treatment of fractures of the upper end of the humerus. J. Bone Joint Surg., *16*:1, 134.

Mann, T. S.: Prognosis in supracondylar fractures, J. Bone Joint Surg., *45B*:516, 163.

Maylahn, D. J., and Fahey, J. J.: Fractures of the elbow in children; a review of three hundred consecutive cases. JAMA, *166*:220, 158.

McLearie, M., and Merson, R. D.: Injuries to the lateral condylar epiphysis of the humerus in children. J. Bone Joint Surg., *36B*:84, 1954.

Milch, H.: Fractures of the external humeral condyle. JAMA, *160*:641, 1956.

Mitchell, N. J., and Adams, J. P.: Review of 83 children with supracondylar fractures of humerus. JAMA, *175*:573, 1961.

Neer, C. S., Brown, T. H., and McLaughlin, H. L.: Fracture of the neck of the humerus with dislocation of the head fragment. Am. J. Surg., *85*:252, 1953.

Neviasser, J. S.: Complicated fractures and dislocations about the shoulder joint (An instructional course lecture of the American Academy of Orthopedic Surgeons). J. Bone Joint Surg., *44A*:984, 1962.

Smith, F. M.: Medial epicondyle injuries. JAMA, *132*:396, 1950.

Smith, F. M., and Joyce, J. J.: Fractures of the lateral condyle of the humerus in children. Am. J. Surg., *87*:334, 1954.

Vivian, D. M., and Janes, J. M.: Fractures involving the proximal humeral epiphysis. Am. J. Surg., *87*:211, 1954.

Wray, J. B. Management of supracondylar fracture with vascular insufficiency. Arch. Surg., *90*:279, 1965.

Pulled Elbow

Green, F. M., and Gay, F. H.: Traumatic subluxation of radial head in young children. J. Bone Joint Surg., *36A*:655, 1954.

Magill, H. K., and Aitken, A. P.: Pulled elbow. Surg., Gynec Obstet., *98*:753, 1954.

Sweetnam, R.: Manipulation for pulled elbow. Practitioner, *182*:487, 1959.

Elbow Dislocations

Lavine, L. S.: A simple method of reducing dislocations of the elbow joint. J. Bone Joint Surg., *35A*:785, 1953.

Parvin, R. W.: Closed reduction of common shoulder and elbow dislocations without anesthesia. Arch. Surg., *75*:972, 1957.

Fractures and Dislocations of Head and Neck of the Radius

Leriche, R., and Fontaine, R.: Fracture de la tête radiale' traitée par les infiltrations locales repétées; guérison avec récupération fonticionelle intégrale. Rev. Chir., *75*:761, 137.

London, P. S.: Observations on the treatment of some fractures of the forearm by splintage that does not include the elbow. Injury, *2*:252, 1971.

Moser, H.: The treatment of fractures and of epiphysiolysis of the head of the radius. Arch. Klin. Chir., *277*:508, 1954.

Postlethwait, R. W.: Modified treatment for fractures of the head of the radius. Am. J. Surg., *67*:77, 1945.

Quigley, T. B.: Aspiration of the elbow joint in the treatment of fractures of the head of the radius. New Eng. J. Med., *240*:915, 1949.

Ramsey, R. H., and Pedersen, H. E.: The Monteggia fracture-dislocation in children. JAMA, *182*:1091, 1962.

Reidy, J. A., and VanGorder, G. W.: Treatment of displacement of the proximal radial epiphysis. J. Bone Joint Surg., *45A*:1355, 1963.

Fractures of the Olecranon

Adler, S., Gardner, F. F., and MacAusland, R. W., Jr.: Treatment of olecranon fractures. J. Trauma, *2*:597, 1962.

Bakalim, G., and Wilppula, E.: Fractures of the olecranon; I—analysis of 109 consecutive cases. Ann. Chir. Gynec. Fenn., *60*:95, 1971.

Fractures of the Shafts of the Ulna and Radius

Adler, J. B., Doherty, J. H., Skudder, P. A., and Wade, P. A.: Adult forearm fractures— principles of management. J. Trauma, *5*:319, 1965.

Altner, P. C., and Hartmann, J. T.: Isolated fractures of the ulnar shaft in the adult. Surg. Clin. N. Am., *52*:155, 1972.

Bairov, G. A., Bogopol' skiĭ-Bol'ski, and Gorenshtein, A. I.: Monteggia fractures in children. Vestn. Khir. *107*:74, 1972.

Bohler, L.: The Treatment of Fractures. ed. 5. New York, Grune & Stratton, Vol. I—1956, Vol. II—1957, Vol. III—1958.

Carr, C. R., and Tracy, H. W.: Management of fractures of the distal forearm in children. Southern Med. J. *57*:540, 1964.

Hughston, J. C.: Fracture of distal radial shaft; mistakes in management. J. Bone Joint Surg., *39A*:249, 1957.

——: Fractures of the forearm in children. An instructional course lecture, The American Academy of Orthopedic Surgeons. J. Bone Joint Surg., *44A*:1678, 1962.

Pavel, A., Pitman, J. M., Lance, E. M., and Wade, P. A.: The posterior Monteggia fracture, a clinical study. J. Trauma, *5*:185, 1965.

Ramsey, R. H., and Pedersen, H. E.: The Monteggia fracture-dislocation in children. JAMA, *182*:1091, 1962.

Fractures of the Distal End of the Radius

Brindley, H. H.: Wrist injuries. Clin. Orthop., *83*:17, 1972.

Flandreau, R. H., Sweeney, R. M., and O'Sullivan, W. D.: Clinical experiences with a series of Smith's fractures. Arch. Surg., *84*:288, 1962.

Geckeler, E. O., and Gross, D. J.: Colles' fractures; classification and treatment. Penn. Med. J., *61*:486, 1958.

Lewis, R. M.: Colles' fracture—causative mechanism. Surgery, *27*:427, 1950.

Milch, H.: Torsional malalignments in transverse fractures of lower end of the shaft of the radius. Surgery, *55*:396, 1964.

Older, T. M., Stabler, E. V., and Cassebaum, W. H.: Colles' fracture: evaluation and selection of therapy. J. Traumz, *5*:469, 1965.

Small, G. B.: Long-term follow-up of Colles' fracture. J. Bone Joint Surg., *47B*:80, 1965.

General References

Böhler, L.: The Treatment of Fractures. ed. 5. New York, Grune & Stratton, Vol. I—1956, Vol. II—1957, Vol. III—1958.

Key, J. A., and Canwell, H. E.: The Management of Fractures and Sprains. ed. 5. St. Louis, E. V. Mosby, 1951.

Quigley, T. B., and Banks, H.: Progress in the treatment of fractures and dislocations, 1950–1960. New Eng. J. Med., *263*:495, 1960.

Watson-Jones, R.: Fractures and Joint Injuries. ed. 4. Baltimore, Williams & Wilkins, Vol. I—1952, Vol. II—1955.

24

Hand and Fingers

Part I—Soft Tissues

Mark W. Wolcott, M.D.

INFECTIONS

PARONYCHIA

Acute Paronychia

Etiology. Paronychia is probably the simplest type of infection that involves the distal phalanx. It appears along the edge of the nail near the base (Fig. 24-1). Most often the infecting organism gains entrance into the space between the skin surface and the nail as a result of the pulling away or the biting off of hangnails or as a result of other trauma, such as that received in manicures. Almost invariably, the infecting organism is the *Staphylococcus aureus.*

Progress of the Infection. For the first 2 or 3 days, the infection remains at the site of the original entrance of the infecting organism. An increasingly painful swelling forms and extends into the soft tissues at the side of the nail. As time goes on, the infection progresses proximally underneath the eponychium, thence across the base of the fingernail to the opposite side. At first, the infection lies between the overhanging eponychium and the nail. It extends to undermine the nail at its base; a subungual collection is formed, with considerable swelling involving the tissues at the base of the nail and on each side (Fig. 24-2).

Treatment. If the lesion is noted early, abscess formation may be aborted by the use of antibiotics to which the staphylococcus is sensitive. Since often no culture or sensitivity tests are available, the choice may be made among penicillin, tetracycline, and erythromycin. Once an abscess has formed, early drainage of the primary focus of infection will permit a rapid subsidence of the inflammatory process and healing within a day or two. Reliance on antibiotic therapy may delay the primary treatment, which is surgical drainage.

When there is definite swelling along the edge of the nail, the mistake often is made of incising the soft tissues at the side of the finger. The patient experiences no relief after such incisions.

An understanding of the course of the infection makes it plain that drainage is obtained in the early cases simply by lifting up the skin edge from the nail (Fig. 24-3). This can be accomplished easily without anesthesia by inserting the tip of the scalpel carefully along the edge of the nail at the site of the swelling. A drop of pus escapes, and the patient experiences almost immediate relief of pain. The point of the knife should be carried along

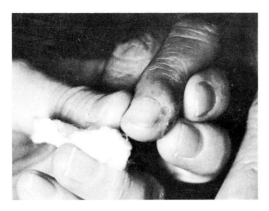

Fig. 24–1. Paronychia underneath the eponychium on the lateral side of the nail.

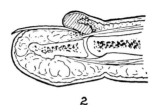

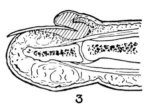

Fig. 24–2. Paronychia. (1) The site of the abscess at the side of the anil. (2) The infection has extended round the base of the nail. It has raised the eponchium but has not penetrated under the nail. (3) End stage of paronychia with a subeponchial and subungual abscess.

the nail to separate the skin over the tiny abscess sufficiently to provide adequate drainage. As a rule, a tiny pocket about as big as a match head will be found. The overhanging superficial skin may be cut away with the knife edge without causing pain or bleeding. A sliver of rubber dam is inserted into the abscess pocket to permit continued drainage. Hot wet compresses for 24 hours usually suffice to permit discharge of any remaining purulent material. At the end of this time, the drain may be removed, and simple dry dressings are applied until healing takes place. Usually, all bandages may be removed in 3 or 4 days when symptoms have disappeared.

When the paronychia has extended underneath the eponychium at the base of the nail, the same procedure may be carried out. If, however, the infectious process has extended to invade the subungual space, adequate drainage cannot be obtained without excising the base of the nail (Fig. 24-4). To accomplish this, incisions must be made through the eponychium parallel to the lateral edges of the nail. This can be accomplished using a digital nerve block, and a rubber band tourniquet gives a bloodless field. These incisions are carried downward to permit the eponychium to be turned back to expose the nail base. As much of the nail base as is undermined with pus is excised, the scalpel or scissors being used.

The abscess pocket under the eponychium is packed with petrolatum gauze, and a voluminous dressing is applied. Hot moist solutions are applied by dipping the finger in a cup or glass with the dressing still in place; this promotes continued drainage. The dressings should not be changed until the second day, when the packing may be removed and the eponychium permitted to fall back in place. The distal portion of the nail should not be removed, since it offers good protection and gradually it is pushed off as the new nail grows in place. This takes several weeks.

In a few cases, infective hypertrophic granulations appear at the site of the abscess underneath the eponychium. These are extremely painful, and they can be prevented by snug bandaging. When

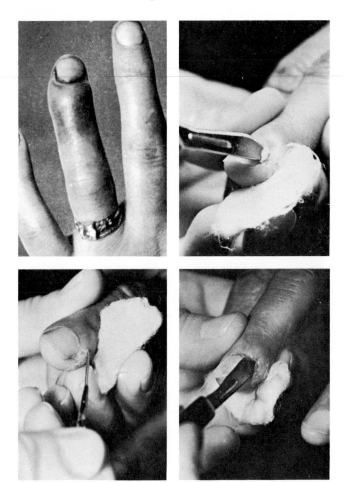

Fig. 24–3. (*Top, Left*) Typical swelling of the soft tissues at the base of the nail in a paronychia that has extended into this area.

(*Top, right*) Drainage of a paronychia without anesthesia by inserting the tip of a knife along the nail edge and lifting away the eponchium from the nail. A drop of pus is evacuated from the abscess pocket.

(*Bottom, left*) Drainage of a paronychia. The tip of a knife is used to lift away the skin edge. Note the site of the abscess cavity at the side of the nail.

(*Bottom, right*) Drainage of a paronychia. A small sliver of rubber dam is inserted into the abscess cavity with the tip of a knife.

they occur, pressure bandages will flatten down the granulation and healing will take place, except in a few cases in which it is necessary to excise a little more of the nail because its edge is cutting into the overhanging granulation and causing discomfort.

Chronic Paronychia

Etiology and Symptoms. This is another common infection of the nail border; it produces a sluggish inflammation of the eponychium that gradually crosses the nail and involves the soft tissues on both sides. The eponychium becomes red and swollen and separates slightly from the nail. Beneath it appears a drop or two of seropurulent exudate, which dries and often crusts, causing slight discomfort.

The cause of this lesion may be either a low-grade staphylococcal infection or ringworm. The long-continued infection underneath the eponychium produces an inflammatory reaction in the nail matrix, so that the nail is often roughened and pitted, and in cases of ringworm it may have a moth-eaten appearance (Fig. 24-5).

Treatment. The inflammation may subside with home treatment, hot soaks being used, but almost invariably it recurs. Usually, the patient does not seek treatment until home therapy has been tried unsuccessfully for several weeks.

In a few cases seen during the first week or two, antibiotics and hot moist applications may be tried for a time, but these usually are unsuccessful in effecting a cure. In those cases of such long standing that there is necrosis of the base

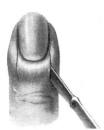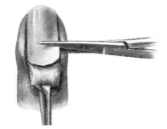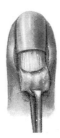

Fig. 24–4. Operation for drainage of a paronychia in which the infection has extended under the base of the nail. Lateral incisions are made through the eponychium, which is dissected away from the nail and turned back. The base of the nail is cut off with the knife or scissors to drain adequately the subungual abscess.

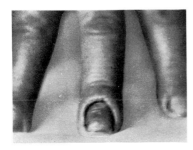

Fig. 24–5. Chronic paronycia. Note the thickening of the tissues of the eponychium and the roughened appearance of the nail.

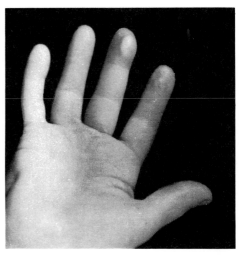

Fig. 24–6. Dermatitis repens of the palmar surface of the index and the middle fingers. Note the blister-like swelling distended with purulent fluid and the slight amount of hyperemia around the edge of the blisters.

of the nail, conservative therapy is no longer of any value. The necrotic nail base acts as a foreign body and produces a continual exudation that cannot be relieved except by excising the nail base. This operation is the same as that described for acute paronychia. In cases in which the chronic paronychia is due to ringworm, removal of the entire nail is necessary. Some cases of ringworm of the nails respond to treatment with Griseofulvin, 0.5 g. daily for 4 to 6 months or longer. These patients are best referred to a dermatologist for definitive laboratory diagnosis and advice as to treatment.

DERMATITIS REPENS

Etiology and Symptoms. Dermatitis repens is the name given to a recurring pyogenic infection that occurs most frequently on the dorsum of the distal phalanx around the nail. It is seen also on the palmar surface of the fingers and the hand. It is characterized by a blisterlike elevation of the superficial layer of skin containing a purulent exudate (Fig. 24-6). Culture of the pus most often shows a nonhemolytic streptococcus, although staphylococcus also may be found. When the superficial layer of the blisterlike swelling is removed, a small amount of thin liquid pus escapes, and the underlying unbroken true skin is seen to form the base of the lesion. Rupture of the blister does not permit healing. The process tends to extend peripherally, with varying degrees of pain and swelling, and it may involve the skin of the dorsum of the finger from the nail to the proximal interphalangeal joint. On the palmar surface of the finger, the infection starts most often around the tip near the nail, in the same sort of blisterlike swelling. Because of the rich nerve supply to this area, tenderness is a common symptom.

Treatment. The important primary therapeutic measure for this type of infection is to obtain adequate and complete drainage by cutting away the entire detached area of superficial skin. Any overhang of epidermis left will permit the progression of the infection, which probably is an anaerobic one and which tends to extend underneath the protective layer of dead skin.

The prognosis for these cases is good. It is probable that the infection is self-limiting, but often it is slow in healing and is the cause of considerable discomfort to the patient and of anxiety to the surgeon. Systemic antibiotic therapy may be used, and, as a local application, bacitracin in a concentration of 1,000 units per ml. may be tried. Culture and sensitivity tests permit the choice of the most effective antibiotic.

FURUNCLES OF THE DORSAL SURFACE OF THE PROXIMAL PHALANX

Etiology. The hair follicles and the sebaceous glands of the dorsal surface of the proximal phalanx are common sites of origin for furuncles. Often these are caused by wearing dirty gloves, the infecting organisms being ground into the hair follicles and the gland openings. The infection begins as a small, red, tender area and extends to the subcutaneous tissues. Usually, pain and swelling are considerable. Not only does the infection involve the dorsal surface of the proximal phalanx, but it extends also to the adjacent loose tissues of the dorsum of the hand.

Treatment. As a rule, conservative therapy is of value, at least until definite pointing takes place. Almost always, the infecting organism is a staphylococcus, which tends to produce a localized inflammation if the part is immobilized and hot moist dressings are applied. Therefore, the application of a finger splint and of sufficient gauze dressing overlaid with waxed paper to give almost constant heat is indicated. The hand is elevated in a sling, and the dressings are moistened at intervals of 2 or 3 hours with warm saline solution. At the end of 24 or 48 hours, definite localization usually occurs. The edema of the dorsum of the hand disappears, and in many cases it may be possible to delay any surgery until spontaneous separation of the necrotic core takes place. If this method of therapy is decided upon, splinting and hot moist dressings are continued for another day or two, at the end of which time drainage of the furuncle will take place spontaneously and the central area of necrosis may be picked out with forceps. Hot moist dressings are continued for another 48 hours, after which a simple dressing without splinting is all that is necessary.

Since this is an ordinary furuncle caused by the staphylococcus, it would be expected to show a rapid response to antibiotic therapy, and this is true. Penicillin obviously is the antibiotic of choice, and it is given best as aqueous penicillin, 500,000 units, 3 to 4 times daily, until the inflammatory reaction has subsided. If the infecting organism appears to be resistant to penicillin, sensitivity tests should be done to determine the appropriate antibiotic. In the experience of the author, effective results are usually obtained from large initial doses of penicillin. If a change of antibiotic seems to be indicated, erythromycin is preferred. The availability of the antibiotics and their great help in the treatment of infection does not mean that the methods of therapy previously used can be abandoned. If the antibiotics are used early, they may abort the infective process and

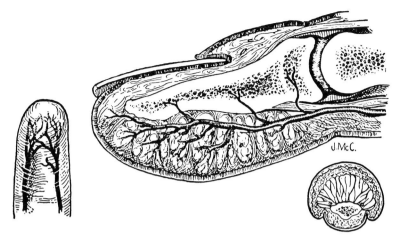

Fig. 24–7. (*Top and left*) Longitudinal section of the distal closed space, showing the blood supply. Note that the distal portion of the pulp of the finger is enclosed in a more or less definite fibrous capsule. One vessel enters the epiphysis of the phalanx; this portion of the bone almost never undergoes necrosis. Note also the location of the flexor tendon, which is involved very late, if at all, in infections of the distal closed space. (*Lower right*) Cross section of the distal closed space, showing the formation of the fibrous tissue septa, in which are located pockets of fatty tissue.

prevent necrosis and suppuration. When they are not used until necrosis and pus already are present, incision and drainage still are necessary.

If incision and drainage are decided upon, general or local anesthesia may be used. If local anesthesia is chosen, cutaneous injections are made in longitudinal and transverse lines across the center of the infected area. Care should be taken not to apply pressure as the incision is made, otherwise considerable pain may be produced. A cruciate incision is made, and whatever loose necrotic tissue is present is picked away with forceps. In spite of its appearance, none of the skin should be cut away. The wound may be packed with petrolatum gauze. Hot moist dressings are continued until all the sloughing tissue has come away, after which pressure dressings held in place with adhesive are all that is necessary.

Furuncles of the dorsum of the proximal phalanx are similar to furuncles that occur elsewhere on the body. They practically never involve the underlying tendon, although at times they extend laterally in the soft tissues of the finger. There is never any reason to incise the swelling on the dorsum of the hand.

INFECTION OF THE DISTAL CLOSED SPACE (FELON)

Anatomy and Pathology. The palmar surface of the distal half or two-thirds of the distal phalanx is spoken of as the distal closed space. It is given this name because of the peculiar formation of the pulp of the distal phalanx (Fig. 24-7). Fibrous tissue septa extend from the skin to the periosteum of the phalanx in a manner which more or less shuts off the portion of the phalanx distal to the epiphyseal line from the remaining portion of the finger. The fibrous tissue septa enclose large globules of fatty tissue that pad and protect the distal phalanx and form the rounded portion of the fingertip. Included in this tissue are numerous small glands. The fibrous tissue septa are so arranged as to divide the fatty pulp of the finger into pockets, more or less definite in themselves and at least partially shut off from one another. Although it is not anatomically correct, from a practical point of view one may consider the pulp of the fingertip as looking something like an orange that has been cut transversely, the center of the orange representing the bone and the orange skin representing the skin of the finger. The divisions between the orange sections represent the fibrous tissue septa, and the pulp of the orange represents the fatty tissue included between them.

This conception of the distal closed space offers anatomic explanations for various clinical and pathologic findings in infections of this area. Infection of the distal closed space rarely, or only in the late stage, involves the flexor tendon sheath, which inserts at the epiphysis, that is, at the base of the phalanx and, therefore, proximal to the distal closed space. The joint and the epiphyseal part of the bone are rarely involved, except late in the process of an infection of the distal closed space. The enclosure of the distal portion of the soft tissues of the finger in a more or less definite fascial space explains the extreme pain produced by inflammatory swelling in the early stages of infection in this area; and it also explains the fact that tension produces an early obliteration of the blood supply, not only to the soft tissues, but also the the diaphyseal portion of the phalanx, producing rapid necrosis of both the soft tissues and the bone. It is for this reason that early incision, which relieves tension, is important in the treatment of infections of this area.

Symptoms and Progress of the Infection. The usual source of infection is some minor injury, such as a pinprick, although frequently no injury is remembered by the patient. The infecting organism usually is the staphylococcus or the streptococcus. As a rule, 2 or 3 days elapse between the time of the injury and the appearance of a sticking sensation when the fingertip is touched. This gradually progresses to a constant pain, at first minor nature, then becoming constant and throbbing in character. The throbbing is more marked when the finger is dependent, so that the patient goes about with the hand elevated. The pain is usually sufficiently marked to prevent sleep at night, and it continues until the death of the nerve supply to the fingertip, when the throbbing pain stops suddenly and a simple soreness takes its place. This is a late stage of felon and indicates extensive necrosis of the tissues of the distal closed space.

Diagnosis. On examination of the finger in the earlier stages, one finds a swelling of the distal phalanx as compared with the normal finger on the opposite side. The distal phalanx is dusky red in color, and, if the finger is examined with the point of a pencil or some other blunt object, there usually is one area in which pressure gives exquisite tenderness. This represents the area of skin that overlies the infected portion of the finger pulp. As the process goes on, this area of tenderness becomes less definitely localized, and, in the late stages, a sac of pus may be found underneath the skin of the distal phalanx. There is usually only slight swelling of the remaining portion of the finger and no involvement of the tendon, as is evidenced by the ability to move the finger without marked pain.

Treatment. Early and adequate incision is the key to the prevention of finger deformity and disability. In the early stages, when there is only a slight sticking sensation or tenderness at the site of infection, abortive therapy may be attempted by the use of antibiotic drugs (penicillin, erythromycin), elevation, and hot moist soaks. If the drugs are to be effective, they should be used in large doses, so as to obtain an early high blood concentration. This may be continued for from 12 to 24 hours, but the finger should be seen and examined at least once during this period. An incision for drainage is warranted in the case of any patient who exhibits a point-pressure tenderness after a sleepless night or who is not much improved in this time frame.

The operation is performed under local anesthesia, using a finger block technique. A rubber tourniquet then is applied around the base of the finger. In

Fig. 24–8. Incisions for drainage of an abscess of the distal closed space. (*A*) Hockey-stick incision, which can be employed when the abscess is demonstrated definitely to lie in the lateral side of the space; it should not be used unless the abscess can be located accurately. (*B*) Fishmouth, or horseshoe, incision, which gives the most adequate drainage. Although it may seem to be radical, nevertheless it gives excellent results. The soft tissues of the finger should be incised directly in front of the bone, as noted in the illustration; the incision should not be carried below the distal closed space because of the danger of entering the sheath of the tendon. (*C*) Through-and-through type of incision for drainage of the distal closed space. In the author's opinion, this incision does not give adequate drainage; therefore, for general use, it is not as safe as is the fishmouth incision.

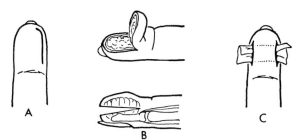

operating under local anesthesia, the common fault is to incise too quickly, that is, before the anesthesia is complete. A period of 10 to 15 minutes or longer should be allowed to elapse between the injection and the application of the tourniquet and the incision. One of several types of incision may be used, depending upon the site of involvement of the finger pulp.

Hockey-Stick Incision. If the area of infection appears to lie to one side or the other of the fingertip, a hocky-stick incision may be made; it should extend halfway across the finger, just in front of the nail, and downward along the side of the phalanx (Fig. 24-8, *A*). After waiting for a few minutes to sponge away the few drops of blood that have remained in the finger, the edges of the wound are separated sufficiently with Allis forceps or tiny rake retractors to visualize the yellowish area of necrosis at the site of the infection. If any necrotic tissue is loose, it is removed with forceps. A small piece of petrolatum gauze is inserted for drainage.

Through-and-Through Incision. Another incision recommended by many surgeons is the through-and-through type. An incision is made on each side of the finger, and these two incisions are connected by severing the connective tissue septa between the skin and bone. A rubber drain is inserted through the opening thus made (Fig. 24-8, *C*).

Horseshoe, or Fishmouth, Incision. In spite of many objections found in the literature, the author believes that the more radical, curved, horseshoe, or fishmouth incision made just anterior to the nail is the safest one for general use in infections of the distal closed space (Fig. 24-8, *B*). The objections to it are that the wound takes a long time to heal, and that the incision produces a deforming scar of the fingertip, which is sensitive and therefore, disabling for a short time. These objections seem to be more theoretical than real. If the packing or the drain is removed from a fishmouth incision in 2 or 3 days and the tissues are allowed to fall together, healing takes place with a minimum of scarring and almost as rapidly as is the case with the less radical incisions. The resulting deformity of the finger depends not so much upon the type of incision as upon the extent of the infectious necrotic process.

This incision gives the most adequate drainage, which is the important requisite and the neglect of which is the chief fault in the handling of fingertip infections. When the fishmouth incision is made, it is carried downward for about two-thirds of the distance to the distal flexion crease. When the resulting flap is turned back, the area of necrosis in the pad of the fingertip is exposed. Necrotic tissue may be removed in large measure, and a strip of rubber dam or petrolatum gauze is inserted across the phalanx and a firm dressing is applied. In felons, although the infection extends early to the bone, usually there is no necessity for scraping or curetting the bone in the early or even the moderately advanced cases.

No matter what incision has been made, a snug finger bandage is applied, and a hairpin splint is used to immobilize and protect the area of inflammation. After 2 or 3 days, the packing is removed, and the tissues are permitted to fall together. The dressings are somewhat painful until the slough is separated and granulation begins to form. Nevertheless, mechanical cleansing is the essential therapeutic measure. This can be done gently by irrigation with boric acid solution or saline in a syringe. What loose tissues appear to remain attached may be removed with forceps and scissors without great discomfort. Warm boric acid or saline solution is applied to the dressing every 2 or 3 hours until the slough is separated completely. In the later stages of the treatment, snug dressings are of considerable help in preventing swelling and edema and in promoting healing without excess granulation and scarring. Antibiotic therapy is continued in adequate dosage, even though incision has been performed.

In the late stages of an acute felon, the entire pulp of the fingertip appears to be a mass of necrotic tissue and pus (Fig. 24-9). The bone often lies free in this abscess cavity, and in children the entire diaphysis may be raised from the epiphysis. If the bone is loose, it should be removed, but no effort should be made to curette or rongeur away any bone that is firmly attached. Without exception, the incision of choice in this type of case is the fishmouth. After the necrotic material has been removed, a petrolatum pack is inserted. It is wise to avoid the excision of any skin tissue, except the thickened outer layer, which often becomes loose during the succeeding days of hot soaks.

It is surprising to see the amount of regeneration that takes place following drainage of a distal closed space. In many

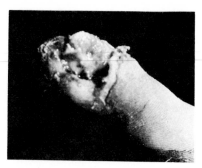

Fig. 24–9. Neglected felon, showing loss of almost all the tissues of the distal phalanx.

patients, even those with marked necrosis of the soft tissues and with definite osteomyelitis, as shown by roentgenograms, regeneration takes place to such an extent that a phalanx with almost normal function may be expected.

COLLAR-BUTTON ABSCESS

The collar-button type of abscess denotes a definite infectious process that occurs almost entirely on the hands and the feet. The name is given the lesion because of the similarity of its shape to that of a collar button. It is composed of a superficial abscess lying between the layers of the skin, usually underneath a callus, and connected by a small sinus through the true skin to a subdermal abscess in the subcuticular areolar tissue. This type of abscess occurs wherever there is a thick layer of superficial skin, such as that occasionally seen on the finger, but it occurs more commonly under the calluses in the distal part of the palm at the base of the fingers.

Etiology. The focus of infection may be an injury, but more often one is not found. The infecting organism probably entered the skin through a small crack or abrasion which was unnoticed by the patient. The infecting organism usually is the staphylococcus or the streptococcus.

Symptoms and Course of Infection. A small intradermal abscess forms primarily. This occasions slight soreness but relatively few symptoms, at least at first. The hard thick layer of skin above the

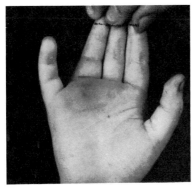
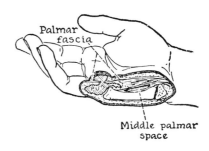

Fig. 24–10. (*Left*) Collar-button abscess under a callus at the base of the ring finger. Note the surrounding swelling with extension into the web of the finger. (*Right*) Collar-button abscess in cross-sectional view. The abscess between the layers of the skin has perforated through the true skin and has extended into the loose connective tissue space in the web of the fingers. It tends also to extend along the lumbrical canal toward the palmar space.

infected area does not permit the escape of purulent material, and, as a result, the infection tends to perforate through the deeper layers of skin and form a subcutaneous abscess. With this extension of the infection, which usually is in the web of the finger, there is a swelling between the fingers and in the dorsum of the hand adjacent to the abscess (Fig. 24-10). Pain is experienced when the hand is used, and the fingers are held in flexion, but the fingers can be moved actively and passively without pain except in the extremes of flexion and extension, when tension is placed upon the area of inflammation.

Then, the patient begins to complain of tenderness and soreness, but not of the excruciating pain noted in distal closed space infection, although the hand becomes relatively useless because of tenderness in the palm. If the process is allowed to progress, the infection extends along the lumbrical canals to the middle palmar space or, less frequently, to the thenar space (Fig. 24-10).

Treatment. The treatment of collar-button abscess is relatively simple if operation can be performed at an early date, that is, before the fascial spaces of the palm are invaded. With a tourniquet controlling the blood flow, usually under general or a local block anesthesia, the thick superficial skin overlying the intradermal abscess is excised (Fig. 24-11). When the pus has been sponged away, gentle pressure is made around the floor of the abscess, and a drop or two of pus may be seen escaping through the sinus which pierces the true skin. Using this sinus as a guide, a pointed hemostat is inserted and spread as it is removed. Usually, a considerable amount of thick material escapes, and when it is sponged away, the extent of the abscess may be seen. Often it is advisable to incise the skin of the web of the finger to open the abscess pocket completely.

The wound may be packed gently with petrolatum gauze to control bleeding. A firm dressing and a splint to immobilize the palm and fingers complete the dressing.

As a rule, the dressing is not changed for 2 or 3 days; then the packing may be removed and a simple dressing applied; splinting should be maintained for 4 or 5 days longer. Hot solutions of saline applied to the dressing prevent crusting and permit the drainage of pus to continue.

In simple collar-button abscesses, healing usually occurs rapidly and without complication. The important thing is to

Superficial abscess evacuated, skin cut away. Pus expressed from underlying abscess.

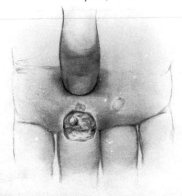

Approx. extent of deep abscess

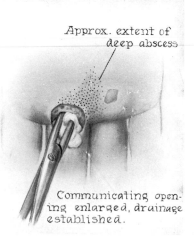

Communicating opening enlarged, drainage established.

Fig. 24–11. Drainage of a colar-button abscess. The callus has been cut away, which has unroofed the superficial, or epidermal, abscess. Pressure has produced a drop of pus at the site of perforation of the true skin. Drainage is accomplished by inserting a hemostat through this tiny opening to enlarge it and evacuate the deeper abscess.

make sure that the infection has not involved the middle palmar space. Such involvement is indicated by tenderness over the palm. When pressure is exerted over the area of the middle palmar space while the abscess is being re-dressed, the appearance of pus from the depth of the wound indicates that the infection has extended to the fascial space, and frequently a more adequate drainage is necessary. It is usually better to ensure adequate and complete drainage at the first operation; therefore, this investigation of the abscess cavity should be made at the time of the original incision. However, a close watch must be maintained to make sure that this extension of the infection does not occur at a later date.

Antibiotics are to be used in conjunction with, and not instead of, surgical therapy. They contribute to a more rapid subsidence of the inflammation and are worthwhile as prophylactics against spread of the infection to the palmar spaces.

INFECTIONS OF THE FASCIAL SPACES OF THE PALM

Anatomy. To understand the infections of the fascial spaces of the palm, it is necessary to review the anatomy of the palm briefly (Fig. 24-12). The skin of the palm is closely attached by fibrous tissue septa to the underlying palmar fascia. Between these septa lie collections of fat, which are most numerous at the distal part of the palm, just proximal to the bases of the fingers. Beneath the skin lies the fanlike extension of palmar fascia, which is most dense over the middle of the palm and which sends a projection to the proximal phalanx of each finger. From its deep surface there extends a fascial connection, which is attached along the length of the middle metacarpal bone.

This fascial attachment of the palmar fascia is important because it outlines the division between the major palmar spaces of the hand. Lying to the ulnar side of it are the flexor tendons of the middle, the ring, and the fifth fingers, whereas the flexor tendons of the index finger lie to the thumb side. In this same plane with the tendons lie the vessels and the nerves of the hand. Between this layer of tendons and vessels and the interosseous muscles that lie between the metacarpal bones on the ulnar side of the hand, is the middle palmar space. Medially, this space is bounded by the fascial attachment of the palmaris longus along the middle meta-

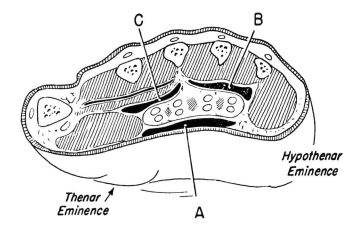

Fig. 24–12. Schematic cross section of palm of hand. (*A*) Pretendinous space of Iselin. (*B*) Middle palmar space. (*C*) Thenar space. (Byrne, J. J.: Am. J. Surg. *88*:439, 1954)

carpal bone. Laterally, it extends to the hypothenar muscles; distally, to within a thumb's breadth of the bases of the fingers; and proximally, to the base of the palm.

Lying to the thumb side of the fascial attachment of the palmar fascia to the middle metacarpal bone is the thenar space; it is between the tendons and the anterior surface of the adductor pollicis muscle. This muscle also takes its origin along the middle metacarpal bone, and the space then lies between it and the fascial attachment to the bone and extends toward the thumb through the tissues of the web of the thumb. These are the major spaces of the palm, and they are most significant from the surgical point of view.

Middle Palmar Space Infection

Etiology. The middle palmar space may become infected as the result of an extension of a tenosynovitis from the middle or the ring finger, in which case the infection invades the space by rupture of the proximal portion of the tendon sheath and extends along the lumbrical muscle to the palmar space. Infection of the tendon sheath of the fifth finger rarely produces an infection of the palmar space, since it extends along the tendon sheath to the ulnar bursa. Infection of the space may result also from injuries to the palm, such as lacerations or compound fractures, or from extension of collar-

button abscesses. Finally, in neglected cases, the pus may rupture from an infection of the thenar space through the fascial plate separating the two spaces.

Symptoms and Diagnosis. Usually, the symptoms of infection of the middle palmar space are quite typical; if one remembers the routes by which infection may travel to this space, the history is often helpful in making the diagnosis. On inspection, the fingers, especially the middle and ring fingers, are held in partial flexion, although, except in cases of an extension from a tenosynovitis, fixed flexion is not present. Swelling is characteristic; there is a loss of the cavity of the palm, especially on the ulnar side, with swelling most marked at the distal portion of the palm between the middle and the ring fingers. This area of swelling represents the extension along the lumbrical muscle to the loose connective tissues in the web of the fingers. There is always a very marked edema of the loose tissues of the dorsum of the hand. This edema is soft, it pits easily, and it is due to the fact that the lymphatic drainage is from the palm to the dorsum by the shortest possible route. This edematous swelling should never be incised with the mistaken idea that the purulent process lies on the dorsum. Finally, tenderness is acute on slight pressure over the outline of the middle palmar space.

Treatment. To drain an infection of the middle palmar space, an incision is made in the distal palm between the middle and

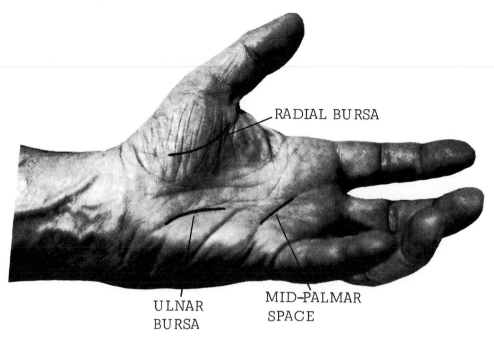

RADIAL BURSA

ULNAR
BURSA

MID-PALMAR
SPACE

Fig. 24–13. Lines of incision for drainage of the mid-palmar space and the radial and ulnar bursae.

the ring fingers or between the ring and the fifth fingers (Fig. 24-13). A curved hemostat, inserted with its point down, can be advanced over the head of the metacarpal bone into the middle palmar space, which can be drained easily be spreading the hemostat. The incision is carried far enough into the palm to permit adequate drainage, and a rubber dam or, better, petrolatum gauze is inserted into the opening.

The wound is dressed with voluminous gauze compresses, and the hand and the wrist are placed on a splint, the hand being so padded that the fingers are held in partial flexion (Fig. 24-14).

In the postoperative care, elevation and hot wet dressings are the principal measures. The wound is dressed 2 or 3 days after incision, then at intervals of 2 days, the wound being irrigated with normal saline to remove slough. Usually, packing is not reinserted after the first or second dressing.

Antibiotic therapy, usually penicillin in massive doses, is employed as an adjunct to surgical therapy, and occasionally bac-

itracin, 1,000 units per ml., is instilled into the space after drainage.

Thenar Space Infection

Etiology. The thenar space may be infected by an extension of an infection from the tendon sheath of the index finger. It occurs only rarely from an infection of the tendon sheath of the thumb, because this extends along the tendon sheath and involves the radial bursa. A collar-button type of abscess lying between the middle and the index fingers, if it is neglected, extends along the lumbrical canals and invades the thenar space. Finally, a direct implantation or a compound fracture may be the source of infection.

Symptoms and Diagnosis. The diagnosis may be made from the history if the sources of infection of this space are borne in mind. On examination, the index finger and, to a lesser extent, the thumb are held in partial flexion, but they are not rigid unless there has been a previous tenosynovitis of the index finger. There

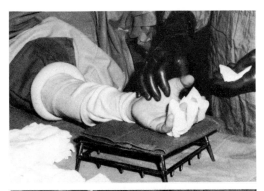

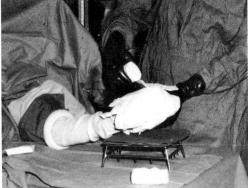

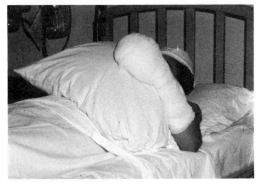

Fig. 24–14. (*Top*) Application of a bulky dressing for hand infections. Note gauze between fingers. Hand in position of function. (*Center*) Palmar space and hand covered with fluffed gauze, and roller bandage of loose-weave, 3-inch gauze being applied with slight tension only. (*Bottom*) Dressing completed, arm in elevation.

is marked swelling of the radial side of the palm, as well as marked edema of the dorsum of the hand. The most characteristic observation is that of the ballooning out of the tissues of the web of the thumb, which process appears to push the thumb

as far away from the palm as possible. The swelling in the web is more marked perhaps on the dorsal than on the palmar side. An infection of the latter extends along the palmar surface of the adductor pollicis and invades the loose areolar tissue of the thumb. Tenderness is marked over the area of the thenar space.

Treatment. Drainage of the thenar space is accomplished easily by incising the bulging tissues in the web of the thumb. The incision is made somewhat on the dorsum, a little to the thumb side of the second metacarpal bone and almost aprallel to it. The operation is performed under general anesthesia using a blood-pressure tourniquet. As soon as the skin opening is made and any purulent material is sponged away, the extension of the infection may be seen passing anterior to the adductor pollicis into the thenar space. A petrolatum-gauze drain inserted along the anterior surface of the adductor pollicis and underneath the tendon provides excellent drainage. Voluminous dressings, immobilization with a splint, intermittent application of hot solutions, and elevation of the arm usually result in a rapid subsidence of the infection. The drain should be allowed to remain in place for only 3 or 4 days; thereafter, the splint is continued until purulent drainage ceases. Maintenance of elevation throughout the period of treatment reduces edema and permits earlier healing. The antibiotics, usually penicillin, are invaluable adjuncts to surgical treatment.

INFECTIONS OF THE
DORSUM OF THE HAND

*Subcutaneous
Dorsal Space Infections*

Anatomy and Etiology. There are two ill-defined fascial spaces on the dorsum of the hand. One is superficial and is called the subcutaneous space. It is composed of loose areolar tissue. Infection of this area arises most often by direct implantation, although frequently an abscess appears as a result of cellulitis or lymphangitis. In diagnosing this infection, one should note that the swelling is more definitely an induration than is the soft, pitting edema usually seen in infections of the palm.

Treatment. Simple incision and drainage are all that is necessary in treating a subcutaneous fascial infection. Splinting, hot wet dressings, elevation, and antibiotics comprise the postoperative treatment.

Subaponeurotic Dorsal Space Infections

Anatomy and Etiology. The other space on the dorsum of the hand lies between the metacarpal bones and the aponeurotic plate, including the extensor tendons. Infection here is relatively rare, except from direct implantation from wounds over the dorsum of the hand. One of the common sites of infection from bite wounds following a blow on the knuckles is this space.

Symptoms. Symptoms of this infection are usually recognized easily, since the history of the injury and the appearance of the wound point definitely to a lesion on the dorsum of the hand. Swelling and edema of the dorsum are marked, but the absence of induration in the swelling, which is seen in subcutaneous infections, makes the diagnosis of subaponeurotic abscess more likely. Frequently it is difficult to distinguish between these two infections, and often both spaces may be involved in wounds of the dorsum of the hand.

Treatment. Incision under general anesthesia, with a tourniquet applied and followed by drainage, splinting, hot wet dressings, antibiotics, and elevation, usually produces rapid subsidence of the infection.

TRAUMATIC LESIONS

WOUNDS

The Fingers

Wounds of the fingers vary from simple cuts or punctures that involve only the skin and the subcutaneous tissues to ex-

tensive lacerations that involve the underlying tendons, bones, and joints. Frequently they lead to minor or serious infections, and their prophylactic care should be a matter of serious consideration.

Treatment. Tiny puncture wounds, such as needle punctures, pinpricks, and so forth, are not often followed by serious difficulties.

A larger potentially infected wound is treated as is any open traumatic wound elsewhere in the body. In the first-aid treatment, it is unwise to apply irritating antiseptics. The wound should be covered with sterile gauze dressings and the patient transported to a dispensary or hospital where appropriate first aid can be given.

Thorough cleansing of the surrounding tissues with soap and water and, finally, irrigation of the wound itself with sterile saline permit closure with a minimal danger of infection. Devitalized tissues are cut away, but conservatism should be the rule in excising tissues of the finger. If the patient can be seen within the first 12 hours after injury, tendons that are divided should be sutured and the wound should be closed. The author has found that alloy steel wire is of particular value for such sutures, because it may remain in place for as long as 10 or 12 days without fear of reaction round it. As a rule, pressure dressings are sufficient to control hemorrhage from the wound. Splints made of hairpins enclosed in adhesive are of value in immobilizing the finger while healing takes place. Commercially produced splints are available.

If the wound is seen after the period of contamination, it is better not to attempt primary suture. Antibiotics, usually penicillin, are given in generous doses. The wound is cleansed as described above, its edges are pulled together with adhesive strips, and a splint is applied. If the wound becomes infected, it is opened and cared for easily, hot wet dressings being used. No attempt should be made to suture tendons if tissue is avulsed or crushed and the wound cannot be debrided completely.

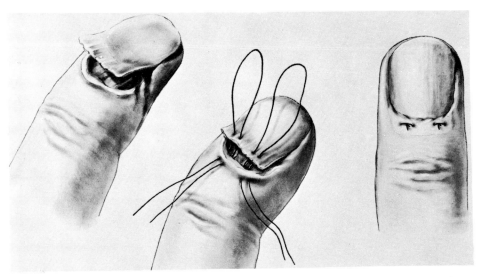

Fig. 24–15. Method of replacing avulsed nail matrix, using mattress sutures of 5-0 catgut. Usually local infiltration anesthesia is used. (Kleinert, H. E.: Am. Surg., *25*:41, 1959)

Crush Wounds
of the Distal Phalanx

Etiology and Symptoms. Crush wounds of the distal phalanx, with fracture of the phalanx and partial or complete avulsion of the nail, are common, not only in industry but also in civil life, the fingertip having been caught between objects or in house or automobile doors. The injury is usually quite characteristic: the proximal portion of the nail is ripped from its position under the eponychium and may lie on top of the eponychium, the entire base of the nail being exposed. A roentgenogram usually shows a fracture of the distal phalanx. If the crush has involved the palmar surface of the tip, there is a contused, jagged wound.

Treatment. The treatment of such an injury is usually simple and successful if it can be accomplished within a few hours of its occurrence. The area is cleansed thoroughly with soap and water. Penicillin is given as a prophylactic measure. The avulsed nail is cut away, usually without anesthesia, or is pulled back in place with two mattress sutures of 5-0 catgut (Fig. 24-15). When the injury produces a longitudinal laceration of the fingertip, often involving the bone, the tissues are replaced as well as possible by suturing through nail and soft tissue (Fig. 24-16), and the wound is covered with a layer or two of sterile petrolatum gauze. The entire dressing is then enclosed in a plaster thimble made with 4 or 5 layers of plaster rolled into a cylinder, put on the finger, and then moistened with sterile water. The plaster is molded to conform to the shape of the finger and the fingertip, and is permitted to harden (Fig. 24-17). If this dressing is applied properly, it need not be changed until it is removed in about 10 days to 2 weeks. By this time, the wound usually has healed. When there is a fracture, it is wise to maintain the dressing for a longer period by the reapplication of a plaster thimble. By this method of therapy, pain is relieved, and the protection offered by the plaster thimble permits the use of the finger.

The Hand and the Fingers

Wounds of the hand and the fingers are extremely common in industry. They are very important because even small wounds may produce serious disability if they are complicated by tendon, nerve, or

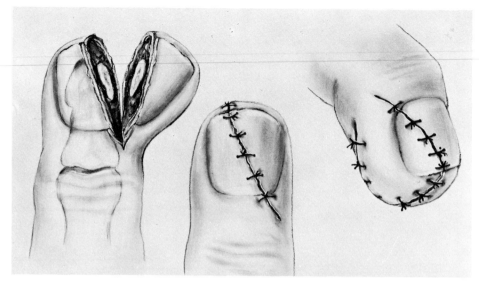

Fig. 24–16. Longitudinal laceration of fingertip involving bone and nail. Repair by suture. (Kleinert, H. E.: Am. Surg., *25*:41, 1959)

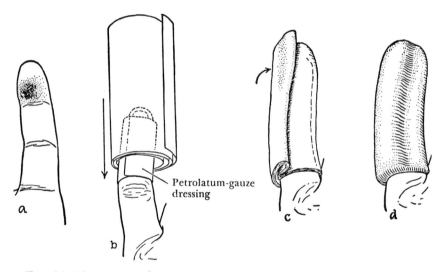

Fig. 24–17. Dressing for crush wounds (*a*) of the distal phalanx of the finger. After the wound has been cleansed thoroughly, it is protected with petrolatum gauze, and a cylinder of plaster is placed over the finger (*b*). This then is wet with sterile water and molded to form a plaster thimble (*c* and *d*), which is allowed to remain in place for about 3 weeks. This dressing is borne easily and permits the patient to use the hand without pain from trauma to the finger.

bone injury or by tissue necrosis or infection. With such an injury, the patient is almost always ambulatory, and he may be seen for the first treatment in an office or a plant dispensary. The patient's best interests will be served if the wound is covered as soon as possible with a sterile dressing, if exploration of the wound is avoided, if antiseptic applications are withheld, and if simple cleansing with soap and water around the covered wound is the only first-aid treatment.

It is most important to evaluate the wound for deep injury (to bone, tendon, or nerve). Wounds involving only skin and subcutaneous tissue may be treated in an office or a dispensary with proper facilities. In the case of more serious injuries, involving loss of skin, open fractures, or tendon and nerve injuries, the patient should be hospitalized to obtain the benefits of adequate anesthesia, instruments, assistance, light, etc.

Mason has outlined the important steps in the treatment of hand wounds. He emphasizes the importance of preserving all viable tissues, obtaining hemostasis, and effecting primary closure of the wound, if necessary by skin graft. The hand should be dressed with a compression dressing and splinted in the position of function (slight dorsiflexion of the wrist, with the fingers in partial flexion) (Fig. 24-14). Antibiotics are given prophylactically as a rule.

For skin suture, it is our choice to use fine alloy steel wire. The lack of reaction in the tissues makes it possible to leave these sutures in place for as long as 2 or 3 weeks.

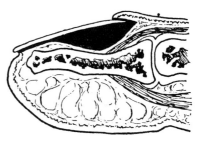

Fig. 24–18. Diagram of subungual hematoma. Note the location of the blood in an unyielding space bounded, above, by the nail and, below, by the dorsum of the phalanx. This accounts for the excruciating pain from this relatively minor injury.

SUBUNGUAL HEMATOMA

Etiology and Symptoms. Blows on the fingernail produce a hemorrhage under the nail. Although relatively minor, this injury causes excruciating pain because there is marked tension in the unyielding space bounded by the firm nail above and the bone below (Fig. 24-18). Most carpenters know better than most physicians that relief of tension in this area will permit relief of pain.

Patients usually seek treatment with the story that the finger was struck by a hammer, following which there was marked swelling and pain. On examination, there may be only an area of dark, bluish discoloration at the base of the nail, or, in more severe cases, marked swelling with distention of the eponychium.

Treatment. Rapid relief of pain is obtained by permitting the escape of the blood. Early accomplishment of this is best, when the blood still is fluid. In those cases in which the eponychium is dis-

tended, the knife edge may be inserted between the eponychium and the nail, which permits blood to escape and relieves tension. When the hematoma lies entirely under the nail, it is necessary to make a small opening in the base of the nail to permit the escape of the blood. This is a somewhat painful procedure if much pressure is placed on the nail, because such pressure increases tension and, consequently, pain. If, however, one makes an incision with the scalpel, cutting more or less across the nail without much pressure, little pain is experienced, and blood escapes in a large drop as soon as the nail is punctured. As a rule, a bit of the nail can be cut out by making two oblique incisions across its base. This permits continued drainage of blood and serum, and it prevents subsequent tension. A small pressure dressing consisting of a Band-Aid is all that is necessary.

In occasional cases the hematoma may extend toward the finger tip. In such cases the careful insertion of the tip of a pointed scalpel just under the nail will permit drainage of the hematoma without anesthesia.

TENDON INJURIES AND TENDON SUTURE

Injuries to the hand and the fingers, especially those producing cuts of the skin, are likely to divide the underlying tendons. The wound itself may be in-

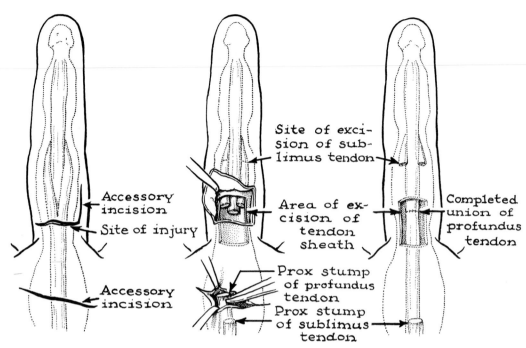

Fig. 24–19. Method of repair of flexor tendons of the finger. With division of both flexor tendoms in the finger, the profundus tendon only should be sutured. The original wound is enlarged to permit excision of the distal sublimis stumps and to allow sufficient room for tendon suture. The proximal stump of the profundus is picked up through an accessory incision in the palm and is led back through the tunnel into the finger, and repair is accomplished. A square segment about 1 cm. long is then excised from the fibrous sheath over the site of tendon repair. When the skin is closed, this square window is covered by the subcutaneous fat, which will permit gliding of the tendon after healing. (After Mason, M. L.: Surg., Gynec. Obstet., *70*:392, 1940)

significant, a small cut with a knife or a piece of glass, but examination always should be made at the first inspection for evidence of a tendon injury. When a tendon division is demonstrated, suture should not be attempted without adequate facilities, which are usually to be found only in a hospital operating room. However, the patient may be ambulatory with a splint after operation.

Mason taught that, to be successful, primary suture of a divided tendon should be performed within 2 hours after injury and only after very careful preparation of the wound, which consists of excision of nonviable tissue after meticulous skin cleansing and wound lavage. It is probable that by using antibiotics, this time limit may be lengthened. A bloodless field produced by an inflated blood-pressure cuff acting as a tourniquet makes rapid and careful work possible. In a bloodless wound irrigated frequently with saline, nonviable tissue is excised with forceps and a knife, but wide wound excision is usually not performed. Often, in the case of small wounds of the fingers and the hands made by sharp objects, such as a chisel or a piece of glass, no tissue need be sacrificed. Tendons, nerves, and blood vessels must be carefully protected.

To obtain exposure of the severed tendons, the incision may have to be enlarged, or a second incision may be necessary to locate a retracted tendon. Such

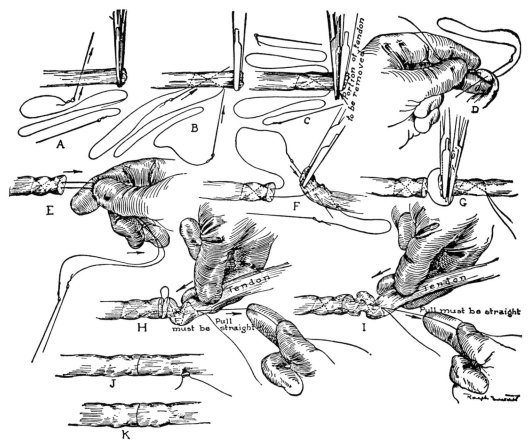

Fig. 24–20. Suture of tendon with silk technique. (*A-D*) With each of 2 needles, the suture is placed to traverse the tendon from 2 to 4 times and emerge through the end. (*E*) All slack is drawn out. (*F-G*) In the same way, the suture is continued up the other tendon. Both ends are brought out at the same spot. To prevent spearing the thread, the 2 needles should be thrust through the tendon at the same time. (*H-I*) To prevent the tendon ends from separating under strain, the slack is removed from the second tendon. To do this, 1 suture is pulled at a time as the tendon is shoved along it to snug against the other tendon end. (*J-K*) There is only 1 knot; when tied, it sinks into the tendon, and at a place at which it receives the least strain, as knots are the weakest parts of a tendon suture. (Boyes, J.: Bunnel 11's Surgery of the Hand. ed. 4. Philadelphia, J. B. Lippincott, 1964)

incisions should be made in flexion creases and along the sides of the fingers to avoid scar contracture and adhesions.

In preparing the tendon for suture, the traumatized end is excised conservatively; in clean cuts, no excision at all may be necessary. When the flexor tendons of the finger are divided, it is usually best to sacrifice the sublimis tendon, from its attachment to the base of the middle phalanx to a point well proximal to the point of division (Fig. 24-19). The nerves should be identified, and if they are sev-ered, they should be prepared for suture in the same way as are the tendons. After thorough preparation of the wound, the tourniquet is released temporarily while all bleeders are ligated with fine silk.

Tendons should be sutured with material that produces the least reaction in the tissue and the least bulk at the suture line. Fine silk (Fig. 24-20) and fine alloy steel wire (Fig. 24-21) fit these requirements best. Mason and Allen approximate the cut ends with transverse stay sutures of silk, uniting the peritendinous tissues

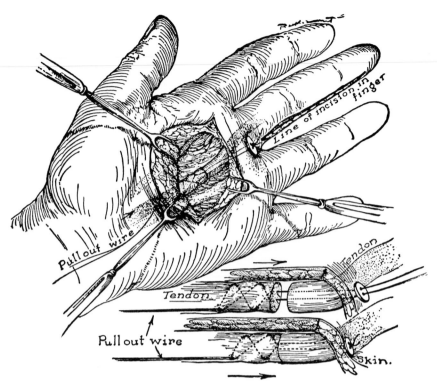

Fig. 24–21. Suturing a tendon in the palm with removable stainless-steel wire. In 3 weeks the tendon will have joined, and, after being cut, the suture beneath the button may be withdrawn backward by the pull-out wire, which is looped about it. (Boyes, J.: Bunnell's Surgery of the Hand. ed. 4. Philadelphia, J. B. Lippincott, 1964)

with interrupted sutures of the same material. When the tendons are divided in a tendon sheath, a segment of the sheath overlying the suture line should be excised, or the tendon sheath should be split its length along the lateral attachment to the phalanx.

When divided nerves are found in association with tendon injuries, they should be approximated carefully by placing fine sutures in the fibrous tissue surrounding them.

After careful skin closure, a firm pressure dressing is applied before the tourniquet is removed, and the part is splinted in such a position as to produce maximum relaxation of the sutured tendon. Unless some complication appears, the wound should not be dressed for 2 weeks at least. Mason and Allen have shown that ten-

dons heal better if complete immobilization is maintained for 14 days at least. During the third and fourth weeks, restricted use of the tendon "may be expected to lead to only a slight increase in reaction and to a rapid increase in tensile strength of the union." Unrestricted use may be permitted 4 to 5 weeks after tendon suture.

CONTUSIONS OF THE DORSUM OF THE HAND (WRINGER INJURY)

Contusions of the dorsum of the hand are seen frequently, particularly in women and children whose hands have been caught in a clothes wringer. Rupture of some of the vessels of the dorsum produces rapid swelling and, sometimes, hematoma formation.

Treatment. If the patient is seen early, an excellent form of treatment is to apply a pressure bandage incorporating fluff gauze or mechanic's waste and to place the hand on a splint. If there is a hematoma, in spite of the fact that fluctuation may be present, aspiration is of no value. Incision and drainage permit evacuation of the clot, which results in more rapid and complete subsidence of the swelling. In cases untreated for a long time, the fibrosis that results from prolonged edema of the dorsum of the hand may give discomfort and some disability. Little can be done in the way of therapy except to prevent edema by pressure and elevation. The swelling and the discomfort disappear gradually, but it sometimes takes several weeks, even months, for complete subsidence of the process. In some patients with persistent disability, some authors have recommended excision of the hard mass of scar tissue. This has never been necessary in our experience.

Traumatic Amputation of the Soft Tissues of the Distal Phalanx

Knife, razor, and glass injuries to the distal phalanx often result in the traumatic amputation of the soft tissues of the finger, and frequently the bone is exposed. In such cases, if healing is allowed to take place, the result is a scar deformity of the distal phalanx, which is tender and often produces marked disability. This is especially true if the tip of the bone lies directly under the scar. It should be emphasized that fingertip injuries are serious wounds whose importance to the individual far exceeds the extent of tissue damage. In the treatment of these injuries maximum conservation of tissue and of finger function must be constantly in the mind of the surgeon.

In a few cases, the amputated bit of skin and soft tissues is at hand or is hanging by a mere shred of tissue. When this is so, the wound should be cleansed thoroughly with soap and water and the detached portion of the skin and the soft tissues sewn in place with fine silk or dermal sutures. It is important to use only a few sutures.

If the wound of the fingertip does not expose the bone and is less than 1 cm. in diameter, the area is carefully cleansed, covered with a strip or two of petrolatum gauze, and dressed with a protective splint. During re-dressings, the petrolatum gauze should be left in place. It will come away when the wound has epithelialized in 12 to 14 days.

If the wound is larger but the bone is not exposed, the area may be covered with a graft removed from the forearm or the thigh. This should be cut accurately to fit the site. The edges of the graft should be free of any subcutaneous fat, but the middle of the graft often may contain a small amount of fatty tissue to advantage. The graft is sewn in place with fine silk sutures, and a dressing of paraffin gauze with a snug bandage and a splint is applied. Unless there is some reason to suspect that the graft is not taking or unless infection is present, it is wise not to change the dressing for a period of from 10 to 14 days. At this time the sutures may be removed and a protective dressing applied until firm healing takes place.

When there is complete loss of the fingertip, including bone, depending on the amount of other injury, one of three methods of treatment is available.

1. Amputation More Proximal. Sufficient bone is removed with a rongeur to permit the soft tissue to be approximated over the tip of the finger without tension. If the finger has been amputated near the base of the nail, the nail matrix should be completely excised, to avoid the growth of a small painful nail fragment (Fig. 24-22).

If the amputation is below the distal phalanx, or through the distal interphalangeal joint, amputation more proximal is often done. In such cases, the condyles of the middle phalanx with their articular cartilage are scraped away with a rongeur as far as necessary to allow soft tissue approximation over the stump without tension. Traction is applied to the

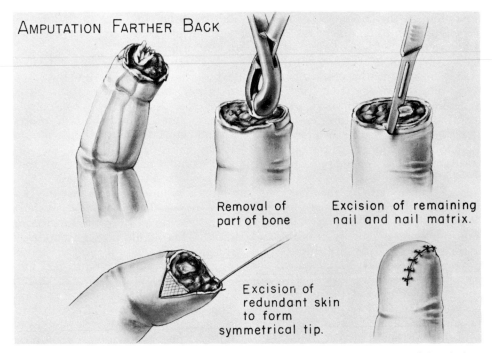

AMPUTATION FARTHER BACK

Removal of
part of bone

Excision of remaining
nail and nail matrix.

Excision of
redundant skin
to form
symmetrical tip.

Fig. 24–22. Soft-tissue covering of amputation of fingertip by amputation of the phalanx farther back. This shortens the phalanx somewhat but gives good coverage with few complications. (Kleinert, H. E.: Am. Surg., *25*:41, 1959)

tendons, flexor and extensor, and they are exposed and cut off so that they will retract. Skin closure with fine wire sutures is carred out, and the wound is covered with petrolatum gauze and guarded by a hairpin splint. Sutures are removed in about 2 weeks.

2. Local Revision. Several methods of revision of the fingertip wound have been designed to provide a soft-tissue covering for the amputated bone. Kutler made a V-shaped incision on each side of the amputated stump, sliding the V-shaped areas of skin and fibrofatty tissue upward to cover the bone (Fig. 24-23). Kleinert slides the remaining fibrofatty pad upward to cover the end of the bone and covers the exposed pulp with a heavy split-thickness skin graft (Fig. 24-24).

3. Reconstructive techniques. A palmar flap fashioned from skin, usually of the thenar eminence, is sometimes used to cover an amputated finger tip (Fig. 24-25). The flap is separated from its position in 14 to 18 days. The results are good as far

as function is concerned, but the procedure is complicated, and it takes 6 to 8 weeks before function can be resumed.

Cross Finger Flaps in the Treatment of Injuries to the Fingers

It is recognized that preservation of a functioning finger and hand is invaluable. In an effort to preserve as much as possible of the length of the finger and to prevent a painful scar in which bone is included, a flap of skin has been fashioned from an adjacent finger and rotated to permit covering of the bare stump of an amputated finger. Many authors believe this to be the best method of treatment of fingertip injuries.

The cross finger flap covering of a denuded finger necessitates a two-stage procedure, but as much as possible of the finger is preserved and the results as far as a functioning finger are much better than they are by other methods of repair.

The flap may be based proximally (Fig.

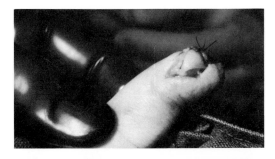

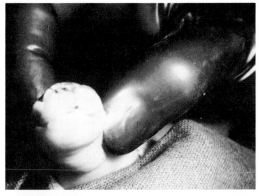

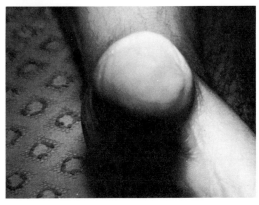

Fig. 24–23. Kutler's technique to provide a soft-tissue cover for an amputated fingertip. (*Top*) A V-shaped incision is made on each side, the tissues are slid together (*Center*) and sutured with a few fine sutures. (*Bottom*) End result is a soft, well-padded tip.

24-26) or distally (Fig. 24-27) or may be hinged longitudinally (Fig. 24-28). The blood supply to the flap is good and is not impaired by slight kinking of the flap. The area from which the graft was taken is covered by a split-thickness graft, cut from the forearm of the same limb. This leaves the other arm without wounds.

The dressing includes a palmar pad of sterile fluff gauze, gauze between the apposed fingers, a bandage or adhesive to hold the apposed fingers together, a firm fixed dressing over the skin graft, a bandage of stretch gauze, and a light plaster covering over all.

The hand should be kept elevated in a sling. The second stage is performed 2 to 3 weeks later. The flap is shaped to cover the defect and is sutured in place; the unused portion of the flap may be returned to the site from which it was taken. Sutures are removed in 7 to 10 days. Patients are allowed to return to light work 3 weeks after the second operation.

PRESSURE GUN INJURIES

This is a relatively new type of injury which can involve any area of the body, but often involves the finger or the hand. It is usually an inadvertant injury, caused by the accidental firing of the pressure gun when it is in contact with the skin. The most common causes are grease guns, hot steam-cleaning guns, or paint guns.

Symptoms. The symptoms are immediate pain and swelling of the part, and, depending upon the agent in the gun, discoloration. The point of injury is often quite small (Fig. 24-29, *top*).

Treatment. The treatment of this condition is immediate fasciotomy along the side of the finger, extending from the distal flexion crease to the proximal flexion crease, with great care being taken to avoid injuring the nerve or blood vessel, if possible. Careful cleaning and débridement, plus irrigation and the picking out of foreign bodies, must be carried out. Usually this will require general anesthesia, although an axillary block is sometimes satisfactory if the injured part is a finger. Following this, the wound should be left open, a dressing should be applied, and the lesion should be treated with hot moist soaks, elevation, and antibiotics.

Although the results of fasciotomy and débridment may not be totally successful (Fig. 24-29), *center* and *bottom*), these measures can result in the saving of all or part of a finger.

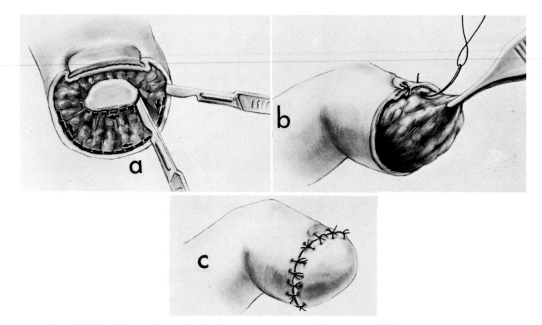

Fig. 24–24. Kleinert's method of covering stump of amputated distal phalanx. (*a*) Pulp is separated from the skin and bone for a distance of 1 cm. (*b*) Pulp is slid forward and sutured to nail bed, covering exposed bone. (*c*) Full thickness or heavy split thickness skin graft applied over pulp. (Kleinert, H. E.: Am. Surg., *25*:41, 1959)

PRACTICAL POINTS IN THE TREATMENT OF INJURIES OF THE FINGERS

Some surgeons may feel that hospitalization is required for the treatment of all hand and finger injuries. This is true for extensive injuries. Minor injuries, however, can be cared for easily in an ambulatory patient.

Practically all injuries of the finger can be treated after a local anesthetic has been injected to block the nerves at the base of the finger or in the distal palm. In most cases, it is wise to inject the anesthetic before attempting to cleanse the part; thus the anesthesia begins to take effect while the area around the wound is being cleaned. By the time the wound itself is cleaned, the finger is insensitive to pain. The new short-acting general anesthetics make possible the use of general anesthesia for ambulatory hand surgery, and many times they are preferred by both the patient and the surgeon.

A blood-pressure cuff used as a tourniquet prevents bleeding during the care of the finger.

As a rule, it is not necessary in most of these injuries to ligate the vessels. Pressure bandages are usually sufficient to produce hemostasis.

TENDON INJURIES

Mallet Finger
(Baseball Finger, Drop Finger)

Etiology. Mallet finger and drop finger are names given commonly to the deformity of the distal phalanx that results when the extended finger is struck end on. A forcible flexion of the distal phalanx on the middle phalanx occurs. This accident occurs often in sports, when a baseball or a football is caught on the end of the finger.

Symptoms. In some cases, the injury is so trivial that it is disregarded. On the other hand, the patient may feel or hear a

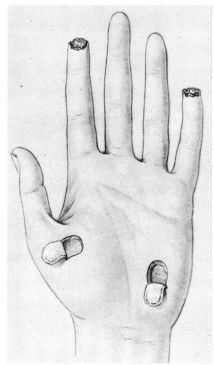

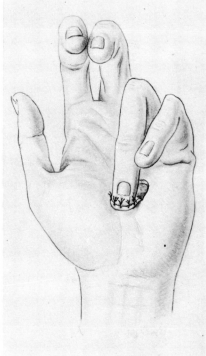

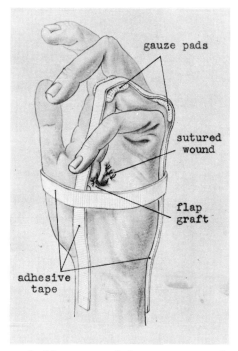

Fig. 24–25. (*Top Left*) Lateral and proximal types of pedicle flaps. (*Top Right*) Method of suturing flap to defect on fingertip. Kinking of flap should be avoided. (*bottom right*) Completed operation. The wound in the palm has been sutured after uniting the flap to the fingertip. (The author has also covered the palmar defect with a free graft in several cases.) An adhesive support is applied before bandaging. (Jones, R. A.: Am. J. Surg., 55:331, 1942)

snap and experience sharp pain in the region of the distal interphalangeal joint. As a rule, swelling occurs in the joint region, and there is some soreness, but the chief symptom is an inability to extend the distal phalanx. Swelling and tenderness sometimes mask this important symptom, and the true disability is disregarded in the early phases of treatment.

The trauma producing mallet finger may result in several different kinds of injury, the most frequent of which is probably a tear of the extensor tendon at its insertion on the dorsum of the base of the distal phalanx. In some cases, there may be an associated sprain fracture—a

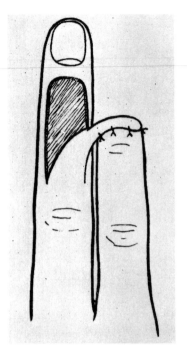

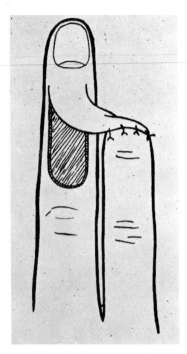

Fig. 24–26. Cross finger flap based proximally. (Tempest, M. N.: Plast. Reconstr. Surg., *9*:205, 1952)

Fig. 24–27. Cross finger flap based distally. (Tempest, M. N.: Plast. Reconstr. Surg., *9*:205, 1952)

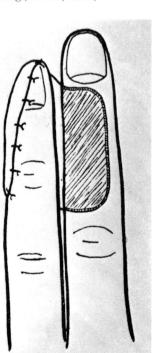

tearing away of bone at the insertion of the extensor tendon.

A large majority of these injuries go without adequate treatment, and, as a result, there is a gradual subsidence of the swelling and the pain in the region of the distal interphalangeal joint, but the thickening of the joint and the inability to extend the distal phalanx remain as a disfiguring and somewhat disabling deformity (Fig. 24-30).

Treatment. Successful treatment of mallet finger depends on the early recognition of the lesion and the early institution of appropriate therapy. It is a wise precaution to do a roentgen examination to ascertain if there is a fracture of the base of the distal phalanx and, if there is,

Fig. 24–28. Cross finger flap hinged longitudinally, (Tempest, M. N.: Plast. Reconstr. Surg., *9*:205, 1952)

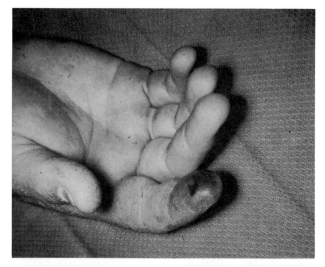

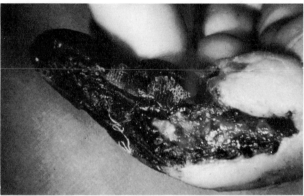

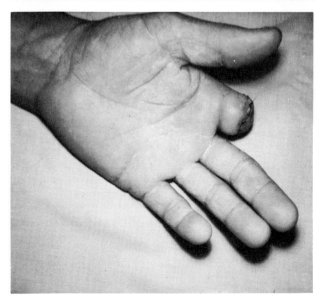

Fig. 24–29. (*Top*) Pressure (grease) gun injury of tip of index finger. (*Center*) Fasciotomy has been done and gangrene has occurred at the distal half of finger. (*Bottom*) Proximal amputation and closure.

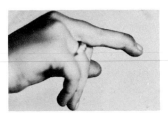

Fig. 24–30. Recent mallet finger. Note the inability to extend completely the distal phalanx.

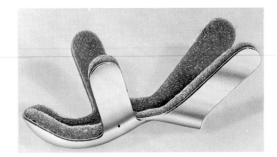

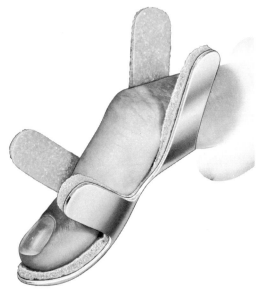

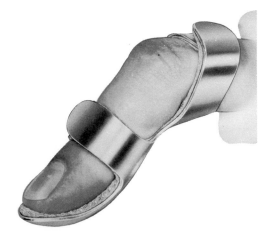

to determine its type. In those cases without fracture, the supposition is that the disability is due to a tear of the extensor tendon, and an examination should show whether the lesion is at the distal interphalangeal joint, which is commonly the case.

Treatment may be conservative or operative. Conservative treatment consists in immobilizing the finger, especially the distal interphalangeal joint, in hypertension. This is done by splinting (Fig. 24-31) or, more successfully, by applying a plaster cast. Four or five layers of a plaster bandage are rolled into the form of a cylinder; this is then applied over the involved finger, which then is dipped into water, and the plaster is molded firmly to the finger. The patient himself holds the distal phalanx in hyperextension and the proximal interphalangeal joint in flexion by pressing the finger involved against the thumb (Fig. 24-32). In this way, the extensor tendon is relaxed, and thus the distal phalanx is held in the position in which healing of the ruptured tendon is most likely to occur. This dressing is allowed to remain in place for 5 weeks at least. There is no difficulty from pressure in such a dressing, and most patients are able to pursue their usual occupation with the cast in place.

We have used the same method of therapy in many cases in which there was a triangular fracture at the base of the distal phalanx. If postreduction roentgenograms show the fragments to be in good position, nothing further is necessary to obtain good union and a good result. Various other methods for the

Fig. 24–31. Malleable aluminum splint for mallet finger injuries to hold distal phalanx in extension. (*Top*) Splint lined with soft plastic material. (*Center*) Before adjusting splint. (*Bottom*) Splint in place on finger. (Richards Mfg. Co.)

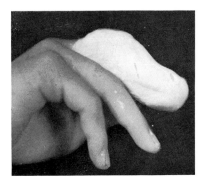

Fig. 24–32. Plaster thimble for treatment of mallet finger. Three or four layers of 3-inch plaster bandage are rolled into a cylinder; this is slipped over the finger, and the finger is dipped in a vessel of water. While the plaster is wet, it is molded to the finger while the distal phalanx is held in hyperextension and the proximal phalanx is held in flexion by the patient; this relaxes the extensor tendon to the distal phalanx.

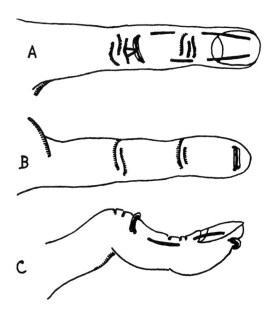

Fig. 24–33. Silk suture method of holding distal phalanx in extension suggested by Hillman for mallet finger and fracture of the articular surface of the distal phalanx. (Hillman, F. E.: JAMA, *161*:1135, 1956)

treatment of mallet finger have been suggested, because there is the belief that the cast becomes loose and is not effective in holding the distal phalanx in extension while the proximal interphalangeal joint is held in flexion. Fowler and Spiegelman have devised splints and slings for this purpose. Hillman has suggested a suture method to hold the distal phalanx in extension (Fig. 24-33). He places a silk or wire suture from the palmar side of the finger tip through the nail, then twice through the soft tissues at the side of the finger to end on the dorsolateral side of the middle phalanx. The other end of the suture is passed through a short segment of narrow vinyl tubing and is placed in a similar fashion on the other side of the finger. One end of the suture is threaded through another short segment of vinyl tubing, and the two ends are pulled taut and tied. A sterile gauze dressing is applied and is held in place with a bandage. Slight pain is relieved by salicylates or codeine for 2 or 3 days. The bandage is changed every 5 to 7 days, and the suture is removed in 4 to 6 weeks.

Operative therapy is recommended as the treatment of choice by Mason, Kap-

lan, and others. Mason believes that, in cases of complete rupture, fragments of the torn tendon may fall into the joint space, preventing normal healing of the tendon and producing disability in extension of the joint. Kaplan feels that replacement of the fractured fragment at the base of the distal phalanx is necessary to obtain a normal articular surface and a good result in cases in which a definite fracture is demonstrated.

Certainly, in all cases of old injury, little can be expected from conservative treatment, and operation is the only method of improving the result. This may be performed with the use of local block anesthesia at the base of the finger. A U- or an L-shaped flap is made, the flap being turned away from the distal phalanx, as recommended by Mason and Smillie, or toward the distal phalanx, as recommended by Kaplan. Through either type of incision, the extensor tendon is exposed. The site of the tear in the tendon can be recognized easily, and the two ends are approximated with fine silk sutures mounted on a small curved cutting-edged needle. In old cases, the area of the tear often is united by scar tissue, which must be excised, and the tendon ends must be approximated if normal extension of the distal phalanx is to be obtained. After the wound has been sutured, sterile petrolatum gauze is placed over it, and the wound is encased in a plaster cylinder (Fig. 24-32). This dressing is allowed to remain in place for from 4 to 5 weeks. If the sutures are of fine alloy wire, they may be left in place for this length of time without difficulty.

The prognosis for a complete resumption of extension in the injured phalanx is good if early treatment is instituted. A good functional result may likewise be obtained in old cases if tendon rupture is the cause of the disability. However, in old cases of fracture of the base of the distal phalanx, the prognosis is not very good, and frequently little improvement can be obtained by operation because of the bony deformity in the joint.

Buttonhole Rupture of the Extensor Tendon Over the Proximal Interphalangeal Joint

Anatomy. Another, less common, tendon rupture of the finger is that of the aponeurosis of the extensor tendon over the proximal interphalangeal joint. To understand this injury, it is necessary to be conversant with the anatomy of the extensor tendon in this area. In approaching the metacarpophalangeal joint, the extensor tendon spreads fanlike over the proximal phalanx and separates into two lateral bands and one central band. The central band inserts at the base of the middle phalanx and has to do with the extension of that phalanx on the proximal phalanx. The lateral bands have the tendinous insertions of the interosseous muscles attached to them. They extend lateral to the proximal interphalangeal joint and thence unite over the middle phalanx to insert at the base of the distal phalanx (Fig. 24-34).

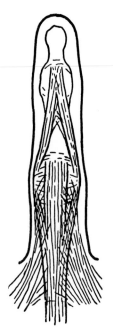

Fig. 24–34. Diagrammatic drawing of the extensor tendon of the finger. Note the central slip, which inserts at the base of the middle phalanx, and the two lateral slips, which pass to join and insert at the base of the distal phalanx.

Etiology. The injury causes a tear of the central band of the extensor tendon (Fig. 24-35). It may occur indirectly as the result of a forceful flexion of the distal and the middle phalanges on the proximal phalanx while the finger is being held in extension. Thus, in sports, the finger is often struck on the back of the middle phalanx while it is being held in extension. The injury often occurs directly from a blow over the proximal interphalangeal joint, the tendon being sheared off by the traumatizing force acting against the head of the proximal phalanx.

Symptoms. The finger becomes swollen and painful. On examination, there is inability to extend the middle upon the proximal phalanx, the finger thus being held in partial flexion. Efforts to extend it result in hyperextension of the distal phalanx and extension of the proximal phalanx, the middle phalanx remaining in flexion (Fig. 24-36). In chronic cases, the

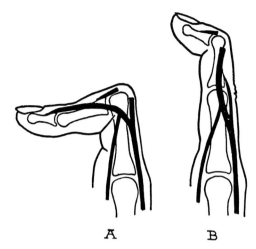

A   B

Fig. 24–35. Diagrammatic representation of ruptures of the extensor tendon of the finger. (*A*) Rupture of the central slip, which inserts at the base of the middle phalanx; this is commonly called a buttonhole rupture. On flexion, the head of the proximal phalanx passes between the lateral slips of the extensor tendon and is caught there when attempts are made to extend the finger. (*B*) Diagrammatic representation of mallet finger, that is, rupture of the extensor tendon, which inserts on the base of the distal phalanx.

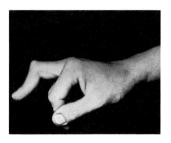

Fig. 24–36. Buttonhole rupture of the extensor tendon. The patient is attempting to extend the finger. Note the hyperextension of the distal phalanx, the middle phalanx remaining in flexion. The prominence of the head of the proximal phalanx may be noted.

patient learns that he can extend the finger passively with the other hand more easily if he does not contract the extensors actively. This disability results from the fact that the tear of the central slip of the extensor tendon, which normally inserts at the base of the middle phalanx, permits the head of the proximal phalanx to extend upward through the buttonholelike opening that results when the finger is flexed. When efforts are made to extend the finger, the lateral slips of the extensor tendon going to the distal phalanx prevent extension by tightening around the head of the proximal phalanx. The harder the patient tries to extend the finger, the more tightly is the head held between the lateral slips of the tendon.

Treatment. Usually this injury responds well to operative repair of the ruptured tendon. An L- or a U-shaped incision is made over the proximal in-

terphalangeal joint. The tear in the tendon exposes the joint, and when the finger is flexed, the head of the proximal phalanx presents in the wound. While the finger is held in extension, the ruptured tendon is sutured in place with fine silk sutures, a very small cutting-edged needle being used. The skin wound is closed with fine silk sutures, and the finger is fixed in full extension in light plaster for 3 weeks. The operation may be performed under local anesthesia.

The prognosis for complete recovery of function is good. The earlier the operation is performed, the better the final result.

Rupture of the Extensor Pollicis Longus Tendon (Drummers' Palsy)

Etiology. Rupture of the long extensor tendon to the thumb is a relatively uncommon lesion. It is frequently spoken of as a spontaneous rupture, although the probability is that usually a long-continued trauma, such as that which occurs in some industries, or occasionally a single trauma may be a factor. Most often the rupture occurs some time after a fracture of the lower radius. The cause of the rupture is probably an interference with the blood supply of the tendon, with a resulting gradual aseptic necrosis of the tendon fibers. The long and rather oblique course of the tendon across the dorsum of the wrist and the firm fixation of the tendon in the dense osseoligamentous tunnel are factors that are suggested as the causes of the gradual fraying and the eventual rupture of the tendon. The injury occurs more frequently in males than in females, and in about 80 percent of the cases, it is the right thumb that is involved. The rupture always occurs at the distal end of the dorsocarpal liagment.

Symptoms. The patient gives a history of sudden, usually painless, loss of function of the thumb. Mason states that only slight swelling appears, but that the functional loss is quite typical. The prominent dorsal border of the anatomic snuffbox is lost. The distal phalanx of the thumb is flexed and cannot be extended unless the thumb is adducted.

Treatment. The only method of therapy is surgical. Operation may be performed under local anesthesia, but the frayed ends of the tendon can rarely be approximated. In some instances, the stumps may be sutured to an adjacent tendon. When they have united with the adjacent tendon, a second operation is performed, and a longitudinal strip of the host tendon is excised to fill in the gap between the tendon ends. Mason suggests as the best method of therapy a tendon transplant from one of the dorsal tendons of the foot. Other authors believe that early operation may permit immediate suture of the ends of the tendon.

After any of these tendon repairs, the thumb must be supported in complete extension for at least 5 weeks, followed by a guarded resumption of function.

Traumatic Tenosynovitis (Peritendinitis Crepitans)

Etiology. So-called traumatic tenosynovitis is an affection seen frequently by industrial surgeons and less often in private and dispensary practice. The usual history is that the patient, after having led a more or less sedentary life, indulges in prolonged or strenuous muscular exertion. Thus we have seen this lesion in a college professor who played

five sets of tennis (on an indoor court) in one day during the winter. It may appear in those who step up their normal activity. Finally, the condition occurs in those carrying out their normal work following trauma.

Pathology. Howard has demonstrated the pathology of the affection by incision and pathologic specimens. He found a jellylike edema of the areolar tissue about the musculotendinous junction, thrombosis of the veins, and an interstitial fibrous deposit. The muscle is shown to have lost its glycogen, and there is even muscle-fiber destruction. Howard believes that the condition arises from fatigue and exhaustion of a definite muscle group. He points out that, in reality, the condition is not a tenosynovitis, because that portion of the tendon having a synovial sheath is unaffected. He believes that the primary change is in the muscle.

Symptoms. The symptoms are quite typical. There is localized swelling, usually on the dorsum of the forearm and the wrist. There are often edema, slight hyperemia, and pain on movement of the involved muscles, usually the extensors of the wrist or of the fingers or the thumb. The characteristic symptom, on which the diagnosis may be based, is a definite crepitus along the wrist and the lower forearm when the muscles and the tendons involved are used. With a stethoscope placed over the tendon involved, a definite crunching and even squeaking, such as that obtained by twisting leather, may be heard. The crepitus is often described as the sensation obtained by crunching snow in the hand.

Treatment. The treatment of crepitating peritendinitis is rest of the muscle groups involved. In the wrist, this usually signifies rest not only of the wrist but also of the fingers. This is accomplished best by a light plaster or other type of molded splint which includes the thumb. Howard reports an average period of disability of 11.6 days in patients treated by complete immobilization, and the author has confirmed this observation in many cases. As a rule, baking, massage, and pressure dressings do not effect a cure. In some cases cortisone preparations injected into the sheath give immediate and often complete relief. In a few patients it may take a day or two before complete relief is obtained.

TENOSYNOVITIS STENOSANS

(Trigger Finger or Snapping Finger)

These names are given to a finger disability in which the patient notices a snapping or a jerking sensation over the area of a tendon of a single finger as it is flexed or extended actively or passively.

Pathology. An understanding of the pathology is necessary to obtain a clear-cut picture of the symptoms. There is fusiform thickening of the flexor tendon in the region of the metacarpophalangeal joint. The sheath of the tendon in this area is not elastic. Constant irritation to both the tendon and the tendon sheath, due to the passage of the fusiform swelling of the tendon through the inelastic sheath, produces an actual thickening of the sheath, with gradual constriction and narrowing of its lumen. This produces a more marked irritation, accompanied by increased thickening, of the tendon itself. As the finger is extended and the tendon passes through the narrowed area, more and more force must be employed to pull the enlarged area of tendon through the constricted portion of the sheath. When this is finally accomplished, the finger snaps into extension. The reverse of this procedure occurs when the finger is flexed, and the fusiform swelling must be pulled back through the stenosed portion of the sheath.

Etiology. Trigger finger is seen occasionally in childhood. It is due to a congenital inequality between the tendon sheaths and the tendons. The lesion is more common in adult life, and, as a rule, it follows a trauma in the region of the metacarpophalangeal joint. The flexor tendon of the thumb is involved more often than are the flexor tendons of the other fingers.

Treatment. Treatment of this lesion by surgery is very simple. By palpation, one feels the enlarged portion of the tendon where it slips through the stenosed area of the tendon sheath. Under local infiltration anesthesia, with hemostasis controlled by a tourniquet, a transverse incision is made over the bulbous area of the tendon. The patient can flex and extend the finger under local anesthesia, and the pathology may be visualized. Incision of the stenosed area of the tendon sheath permits the enlarged area of tendon to move without obstruction. After the wound has been closed, a simple pressure dressing is applied without splinting. The patient is encouraged to use the finger from the very first, to prevent adhesions between the tendon sheath and the tendon. A cure results as soon as the tendon sheath is incised.

Hydrocortisone has been used locally to produce a local inhibition of inflammatory reaction, and this has been tried in the treatment of trigger finger. Several authors have injected from 0.1 to 0.5 ml. (25 mg. per ml.) into the tendon and the sheath involved, and they report relief of pain and disappearance of trigger symptom. From 1 to 3 weekly injections were given. This method of therapy has proved very successful in the hands of the author. I have not operated upon a single case since using it. If it fails, operation can be performed.

STENOSING TENOSYNOVITIS AT THE RADIAL STYLOID

(De Quervain's Disease)

Pathology. De Quervain first described this lesion as a narrowing of that part of the tendon sheath lying over the styloid process of the radius and through which pass the tendons of the extensor pollicis brevis and the abductor pollicis longus. The pathologic change consists of a serous effusion within the sheath of the tendon, with edema and marked thickening of the dense fibrous layer of the tendon sheath. The thickening leads to a constriction that may be almost cartilaginous in consistency. At the same time, there may be fusiform enlargement of the tendon beyond the point of constriction.

Etiology. The disease is usually due to some form of trauma, more often chronic than acute, although in many cases it has followed some single acute injury. Most often, activities that require ulnar deviation of the hand and the wrist while the thumb is fixed on some object are found to produce this lesion. It is seen much more commonly in women than in men, and it seems to follow sewing, typewriting, knitting, golfing, and piano playing.

Symptoms. The usual complaint is of pain about the styloid of the radius that radiates up the forearm and into the thumb. Swelling may or may not be present. On examination, there is definite tenderness over the styloid process of the radius, and if the patient's thumb is grasped and the hand is abducted quickly toward the ulna, pain over the tip of the styloid process is marked. In most cases, on deep palpation there is a thickening, if not a hard mass, in the region of the radial styloid.

Treatment. Immobilization usually results in a cure in a period of 5 to 6 weeks, but a much more satisfactory and rapid cure results from operation under local anesthesia. With a tourniquet controlling bleeding, an incision is made over the radial styloid to expose the sheath overlying the extensor pollicis brevis and the abductor pollicis longus. The hard, thickened sheath is incised, and frequently a portion of it is excised. The wound is closed loosely, and a dressing is applied with moderate pressure. No splint is required because early active and passive motion is employed in the postoperative care.

Operative therapy gives almost immediate relief of the pain in the region of the radial styloid, and practically normal function of the thumb is permitted within a few days.

Hydrocortisone (25 mg. per ml.) has been injected in amounts of from 0.3 to 0.5 ml. into the painful tendon sheath. In many cases it gave rapid relief of pain (within 12 hours) and permitted the patient to be symptom free and working within 24 hours. Howard, Pratt, and Bun-nell believe that patients so treated "may have recurrence and eventually need surgical correction." However, symptomatic relief apparently can be obtained in a short time by the use of local hydrocortisone injections.

Stenosing tenovaginitis may affect any of the other dorsal and volar compartments of the wrist. The treatment, by rest, operation, or hydrocortisone injections is the same as that for DeQuervain's disease.

CONTRACTURE OF THE PALMAR FASCIA

(Dupuytren's Contracture)

Pathology. The palmar fascia represents the palmar insertion of the palmaris longus muscle. It is of surgical importance because it frequently becomes involved in a process of hypertrophy and contraction. This hypertrophy usually begins as a nodular thickening along that portion of the palmar fascia overlying the flexor tendon to the ring finger. As the disease progresses, nodules appear also over the flexor tendons of the fifth and the middle fingers and may indeed involve also the index finger. With the hypertrophy, there is a gradual contraction of the portion of the fascia involved. Because of those vertical fibers of the palmar fascia that insert in the undersurface of the skin, there is early involvement of the palmar integument, with at first a dimpling and then a gradual thickening (Fig. 24-37).

The longitudinal fibers of the palmar fascia extend to the sides of the proximal phalanges, and the contracting process involves these extensions and also the fascia of the finger. As the hypertrophy and the later contraction progress, there is a gradual shortening of the longitudinal fibers of the palmar fascia, with a resulting flexion contracture of the proximal phalanx on the metacarpal bone. Gradually, the contracture involves also the middle phalanx, until the entire finger is drawn down to such an extent that often it touches the palm.

Although the fascia extending to the ring finger is most frequently involved,

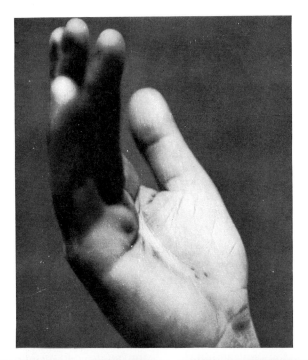

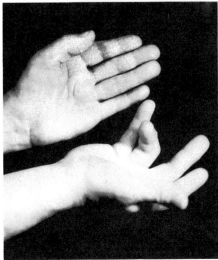 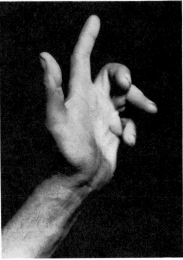

Fig. 24–37. Stages in the development of Dupuytren's contracture. (*Top*) Note the thickening and the dimpling of the palmar skin in the distal flexion crease, with the typical involvement of the fourth finger. (*Left*) Typical bilateral involvement, with more marked contracture of the right fourth finger and beginning involvement of the left hand. (*Right*) Advanced stage of Dupuytren's contracture, with involvement of the middle, the ring, and the fifth fingers. The first two patients underwent surgery as ambulatory cases.

the fascia to the fifth and the middle fingers also is a part of the contracture. The process also extends toward the wrist, and the thickened portion of the palmar fascia may be palpated and often seen as a ridge of hard tissue extending to the base of the hand. The disease is often a bilateral one, and occasionally there appears to be a definite hereditary tendency.

Etiology. As to the etiology, there is some division of opinion. Most writers on the subject feel that trauma is not an important factor in the production of the contracture, since it occurs with almost equal frequency in those who use their hands and in those who do not, such as lawyers, clergymen, physicians, and bankers. However, there are those who feel that trauma plays an important role and others who think that trauma plus foci of infection are the important etiologic mechanisms. In a study of our own cases, trauma has not appeared to be an important factor, and we are inclined to agree with Kanavel, Koch, and Mason that a "hereditary tendency stands out as the most definite and tangible factor in the development of the disease."

Symptoms. The symptoms that occur with Dupuytren's contracture are few, except those due to the contraction. Frequently, in the early stage of the disease, there is slight pain in the region of the nodules that appear, but usually this disappears rapidly, and the nodules may remain without any progression of the disease for months, and even years. There is usually no difficulty in diagnosing this lesion once it is seen.

Treatment. In treating Dupuytren's contracture, it is essential to recognize that the disease involves only the palmar fascia; it does not affect the underlying tendons. Therefore, exision of the fascia permits normal extension and flexion of the fingers involved, because the tendons still are able to function in a normal manner. Operation for excision of the palmar fascia may be performed in ambulatory patients when the process is not too far advanced. However, when the dissection involves an excision of the contracted band along several fingers, and skin transplants are necessary, the patient is hospitalized for treatment.

We have performed excision of the palmar fascia in numerous ambulatory patients under local anesthesia. A block of the median and ulnar nerves at the wrist is not too difficult a procedure, and when future anesthesia is needed, local infiltration is added. A blood-pressure cuff is used as a tourniquet to permit careful and rapid dissection of the fascia. An incision is made along the distal palmar crease, and with small forceps and tiny rake retractors, the contracted fibrous extensions from the palmar fascia to the skin are divided to expose the underlying hypertrophied fascia. The incision must be from $1\frac{1}{2}$ to 2 inches long to permit the dissection to the carried downward far enough to excise the proximal portion of the contracted fascia. When this has been divided, the dissection is carried distally; the skin is dissected from the palmar fascia, and the extensions of the palmar fascia to the metacarpal bone and the interosseous fascia are divided. As the dissection is carried upward to the proximal phalanx of the finger, care must be taken to identify and avoid the digital nerves and vessels that lie embedded in the contracted fascia along the sides of the finger.

Occasionally it is necessary to make a second transverse incision at the crease between the palm and the finger, but this is made only after the dissection has been carried upward from below to the base of the finger. As the dissection progresses, cut vessels can be seen in the cadaveric hemostasis produced by the blood-pressure cuff tourniquet, and these are caught and tied. After the contracted portion of the palmar fascia has been excised, the tourniquet is released, in order to identify any small bleeders that have not been recognized.

After adequate hemostasis has been obtained by ligating the blood vessels with fine silk ligatures, the divided skin is united with fine alloy steel wire sutures. It is important to obtain accurate apposition of skin edges; the sutures are placed close to one another, and often vertical mattress sutures, alternating with interrupted sutures, are inserted. A pressure bandage, in which is incorporated sterile mechanic's waste or a soft rubber sponge, prevents serum collection and capillary ooze. A palmar splint usually is applied, and the patient is given a sling. The pressure bandage should be inspected in 24 hours. However, the dressing is not changed and the sutures are not removed for from 7 to 10 days, unless there is reason to suspect trouble in the wound. The author has never had an infection occur in an ambulatory patient following excision of the palmar fascia for a Dupuytren's contracture. Occasionally there is a slightly imperfect healing of the skin where it has been dissected away from the nodular thickening of the palmar fascia, but this usually heals by conservative treatment without scarring or difficulty.

The prognosis for normal function is excellent, especially in the earlier cases. As a rule, all dressings are discarded within a period of 2 to 3 weeks, and no special postoperative physiotherapy or exercises are necessary to obtain a good result.

Kelly and Clifford have proposed and used a more conservative treatment for Dupuytren's contracture: a subcutaneous division of the contracted palmar fascia (fasciotomy). This therapy is especially indicated when the contracture is limited to a single cordlike deformity affecting one finger and in poor-risk elderly patients in whom the more radical excision of the palmar fascia might produce prolonged disability.

The operation is performed under local or regional anesthesia; the hand is drained of blood, and a blood-pressure cuff is applied as a tourniquet. Four or five small incisions are made through the skin along the ulnar side of the hand, and a small scalpel (#15 Bard Parker) is inserted between the fascial band and the skin. With sweeping cuts the fascia is freed from the densely adherent skin. As the affected finger is extended and the fascial cord placed on tension, the knife is rotated so that the cutting edge impinges on the tense band. By exerting pressure on the knife blade through the overlying skin, the band is divided. Sawing motions are avoided to prevent injury to the underlying nerves and tendons (Fig. 24-38).

This subcutaneous division is repeated through each of the incisions from the base of the finger to the proximal palm.

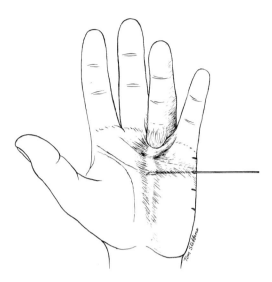

Fig. 24–38. Subcutaneous fasciotomy for Dupuytren's contracture (see text). (Kelly, A. P., Jr., and Clifford, R. H.: Plast. Reconstr. Surg., *24*:505, 1959)

Each incision is closed with a single suture, and, after a pressure dressing of fluffed gauze and elastic bandage has been applied, the arm is elevated and the tourniquet released. The hand is maintained in the elevated position until the hyperemia subsides.

After 48 hours, a smaller gauze and elastic bandage dressing is applied, and use of the hand is encouraged. All dressings and sutures are removed in a week, and passive stretching of the involved finger is encouraged.

Kelly and Clifford report that fasciotomy permits the involved finger to return to the neutral position in about 90 percent of the cases, with very little postoperative disability, but they acknowledge that the nodular segments of the contracture are not removed by fasciotomy, and these may be annoying to the patient. They report a recurrence rate of about 20 percent. This procedure may easily be performed on ambulatory patients.

The author has not seen any worthwhile results due to the use of vitamins or corticosteroids in the usual case of Dupuytren's contracture.

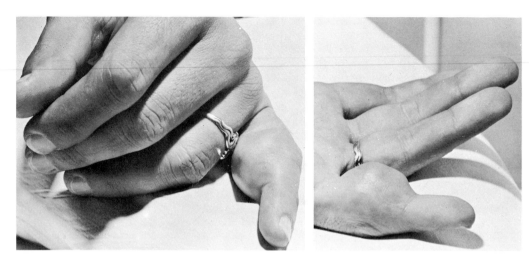

Fig. 24–39. Xanthoma of the finger.

CYSTS AND TUMORS

XANTHOMA

Etiology and Pathology. Xanthoma, or giant-cell tumor, of the tendon sheath is a nodular, coarsely lobulated, slow-growing swelling that occurs most frequently on the palmar surface of the fingers. It may occur also in the hand and the wrist. The tumor is usually not large or painful.

In appearance, xanthomas are mottled yellow-brown-gray in color, and usually they are not as well encapsulated as are cysts. On microscopic examination they are found to contain numerous types of cells, including spindle cells, large round cells, and, most characteristically, large giant cells and collections of large lipoid-containing foam cells.

Treatment. Excision is performed for either cosmetic or functional reasons. The true nature of the tumor is often not suspected until it is exposed following incision, when, because of its distinctive color, it is diagnosed easily.

Removal by blunt dissection usually is simple (Fig. 24-39). Care must be taken to remove all of the tumor; otherwise it may recur.

TUMORS OF THE PERIOSTEUM AND BONE

Chondromas of the Periosteum of the Phalanges

Description. The less common type of chondroma springs from the periosteum of the phalanges. It occurs as a hard round tumor of considerable size that produces deformity and disability. A roentgenogram usually shows some deformity of the underlying phalanx, but not an involvement of the bone proper (Fig. 24-40).

Treatment. Excision of this tumor under local anesthesia is usually a simple matter. It is well encapsulated, and it is unlikely to recur after it has been removed.

Chondromas of the Metacarpal Bones and Phalanges

Pathology. Probably the more common type of chondroma is that which occurs in the shaft of a metacarpal bone or a phalanx. The cortex is expanded markedly over one-half to two-thirds of the circumference of the bone, and the tumor usually remains within the cortex. Frequently,

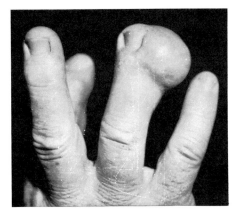
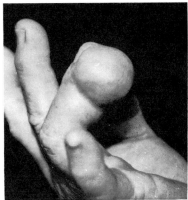

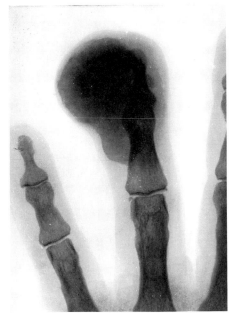

Fig. 24–40. Chondroma of the distal phalanx, removed under local anesthesia. When this tumor was removed, only a shell of skin remained, but as excellent cosmetic and functional result was obtained.

there is some pain due to pressure on nerves that are stretched over the expanding tumor mass.

Diagnosis. The roentgenogram shows a characteristic enlargement of the bone without the definite trabeculations seen in giant-cell tumor, which is the only tumor likely to be confused with chondroma.

Treatment. This consists of complete removal of the tumor tissue with a curette, and Mason recommends chemical sterilization of the cavity with Zenker's solution of 50 percent zinc chloride. This operation may be performed under local block anesthesia with tourniquet hemostasis.

Giant-Cell Tumors

Symptoms and Diagnosis. This tumor occurs in the phalanges of the fingers. It produces a swelling and an enlargement of the phalanx involved. There are few other symptoms, except an occasional pain due to pressure on adjacent nerves. A roentgenogram makes the diagnosis easy, demonstrating frequent trabeculations throughout the tumor mass (Fig. 24-41).

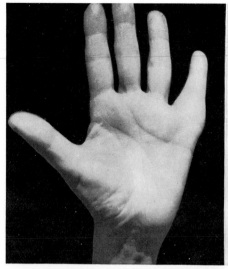
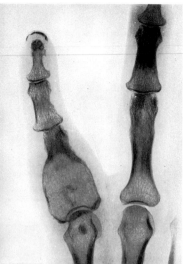

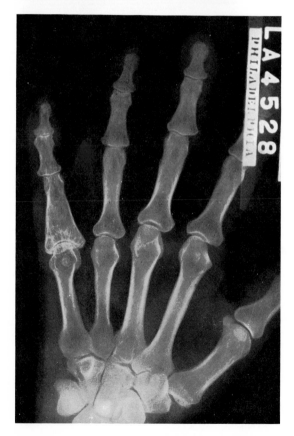

Fig. 24–41. Giant-cell tumor of the proximal phalanx of the fifth finger. Note the marked enlargement of the phalanx and the appearance of the film. The patient had rather marked pain due to pressure of the bone upon the digital nerve along the inner side of the finger. The nerve was exposed and injected with alcohol, and the tumor was treated by roentgen-ray therapy. The lower film was made 7 years later. The finger now is only slightly larger than the fifth finger on the opposite side.

Treatment. Mason recommends complete local excision with a curetter, followed by chemical cauterization of the cavity. He believes that irradiation is of uncertain value.

SUPERNUMERARY DIGITS

Extra fingers are seen occasionally, and frequently they are bilateral. At times, they are attached by only a small fibrous

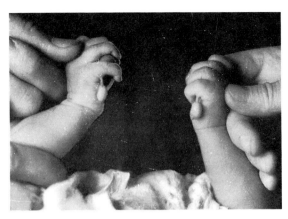

Fig. 24–42. Supernumerary digits attached by small pedicles. These can be removed very easily in infants under local anesthesia. It must be remembered that these pedicles always contain a small central vessel, which must be ligated or sutured carefully.

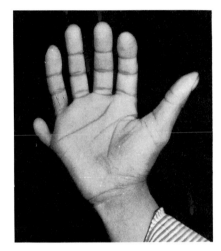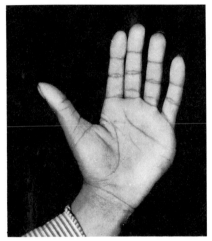

Fig. 24–43. Supernumerary digits. This boy had an extra digit on each hand as shown (*left*). (*Right*) The result on the left hand 3 weeks after exicison of the accessory digit under local anesthesia.

pedicle (Fig. 24-42); at other times, true bony connection is noted. In many cases, especially when the supernumerary finger springs from a metacarpal bone, simple excision of the finger and of the outgrowth of bone from the metacarpal is all that is necessary to obtain a good result. The operation may be performed under local anesthesia (Fig. 24-43).

REMOVAL OF RING FROM SWOLLEN FINGER

Occasionally the surgeon is called upon to remove a ring from a swollen finger. Attempts at removal by the use of soap or oily preparations having failed, the temp-

tation is to try to cut the ring. Often this will prove to be difficult if the finger is much swollen, and especially if the patient is a child.

A piece of stout string about 50 inches long may be used to remove even a tight ring. Soap the string and then thread about 2 inches of it under the ring toward the wrist. This end of the string is held tight while the remaining string is wrapped snugly around the finger, one wrap next to the other, until the finger is covered beyond the proximal interphalangeal joint. The distal end is then held tight. The ring is removed by pulling upward on the end threaded through it. As the string is unwound from the bottom, the ring is removed gradually, advantage being taken of the fact that the tightly wound string has compressed the soft tissues over the joint.

BIBLIOGRAPHY

Tendons and Tenosynovitis

Bunnell, S.: Treatment of tendons in compound injuries of the hand. J. Bone Joint Surg., *23*:240, 1944.

Byrne, J. J.: Hand surgery. Am. J. Surg., *88*:431, 1954.

Howard, N. J.: A new concept of tenosynovitis and the pathology of physiologic effort. Am. J. Surg., *42*:723, 1938.

———: Peritendinitis crepitans, a muscle-effort syndrome. J. Bone Joint Surg., *19*:447, 1937.

Hartwell, S. W., Larsen, R. D., and Posch, J. L.: Tenosynovitis in women in industry. Cleveland Clin. Quart., *31*:115, 1964.

Lamphier, T. A., Pepi, J. F., Brush, C., and Ostroger, J.: Characteristics and treatment of Quervain's disease. J. Int. Coll. Surg., *31*:192, 1959.

Lipscomb, P. R.: Management of tenosynovitis of the hand and wrist. Clin. Orthop., *13*:164, 1959.

Mason, M. L.: Rupture of the tendons of the hand, with a study of the extensor tendon insertions in the fingers. Surg., Gynec. Obstet., *50*:611, 1930.

Mason, M. L., and Allen, H. S.: The rate of healing of tendons. Ann. Surg., *113*:424, 1941.

Roemer, F. J.: Hyperextension injuries to the finger joints. Am. J. Surg., *80*:295, 1950.

Hydrocortisone Injections

Boyes, J. H.: Bunnell's Surgery of the Hand. Philadelphia, J. B. Lippincott, 1964.

Hollander, J. L.: Intra-articular hydrocortisone in the treatment of arthritis. Ann. Int. Med., *39*:735, 1953.

Howard, L. D., Jr., Pratt, D. R., and Bunnell, S.: The use of compound F (hydrocortisone) in operative and nonoperative conditions of the hand. J. Bone Joint Surg., *35A*:994, 1953.

Wounds, Injuries

Farrington, G. H.: Treatment of subungual hematoma. Brit. Med. J., *1*:742, 1964.

Flatt, A. E.: The Care of Minor Hand Injuries. St. Louis, C. V. Mosby, 1963.

Grabb, W. C., and Dingman, R. O.: Repair of fingertip injuries. Mich. Med., *63*:55, 1964.

Jones, R. A.: A method for closing a traumatic defect of a finger tip. Am. J. Surg., *55*:326, 1942.

Kleinert, H. E.: Management of finger tip injuries. Am. Surg., *25*:41, 1959.

Kutler, W.: A method for the repair of finger amputation. Ohio Med. J., *40*:126, 1944.

Mason, M. L.: Hand injuries. Indust. Med. Surg., *22*:378 1953.

———: Principles of management of open wounds of the hand. Am. J. Surg., *80*:767, 1950.

Metcalf, W., and Whalen, W. P.: Repair of injured distal phalanges. Clin. Orthop., *13*:114, 1959.

Reed, J. V., and Harcourt, A. K.: Immediate full thickness grafts to finger tips. Surg., Gynec. Obstet., *68*:925, 1939.

Sturman, M. J., and Duran, R. J.: Late results of finger tip injuries. J. Bone Joint Surg., *45A*:289, 1963.

Infections

Byrne, J. J.: Hand surgery. Am. J. Surg., *88*:431, 1954.

Entin, M. A.: Management of infections of the hand. Surg. Clin. N. Am., *44*:981, 1964.

Kanavel, A. B.: Infections of the Hand. ed. 7. Philadelphia, Lea & Febiger, 1937.

Meleny, F. L., and Johnson, B.: The prophylactic and active treatment of surgical infections with zinc peroxide. Surg., Gynec. Obstet., *64*:387, 1937.

Fingernails

Panzer, H. H.: Griseofulvin. Penn. Med. J., *67*:27, 1964.

Rosenberg, E. W.: Curing nail infections—more than ever a sure thing. Consultant, *4*:26, 1964.

Wechsler, H. L.: Low-dosage treatment of dermatomycoses. Penn. Med. J., *64*:364, 1961.

Congenital Deformities

Meyerding, H. W., and Dickson, D. D.: Correction of congenital deformations of the hand. Am. J. Surg., *44*:218, 1939.

Mallet Finger

Boyes, J. H.: Bunnell's Surgery of the Hand. ed. 4. Philadelphia, J. B. Lippincott, 1964.

Cascells, S. W., and Strauge, T. B.: Intramedullary malfunction of mallet finger. J. Bone Joint Surg., *39A*:521, 1957.

Fowler, F. D.: New splint for treatment of mallet finger. JAMA, *170*:945, 1959.

Hall, T. D., and Alves, A. B.: Treatment of mallet finger. Surg. Gynec. Obstet., *106*:233, 1958.

Hillman, F. E.: New technique for treatment of mallet fingers and fractures of distal phalanx. JAMA, *161*:1135, 1956.

Kaplan, E. B.: Mallet or baseball finger. Surgery, *7*:784, 1940.

Marble, H. C.: The Hand. Philadelphia, W. B. Saunders, 1960.

Mason, M. L.: Rupture of the tendons of the hand, with a study of the extensor tendon insertions in the fingers. Surg., Gynec. Obstet., *50*:611, 1930.

Roemer, F. J.: Hyperextension injuries to the finger joints. Am. J. Surg., *80*:295, 1950.

Smillie, I. S.: Mallet finger. Brit. J. Surg., *24*:439, 1937.

Spiegelman, L.: New splint for management of mallet finger. JAMA, *153*:1362, 1953.

Stark, H. H., Boyes, J. H., and Wilson,,J. N.: Mallet finger. J. Bone Joint Surg., *44A*:1061, 1962.

Dupuytren's Contracture

Freehofer, A. A., and Strong, J. M.: The treatment of Dupuytren's contracture by partial fasciectomy. J. Bone Joint Surg., *45A*:1207, 1963.

Kanavel, A. B., Koch, S. L., and Mason, M. L.: Dupuytren's contraction. Surg., Gynec. Obstet., *48*:145, 1929.

Kelley, A. P., Jr., and Clifford, R. H.: Subcutaneous fasciotomy in the treatment of Dupuytren's contracture. Plast. Reconstr. Surg., *24*:505, 1959.

Meagher, S. W.: The Dupuytren contracture controversy—a presentation of the facts. JAMA, *180*:138, 1962.

Weckesser, E. C.: Results of wide excision of the palmar fascia for Dupuytren's contracture. Am. Surg., *160*:1007, 1964.

Anesthesia

Bradfield, W. J. D.: Digital block anesthesia. Brit. J. Surg., *50*:495, 1963.

Chase, R. N., Macomber, W. B., and Wang, M. K. H.: Peripheral nerve block for hand surgery. Plast Reconstr. Surg., *24*:255, 1959.

24

Hand and Fingers

Part II—Fractures

Andrew C. Ruoff, M.D.

FRACTURES OF THE CARPAL
NAVICULAR (SCAPHOID)

Etiology and Pathology. The navicular may be fractured by a fall on the hand, a blow on the wrist, or torsion of the wrist. These fractures may be divided into two main groups: (1) fractures of the body of the bone, which are intra-articular and represent a disruption of the proximal carpal arch (Fig. 24-44, *left*); and (2) those of the tuberosity (Fig. 24-44, *right*), which are sprain fractures and are extra-articular (Fig. 24-45).

The surface of the scaphoid is covered largely by articular cartilage and is avascular except for small dorsal and lateral areas, through which its main vessels enter. If the fracture lies in the proximal portion of the bone, the proximal fragment may lose its blood supply (Fig. 24-45). In these cases, healing depends on revascularization of the fragment by an ingrowth of vessels from the distal fragment. The loss of blood supply may be recognized in the roentgen films after 4 to 6 weeks; the proximal fragment fails to decrease in density as does the distal. Displacement of the fragments is usually minimal.

Diagnosis. The patient usually complains of pain in the wrist localized in the area just beyond the radial styloid. Grasping with the hand and dorsiflexion of the wrist aggravate the pain. Swelling and

acute tenderness are present in the anatomic snuffbox just distal to the radial styloid. Pressure or percussion in the long axis of the extended thumb causes pain at the site of fracture. This pressure causes no increase of pain in simple sprains.

Roentgen examination is warranted in any patient with signs of sprain of the wrist. Simple sprain of the wrist is an uncommon lesion. Several points concerning roentgen diagnosis of this fracture deserve emphasis. Routine anteroposterior and lateral views may not demonstrate the fracture. Oblique views should be made in every suspicious case, and the films should be carefully inspected. If there is well-localized pain without roentgen findings, it is safest to apply a cast and to repeat the roentgen examination in 10 to 14 days. If pain and motion and localized tenderness are still present, even though the roentgen examination is negative, a cast should be reapplied for another 2 weeks and another reontgen examination made. Some fissure fractures of the navicular may not be noticeable until after a little decalcification has occurred at the fracture line, and this may take 3 to 4 weeks.

Treatment. Prolonged and uninterrupted immobilization is required. Operative exposure of a number of fresh fractures has indicated that the fracture often is unstable. A cast should be applied from the knuckles to the elbow, with the hand

440

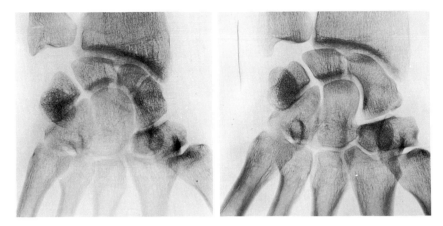

Fig. 24–44. (*Left*) Fracture of the body of the navicular. (*Right*) Fracture of the tuberosity of the navicular. (Ferguson, L. K.: Surg. Clin. N. Am. *17*:1603, 1937)

Fig. 24–45. Types of fracture of the navicular and the blood supply. (*A*) Fracture of the tuberosity of the navicular, extra-articular; (*E*) good blood supply, unites without trouble. (*B*) Fracture through the middle; both fragments receives a good blood supply (*F*). Healing usually is good. (*C*) Fracture through the proximal portion, which becomes avascular (*G*). Healing is delayed until vessels grow in from the distal fragment. (*D*) Fracture close to the middle that has destroyed the dorsal blood supply (*H*). The condition is similar to that in (*G*). (After Lexer by Schnek)

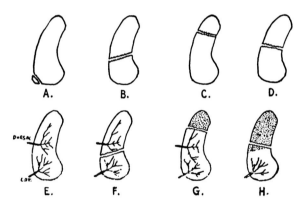

dorsiflexed slightly and the thumb extended moderately (Fig. 24-46). The circular cast should extend to the interphalangeal joint of the thumb. The plaster should be molded snugly in the palm and about the lower radius to secure maximum immobility of the wrist joint, and should be trimmed in the palm to allow full flexion of the fingers. If the cast is molded well, the metacarpals should not pull away from the dorsum of the cast when the fingers are flexed. This cast provides adequate immobilization and permits active use of the hand; the patient is instructed to use the hand as much as possible.

Fractures of the tuberosity require only 4 weeks of immobilization. Fractures of the body require at least 8 weeks. Films are made immediately after the cast is removed. If union is absent or incomplete, a new cast is applied for a further period of at least 6 weeks. Immobilization in a cast should be continued until the fracture is solidly healed, which may take several months. In occasional older patients who do not anticipate strenuous use of the wrist and for whom prolonged wearing of a cast after 10 to 12 weeks is a burden, active use without a cast may be permitted if it is painless, since adequate fibrous union has probably occurred, even though no union may be demonstrable by x-ray examination.

OLD UNTREATED FRACTURES
OF THE NAVICULAR

Pathology. If the bone has not been immobilized completely or if immobilization is discontinued too early, the fragments move on each other, and the vessels growing across the fracture line tear. Of course, this happens also in untreated cases. After 6 or 8 weeks, the films show widening of the fracture line and perhaps decalcification of the distal fragment where it impinges on the proximal, while the proximal fragment remains unchanged or shows a spotty appearance (Fig. 24-47). The bones of the hand show a uniform decalcification due to disuse. The patient complains of weakness of the hand and pain on motion.

After a year or two, both fragments become dense, and arthritic changes appear, usually indicated by irregular proliferation at the tip of the radial styloid; still later, both fragments undergo necrosis.

Treatment. Within the first 6 to 12 months, prolonged immobilization in a lightly padded cast for 4 to 8 months or longer, aided by vigorous active use, may bring about union. The cast is changed as often as necessary. Open reduction should be considered after a reasonable trial of closed treatment. As mentioned above, however, active or operative treatment of every nonunion may not be indicated, especially in patients who do little manual work, and whose symptoms are slight.

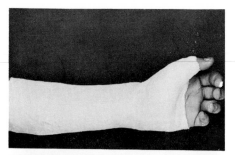

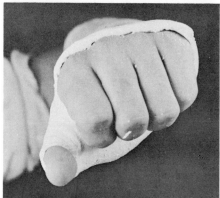

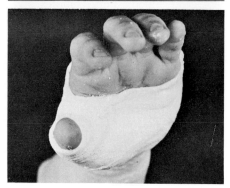

Fig. 24–46. Cast for immobilizing fractures of the carpal navicular. Note that the cast hugs the dorsal surface of the metacarpal heads when the fingers are flexed; note also the accurate molding to fit the palmar concavity. (Ferguson, L. K.: Surg. Clin. N. Am., *17*:1603, 1937)

DISLOCATIONS
OF THE CARPUS

The whole carpus may be dislocated toward the dorsal or the palmar side. The injury is practically always complicated by a fracture of the dorsal or the palmar lip of the articular surface of the radius and by a fracture of the radial or the ulnar styloid. The dislocation is reduced as described below for dislocation of the lunate. Further treatment, as for similar fractures of the radius and ulna, is instituted. Immobilization in a cast for 6 weeks is usually necessary.

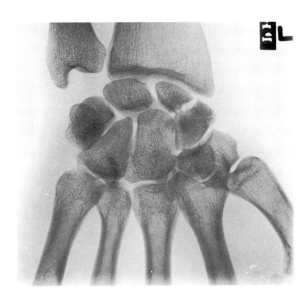

Fig. 24–47. Old fracture of the carpal navicular. Note the marked decalcification at the fracture line.

The distal row of carpals may be dislocated on the proximal row, either forward or backward; rarely are the metacarpals dislocated on the distal row of carpals. The dislocations may be complicated by fractures. Treatment is similar to that described for dislocations of the lunate except that immobilization may need to be prolonged.

DISLOCATIONS OF THE LUNATE

Etiology. Dislocation of the lunate is usually preceded by dorsal dislocation of the carpus, the lunate remaining attached to the radius, and the capitate and the surrounding bones lying dorsal to the lunate (Fig. 24-48). When the dorsal radiocarpal ligament tears, the lunate is pressed down and rotated out of its bed from 90° to 270°, coming to rest on the palmar side of the wrist beneath the flexor tendons and the median nerve. The head of the capitate moves toward the radius. The lunate also may be rotated in the long axis of the extremity (Fig. 24-49).

Sometimes the proximal portion of the navicular remains attached to the lunate and dislocates with it, the result being a "transnaviculo-perilunate dislocation." Fractures of the radial and the ulnar styloids may also be present.

Diagnosis. After an injury to the wrist, the patient finds the area swollen and painful, and he has difficulty in flexing and extending the fingers and the wrist. Paresthesias may be felt in the distribution of the median nerve. Examination shows not only tenderness and swelling but also a distinct bulge on the anterior aspect of the wrist, marked limitation of palmar flexion, and painful and limited extension and flexion of the fingers. This simulates dorsiflexion fracture. However, in fracture, the tenderness is more proximal, the distal end o f the radius rather than the carpus is the site of the deformity, and marked limitation of finger motion is rare, except in neglected cases.

Treatment. Recent dislocations or fracture-dislocations are often reduced easily (Fig. 24-49). Replacement of the bone is verified by roentgenograms. Manipulative reduction sometimes is successful even 2 to 3 weeks after injury. If swelling is not excessive, a cast is applied immediately; otherwise, a dorsal splint and a pressure dressing are used for the first few days. The cast remains in place for approximately 6 weeks. The patient should begin active use of the fingers, elbow, and shoulder immediately after reduction.

If the dislocation cannot be reduced, open reduction is required.

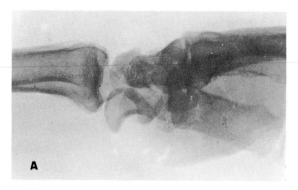

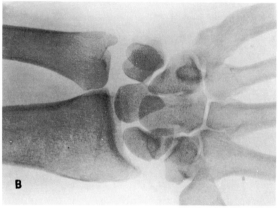

Fig. 24–48. Dislocation of the lunate. Lateral (*A*) and anteroposterior (*B*) views.

FRACTURES OF THE OTHER CARPAL BONES

Fractures of the other carpal bones are caused by crush injuries or by forcing the wrist beyond its normal range of motion. The bones being bound together by dense ligaments, substantial displacements are rare. The diagnosis may be suspected because of unusual tenderness and swelling, but it can be made only by roentgen films.

A padded dorsal splint and pressure bandage are applied at first. Later, a snug cast is applied for 4 to 6 weeks. When the greater multangular is fractured, the cast should extend to the distal joint of the thumb (Fig. 24-46).

FRACTURES OF THE METACARPALS

Anatomy. The metacarpals are short and thick; the dorsal surface is straight, while the palmar surface is concave, and the weakest portion lies just behind the head. Motion of the metacarpophalangeal joints is mainly in the anteroposterior plane, secondly in limited abduction and adduction from a line between the 3rd and 4th metacarpals, and, finally, in a little rotation of the fingers on the long axis. These joints are rather loose, the capsules being strongest where they are reinforced by ligamentous thickenings at the sides, which are tense in flexion and relaxed in extension. With the hand closed, the prominence of the knuckle represents the head of the metacarapal, the proximal phalanx lying anteriorly. Flexion is the most powerful motion of the fingers; extension is weaker. The flexor-extensor arrangement is shown in Figure 24-50).

FRACTURES OF THE FIRST METACARPAL

Bennett's Fracture

The first metacarpal moves freely in two planes due to its saddle-shaped proximal articular surface, which is concave as seen from the side and convex at a right

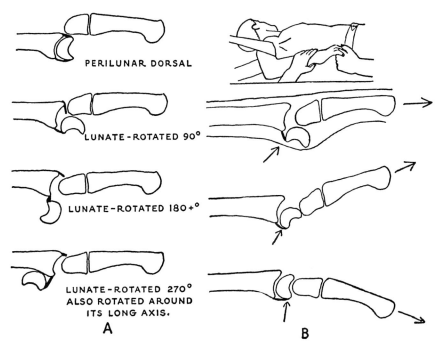

PERILUNAR DORSAL

LUNATE-ROTATED 90°

LUNATE-ROTATED 180+°

LUNATE-ROTATED 270°
ALSO ROTATED AROUND
ITS LONG AXIS.

A

B

Fig. 24–49. (*A*) Dislocation of the lunate. The primary lesion probably is a dorsal dislocation of the carpus over the lunate. When the carpus springs back, the dorsal radiocarpal ligament is torn, and the lunate is displaced forward. The lunate may rotate on its long axis as well. This probably requires open reduction. (Redrawn from Böhler) (*B*) Reduction of dislocated lunate. The patient is arranged as shown after 20 cc. of 1 percent procaine solution has been injected about the bone. An assistant makes powerful traction on the slightly dorsiflexed hand for from 5 to 15 minutes, so as to make room for the lunate. The surgeon grasps the wrist so that his thumb or thumbs press the lunate distally and upward as the dorsiflexion is increased. When the pressure is maximal, the hand may be brought into palmar flexion. In very recent dislocations, the surgeon may make the traction with one hand and the thumb pressure with the other. (Kaplan, L.: Surg. Clin. N. Am., *20*:1695, 1940)

angle to this. A blow on the long axis or on the dorsum of the thumb is the common cause of the so-called Bennett's fracture (Fig. 24-51). This is really a fracture-dislocation, since the small articular fragment on the palmar side remains in normal position, while the base of the metacarpal is displaced dorsally over the multangular.

Diagnosis. Swelling and acute tenderness occur over the proximal end of the bone, and there is distinct deformity due to the dorsolateral dislocation. Crepitus, marked pain on motion, and inability to extend the thumb usually are present. When the fracture is incomplete, localized tenderness and pain on percussion of the thumb in the long axis suggest the diagnosis.

Treatment. Full motion of the thumb depends on the preservation of a normal carpometacarpal joint. Abduction-adduction and opposition become limited, and a deformity results if the joint remains distorted. A well-padded wood or aluminum splint is applied immediately and covered by a snug bandage (Fig. 24-52). Roentgen films are made and inspected. In the absence of severe comminution, the patient keeps the hand elevated and applies an ice bag for from 24 to 48 hours.

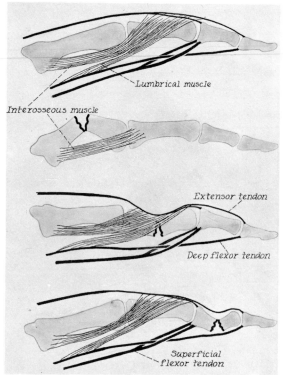

Lumbrical muscle

Interosseous muscle

Extensor tendon

Deep flexor tendon

Superficial
flexor tendon

Fig. 24–50. (*A*) The normal arrangement of the muscles and the tendons. (*B*) Fracture of a metacarpal; the interosseous muscle flexes the distal fragment on the proximal. (*C*) Fracture of a proximal phalanx. The interosseous muscles flex the proximal fragment while the lumbricals and the extensor tendon hyperextend the distal. (*D*) Fracture of a middle phalanx; the bifurcated portion of the superficial flexor tendon flexes the proximal fragment, and the distal is hyperextended by the extensor tendon.

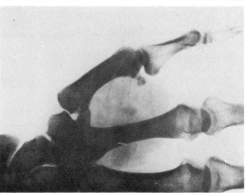

Fig. 24–51. Fracture of the first metacarpal. Bennett's fracture, actually a fracture dislocation.

If the fragments are in good position, the splint may remain in place for 3 or 4 weeks. It is better to discard the splint as soon as swelling has subsided and replace it with a cast (Fig. 24-53). This permits active use of the hand without danger of displacing the fragments.

If the usual displacement is present, the fracture remains undisturbed for 3 or 4 days until the swelling subsides. Reduction is performed under local anesthesia. While an assistant makes traction on the thumb, countertraction is made above the flexed elbow. After a few minutes, the surgeon presses the prominent proximal end of the bone down into place while he brings the distal end laterally into full abduction (Fig. 24-53). The displacement will recur as soon as the pressure is released. The cast is then applied from the mid-forearm down to the interphalangeal joint of the thumb. It should cover the knuckles on the dorsum of the hand and extend as far as the flexion crease in the palm. While the cast is setting, the reduction maneuver should be repeated and pressure should be maintained on the dorsal and palmar sides, with some traction, until the plaster hardens. A fair amount of pressure may be used. Roentgenograms should be taken to verify the reduction. If the position is not satisfactory, the cast is removed and manipulation is repeated. Failure to maintain reduction is an indication for continuous traction or

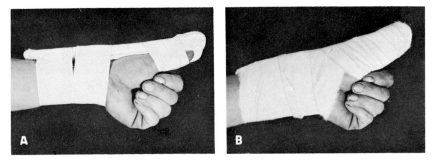

Fig. 24–52. (*A*) Well-padded, tapered dorsal wood splint for fracture of first metacarpal secured snugly with adhesive. (*B*) Firm flannel bandage applied over the splint. The pressure helps to control swelling. (Kaplan, L.: Surg. Clin. N. Am., *20*:1695, 1940)

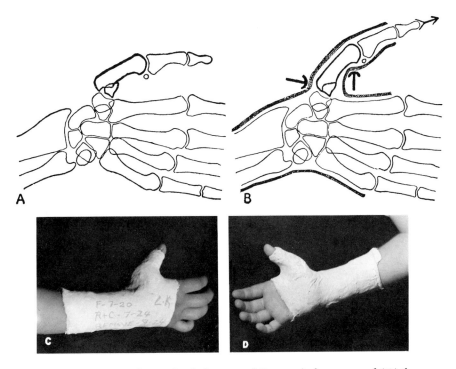

Fig. 24–53. (*A*) Shows the deformity of Bennett's fracture and (*B*) the method of reduction. (*C* and *D*) Show a finished cast. On the dorsum of the hand, the cast should extend to the distal ends of the metacarpals. (Kaplan, L.: Surg. Clin. N. Am., *20*:1695, 1940)

internal fixation with an intramedullary wire (Figs. 24-54 and 24-55).

The patient should be re-examined in 12 to 24 hours. Persistent severe pain at the point of pressure on the dorsum suggests excessive pressure. The cast should be windowed in this area and padded, the window being replaced with additional plaster. Active use of the fingers should begin at once, and no sling is recommended. Roentgen examination should be repeated in one week, and the cast

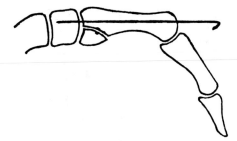

Fig. 24–54. Fixation with intramedullary wire. Sometimes it may be possible to direct the wire through both fragments.

should remain on for from 4 to 6 weeks. Hot soaks and massage, twice daily at home, relieve residual stiffness quickly if active use is reinstituted after the cast is removed.

Intramedullary fixation of these fractures has been found to be useful: with the patient under adequate anesthesia, an assistant flexes the first metacarpophalangeal joint to about 110° and makes gentle traction on the axis of the metacarpal while holding it in the abducted and slightly extended position. If this maneuver does not reduce the displacement completely, direct pressure is made over the dorsal or the dorsolateral surface of the base of the metacarpal. After the position has been verified by

judicious use of the image-intensification roentgenologic technique, a nick is made over the center of the posterior aspect of the metacarpal head, and a medium-sized Kirschner wire is inserted longitudinally, so that it traverses the medullary canal. If the wire is started properly, it goes in easily and enters the center of the greater multangular bone. After roentgen check for adequate penetration of the multangular, the wire is cut off 1 cm. distal to the skin, and a dressing and a plaster cast are applied. The plaster and the wire are removed in 4 to 5 weeks.

FRACTURES OF THE SECOND TO THE FIFTH METACARPALS

These fractures usually result from violence applied to the long axis of the bone, mostly due to the impact of the knuckles of the closed fist against a hard surface. One or more of the metacarpals may be involved. The common site of fracture is at the neck, but the shaft or the base may be involved (Fig. 24–56). The distal fragment is flexed by the action of the interosseous muscles and the lumbricals on the base of the proximal phalanx, the proximal phalanx coming to rest in slight extension.

Diagnosis. Swelling often masks the

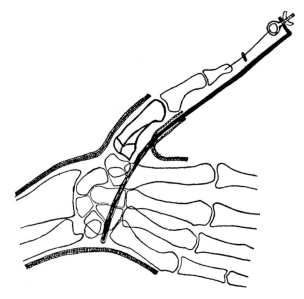

Fig. 24–55. A long bent-wire splint, similar to that shown in Figure 24–60, is twisted at its end to make a loop, and the loop is bent to a right angle with the length of the wire. The splint is incorporated in the wet plaster cast, which is made short in the palm. After the plaster is hard a stainless-steel wire is inserted through the fingertip and attached as shown in Figure 24–61. The amount of traction is controlled by the wing nut. Angulation, especially of phalangeal fractures, may be corrected by bending the wire at the level of fracture. (Kaplan, L.: Surg. Clin. N. Am., *20*:1695, 1940)

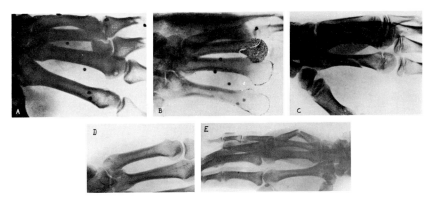

Fig. 24–56. (*A*) Fracture of the neck of the fourth metacarpal. (*B*) After reduction (retouched); the cast is shown in Figure 24–58, *A*. (*C*) Fracture of the shaft of the second metacarpal. (*D*) Fracture of the base of the fifth metacarpal. (*E*) Fracture of the shaft of the fifth metacarpal with marked angulation. (Kaplan, L.: Surg. Clin. N. Am., *20*:1695, 1940)

characteristic deformity: the flat dorsal surface becomes convex and perhaps irregular, the dorsal prominence of the knuckle is lost (Fig. 24-57), and the head of the metacarpal becomes more prominent in the palm. When the fracture is incomplete, localized tenderness and pain on percussion in the long axis aid in the diagnosis. A roentgen examination is made to verify the diagnosis, to determine the displacement, and to search for additional fractures.

Displacement. The distal fragment is flexed, and there is angulation open toward the palm. Slight shortening also occurs. The heads of the second and the fifth metacarpals may deviate medially or laterally, or they may rotate.

Treatment. The first dressing is a well-padded splint extending from the lower third of the forearm to the middle phalanx.

When the fragments are in good position, the splint may be used for 3 to 4 weeks of immobilization.

When the fragments are displaced, they should be reduced. For the most part, this can be done without anesthesia. If the patient cannot tolerate the pain, a small amount of local anesthetic may be injected into the fracture site.

The fracture may be reduced by placing the thumb in the palm just behind the metacarpal head and pressing it distally and toward the dorsum. If it is stable in a reduced position, it may be splinted in some moderate flexion and protected during its healing phase. However, a more satisfactory method of reduction is to apply a short arm cast with the wrist in

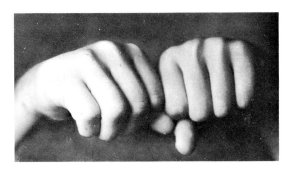

Fig. 24-57. Deformity after fracture of the fifth metacarpal of the left hand. The prominence of the knuckle has disappeared.

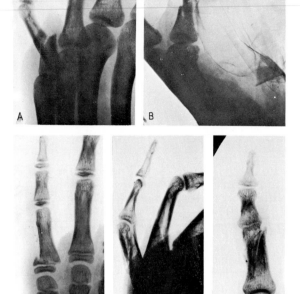

Fig. 24–58. Fractures of proximal phalanges. (*A*) Characteristic angulation. (*B*) Incomplete reduction over a roller bandage in the palm, a very poor dressing. (*C*) Fifth finger, displacement and angulation of shaft. (*D*) Oblique fracture united. Angulation corrected, but shortening allowed the sharp edge of the proximal fragment to come down beyond the joint. Skeletal traction would have given a better result. (*E*) Anteroposterior view of the same fracture. (Kaplan, L.: Surg. Clin N. Am., *20*:1695, 1940)

moderate dorsiflexion and a small piece of felt over the proximal portion of the metacarpal at the fracture site. When this portion of the cast has set firmly, the finger is flexed at the metacarpophalangeal joint to beyond 90°, and then the proximal phalanx is forced against the metacarpal head, pushing it up into place. The finger can then be padded with some sheet wadding or a small piece of felt, and a plaster splint can be applied over the dorsum of the cast and over the finger. The proximal phalanx is held while the plaster sets to keep pressure on the metacarpal head, care being taken to avoid excessive pressure over the middle phalanx. When this plaster has set, the cast may be completed with a small circular bandage, and the remaining fingers may be allowed completely out of the cast. This immobilization should be continued for 3 to 4 weeks.

Kirschner-wire fixation in any simple or complicated fracture of the metacarpals is often very satisfactory. The technique for the introduction of these wires is as previously described.

The heads of the second and fifth metacarpals may deviate to one side or they may rotate, resulting in overlapping of the fingers when the hand is closed if the displacement is not corrected. An excellent method of avoiding this rotary deformity is to splint the affected finger to its neighbor and also to be sure that the flexed fingers are pointing toward the area of the pisiform.

FRACTURES
OF THE PHALANGES

Following an injury to the fingers, swelling and tenderness are considerable. Deformity and crepitus, when present, make the diagnosis. Often, however, the only definite signs of fracture are well-localized tenderness and pain on percussion on the end of the extended finger. Fractures into the joints often simulate

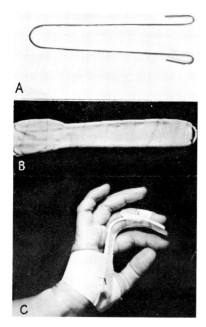

Fig. 24–59. (*A*) Ordinary coat-hanger wire was used to make this finger splint. (*B*) The splint should be wrapped in several thicknesses of adhesive. (*C*) The splint is bent enough for correction at the level of angulation and is secured snugly with adhesive. The adhesive strapping shown is not yet complete. (Kaplan, L.: Surg. Clin. N. Am., *20*:1695, 1940)

sprains and cannot be excluded, except by means of films, when the finger joints are acutely tender and swollen.

FRACTURES OF THE
PROXIMAL PHALANGES

The types of fractures are shown in Fig. 24-58. When the fracture is complete, the interosseous muscles flex the proximal fragment, while the lumbricals and the extensor tendon hyperextend the distal fragment, so that the fragments form an angle open toward the dorsum (Fig. 24-50).

Treatment. A well-padded splint is applied on the dorsum from above the wrist to the end of the finger. This may be secured with adhesive straps, and the dressing completed with a firm bandage. Films are made.

Treatment of Fractures with No Displacement. If no displacement has occurred, the splint may remain in place for 3 to 4 weeks. Since immobilization in extension leads to stiffness and contracture of the lateral ligaments, it is preferable to immobilize the finger in moderate flexion, in which position the lateral ligaments of the metacarpophalangeal and interphalangeal joints are not permitted to contract. A bent-wire or a metal splint is light and comfortable and does not interfere with the motion of the other fingers. A short cast incorporating the splint often aids immobilization.

After 3 or 4 weeks, the splint or the cast may be removed and the affected finger splinted to the adjacent finger with elastic adhesive bandage, with a little sheet wadding between the fingers as protection, for approximately 1 week. This dressing helps control rotation while allowing gradual mobilization in flexion and extension.

It is extremely important to exercise the uninvolved fingers fully and to continue the fullest possible use of the hand, the arm, and the shoulder during the period of immobilization. Disuse leads to stiffness, pain, and atrophy. In the elderly, the disability resulting from disuse may be much greater than that from the original injury.

Treatment of Fractures with Displacement. Displacement requires reduction. When the fracture is transverse, this may be accomplished by direct pressure. The deformity recurs unless the finger and the hand are firmly fixed to a splint in moderate flexion with the arch of the bend lying at the point of angulation (Fig. 24-59). A cast makes a very good dressing. For this method, it is important to wait 3 or 4 days until the swelling subsides. Elevation and ice bags will expedite this. The fracture is reduced by applying cross pressure, with the finger flexed moderately, and it is held reduced until the plaster sets.

Full active use may be resumed as soon as the plaster has set. The position of the fragments is checked by roentgen examination, so that reduction may be re-

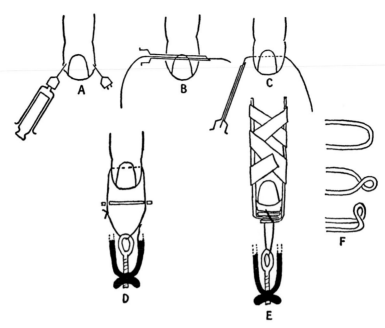

Fig. 24–60. Method of producing traction for finger and metacarpal fractures. (*A*) Each side of the fingertip is anesthetized with procaine, a 20-or a 22-gauge needle is passed through the phalanx, and (*B*) a heavy stainless-steel wire is inserted through the needle. (*C*) The needle is withdrawn. (*D*) A wood or a metal spreader is incorporated, and the wire is tied through the opening of the traction screw. (*E*) Adhesive traction may be used. (*F*) Bending the loop. (Kaplan, L.: Surg. Clin. N. Am. *20*:1695, 1940)

peated if necessary. The cast is removed in 4 or 5 weeks and the degree of union is determined. If union is not solid, it is best to reapply a cast or a splint. Otherwise, the continuous muscle pull may cause a recurrence of the deformity.

Some oblique and comminuted fractures may be held reduced by this method. If good position is not maintained, continuous traction may be required. This is done readily by use of a stainless-steel wire inserted through the distal portion of the finger after a cast has been applied from the lower forearm to the knuckles (Fig. 24-60). A bent coat-hanger wire is added on the palmar side of the cast after a loop has been made in the distal end. The stainless-steel wire is led through a spreader and fastened to a screw traction device. The position of the fragments then may be adjusted by bending the splint and tightening or loosening

the traction as necessary. Adhesive traction may also be used. X-ray control is required.

The fragments are checked frequently during the first 2 weeks. Overtraction must be avoided to prevent delay in union. The cast should be removed when the films indicate firm union, in about 4 or 5 weeks. The affected phalanx may be protected by wrapping it with elastic adhesive bandage; unnecessary limitation of the joint motion must be avoided.

Intramedullary fixation with a Kirschner wire has had increasing usefulness. It permits immediate active use of the hand. With the patient under suitable anesthesia, the fracture is reduced and held reduced while a Kirschner wire is inserted with a hand chuck, with the joint flexed to 90° to facilitate reduction of the fracture and to allow flexion of the finger subsequently (Fig. 24-61). The pin must

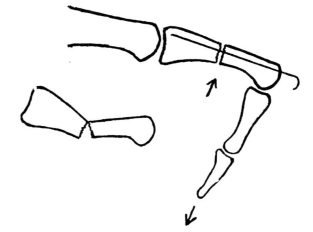

Fig. 24–61. Reduction maintained by insertion of a Kirschner wire. After skin preparation and anesthesia, the fracture is reduced and is held reduced by an assistant while a Kirschner wire (0.062 gauge) is drilled through the articular surface of the fractured phalanx. The finger must be fixed in flexion, as shown, by application of a splint.

be inserted almost to the proximal joint line to insure stability. The position should be checked by roentgen examination. The end of the wire that remains protruding is bent and covered with a collodion dressing. The wire should remain in place for 4 to 6 weeks. Full extension usually returns in a few weeks.

Open fractures are very common. They are treated by débridement and continuous wire traction, as described above. The hand should be kept elevated for the first week or two.

FRACTURES OF THE MIDDLE PHALANGES

After fracture of the shaft of a middle phalanx, the bifurcated tendon of the flexor digitorum sublimis flexes the proximal fragment, while the distal fragment goes into hyperextension. The angle opens toward the dorsum. When the fracture is close to the proximal end, the distal fragment may be flexed by the flexor sublimis, and the angle opens toward the palm.

Treatment. If no displacement has occurred, a bent-wire splint is applied on the palmar side from the knuckle to the fingertip with the finger in moderate flexion.

When there is an angle open toward the dorsum, it can be reduced by flexion over a bent-wire splint alone (Fig. 24-60), or it can be incorporated in plaster. The fracture is reduced while the plaster is soft and is held in position until it sets. Full active use of the uninvolved fingers may be resumed as soon as the plaster is hard. Intramedullary fixation, as described above, may be used, especially when maximum immediate function is desired.

When the angle opens toward the palm, either a plaster dressing may be applied, appropriate pressure being made to secure reduction, or a straight dorsal splint from knuckle to fingertip may be used if preferred. The fracture is reduced, and the finger is strapped firmly to the splint.

Union is not rapid in these fractures; from 4 to 5 weeks of immobilization is required usually.

Oblique and comminuted fractures are treated as are similar fractures of the proximal phalanx.

FRACTURES OF THE TERMINAL PHALANGES

Fractures of a terminal phalanx are usually caused by crush injuries or by blows on the extended finger (Fig. 24-62).

The shaft of the phalanx may show transverse, longitudinal, or comminuted fractures. Usually, swelling and pain are considerable. Fractures close to the base may show a marked tilt of the distal portion, which should be reduced.

Treatment. Fractures without displacement may be immobilized in a splint and covered with a small firm bandage, or a

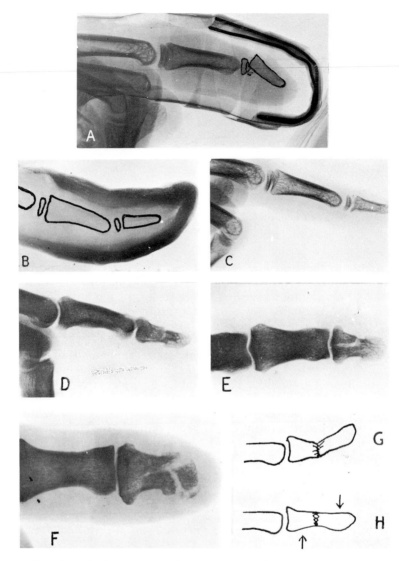

Fig. 24–62. Fractures of the terminal phalanges. (*A*) Compound epiphyseal separation with avulsion of nail from its bed. Dressed with hairpin splint. The hairpin should have been longer. (*B*) Reduction, after infiltrating base of finger with procaine, by forced dorsiflexion, which was repeated after applying a plaster thimble up to the base of the finger. (*C*) Result 3 weeks later. (*D* and *E*) Fracture into the joint space requiring simple but prolonged immobilization. (*F*) Crush fracture: to be treated as was (*E*). (*G*) Compression fracture with angle open toward dorsum. This may be reduced by cross pressure (*H*) and held in a plaster thimble. (*A, B,* and *C*—Kaplan, L.: Surg. Clin. N. Am., *20*:1695, 1940)

plaster finger thimble may be made (Fig. 24-63). After extensive comminution, the fragments sometimes may be molded into position in plaster after a few days of elevation. About 4 weeks of immobilization is usually required. Open fractures

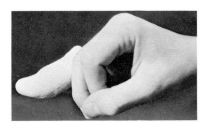

Fig. 24–63. Plaster thimble for certain fractures of the terminal phalanx. (See fig. 24–63, *B, G,* and *H.*)

are cleaned thoroughly, sutured when necessary, and treated with a plaster thimble as are simple fractures.

Fractures Involving the Joint Surfaces

When the end of the extended finger is struck, a fracture may occur at the proximal end of any of the phalanges. Sudden violent hyperextension or flexion may result in a fracture commonly known as a "baseball finger" or "mallet finger" (Fig. 24-64, *G*). A small portion tends to split off the proximal concave articular surface on the palmar or dorsal side. When the fragment is large, dislocation may also be present. Fixation in extension, as shown in Figure 24-64, may be obtained by forcing the terminal phalanx into full extension. The proximal interphalangeal joint should be kept moderately flexed.

Blows on the sides of the fingers may cause longitudinal fractures through the joint surface, sometimes accompanied by lateral subluxation.

Treatment. A dorsal splint and a pressure bandage are first applied. The splint should be long enough to immobilize the affected joint adequately. Displacement is determined by roentgenograms. Many of these fractures may be reduced and held in plaster, angulation and direct pressure on the soft plaster being used to secure apposition of the fragments. When joint involvement is considerable and when subluxations complicate the fracture, continuous traction may be necessary. Internal fixation with a small wire may be

more satisfactory if a fragment is moderately displaced or is large enough to hold a wire.

Finger exercises and active use are begun immediately when possible. After 4 to 5 weeks, the cast is removed and the joint is supported by a splint or by adhesive strapping. Pain may persist for several months, and the joint support is continued during this period. Physiotherapy, such as baking and massage, often increases pain and stiffness and usually should not be considered.

Complications. Failure to immobilize adequately and for a sufficiently long time may result in a chronically swollen, stiff, and painful joint (Fig. 24-65, *A*). Open fracture is very frequent. Failure to reduce fracture-dislocations accurately may necessitate open reduction.

DISLOCATION OF THE FINGER JOINTS

Dislocations of the metacarpoflphalangeal and finger joints usually follow hyperextension (Fig. 24-65 *A*). The distal bone rests on the dorsum of the proximal. These dislocations can often be reduced by traction without anesthesia. The joint is immobilized in at least partial flexion with a wire splint or a cast after films have been made to exclude fractures. Immobilization for 2 to 3 weeks is usually sufficient.

Dislocation of the metacarpophalangeal joint of the thumb (Fig. 24-65, *B*) also follows hyperextension. The head of the metacarpal may protrude through the capsule of the joint and lie between the short flexor tendons of the thumb. Longitudinal traction tautens these structures about the metacarpal head and makes reduction difficult to impossible. Reduction is best accomplished by increasing the hyperextension and making direct pressure on the dorsum of the base of the distal bone while making counterpressure on the metacarpal head. The phalanx is then flexed slowly on the metacarpal. When this maneuver fails, reduction may be effected by pressing the hyperextended phalanx firmly toward the

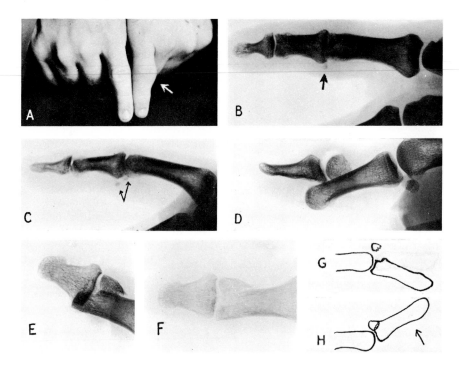

Fig. 24–64. Types of articular fractures of the finger. (*A*) Four months after a fracture into the joint space: marked thickening, stiffness, and pain. (*B*) A displaced ununited fragment on the side of the thickening. (*C*) Another fragment on the palmar side. (*D* and *E*) Compound fracture-dislocation of proximal phalanx of thumb. Débridement; reduction by traction and lateral pressure; immobilization in plaster splints for 6 weeks. (*F*) Good result. (*G*) Terminal phalanx compression fracture of the dorsal margin of the articular surface: the extensor tendon retracts the small fragment; the flexor tendon may flex the main fragment, causing a characteristic deformity. Reduction is obtained by applying a plaster thimble similar to that used in Figures 24–63, *B* and 24–64 and maintaining extreme dorsiflexion until the plaster hardens (*H*). If more of the articular surface is broken off, the phalanx may be dislocated and skeletal traction may be required to maintain position. (Kaplan, L.: Surg. Clin. N. Am., *20*:1695, 1940)

ulnar side and then swinging it into flexion as the downward pressure is made on the base of the phalanx and upward pressure is made on the metacarpal head. Keeping the wrist flexed during these procedures relaxes tension on the flexor tendons. After reduction, a cast is applied from the lower forearm to the distal joint, with the finger held in moderate flexion; this is maintained for approximately 3 weeks. Full use of the hand should be encouraged while the cast is worn.

This dislocation is often irreducible and requires operation.

Dislocation at the carpometacarpal joint of the thumb is less rare than it is in other fingers at this level. The deformity simulates that of Bennett's fracture, but it is reduced by traction and pressure and is fixed in a cast for 3 weeks.

IRREDUCIBLE DISLOCATIONS OF THE FINGER JOINTS

In some cases, a finger joint dislocation is reduced and the displacement recurs immediately, either completely or incompletely. When this is the case, the but-

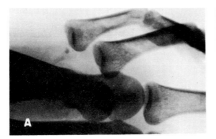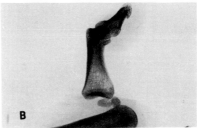

Fig. 24–65. (*A*) Compound dislocation of fourth and fifth meta-carpophalangeal joints caused by a 10-foot fall, the patient landing on his hand. The heads of the fourth and the fifth metacarpals protruded through the skin of the palm. Immediate débridement, reduction, skin sutures only, anterior and posterior plaster splints from elbow to fingertips. Wound healed by first intention. Patient was discharged 3 weeks after injury in excellent condition. (*B*) Metacarpophalangeal dislocation of the thumb. (Kaplan, L.: Surg. Clin. N. Am., *20*:1695, 1940)

tonhole type of dislocation has occurred, and reduction of the displacement has caused the capsule to fold in between the bones. Repeated attempts at reduction are useless, and operation is required. In every case, it is important to make a roentgen examination after reduction of a dislocation.

BIBLIOGRAPHY

Dueben, W.: The question of operative or conservative plaster-cast treatment of old fractures of the navicular bone. Chirurg, *25*:63, 1954.

Gasser, H.: Delayed union and pseudarthrosis of the carpal navicular: treatment by com-pression-screw osteosynthesis. J. Bone Joint Surg., *47A*:249, 1965.

Lipscomb, P. R.: Hints for handling hand fractures. Am. Surg., *29*:277, 1963.

London, P. S.: Sprains and fractures involving the interphalangeal joints. Hand, *3*:155, 1971.

Lord, R. E.: Intramedullary fixation of meta-carpal fractures. JAMA, *164*:1746, 1957.

Mazet, R., Jr., and Hohl, M.: Fractures of the carpal navicular. J. Bone Joint Surg., *45A*:82, 1963.

Peacock, E. E., Jr.: Management of conditions of the hand requiring immobilization. Surg. Clin. N. Am., *33*:1297, 1953.

Robins, R. H.: Injuries of the metacarpo-phalangeal joints. Hand, *3*:195, 1971.

Russe, O.: Fracture of the carpal navicular. J. Bone Joint Surg., *42A*:759, 1960.

Schneewind, J. H.: Surgical emergencies of the hand. Surg. Clin. N. Am., *52*:203, 1972.

Stewart, M. J.: Fractures of the carpal navicu-lar (scaphoid)—a report of 436 cases. J. Bone Joint Surg., *36A*:998, 1954.

Swanson, A. B.: Fractures involving the digits of the hand. Orthop. Clin. N. Am., *1*:261, 1970.

Wiggins, H. E.: and Bundens, W. D., Jr.: A Method of treatment of fracture-dislocation of the first metacarpal bone. J. Bone Joint Surg., *36A*:810, 1954.

Wiley, A. M.: Instability of the proximal in-terphalangeal joint following dislocation and fracture-dislocation: surgical repair. Hand, *2*:185, 1970.

25

Lower Limb

Part I—Soft Tissues

Mark W. Wolcott, M.D.

CALCAREOUS TENDINITIS AND BURSITIS ABOUT THE GREATER TROCHANTER

Symptoms and Diagnosis. Without any injury, or after a trifling one, there is an onset of pain about the greater trochanter that rapidly becomes worse and is so severe that it prevents walking. Examination discloses acute tenderness over the greater trochanter. Roentgenograms show the characteristic calcareous areas (Fig. 25-1); the asymptomatic side may show similar areas.

Treatment. Injection of from 20 to 30 ml. of 1 percent procaine, using a large-bore needle, is particularly efficacious. This may be repeated several times if necessary. Injection of 6 to 8 ml. of 1 percent Xylocaine with 35 mg. of hydrocortisone often works well also.

INGUINAL ADENITIS

Primary infection in the foot or leg or perineum frequently involves the inguinal lymph nodes. The nodes are tender, and walking usually causes pain in the region. Swelling is present in the upper part of the thigh.

If the patient is seen early, local moist heat, combined with effective treatment of the primary infection and antibiotic therapy with the appropriate agent, usually permits the infection to subside. These infections usually are caused by a staphylococcus or a streptococcus, organisms that are controlled readily by penicillin. The adenitis is characterized by redness, tenderness, and temperature elevation, and, as time goes on, fluctuation may appear. When there is fluctuation, or when the duration of the infection in the group of lymph nodes suggests that pus has formed, incision and drainage are indicated. This is accomplished under general anesthesia in cases in which there is no superficial fluctuation, but when there is a definite fluctuant swelling, the incision may be made under local anesthesia. After removal of the pus by sponging or by aspiration, an iodoform-gauze drain is inserted into the abscess, and a pressure dressing is applied and is held in place with a spica-type bandage. Then the patient may be treated at home with hot wet dressings and may return to the clinic or the office for treatment at intervals of 2 or 3 days. As soon as the slough has been removed completely, the wound is permitted to heal by granulation.

CONTUSIONS OF THE THIGH

The thigh is one of the most frequent sites of contusion. This area is bruised

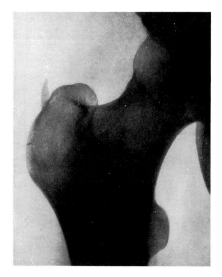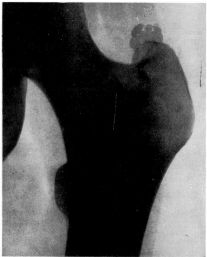

Fig. 25–1. Calcareous tendinitis at the greater trochanter. (*Left*) Shows a small calcareous area on the asymptomatic side. (*Right*) Shows 2 areas on the acutely painful side. Complete relief followed 2 injections of procaine; no treatment was given the painless side. (Kaplan, L.: Penn. Med. J., *45*:37, 1937)

frequently in all types of contact sports, especially football, and also in various forms of industrial and civil accidents.

Treatment. If the injury is treated early, the application of cold for an hour or more is beneficial, but by far the most important therapeutic measure is the application of a firm pressure bandage. Elastic adhesive applied in a spiral manner from the knee up to the groin is very effective, and the earlier it is applied, the less the hemorrhage, and, therefore, the less the disability (Fig. 25-2). This pressure should be maintained for a week unless the skin under the adhesive begins to show signs of irritation. After 2 or 3 days, the application of heat may be of value, but usually ordinary function may be resumed at this time, and we believe that this is more satisfactory than physiotherapy in dispersing the hematoma and in preventing adhesions between muscle bundles, which produce stiffness and soreness and thus prolong disability due to these lesions.

As mentioned above, this injury occurs frequently in contact sports, especially in football. It is difficult to treat these patients because often they want to continue playing. For these patients, it is worthwhile to protect the injured area with

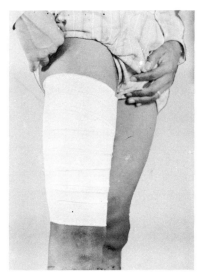

Fig. 25–2. Elastic adhesive bandage of the thigh used in treating contusion. If this dressing can be applied early, hemorrhage and swelling are decreased greatly. It is applied from below upward, the width of one-half each layer being overlapped. The ends must be secured with adhesive strips to prevent rolling.

some hard, unyielding substance padded with sponge rubber. The pad must be large enough to cover completely the area of the primary contusion. If repeated injury can be prevented by this means, it is quite possible for the player to continue at his game.

TRAUMATIC MYOSITIS OSSIFICANS OF THE THIGH

Following trauma, such as multiple trauma of the anterior thigh muscles in playing basketball or football, there may be the development of a solid, indurated, and fixed tumor, not tender, which simulates sarcoma. This is a benign disorder resulting from injury to muscle and fascia and degenerative changes, followed by proliferation of fibrous tissue and, later, ossification. It occurs mostly in teen-age youths. X-ray films taken 2 or 3 weeks after injury may show a diffuse amorphous cloudiness, without a definite border. The calcification gradually becomes more demarcated, ossification occurring parallel to the shaft of the bone. Four to 6 weeks after injury, the films may show a definite bony structure. The mass may attain its maximum density in 6 to 12 weeks. Its appearance on X-ray films may simulate closely that of a malignant tumor, such as osteogenic sarcoma. Even the microscopic appearance of the tissue may simulate malignant tumor, but differentiation may be easier if the possibility of a traumatic process is kept in mind.

If malignancy can be definitely excluded, and biopsy is sometimes necessary to do this, no active treatment is indicated. Rest, minimum activity, and avoidance of trauma are advised. The mass gradually grows smaller, and even the calcification disappears over a period of months or years.

STRAINS AND RUPTURES OF THE ADDUCTOR LONGUS MUSCLE

(Rider's Strain)

Etiology. There are various types of traumatic lesions of the adductor longus muscle, and, since they occur especially in horseback riding, they are mentioned sometimes under the general heading of rider's strain. The muscle may be pulled from its origin on the superior ramus of the pubis, there may be a tendon-muscle strain in the upper part of the muscle, or there may be an actual rupture of the muscle in its belly. All these lesions result from forceful abduction of the leg while the muscle is contracted. In horseback riding, this occurs especially in jumping, when, while the thighs are adducted to hold the rider in his saddle, the saddle is thrust up between the thighs, pushing the legs apart.

Symptoms. The symptoms produced are typical. The patient complains of pain in the upper inner portion of the thigh, and adduction becomes so weak that often he is unable to continue riding.

Diagnosis. On examination, the findings vary somewhat according to the type of injury. In muscle rupture, swelling and ecchymosis of the thigh are definite; at times it is possible to feel an area of depression, which marks the site of the muscle tear. Muscle strains are characterized by tenderness of the adductor muscle in the upper inner part of the thigh when it is palpated between the fingers. A tear of the muscle origin is indicated by marked tenderness along the pubic ramus on palpation. All these muscle injuries cause definite pain when the knees are forced apart while the patient is attempting to hold them together.

Treatment. This is similar for the various lesions. Elastic adhesive bandages, applied firmly to the thigh up to the groin, give good support and frequently relieve most of the discomfort. Applications of heat are of value. As a rule, the patient has little difficulty in pursuing ordinary activities, but motions necessitating forceful adduction of the thigh should be avoided. Recovery eventually takes place, but the muscle may remain painful for 4 to 6 weeks.

RUPTURE OF THE QUADRICEPS EXTENSOR MUSCLE

Etiology. The quadriceps muscle is ruptured occasionally by a violent muscular effort to recover balance. Rupture

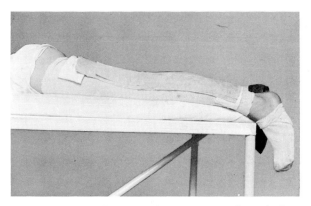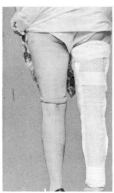

Fig. 25–3. Application of a posterior splint of plaster for immobilization of the knee. Stockinet is drawn up from the ankle to the buttock, and a felt pad is laid at each end. When the splint is hard, the stockinet is turned back and fastened with adhesive. The splint is secured to the leg with wide adhesive straps. Three have been applied. A fourth is placed below the knee. An elastic bandage is wrapped round the knee to control swelling.

occurs when the lower leg is nearly in line with the thigh, whereas the patella is fractured over the condyles of the femur if the same effort is exerted with the knee flexed.

The muscle tears above the patella, and because of the broad expanse of the tendon of insertion of the quadriceps extensor around the patella, usually the entire tendon is not torn.

Symptoms. Usually, considerable swelling is associated with the rupture. This is due to hemorrhage in the area. This marked swelling, in the center of which is a definite depression, is sufficient to make the diagnosis. The patient shows a weakness in extending the leg against resistance, and is often completely unable to do so; and pain is experienced when this motion is attempted.

Treatment. Because of the fact that frequently the rectus femoris portion of the quadriceps is torn, whereas the vasti medialis and lateralis remain intact, it is usually unnecessary to suture the ruptured muscle. The leg is splinted in extension, using a molded plaster splint (Fig. 25-3). After 2 or 3 days in bed, with elevation of the part, the patient may be permitted to walk if the leg is held in complete extension by the posterior splint. A firm elastic bandage is maintained for a period of 2 to 3 weeks at least.

Healing with normal function is the rule, but a period of from 5 to 6 weeks usually is necessary before complete normal function is resumed.

INJURIES TO THE KNEE JOINT

General Consideration

Anatomy. Although the knee joint is exceptionally strong, it is frequently the site of injury due to the great violence exerted on it and due to the length of the tibia and the femur, which act as powerful levers when the extremes of motion are reached. The essential motion of the knee is in flexion and extension. Slight rotation is possible in semiflexion, almost none in full extension. There is practically no sidewise motion.

The knee joint has a strong capsule reinforced anteriorly by the quadriceps tendon, the patella, and the patellar ligament and on the sides by strong collateral ligaments. The collateral ligaments lie toward the posterior portion of the joint; thus they become tense in extension and relaxed in flexion (Fig. 25-4). On the posterior aspect, the expansion of the tendon of the semimembranosus acts as a reinforcement. The joint is strengthened further by the two cruciate ligaments within

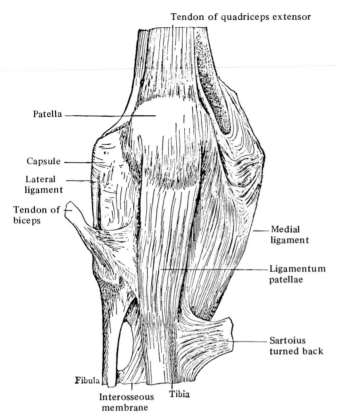

Tendon of quadriceps extensor

Patella

Capsule

Lateral
ligament

Tendon of
biceps

Medial
ligament

Ligamentum
patellae

Sartoius
turned back

Fibula

Interosseous
membrane

Tibia

Fig. 25–4. Right knee joint,
from before. (Piersol)

it. The anterior cruciate ligament runs
from in front of the tibial spine upward,
backward, and outward to insert on the
lateral condyle in the intercondylar notch.
The posterior cruciate ligament runs from
the posterior groove upward, forward,
and inward to insert on the medial condyle in the intercondylar notch (Fig. 25-
5).

Over the plateaus of the tibia lie the
semilunar cartilages. These are C-shaped
fibrocartilages, the thick 6 to 8 mm. outer
margins of which are attached to the tibia
by the coronary ligaments. Their inner
margins are thin and free. The lateral
cartilage moves more freely than does the
medial. Both serve to deepen the slight
concavity of the articular surface of the
tibia. They move forward and backward
to accommodate to the changes in position of articular surfaces of the femur on
the head of the tibia in extension and
flexion.

Examination of the Knee Joint. The
patient's ability or inability to walk gives
the first clue as to the state of the joint.
Serious injuries make walking almost impossible.

With the patient sitting or lying down,
the knees are placed in extension. Deformity, swelling, discoloration, and limitation of extension are seen at a glance.
The joint is palpated carefully for tender
points and for its bony contours. Flexion
is tested, and any pain and limitation of
motion are noted. Mobility mediolaterally
and anteroposteriorly then is determined
(Fig. 25-6).

***Preliminary Treatment of Acute In-
juries About the Knee Joint.*** Acute traumatic synovitis and injuries of the cartilages, the ligaments, bone, and the extensor apparatus have certain effects in common. Pain and swelling develop, with
effusion or hemorrhage into the joint.
Motion is painful, and often there is considerable muscle spasm.

After the initial examination is made,

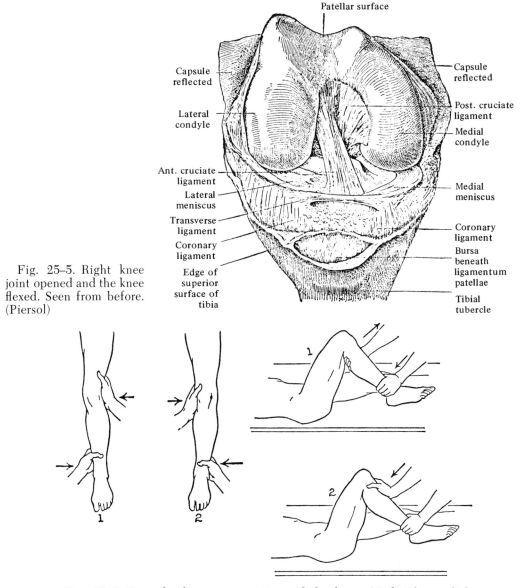

Fig. 25-5. Right knee joint opened and the knee flexed. Seen from before. (Piersol)

Fig. 25-6. Tests for ligamentous injury of the knee. (*Left*) The medial ligament is tested by forcing the leg into abduction on the thigh (1). The lateral ligament is tested by forcing the leg into adduction on the thigh (2). (*Right*) Testing for rupture of the cruciate ligaments. If the upper end of the tibia can be pulled forward (1), the anterior cruciate ligament is torn. If the upper end of the tibia can be pushed backward (2), the posterior cruciate ligament is torn.

aspiration of blood or serous fluid from a tense joint relieves much of the pain and removes a source of irritation and fibrosis. A posterior splint is applied securely. A firm pressure dressing of elastic bandage, or a thick layer of absorbent cotton secured with a muslin bandage, then is applied. This aids in preventing further effusion into the joint. A roentgen study is made. Salicylates and phenobarbital or

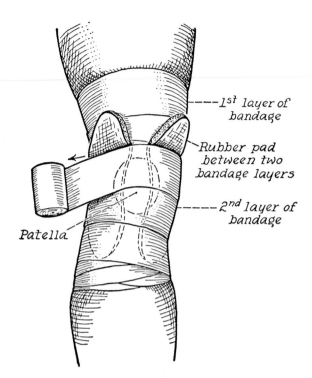

----1ˢᵗ layer of bandage

Rubber pad between two bandage layers

----2ⁿᵈ layer of bandage

Patella

Fig. 25–7. Pressure dressing for the knee. An elastic adhesive bandage is applied from 41/2 in. below the patella to 41/2 in. above it. Rubber pads 8 inches long, 2 inches wide, and 1/4 inch thick are placed in position, and the bandage is continued over them. (Truslow, W.: JAMA, *110*:285, 1938)

codeine are given for pain. Crutches are provided to avoid weight bearing on the injured leg.

HEMARTHROSIS AND EFFUSION INTO THE KNEE JOINT

Etiology and Diagnosis. Effusion and hemorrhage into the knee joint follow injuries to the ligaments, the semilunar cartilages, the articular cartilages and the snyovial lining; and fractures of the femoral condyles, the spines of the tibia and the tibial plateaus. There may be a small or a large collection of fluid. Small amounts are detected by comparing both knees in full extension and observing any fullness of the hollows present normally at the sides of the patella and proximal to it. When there is considerable effusion, the capsule of the joint is distended, and an inverted U-shaped swelling of the joint occurs. The dense patellar ligament prevents distention of the capsule beneath it, so that the swelling has this characteristic shape.

This condition must be differentiated from effusion into the prepatellar bursa. Bursal swelling distends the bursa, which lies mainly over the lower portion of the patella, between it and the skin. Effusion into the joint occurs posterior to the patella, whereas bursal swelling occurs anterior to it. With the knee extended, a large effusion causes the patella to "float," that is, to be lifted away from the femoral condyles. By a sharp thrust of the fingers, the patella may be made to click against the condyles. Complete extension and flexion are often impossible because of the joint tension produced by the effusion.

Distention of the joint by effusion or hemorrhage causes considerable pain and disability. If the exudate or the blood is not removed, it is partly absorbed, but part of it may undergo organization, resulting in the formation of adhesions or bands in the joint.

Treatment. Very small effusions require only a firm pressure dressing of elastic bandage in addition to treatment

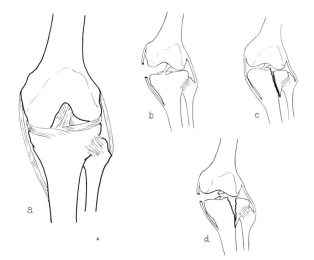

Fig. 25–8. Forced abduction of the leg or forced adduction of the knee may cause the injuries shown in *b*, *c*, and *d*. (*a*) Normal ligament arrangement. (*b*) Rupture of the medial ligament. (*c*) Fracture of the lateral plateau of the tibia. (*d*) Splitting fracture of the lateral plateau, rupture of the medial ligament, and rupture of the anterior cruciate ligament.

of the main injury. When the effusion or the hemorrhage into the joint distends the capsule or causes pain, the joint contents must be removed by aspiration, which relieves pain by relieving tension and removes a source of irritation and fibrosis.

Aspiration of the Knee Joint. After the skin has been cleansed with two applications of 70 percent alcohol, a skin wheal is made with procaine solution 1 cm. medial to the lower half of the patella. A large-bore, 16- to 18-gauge needle, attached to a 10- or 20-ml. syringe, is introduced through the wheal and is directed upward and outward, toward the center of the joint. When the joint is entered, the contents can be withdrawn freely. As much fluid as possible is removed. If pressure is made on the joint and over the suprapatellar bursa, the fluid can often be pushed toward the site of the needle.

An alternate site of aspiration in marked effusion is from the distended suprapatellar portion of the joint capsule lateral to and above the patella. The technique of aspiration is the same as that described above.

Following aspiration, a posterior splint and a pressure bandage are applied. Continuous elastic pressure is obtained by incorporating pads of sponge rubber in the dressing and by applying elastic

bandages (Fig. 25-7). Reaspiration may be performed as necessary.

ACUTE TRAUMATIC SYNOVITIS

Following an injury to the knee, there may be moderate pain on motion and serous or serosanguineous effusion into the joint. When no definite evidence of bone, ligament, or cartilage injury can be demonstrated clinically or roentgenographically, it is assumed that the synovium mainly has been injured.

Treatment. A splint and a pressure dressing are used until pain and swelling have subsided. The splint is removed after about 2 weeks, and the elastic pressure bandage is continued for a week or two longer. Residual stiffness is relieved by heat and massage. A light cylinder cast from the ankle to mid-thigh is very effective and is simpler to maintain.

INJURIES TO THE COLLATERAL LIGAMENTS

MEDIAL LIGAMENT INJURIES

Etiology. Injury to the medial ligament usually is caused by abrupt forced adduction of the knee while the leg is fixed, or by sudden internal rotation of the thigh upon the fixed leg (Fig. 25-8). The ligament tears through its substance or at its

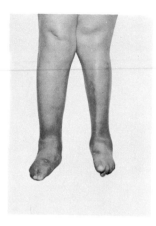
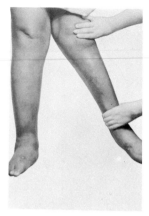

Fig. 25–9. An old neglected rupture of the left medial collateral ligament. The leg can be abducted widely at the knee.

tibial or femoral attachment. The lacerations may be either very slight or very extensive. At the femoral attachment, the laceration may include a portion of the periosteum and the bone into which the ligament inserts. Periosteal injury is manifested later by thickening and persistent tenderness at the medial side of the medial condyle, and, in a few weeks, roentgenograms show calcification along the tender area. This may be a form of the condition known as Pellegrini-Stieda disease.

Diagnosis. In sport injuries it is often possible to make a diagnosis at once by reproducing the mechanism of the trauma before muscle spasm and pain make the maneuver impossible. However, in most cases the diagnosis is based on the history of injury followed by pain and disability at the knee. The patient limps or is unable to bear any weight on the knee. Muscle spasm maintaining slight flexion suggests a cartilage injury, but the flexion spasm subsides on gentle extension and on procaine injection into the painful area. Effusion into the joint, localized tenderness of the medial side of the knee, and pain on forced abduction of the leg usually are present. When the ligament is ruptured, it is sometimes possible to abduct the leg beyond the normal limit (Fig. 25-9). Ligament injuries often accompany other injuries to the knee. Roentgen examination should always be carried out.

Treatment. Infiltration of the acutely painful area with 1 percent procaine solution, from 10 to 20 ml., gives almost immediate relief of pain and muscle spasm. Repeated aspiration of the joint may be necessary. When the injury is mild, a splint and a pressure dressing or a light plaster cylinder cast are continued for from 7 to 14 days, or until the local tenderness subsides. Additional injections of procaine are helpful for persistent pain.

When the injury is severe and actual rupture of the ligament is present, the immobilization must be prolonged to obtain firm healing. Many orthopedic surgeons prefer immediate operative repair of the injured ligaments.

Prognosis. The prognosis varies with the severity of the injury. If treatment is adequate and no other knee injuries have occurred, a satisfactory result may be expected.

LATERAL LIGAMENT INJURIES

The lateral ligament sustains an injury much less often than does the medial. The etiology, the diagnosis, and the treatment of this injury are analogous to those described for medial ligament injuries.

INJURIES TO THE SEMILUNAR CARTILAGES

(Medial and Lateral Menisci)

Etiology. Injuries to the semilunar cartilages are the most common derangements of the knee joint. The medial semi-lunar cartilage is less mobile and is injured much more often than is the lateral. The cartilages are dislocated or torn, the laceration being longitudinal or in the anterior or the posterior portion. Injury to the medial cartilage occurs when the knee is partially flexed and is bearing weight and there is internal rotation of the femur on the tibia, which is fixed by the foot on the ground or the floor. Injury to the medial ligament also follows this violence. Less often, other forms of violence cause cartilage injuries. When a thick portion of the cartilage slips between the femoral condyle and the tibia, the knee locks and cannot be extended fully.

Diagnosis. A history of the typical violence followed by a sensation of "something snapping" or "something giving way" in the joint is usually obtained. There is severe pain on the involved side of the knee and often there is a typical locking of the joint. The diagnosis is simple if the patient's knee is locked at the time of the examination. Or he may describe manipulation of the locked leg by a friend or a bystander that was followed immediately by (1) relief of the acute pain and (2) ability to extend the knee. Later the knee becomes swollen, stiff, and increasingly painful.

Examination may disclose a typical locking of the knee; the patient is able to flex it but is unable to extend it to more than 150° to 160°. If the locking has been reduced prior to examination, there may be only effusion in the joint, acute tenderness at the anteromedial margin of the medial tibial plateau when the medial cartilage is torn, or at the anterolateral margin if the lateral cartilage is torn, and pain on motion. According to Rix:

The patient is examined lying down with the knee in acute flexion. When the leg is internally or externally rotated and slightly extended at the same time, a grating, popping, snapping or crunching may be produced, audible and palpable to the examiner, sometimes consciously felt by the patient, and often associated with pain. Occasionally a knee can actually be locked by manipulation. For exam-

ple, in some medial meniscus tears if the knee is acutely flexed and the leg externally rotated, it cannot be extended. If now the leg is rotated in the opposite direction into internal rotation, the knee becomes "unlocked" and can then be extended freely.

Other injuries to the knee often complicate cartilage lesions.

Treatment. The effusion is aspirated, and if locking is present, it is reduced immediately. Anesthesia is not always necessary, but 10 ml. of a 1 percent procaine solution may be infiltrated at the site of the acute tenderness. In some instances, general anesthesia is needed. With the patient seated on a table so that the legs hang freely over the edge, downward traction is made on the ankle, and, for injury of the medial cartilage, the leg is abducted, rotated externally, and extended rapidly. When the cartilage slips into place, the knee can be extended as fully as the uninjured one.

Lewin uses pentothal anesthesia for the reduction.

The patient is placed in a supine position with a pillow placed lengthwise to maintain flexion of the knee. The surgeon stands on a platform at the side of the patient, at the level of the knee. The maneuvers are simple but precise. They must not be carried out in a jerky or rapid manner. They are effective and nontraumatic. For medial meniscus displacement the knee and hip are hyperflexed, then the foot and knee are forced into the valgus position and the knee and hip slowly and firmly placed in extension. The knee and hip are again hyperflexed; the foot and knee are then forced into the varus position and the knee and hip slowly and firmly placed in extension. For lateral meniscus displacement the knee and hip are hyperflexed; the foot and knee are forced into the varus position and the knee and hip extended; the knee and hip are again hyperflexed; and the foot and knee are then forced into a valgus position and the knee and hip extended. The success of the maneuvers is proved by the attainment of complete extension without the slightest tension.

When reduction has been obtained, or when the patient gives the typical history and has the local signs of cartilage injury without locking, the knee must be immobilized for a prolonged period to obtain good healing and to avoid recurrence.

A cast is applied, the medial border of the heel is wedged up ¹/₈ to ³/₁₆ of an inch, and the patient is permitted to use the leg.

The immobilization is continued for from 4 to 6 weeks. The after-treatment is similar to that for collateral ligament injuries.

When locking cannot be overcome, operation must be done without undue delay.

Recurrent Dislocation. Aside from a repetition of the violence to the knee (as in football), the most common cause of recurrent dislocation is poor healing of the cartilage. Repeated dislocation requires excision of the cartilage; otherwise chronic joint changes take place.

Prognosis. It is questionable whether or not true cartilage tears ever heal, even with adequate early therapy. If there is persistent pain or disability, arthrotomy may be indicated. The patient should be informed that the dislocation is likely to recur and that, in that event, operation may be necessary.

INJURIES TO THE CRUCIATE LIGAMENTS

ANTERIOR CRUCIATE LIGAMENT INJURIES

Etiology. The anterior cruciate ligament, which runs from in front upward, backward, and outward, prevents anterior displacement of the tibia on the femur. It is a factor also in preventing abduction of the tibia on the femur and, to some extent, in preventing internal rotation of the tibia. Injury to the ligament may occur when the normal range of any of these motions is exceeded greatly, as in forcible hyperextension. It is likely to occur when the medial ligament is lacerated extensively, and when there has been a dislocation of the medial semilunar cartilage. Rupture of a cruciate ligament is very rare without other knee injuries.

The site of the injury, or rupture, of the ligament varies. It may be through the substance of the ligament or at the femoral or the tibial attachment. At the latter attachment, the injury is manifested as an avulsion of the spine of the tibia (Fig. 25-10).

Diagnosis. Severe injury to the knee is evident. To test the cruciate ligaments, the patient is seated on a table with the knee flexed at a right angle and the foot on a footstool. The examiner places his hand on the back of the leg below the flexed knee and presses the tibia forward. If the anterior cruciate ligament is torn, the tibia can be displaced forward. Roentgen examination is indicated.

Treatment. Prolonged immobilization is necessary to obtain good union of the torn ligament. Preliminary treatment of the knee (p. 462) is carried out. Repeated aspiration may be necessary. The splint, the pressure dressing, rest, and elevation are continued until the swelling subsides. A plaster cast is then applied with the knee in 15° of flexion. The medial border of the heel is elevated ¹/₈ to ³/₁₆ of an inch. The patient is permitted to use crutches at first, later walking without them. The cast is worn for from 2 to 3 months. When it is removed, an elastic stocking is applied from the toes to the knee, and an elastic bandage is wrapped about the knee. If the knee seems to be at all unstable, a knee brace is worn for 6 months. Early operation is often advisable.

POSTERIOR CRUCIATE LIGAMENT INJURIES

Etiology. The posterior cruciate ligament, which runs upward, forward, and inward, prevents posterior displacement of the tibia on the femur. Injury, which is rare, is caused by hyperflexion or by the tibia's being driven backward when the knee is flexed. The rupture occurs through the substance of the ligament or at the femoral or the tibial attachment. Both cruciate ligaments may be torn at the same time; usually this is associated with dislocation of the knee.

Diagnosis. The patient is seated on a table with the knee flexed at a right angle and the foot on a footstool. The integrity of the posterior cruciate ligament is determined by attempting to displace the tibia

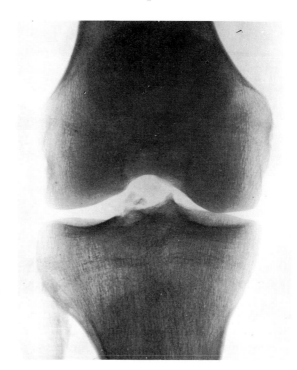

Fig. 25–10. Fracture of the spine of the tibia at the insertion of the posterior cruciate ligament. There also was a tear of the medial ligament. With conservative treatment, this patient played varsity football 10 months later.

backward; when this is possible, the posterior cruciate ligament is ruptured.

Treatment. The treatment is as described for injury of the anterior cruciate ligament (see above), except that the knee is kept fully extended.

INJURY AND HYPERTROPHY OF THE INFRAPATELLAR FAT PAD

Etiology. The infrapatellar, or subpatellar, fat pad fills the space inside the capsule of the knee joint just beneath the patellar ligament. It is bruised frequently and becomes edematous. Repeated injuries produce permanent hypertrophy due to fibrosis. When the fat pad is enlarged, it may be pinched between the bones of the knee in extension.

Diagnosis. Following sudden hyperextension of the knee or direct pressure below the knee, the patient complains of pain beneath the patella and the patellar ligament, especially on going up or down stairs. On examination, an elastic and rather tender fullness of the tissues is found on both sides of the patellar ligament. An effusion may be present in the joint. Full extension of the knee causes pain that is localized beneath the patellar ligament, and often it is impossible because of the edematous mass of synovium in the infrapatellar space.

Treatment. If the symptoms are acute, the preliminary treatment of the knee (p. 462) is given. If full extension causes marked discomfort, from 5° to 10° of flexion may be allowed. Repeated procaine injections into the tender areas are helpful. After the acute symptoms subside, an elastic knee support or a bandage is applied. When the symptoms are persistent in spite of treatment, excision of the fat pad must be considered.

PREPATELLAR BURSITIS

Etiology. The prepatellar bursa is one of the adventitious bursae found commonly. It lies in a subcutaneous position over the knee, usually distal to the patella and over the patellar ligament (Fig. 25-11). The bursa becomes thickened, due to chronic inflammation and trauma. Often it is made prominent due to effusion. Appearing most often in those who work

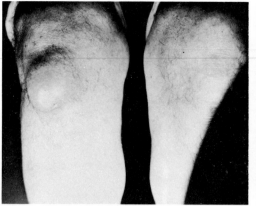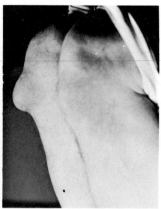

Fig. 25–11. Prepatellar bursitis. This was a chronically inflamed bursa with thick walls. Note the position of the bursa, not over the patella but below it, in the region of the patellar ligament.

upon their knees, this lesion is commonly called housemaid's knee and is considered to be an occupational disease.

Symptoms. The bursa gives symptoms when, due to some recent trauma, it becomes filled with bloody or serous effusion. It then presents itself as a swelling in front of the knee below the patella, usually without marked pain or tenderness. There is little tendency for the fluid to be absorbed spontaneously.

Treatment. Under local anesthesia, the fluid may be aspirated (Fig. 25-12). It is bloody if there has been recent trauma, straw colored if the bursitis is of some duration. After aspiration, movable bodies representing villi and fibrous bands across the bursa may be palpated. These are tender upon pressure.

If reaccumulation of fluid occurs after 2 or 3 aspirations, the bursa may be obliterated by separating the roof from the floor of the bursa through subcutaneous incisions, as described in Chapter 23. The operation may be performed under local anesthesia. A firm elastic bandage should be kept on the knee for from 10 to 14 days.

The bursa may be excised under local anesthesia and the wound sutured. A flap usually is turned, so that the scar does not lie directly over the knee. The area is dressed with a pressure bandage, a rubber sponge and a posterior splint usually being employed.

Infection of the prepatellar bursa occasionally follows furunculosis over the knee. In furunculosis the area becomes tender and swollen, with marked redness. If a posterior splint is applied to immobilize the knee and hot moist dressings are used for 2 or 3 days, the infection usually localizes and points, as does any furuncle or carbuncle. As a rule, further progress of the infection can be prevented by appropriate antibiotic (penicillin) administration. Frequently, however, by contiguity the infection may involve the underlying prepatellar bursa, in which case adequate incision and drainage are necessary and may be carried out under local infiltration anesthesia through a transverse incision. The wound is packed with plain or iodoform gauze, and a posterior splint is applied. With hot moist dressings, splinting, elevation, and antibiotics, the infection usually subsides, and healing occurs as with the uncomplicated furuncle.

MUSCLE-SHEATH HERNIAS

Muscle-sheath hernias appear as small protrusions on the leg. They may or may not be associated with varicose veins, and often they are mistaken for the bulges of varicosities. Frequently they are extremely painful.

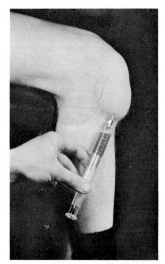
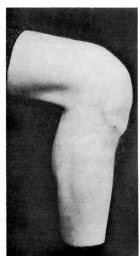

Fig. 25-12. Aspiration of bloody fluid from a prepatellar bursa and appearance following aspiration.

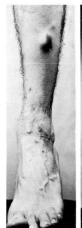
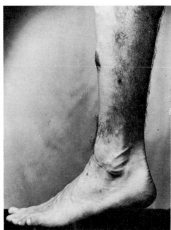
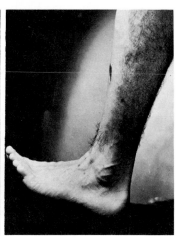

Fig. 25-13. Post-traumatic muscle hernia due to shrapnel injury. Note the prominence of the muscle bulge when the patient stands on his toes and the depression when the weight is borne on his heels. (Official U. S. Navy photograph)

Etiology. These lesions are congenital or traumatic openings in the deep fascia of the leg through which the underlying muscle protrudes. When they occur without any previous history of trauma, they are located often where the nerves perforate the deep fascia to become subcutaneous. The nerves involved most frequently are the sural and the superficial peroneal nerves, on the lateral aspect of the leg.

Diagnosis. A muscle hernia is distinguished easily from a varicose vein by the fact that it protrudes when the patient is standing and becomes even larger when he is standing on his toes. It is less prominent when the patient is not on his feet or when he is standing with the foot dorsiflexed, at which time the protrusion may disappear entirely. In thin people, it may be possible to palpate the fascial rings through which the hernia protrudes (Fig. 25-13).

Treatment. Pain and disfigurement are the usual reasons for therapy in this type of hernia. If the pain is believed to be due to pressure on a nerve at the site through which the hernia protrudes, it is probable that an operation is the best method of therapy.

Under local anesthesia, the hernial opening is exposed; the nerve is found emerging through the deep fascia at the lowermost portion of the hernial opening. In several such cases, the author has enlarged the opening downward so as to have the nerve emerge through a new opening. The fascial defects are then closed by suture. If it sometimes necessary to perform a fascial transplant, removing a portion of the fascia lata and suturing it in the hernial opening. The wounds are closed, and a firm elastic adhesive bandage is applied. Crutches are provided so as to prevent weight bearing on the foot for a period of about 3 weeks.

PERITENDINITIS CREPITANS

(Traumatic Tenosynovitis)

Etiology and Symptoms. This lesion is described in some detail in the chapter on the hand and the fingers. It occurs also in the muscles of the legs, and frequently follows prolonged muscular effort to which the individual is unaccustomed, such as tramping, hiking, or dancing; or it occurs with use following trauma. The symptoms are similar to those described for the so-called traumatic tenosynovitis of the forearm: pain on use of the involved muscles, swelling, and crepitation during muscle function. The Achilles tendon is the one most often affected.

Treatment. Since the tenosynovitis is the result of repeated unusual function of the muscles and tendons involved, rest of the part might be expected to give relief. Injection of the paratenon with hydrocortisone (35 mg. in 6 to 8 ml. of 1 percent Xylocaine) and the application of a firm elastic bandage usually results in a rapid cure.

TENNIS LEG

Tennis leg occurs during activities in which the knee is fully extended and the foot is held in plantar flexion. If the foot is forcefully brought into dorsiflexion, as occurs in coming down on the foot in a tennis serve, the patient experiences a sudden acute pain in the calf of the leg; often this is associated with a snap that is audible to both the patient and those about him. The pain is so sudden and knifelike that the patient turns to see who has thrown a stone or stuck a knife in his leg. Pain and weakness in the leg become so severe that it is necessary for him to discontinue his activities, and soon there is a painful swelling of the calf.

Although tennis leg was for a long time believed to be due to rupture of the plantaris muscle at its musculotendinous junction, further study of this syndrome has shown it to be due to rupture of the medial head of the gastrocnemius muscle from its tendinous attachment to the underlying soleus aponeurosis (Fig. 25-14).

Diagnosis. At first, there is a circumscribed tenderness and swelling on the medial aspect of the calf, midway between the knee and the heel. Careful palpation of the calf reveals a dimplelike depression just medial to the midline of the calf, and in a position corresponding to the musculotendinous junction of the medial belly of the gastrocnemius. This is the site of the most acute tenderness. The most distinctive and diagnostic symptom is pain when the muscle is used against resistance. This is demonstrated by asking the patient to plantar flex the foot while the examiner's hand is placed to resist this motion. As time goes on, a definite ecchymosis begins to appear in the lower part of the leg and extends down to the foot.

Treatment. Almost immediate relief of symptoms may be obtained by the application of a firm supporting bandage or dressing. The easiest to apply is one of elastic adhesive; this is begun at the foot and carried as a spiral bandage up the leg to the knee. Elevation of the heel to relieve tension on the ruptured muscle is worthwhile. In a few cases, a plaster cast may be applied below the knee to hold the foot in plantar flexion. The ball of the foot is left out of the cast to permit weight bearing. The patient may remain ambu-

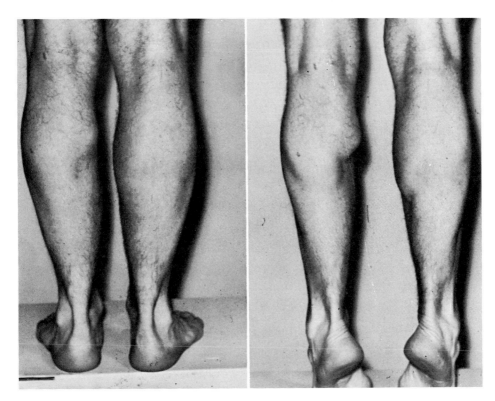

Fig. 25–14. Tennis leg, showing typical deformity of rupture of the medial head of the gastrocnemius. (*Left*) At rest. (*Right*) Standing on tiptoe. (Fahrni, H.: Canad. J. Surg., 7:157, 1964)

latory throughout the treatment with either dressing, which should be continued for 3 or 4 weeks at least. Active function with support gives much more comfort and earlier relief of symptoms than does conservative therapy with rest, diathermy, and other measures.

OSGOOD-SCHLATTER DISEASE

This is a painful enlargement of the tibial tubercle during the years of puberty (Fig. 25-15). It is seen more often in boys than in girls, and is characterized by an enlargement of the tibial tubercle with some pain, especially on extension of the lower leg on the thigh against resistance. Frequently there is a history of direct or indirect trauma, such as kicking a football.

Pathology. Cole made a study of this disease. He believes that it occurs as a result of rapid growth during adolescence, during which period the quad-

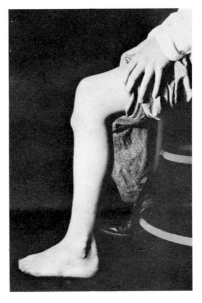

Fig. 25–15. Osgood-Schlatter disease. This appeared typically in a young boy as a painful swelling at the tibial tubercle.

riceps muscles are placed under a great physiologic strain. This produces changes within the patellar ligament due to alterations of the blood supply in the tendon; microscopic section demonstrates fibrocartilaginous areas in the tendon, which later become calcified and ossified. Cole believes that the disability experienced by patients with this disease is due to an increase in intratendinous pressure. As time goes on, if conservative treatment is instituted, the peritenon adapts itself to the increased size of the tendon, and eventually the disability and pain disappear. The enlargement of the tissues in the region of the tibial tubercle is associated with bony changes in this area, and lateral roentgenograms show progressive changes in calcification in the region of the epiphysis of the tibial tubercle. Cole believes that these changes occur in the tendinous insertion of the quadriceps extensor muscle, and that the calcified and the ossified islands appearing in the film occur really in the tendinous tissue rather than in the epiphysis.

Treatment. Since this disease is self-limiting, conservative therapy by means of a light circular plaster cast, incorporating the knee joint and extending from ankle to mid-thigh to relax the quadriceps muscle and tendon, is the treatment of choice. This must be maintained for a period of several weeks, sometimes as long as 5 or 6 weeks, but invariably the condition gradually subsides spontaneously without other therapy.

VARICOSE VEINS

Abnormal enlargements of veins are spoken of as varices or varicosities. These are seen most commonly in the lower extremities, and it is here that they produce symptoms and disability.

Anatomy. To understand the pathology and the treatment of varicose veins, it is important to recall the anatomy of the veins of the leg. The venous blood is transmitted upward to the heart by two sets of veins: the deep veins, represented by the posterior tibial, the anterior tibial, the peroneal, and the popliteal, which go to form the femoral vein; and the superficial veins, represented by the long and the short saphenous veins. These two venous systems are connected by communicating veins, which pierce the deep fascia of the leg (Fig. 25-16).

The veins are supplied with bicuspid valves, which maintain the flow of blood upward and prevent backflow so long as they are competent. Blood is moved onward by a combination of forces, which includes capillary pressure, cardiothoracic aspiration, which is produced by respiration, and especially, perhaps, the force of contracting muscles. In a general way, the flow in the superficial veins is upward, but it is probable that blood reaches the deep circulation by the shortest route and that, in large part, the flow from the superficial circulation is through the communicating veins. The direction of this flow is maintained also by bicuspid valves, which prevent backflow from the deep into the superficial circulation in periods of muscular relaxation.

Etiology. The superficial veins of the leg are particularly subject to dilatation, the causes of which are many. They are placed in the superficial subcutaneous areolar tissue, where they have little perivenous support. In addition, the long saphenous, because of its great length, is subject to a high internal pressure. It is estimated that about 98 percent of varicosities are of the long saphenous.

Various other factors appear to be common in the etiology of varicose veins. Unquestionably, there is a hereditary tendency. Frequently, patients volunteer the information that several members of the family have or have had varicose veins. This suggests the possibility of a weakness of the elastic tissue in the vein walls. Many varicose veins appear to be occupational in origin. Prolonged standing, especially in hot rooms, may predispose to the development of varicosities. Pregnancy is a frequent cause, and it is probable that two etiologic factors play a part in these patients: one is pressure upon the veins of the pelvis by the enlarging uterus; the other is an increase in the intra-

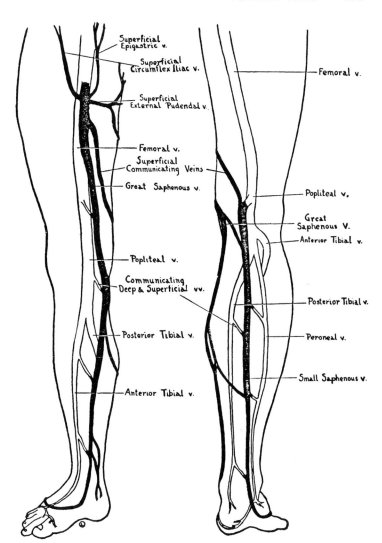

Superficial
Epigastric v.

Superficial
Circumflex Iliac v.

Superficial
External Pudendal v.

Femoral v.

Superficial
Communicating Veins

Great Saphenous v.

Popliteal v.

Communicating
Deep & Superficial vv.

Posterior Tibial v.

Anterior Tibial v.

Femoral v.

Popliteal v.

Great
Saphenous V.

Anterior Tibial v.

Posterior Tibial v.

Peroneal v.

Small Saphenous v.

Fig. 25–16. Anatomy of the veins of the leg. The superficial veins are indicated in solid black, and the deep veins in outline. The great saphenous is also known as the long, or the internal, saphenous; the small, as the short, or the external, saphenous. (Ferguson, L. K.: Ann. Surg., *102*:304, 1935)

abdominal pressure. Both tend to produce partial obstruction of the venous return, with consequent dilatation of the vessels. Phlebitis, whether due to infection or to trauma, may produce partial incompetence of the valves of the vein, with subsequent dilatation of the venous segment in that region. There is no question that, as the vein dilates, more and more valves become incompetent, and, as this occurs, the veins become more dilated, so that a vicious cycle is started.

Pathologic Physiology. It is believed that usually valvular failure involves the saphenous system, but incompetence of

the valves of the communicating veins is also found; this is either congenital in origin or the result of a phlebitis.

The fact should not be overlooked that the dilatation of the superficial veins may be a physiologic one which is due to a block of the deep venous circulation by phlebitis. In these cases, the dilatation may be compensatory, but canalization of the thrombus produced by the deep phlebitis usually takes place at a later date, and the enlarged superficial veins remain then as varicosities.

Symptoms. Many varicosities give no symptoms, escept disfigurement, and, es-

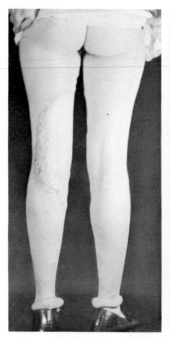

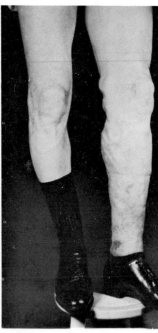

Fig. 25–17. (*Left*) Unsightly veins causing relatively few symptoms. This represents a dilatation of the superficial communicating veins extending from the popliteal to the saphenous vein. (*Right*) Early stage of pigmentation and stasis dermatitis in a patient with large varicose veins.

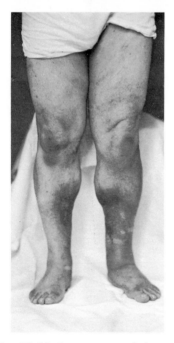

Fig. 25–18. Later stage of degenerative change in the lower leg associated with varicose veins. Note the fibrosis and relative constriction of both legs above the ankle and the ulcerations developing in the fibrotic area.

pecially in the spring months, patients seek medical aid to have their veins obliterated to avoid the embarrassment of revealing unsightly legs when they appear in a bathing suit (Fig. 25-17). More often, however, the patient will complain of heaviness and easy fatigue in the leg involved, and of slight swelling about the ankle after having been on his feet all day. This swelling disappears during the night. Frequently, there are nocturnal cramps which waken the patient. Usually, the cramps occur in the calf of the leg and in the foot. Many female patients complain of soreness in the region of the veins only at the time of the menses, at which time, also, the veins seem to be larger.

As time goes on, various changes occur in the skin and the subcutaneous tissues which are drained by the enlarged vein. There is a brownish pigmentation, often associated with itching, and an eczematoid dermatitis which has been termed stasis dermatitis (Fig. 25-18). When edema is a prominent factor, there is a gradual replacement fibrosis of the subcutaneous fatty tissue, so that a firm induration with a brawny pitting edema replaces the soft subcutaneous tissue of the leg above the ankle. In older patients, pain in the ankles and in the knee joints is quite common.

When cutaneous vessels are dilated, often the skin over them is so thin that the veins are traumatized, with the formation of a thrombus which eventually may ulcerate and bleed. In the erect posture, the high venous pressure permits a spurt of considerable force from the ulcerated vein. This is not dangerous unless it is unrecognized, as may be the case if it occurs at night while the patient is in bed. Of course, it may be controlled easily by applying a firm bandage. The late and the most dreaded complication of varicose veins is the so-called varicose ulcer. This usually results from trauma in an area in which the resistance to infection has been lowered by vascular change and replacement fibrosis. The tissues become hypoxic and therefore have lowered resistance to infection and heal poorly when injury occurs from whatever cause.

Examination of the Patient. The symptomatology of the patient with varicose veins does not always give a clear picture of the type of veins to be found. Disfigurement may be due to enlarged venous radicles or to numerous small cutaneous varices in the thigh and the leg. Pain may be due to edema, to chronic phlebitis, or to simple distention of a group of dilated cutaneous vessels within the skin.

For the examination, the patient should stand on a platform from 12 to 14 inches high. The entire leg, up to the groin, is observed. Notation is made of the site and the size and the position of the veins, that is, whether cutaneous or subcutaneous, and observations are recorded as to edema, replacement fibrosis, pigmentation, ulceration, and so forth.

Tests for Varicose Veins

In the case of large varicose veins, tests for valvular incompetence are important, because the subsequent therapy depends upon the results of these tests.

Schwartz, or Percussion, Test (Fig. 25-19). With the patient standing on a stool and the examiner sitting in front of him, one hand is placed along the inner surface of the upper thigh, and the vein in the calf is tapped gently with the fingers. In dilated veins, a wave of fluid may be palpated by the upper hand, and by means of this fluid wave, the vein can be traced to the saphenous opening. This is the most accurate method of locating the course of the long saphenous vein, and it is always used in determining the site of a saphenous ligation. The Schwartz test does not necessarily demonstrate incompetence of the valves of the veins, but in the author's experience, any vein showing a positive Schwartz test has shown incompetence.

Trendelenburg Test (Fig. 25-20). When the course of the saphenous vein in the upper thigh has been located by means of the Schwartz test, the area is marked, or the hand is held in place, and the patient is asked to lie down. Then the leg is elevated to permit the blood to drain by gravity from the dilated vein. Next, pressure is made and maintained over the saphenous opening while the patient stands. If the veins remain empty for from 30 to 35 seconds after the patient is in the erect posture and then fill up rapidly from above when the pressure is removed from the saphenous opening, the inference is that the valves of the long saphenous are incompetent and permit a backflow from the saphenofemoral junction into the saphenous vein. This is said to be a positive Trendelenburg test. If the veins fill up while pressure is maintained over the saphenofemoral junction during the first 30 seconds after the erect posture is assumed, the inference is that blood is passing from the deep to the superficial circulation through the communicating veins, and that, therefore, the valves of the communicating veins are incompetent. If they fill also from above when pressure is removed from the saphenofemoral junction, it indicates that the valves of the communicating veins *and* the long saphenous are incompetent. This is called a doubly positive Trendelenburg test.

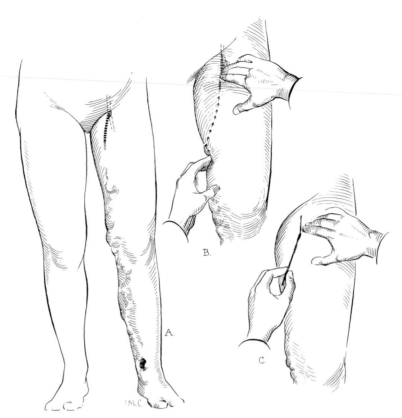

Fig. 25–19. The Schwartz, or percussion, test. (*A*) The patient stands with the weight distributed equally on both feet. (*B*) For the examination of the left leg, the right hand is placed in the region of the groin, and, with the left hand, the vein is percussed gently. A percussion wave, palpated at the upper portion of the saphenous vein, gives the examiner an accurate idea of the location of the vein. (*C*) In preparing the patient for ligation, a colored antiseptic solution is used to mark the course of the vein on the skin.

Perthes' Test. Perthes' test determines the competence of the deep circulation. A tourniquet or a firm bandage is placed below the knee to block backflow in the saphenous vein from above. Walking, or any other motion producing contraction and relaxation of the muscles of the leg, should cause blood to be sucked from the superficial into the deep circulation by way of the communicating veins, so that the veins below the knee are less distended if the deep circulation is competent. This test is somewhat indefinite in its practical applications, and in many cases the patients already have demonstrated competence of the deep circula-

tion by compression of the superficial veins with elastic stockings or bandages. This has proven to be more valuable clinically than Perthes' test in estimating the competency of the deep venous circulation.

Pratt's Test for Incompetent Communicating Branches. To find incompetent communicating branches, Pratt applies elastic bandages from the foot to as high as possible on the thigh, and then a snug tourniquet above the bandage to compress the saphenous vein. With the patient standing, the bandage is removed slowly from above downward. "A sudden protrusion of a collection of veins shows

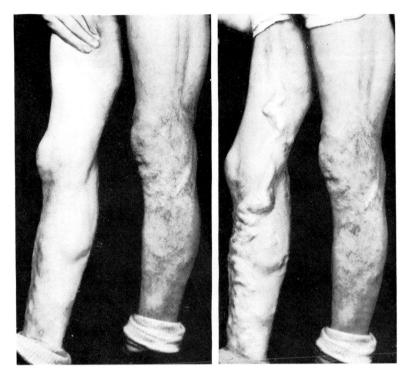

Fig. 25–20. Trendelenburg test. The patient is placed on the examining table, and leg is elevated to empty the blood from the superficial veins. Pressure is made with the hand over the saphenous vein at its uppermost portion, and the patient is asked to stand. (*Left*) The veins are not apparent while the pressure still is maintained. (*Right*) As soon as the hand is removed, the vein fills rapidly from above. This is a positive Trendelenburg test.

the point of incompetence." This site should be marked on the skin. By applying a second elastic bandage from above downward, the upper veins are compressed as the lower bandage is released gradually, and each incompetent perforating branch may be demonstrated accurately and marked, down to the ankle. This method gives the most useful information of any test yet proposed for the demonstration of incompetent communicating veins.

TREATMENT OF VARICOSE VEINS

By high saphenous ligation, multiple ligations at the sites of perforating veins and injection of the remaining veins, most of the offending veins can be removed and the changes caused by venous stasis controlled. It is apparent that new veins may enlarge or injected segments canalize; hence the necessity for any patient under treatment for varicose veins to make biannual visits for injection of veins that appear.

A more complete relief of venous stasis and a more rapid and permanent result can be obtained by removal of the varicose veins by stripping after high saphenous ligation. This operation entails hospitalization for anesthesia and for several days' convalescence, but the patients are ambulatory from the first, and the removal of sutures is an office procedure.

If there is an enlargement of the lesser saphenous vein and if the Trendelenburg test, with the pressure applied at the knee, is positive, ligation of the lesser saphenous vein is performed in the popliteal space. Whatever veins remain 3 to 6 weeks after the time of ligation are treated by injection.

Small, thin-walled varicose veins in young women, enlargement of cutaneous veins, recurrences following ligations and excisions of veins, and veins associated with arthritic pain in the ankle and the knee joint are treated by injection.

Ligation of the Saphenous at the Saphenofemoral Junction. This procedure is indicated in all cases of varicose veins in which studies indicate an incompetence of the valves of the long saphenous vein. The ligation may be performed safely in ambulatory patients; the author has performed many ligations as an ambulatory procedure in an outpatient department. An assistant to hold retractors is, of course, necessary.

In preparation for the operation, the patient is asked to remove his clothes and to put on a gown. The upper thigh and the groin are shaved, and, with the patient standing, the course of the vein is identified by palpation and percussion. The upper portion of the vein and the saphenofemoral junction are marked with a colored solution, such as tincture of Merthiolate, or with an indelible pencil. It is important to localize the vein as well as possible, since this makes dissection easier and lessens the likelihood of causing trauma to fatty tissue in hunting for the vein. The patient is placed on the operating table with the leg turned outward slightly and the knee flexed a little. The field is prepared by washing it several times with 70 percent alcohol.

The incision may be vertical, along the course of the saphenous, or transverse, along the fold of the groin. The line of the incision is infiltrated with 1 percent procaine containing epinephrine. The deeper, subcutaneous, infiltration then is made through the cutaneous anesthetic area. An incision from $1\frac{1}{2}$ to 2 inches long is made through the skin, and small sharp rake retractors are introduced to permit exposure. With a curved hemostat, the fatty tissues are separated to expose the vein, which appears as a bluish structure in the depth of the wound. If the marking before

operation has been accurate, the dissection should come down directly upon the vein. If it is not found at first, it is probably because the incision has been placed too far laterally, and the dissection should be carried into the fatty tissues in the medial part of the wound. The vein is always superficial to the deep fascia of the leg, and it should be found just medial to the pulsation of the femoral artery, which is easily palpable in the wound.

When the vein has been located, the rake retractors are placed more deeply, and, with forceps and curved hemostat, the connective tissue sheath of the vein is divided (Fig. 25-21). It is wise at this time to infiltrate around the vein with the anesthetic solution, because tension upon the perivenous structure sometimes gives slight discomfort. The vein is then lifted up with the forceps, and, with the curved hemostat, it is dissected away from the fatty tissue until 1 cm. or more is entirely free. Two hemostats are placed on the vein, which is divided between them with the scissors. This is one of the most important steps in the operation, because after the vein has been divided, it may be placed on tension with the hemostat and turned backward upon itself, making the dissection much easier and more rapid. The distal end of the vein first is dissected free, the retractors being placed in the lower end of the wound. By pulling down upon the wound and upward upon the vein, a considerable portion of the vein may be exposed. With a curved hemostat placed on the vein as far down as it can be exposed, a ligature is tied about it at the site of the hemostat. A second ligature is usually placed near the first as a safety measure, and then the vein is cut off, leaving a cuff about 0.5 cm. long. The vein tends to retract into the cone-shaped portion of the wound from which it has been dissected.

Retractors are now placed in the upper portion of the wound. The upper portion of the vein, which is in the grasp of the hemostat, is placed on tension, turned up, and dissected free from the underlying connective tissue. As the dissection progresses, numerous branches are met;

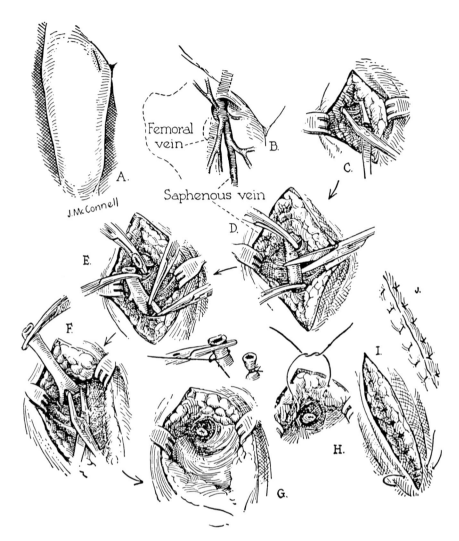

Fig. 25–21. Technique of ligating the saphenous vein at the saphenofemoral junction. (*A*) Line of incision. (*B*) Diagrammatic drawing of the vein and its branches. (*C*) The wound is being dissected bluntly with a curved hemostat. (*D*) The vein has been isolated and clamped with hemostats, so that it may be divided with the scissors. (*E*) The lower portion of the vein is reflected downward; whatever small vessels appear are ligated separately, and the main vein is ligated as far down as possible in the wound. (*F*) Attention then is turned to the upper portion of the vein, which is turned upward and dissected out from below. Each vessel as it appears is clamped and ligated singly. (*G*) The saphenous is ligated doubly at its junction with the femoral vein. (*H*) The ends of the veins are buried with purse-string sutures. (*I*) The wound is closed with interrupted sutures, which encircle the entire base of the wound. (*J*) Mattress sutures of fine wire are used in the skin.

these are not constant by any means, but usually at least two small veins are entering the upper part of the saphenous from the lateral side, two from the medial side, and one from above. As each vein is encountered, it is divided between hemostats and ligated. With adequate retraction and downward or upward traction upon the saphenous, the entire saphenous opening may be exposed, and, after all the vessels entering its upper portion have been ligated, a curved hemostat is placed across the saphenous vein at the saphenofemoral junction, and the vein is ligated doubly at this point with silk. The vein is then divided about 1 cm. below the ligatures.

If the operation has been performed carefully, the wound is completely dry and the ligated ends of the veins have retracted into a cone-shaped area at each extremity of the wound.

Wound closure is effected with fine silk or Dacron sutures, which are placed from just below the skin on one side of the wound to the same point on the other, the fatty tissues being caught at the sides and in the depths of the wound. These sutures, which are placed to obliterate dead space, surround the stumps of the ligated vessel in the upper and the lower angles of the wound. Usually, the upper and the lower sutures are placed and tied first. Both middle sutures are inserted before either one is tied; otherwise it is difficult to place them accurately in the depths of the wound. The skin is closed with mattress sutures of fine alloy steel wire, usually three of them, and occasionally interrupted sutures are inserted between them.

A compression bandage is applied. Usually a 3 x 3 inch dressing folded upon itself is placed directly over the wound, and then a larger dressing is placed over it to form a pyramid of gauze, which is held in place with one or two strips of 1-inch adhesive. The patient then is asked to stand, and further compression is provided with a strip of elastic adhesive. This is started on the upper lateral surface of the thigh and is brought downward just below the groin and round the leg to end upon itself on the medial surface of the thigh. To prevent the ends of the elastic adhesive from rolling, they are secured with two strips of ordinary adhesive.

The patient is allowed to dress at once and is given a prescription for 6 tablets of morphine sulfate, gr. $^1/_6$, with instructions to take one every third hour if needed for relief of pain. He is warned that he will have some pain about an hour after operation, that it will last for about 2 hours, and that after that he can expect some soreness in the area of the wound, which, however, should lessen each day. He is permitted to be about and is urged not to stay in bed. In our experience, patients have less discomfort and there is less likelihood of complication if they are ambulant. The patient may pursue his usual occupation unless it requires strenuous physical exertion, in which case the operation is planned so that he will have 2 or 3 days away from it.

Frequently, there is a thrombosis of the saphenous vein below the site of the ligation, characterized by a painful hard swelling along the course of the vein. The patient is warned of this possibility and is instructed to return if this complication arises; the pain and the disability may be relieved easily by applying a firm elastic adhesive bandage over the vein involved.

If there are no complications, the patient is asked to return 1 week from the day of the operation, when the sutures are removed and a simple dressing is applied, either gauze and adhesive or gauze and elastic adhesive being used. The patient removes this dressing in 4 or 5 days and is asked to return for further observation in 3 weeks, unless pain and soreness in the vein, indicating thrombosis, make an earlier trip necessary.

The complications following this operation are relatively few. Many patients do not take the morphine tablets prescribed, or if they do, it is a matter of only one or two. When they appear for the removal of the sutures, many of the patients volunteer the information that the leg feels much lighter, and that the swelling and the ache have disappeared. Infection has occurred in only 1 of 200 ligations performed as an office procedure. Thrombosis of the vein below the site of ligation occurs in about 1 of every 10 patients.

There have been suggestions in the literature concerning injection at the time of ligation, either into the distal stump of the vein or through a catheter inserted into its distal portion. This produces an excellent thrombosis of the distal segment

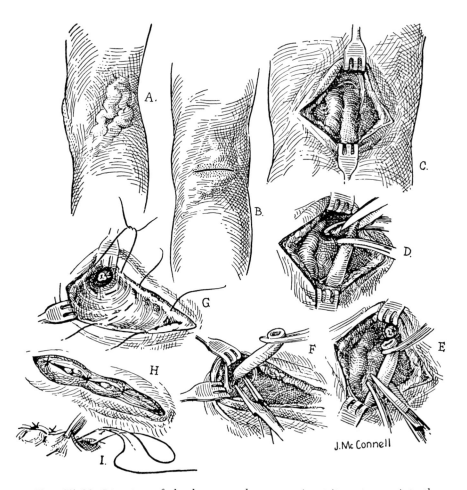

Fig. 25–22. Ligation of the lesser saphenous vein at its entrance into the popliteal vein in the upper popliteal space. Various steps in the operation are shown.

of vein, but the reaction often is quite marked. Many times thrombosis occurs without injection.

Ligation of the Lesser Saphenous Vein at Its Entrance into the Popliteal Vein (Fig. 25-22). When the Trendelenburg test indicates an incompetence of the lesser, or short, saphenous vein, ligation is performed in the upper part of the popliteal space. With the patient standing, the course of the vein is marked on the skin with a colored antiseptic, such as tincture of Merthiolate, and the patient is placed on the operating table in the prone position. The posterior lower thigh and the area of the knee are shaved. Usually, the vein enters the popliteal vein a little

above the highest level at which it can be palpated, because it lies below the fascia at this point. After a transverse infiltration into the skin in the popliteal space, a transverse incision is made, and sharp rake retractors are placed to expose the deep fascia. This is separated with a blunt hemostat after it has been infiltrated with procaine solution. The vein is exposed and divided between hemostats. After the wound has been closed, and with the patient standing, a pressure dressing is applied. The same postoperative instructions are given as are given after ligations at the saphenofemoral junction.

Ligation in the Presence of Ulcers. The ligation of veins is not contraindicated in the presence of varicose ulcers; rather, it is indicated. The ulcer may be treated with compression at the same time that the vein is ligated.

Ligation of Incompetent Communicating Vessels. When the Trendelenburg test is doubly positive, or when there is other evidence of incompetency of communicating veins, it is necessary to ligate the incompetent communicating veins to obtain a successful result. This may be performed wherever the vein is located in the calf or in the thigh.

After the site of operation has been prepared, a local anesthetic is infiltrated in the line of the vein. The skin is incised, and, with sharp retraction, the superficial vein is exposed at its junction with the communicating vein. Usually, it is possible to dissect it free, either above or below the communicating branch. It is divided between hemostats, and the upper and the lower stumps are ligated. When this has been accomplished, the dissected portion of the vein is still attached to the communicating vein, which perforates the deep fascia. This vein may be dissected as far as the deep fascia and ligated at the point at which it perforates this structure. Wound closure with mattress sutures of fine alloy steel wire completes the operation.

Injection Treatment of Varicose Veins

Although preliminary ligation is well recognized as the method of choice in the treatment of varicose veins with incompetence of the valves of the long saphenous vein, many varicosities still remain for which injection treatment is indicated.

Indications for Injection. Chief of these are (1) thin-walled varicose veins in young women without evident changes in the long saphenous vein in the thigh; (2) painful or disfiguring groups of small cutaneous varicosities that appear in the calf and the thigh; (3) recurrent varicose veins that have developed following ligation or the excision, or stripping, operation; (4) varicose veins associated with arthritic pain in the ankle and the knee joint; and (5) the veins that still remain in

the calf following primary high saphenous ligation.

Contraindications to Injection. The chief contraindication of the injection of varicose veins is a recent thrombosis or phlebitis. Thrombophlebitis is a contraindication when it has occurred in the deep veins, because time must elapse before it can be determined whether the varicose veins are compensatory dilatations or true varicosities. There is also the danger that the reaction induced by the injection may reactivate a latent infection. Therefore, extreme care must be taken in injecting the veins of patients who give a history of a previous thrombophlebitis.

Patients with varicosities of the upper thigh and the lower abdomen have usually had a previous partial or complete block of the veins of the pelvis. In such cases, the treatment of varicose veins should be approached with extreme caution because of the fact that the dilated veins frequently are compensatory venous channels.

Varicose veins associated with large uterine fibroids or with other pelvic tumors are best treated conservatively, by the use of supportive bandages or stockings, until the pelvic pathology has been corrected.

Solutions for the Injection of Varicose Veins. Glucose, 50 percent, is an excellent and safe solution for sclerosing tiny cutaneous veins. In our experience, its escape into the perivenous tissues never has caused a slough. The amount injected may be from 1 to 10 ml.

Sodium chloride, 30 percent, and glucose, 50 percent, in equal parts give excellent results in sclerosing the larger varicose veins. From 5 to 10 ml. are used, and injection into the vein should be made very carefully because the escape of the fluid into the perivenous tissues may result in a slough. The injection of this solution is associated with a crampy pain in the part and a spasm of the vein. The cramp lasts from 3 to 5 minutes, and it may extend from the foot to the thigh. This solution is especially valuable for the injection of large varices because of the large amount of solution that may be injected, and it is used in all patients who have pains in the region of the ankle and the knee joints associated with varicose veins.

Various solutions of salts of fatty acids have been found to be extremely valuable in the injection treatment of varicose veins. Perhaps the one that is used most widely is sodium morrhuate, but there are others, such as monoethanolamine morrhuate, monoethanolamine oleate, Sotradecol, and sodium psylliate (Sylnasol), which produce almost the same sclerosing effect. These solutions are injected in amounts of 1 to 5 ml., depending upon the size of the vein. No more than 5 ml. is injected at one time, although this amount may be divided into smaller injections in several areas. These solutions produce excellent thrombosis, with a moderate reaction at the site of injection. They cause no crampy pain at the time of the injection, although there is some discomfort in the region of the vein almost immediately following injection. They produce a definite perivenous reaction if the injected fluid escapes into the surrounding tissues. This is more in the nature of an acute inflammation or cellulitis of the fatty tissues rather than the sloughing that is seen following escape of sodium chloride or quinine and urethane. An occasional patient exhibits an allergic reaction following the injection of sodium morrhuate solution. It is for this reason that the more purified salts of fatty acids, such as monoethanolamine morrhuate, are sometimes preferable. Their sclerosing effects are as good as those of sidium morrhuate.

Technique of Injection. It is easier to find and inject the veins if the patient's legs are dependent. Therefore, the patients stands, or sits upon a table with his foot on the surgeon's knee. If the veins are thin walled and not large, there is no particular value in emptying them before injection. A firm pad of gauze is placed over each injection site and is held in place with 2 strips of ½-inch adhesive.

If the vein is large and thick walled, the sclerosing effect is enhanced by emptying it before injection. The needle is introduced into the vein with the leg in the dependent position. The syringe then is held against the leg, and the patient is asked to lie down and elevate the extremity. In this way, the vein is emptied, and a rubber-tube tourniquet is then placed about the knee or the thigh, depending upon the site of injection. The leg is returned to the horizontal position on the table, and the injection is made into the empty vein. The tourniquet holds the solution in the area of injection for a time and so may increase the amount of sclerosis produced.

It is perhaps unnecessary to say that the injection should not be made until blood is aspirated into the syringe, indicating that the needle tip is in the vein. The injection should be made slowly, and the site of the needle tip should be watched carefully to note the appearance of fluid escaping into the tissues. If there is any question as to whether or not all the fluid is entering the vein, the injection should be stopped at once. *It is a valuable practice to aspirate once or twice during the injection* to make sure that the needle is placed properly within the vein.

After the injection, the patient is asked to remain recumbent for at least 5 minutes. If the leg is kept in the horizontal position, the solution is believed to remain somewhat longer in the segment of vein injected; thus its sclerosing effect is probably enhanced. No bandage other than the adhesive necessary to hold the pad over the injection site is applied. This is removed by the patient the next day.

The injections are made at weekly intervals unless the reaction following the previous treatment is quite marked, in which case the injection is delayed until the reaction has subsided. Often it is possible to inject 2 or 3 sites at the same visit, although it is wise to proceed cautiously and to reinject rather than to overinject.

Effects of Injection Therapy upon Varicose Veins. The purpose of the injection treatment of varicose veins is to set up an inflammatory reaction within the vein lumen. This is accomplished by producing a chemical irritation of the intima of the vein, which in turn leads to a throm-

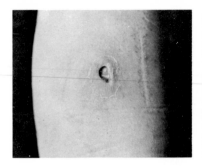 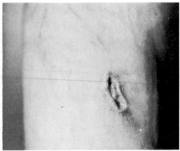

Fig. 25–23. Examples of injection ulcers. Both were treated by excision and primary suture in ambulatory patients.

bosis due to the destruction of the intimal lining of the vessel. The thrombosis occurs only at the site of the intimal destruction, but there is an intravascular clot that extends in both directions from this primary thrombus. As time goes on, the thrombus and the clots become organized, the result being a closure of the venous radicle. If there is a hydrostatic pressure above the area of thrombosis, the thrombus may become canalized, and there may be a reappearance of the varicosity at some later date.

Associated with the thrombosis is a more or less perivenous reaction, characterized by redness, swelling, and tenderness along the course of the vein and in the perivenous areolar tissue. Often this reaction extends throughout the course of the vein and is sufficient to cause the patient considerable discomfort. If a firm elastic adhesive bandage is applied, not only are the patient's symptoms relieved almost completely and immediately, but there is a rapid subsidence of the perivenous inflammation.

In some cases, as the perivenous inflammation subsides, with the purplish discoloration appears along the course of the vein. If left alone, this area often ulcerates, with the escape of a good bit of partially liquefied clotted blood. This relieves the discomfort, and healing takes place. The process may be shortened and the possibility of ulceration avoided by aspirating this partially clotted blood from the portion of the vein involved. If a needle of fair size is inserted into the

discolored portion of the vein, a considerable amount of the material often may be drawn into the syringe. At other times, the blood is so thick that it will not pass through the small bore of the needle; in such cases, the needle is withdrawn, and gentle pressure is made along the course of the vein. The dark semiclotted blood will usually pass through the hole made by the needle, and if a little time is spent in expressing this material, the discomfort and the pain along the vein disappear. A pressure dressing with elastic adhesive is usually maintained until all symptoms are gone.

The most disturbing complication following the injection treatment of varicose veins is the so-called injection ulcer. Usually, this is due to faulty technique, and it especially follows injections of sodium chloride solution in which some of the fluid is permitted to escape into the soft tissues around the vein. The result is a stinging pain in the area, even at the time of the injection, and, as time goes on, there is a definite cellulitis, with a secondary necrosis of the skin over the area and the formation of a deep ulcer with a necrotic base (Fig. 25-23). The ulcers usually are very painful, and, because the injected solution has sclerosed all vessels in the vicinity, healing is extremely slow. We have found that the method of treatment that results in the most rapid healing in such cases is complete excision of the ulcer area. This may be performed under local anesthesia, the ulcer and the surrounding adipose tissue being excised and the wound closed with interrupted sutures. If excision is not permitted or is not advisable, the ulcer can be expected to heal eventually, but it may take several weeks or longer.

Varicose Veins in Pregnancy

Pressure of the enlarging uterus on the pelvic veins, increase in intra-abdominal tension, and increase of circulation in the pelvis, all are probably factors in the well-known association of pregnancy with varicose veins. In many cases, pain and discomfort due to the enlarged veins produce outstanding disability in the latter months of pregnancy. Attempts at relief by the use of elastic stockings and bandages are rarely more than partially successful, and in severe cases the patient may hardly be able to be on her feet at all. Leotardlike elastic supports are now available and provide probably the best support of any elastic garment as yet used. These waist-high elastic leotards are of great value when the varicosities extend into the upper thigh, the groin, and the vulva.

Over the years, a general attitude against the treatment of varicose veins during pregnancy has developed. This has meant that many women have endured unnecessarily the discomfort and the disability of varices with each pregnancy. Some physicians think it is useless to treat varicose veins before the childbearing period is over because of the possibility of the recurrence of varices with each pregnancy.

Our experience has proven the truth of Stalker's statement that "varicose veins should be treated as though the pregnancy were not present." Active treatment, whether by ligation, stripping, or injection, is safe, and it affords rapid and almost complete relief of symptoms. Varicose veins are treated best in the earlier months of pregnancy, but they can be treated safely even during the seventh or the eighth month if the symptoms warrant it. It should be understood that treatment of varices during pregnancy is not for cosmetic purposes. The veins decrease in size and in extent very remarkably after delivery, so that in the puerperium active therapy should be withheld for about 3 months to permit a more accurate evaluation.

STASIS ULCERS OF THE LEG

Ulcerations of the lower leg that fail to heal with the usual therapeutic measures often are termed varicose ulcers. This term implies that venous stasis associated with varicose veins is the basic alteration. This assumption must be modified by the facts. All stasis ulcers of the legs cannot be classified in one group, and an understanding of the underlying pathology is necessary for a logical diagnosis and plan of treatment.

Types of Stasis Ulcers

Varicose Ulcers. In this type of ulcer, the patient's history is quite typical. There are large varicose veins in the leg for some time, with chronic edema of the ankle. Gradually, replacement fibrosis and pigmentation of the skin appear, so that the lower leg, especially on the medial side, becomes hard and discolored and loses most of the subcutaneous areolar tissue. Then some minor trauma produces a break in the skin; secondary infection follows, and the tissues, having a poor resistance to infection, permit an extension of the infective process and the gradual formation of an ulcer. This is indolent, slightly painful, and, in spite of various ointments and powders, continues to enlarge rather than to close (Fig. 25-24, *right*).

Postphlebitic Ulcers. There is a history of previous phlebitis, and the leg is often fat and without marked varicosities. Chronic edema is present in the lower part of the leg. Without any apparent cause, a painful reddened area of low-grade cellulitis develops above the malleolus (Fig. 25-25). The pain is characterized by a burning sensation, which often is worse at night.

As time goes on, the inflammation may subside, leaving an area of fibrosis and

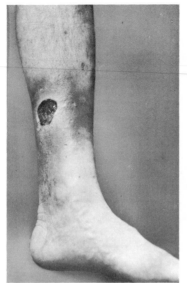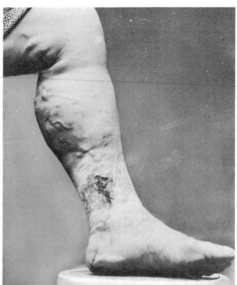

Fig. 25–24. Leg ulcers. (*Left*) Postphlebitic ulcer. Note marked fibrosis and pigmentation of area round the ulcer. (*Right*) Varicose ulcer in usual location.

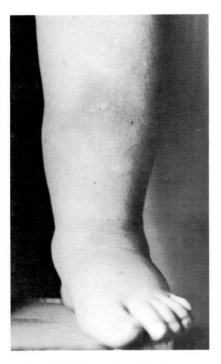

Fig. 25–25. Thrombophlebitic edema with area of painful cellulitis above the ankle.

induration (Fig. 25-26). Recurrence of the inflammatory plaque is seen with each episode of prolonged edema. Ulceration may occur as a result of blistering at the area of localized cellulitis or following minor abrasions or contusions. The surrounding tissues become indurated, and the ulcer may assume a punched-out appearance.

In many of these patients there is no evidence at all of varicose veins; in others, varicose veins are present that at first may have been compensatory dilatations as a result of a deep venous block. As canalization of the thrombi in the deep veins takes place, the enlarged superficial veins remain as varicosities and contribute to the venous stasis.

Between these two commonly seen types of ulcers are many variations.

TREATMENT OF STASIS ULCERS

The aim in the treatment of stasis ulcers is to prevent edema. This may be accomplished in various ways. If the patient can be put to bed with the leg elevated, the

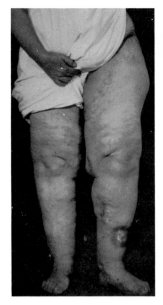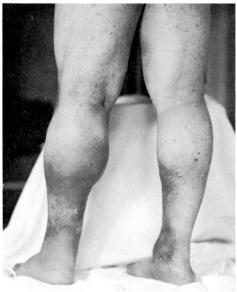

Fig. 25-26. (*Left*) Typical plaquelike area of pigmentation and fibrosis left after the acute phase of the thrombophlebitic process has subsided. (*Right*) Late stage of thrombophlebitic edema, in which there is practically complete loss of subcutaneous fatty tissue, with resulting fibrosis and constriction of the legs above the ankle.

edema will subside and the ulcers will heal. To ligate the varicose veins that produce edema by causing venous stasis will greatly hasten the healing of ulcers, and treatment of varicose veins is not contraindicated in the presence of ulcers. Various types of compression and supporting bandages may be employed in ambulatory patients, and these may also be applied after injecting varicose veins. They prevent venous stasis by obliterating the superficial veins by pressure.

Unna's Paste Boot (Fig. 25-27). In our experience, this has proven to be the most

serviceable supporting dressing. It provides constant compression and protection, permitting rapid subsidence of the edema. Although Unna's paste may be produced in the office,* commercial preparations now are available and are much simpler to handle.

If the Unna's paste preparation is used, the gelatin mixture is warmed in a double boiler until it liquefies enough to be applied with a brush. The entire leg and the dorsum of the foot to the toes are painted, and usually an extra pad of gauze impregnated with gelatin is placed over the ulcer. A gauze bandage is then applied to the leg over the gelatin. This is more satisfactory if it is started along the side of the foot, so that the lowermost turn covers the lowermost portion of the foot. It is carried round the foot and the ankle in figure-of-eight turns until the entire foot and ankle are covered with 1 or 2 layers of gauze. Then it is carried round the leg in circular turns so long as the bandage lies flat. When the conical portion of the leg

---

*Unna's gelatin mixture is prepared in a double boiler as follows:

Gelatin	200 g.
Zinc oxide powder	100 g.
Glycerin	400 cc.
Hot water	375 cc.

Dissolve the gelatin in the hot water. Mix the glycerin and the zinc oxide powder until smooth, then add to the dissolved gelatin. Cook in the double boiler for one half hour. This makes enough paste for 4 or 5 boots.

does not permit circular turns, the gauze is carried upward in spiral turns to the uppermost part of the paste application. There it is reversed loosely and brought down in spiral turns to meet the completed portion of the bandage. Then follow a series of spirals of the leg, reverse turns being made at the top, until the

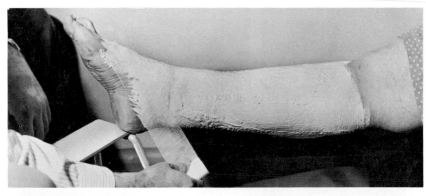

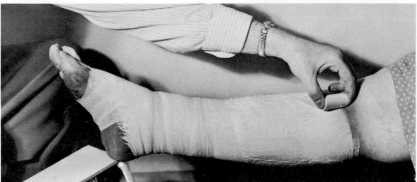

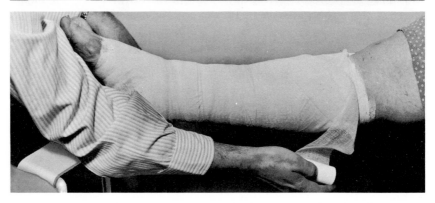

Fig. 25-27. Unna's past boot. (*Top*) The leg is painted with gelatin paste from the toes to the knee. The bandage is started along the lateral side of the foot; 2-inch bandage is used for the foot-and-ankle portion of the boot. (*Center*) After covering the foot and the ankle, the bandage is continued in a circular manner until it must ascend in a spiral turn in order to lie flat on the part. Three-inch bandage now is substituted for the 2-inch bandage to cover the upper part of the leg. (*Bottom*) Reverse turns are made only at the upper part of the dressing.

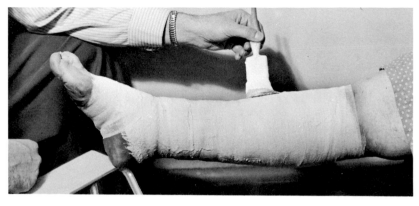

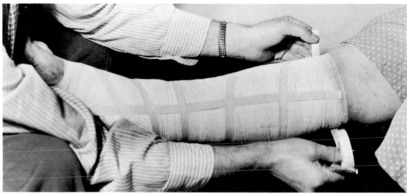

Fig. 25–27 (*cont.*). (*Top*) After the layer of gelatin and bandage has been applied, the entire bandage is painted again with the gelatin mixture. (*Bottom*) The bandage is completed with one longitudinal ¹/₂-inch strip of adhesive on each side, held in place with circular turns.

entire leg is covered with 2 layers of gauze. The bandage is completed with 1 or 2 circular turns at the top. No reverse turns are made on any part of the leg except at the top of the bandage, and each layer must be pulled snug and made to lie absolutely flat upon the part. Care in this particular will prevent pressure due to tight ridges in the bandages. As a rule, 2-inch gauze bandage is most satisfactory for covering the foot and the ankle and for small legs. For large legs, it is better to use a 3-inch gauze bandage for the upper portion of the boot.

After the first layer of paste and gauze has been applied, the leg is painted again with the liquid gelatin, the meshes of the gauze being impregnated generously. A second layer of gauze is applied over the paste exactly as was the first. When there is much discharge, a piece of waxed paper

or Saran Wrap may be incorporated over the ulcer between the first and the second layers of the boot. This prevents subsequent soiling of the clothes. In many cases in which the ulcer is deep, further elastic pressure may be obtained by incorporating a thin layer of sponge rubber over the ulcer between the first and the second layers of bandage.

In using the commercial preparation the procedure is the same except, of course, no painting of the paste on the leg is necessary since the Unna's paste is already incorporated into the bandage.

After the bandage has been completed, ¹/₂-inch adhesive is applied. Longitudinal strips on each side, from the top of the bandage down under the foot and over the dorsum, hold the layers of gauze together, and the whole is anchored by circular turns of adhesive applied about 2 inches apart from the foot to the knee. In performing these circular turns, the middle of a strip of adhesive is applied to the back of the leg, then each end is brought forward round the leg. At the conical part of the leg, the ends must be brought slightly upward, toward the knee, if the adhesive strip is to lie flat on the part.

The frequency of changing the gelatin boot varies with the patient, the amount of edema of the leg, and the amount of secretion from the ulcer. If the boot is applied when there is considerable edema, it should be changed in a week, or even sooner, because as the edema goes down under the boot, a new boot giving more compression should be applied. If there is no edema when the boot is put on, and there is no marked secretion from the ulcer, the boot may be allowed to remain in place for 3 to 4 weeks to advantage. One patient, who failed to keep an appointment, wore her boot for 3 months; when it was removed, the ulcer, which had been present for some years, was healed entirely. As a rule, because the secretion from the ulcer sometimes produces maceration of the surrounding tissues, boots should be changed every 2 or 3 weeks. If secretion has produced maceration and superficial ulceration of the skin round the ulcer, the area should be protected with zinc oxide ointment before a new boot is applied, and the boot should be changed as often as once a week until the secretion decreases.

The support afforded by a gelatin boot, or of a well-fitted elastic stocking, should be continued for at least 4 to 6 weeks after the ulcer has healed. To remove this support too soon often results in a recurrence of the ulcer.

Other Types of Supportive Bandages and Stockings. In the treatment of leg ulcers, elastic bandages do not give the compression that can be obtained from a gelatin boot. Nevertheless, there may be instances in which gelatin is not available or other reasons why a boot cannot be applied. In such cases, elastic bandages or elastic adhesive bandages may be substituted. Several types are available; the 3-inch width is probably the most serviceable.

After the ulcer has healed, elastic bandages or stockings may often be substituted for the gelatin boot. This provides continued support for a time and permits the patient to bathe. The lightweight Lastex type of stocking is recommended; it is not nearly as hot or unsightly as the heavier-weave elastic stockings, and it gives equal support. The best stocking is the custom-fit, two-way stretch stocking made by the Jobst Institute of Toledo, Ohio. This stocking is made to measurement to provide an even pressure of 40 mm. Hg. It is worn from toes to knee.

Local Applications to the Ulcer. It should be understood from the beginning that the basic problems in stasis ulcer are venous stasis and associated edema, and that treatment of these two disturbances is essential to the healing of the ulcer; whatever local applications are made to the leg and/or the ulcer are of secondary importance.

In the belief that infection is a prominent factor in leg ulcer, various types of local anti-infectious applications have been made. Robinson has applied powdered antibiotics to the ulcers. He thought that chloramphenicol, bacitracin, and bacitracin-polymyxin B sulfate gave the best results. The antibiotic powders applied to the ulcer formed a crust that was not removed. Healing took place under the crust. Rutter has used various antibiotics, and he recommends especially a polymyxin ointment for resistant infections with *Pseudomonas pyocyaneus (aeruginosa)*, to be suspected in sluggish and unresponsive ulcers.

Spier and Cliffton recommend for necrotic ulcers local débridement with plasminogen (a fibrinolytic enzyme) to which has been added streptokinase-streptodornase (Varidase) solution. After the ulcer has been cleaned up, hyaluronidase and bacitracin or Terramycin are applied to control infection and cellulitis and to give rapid relief of pain. As soon as redness and edema have subsided, hyaluronidase is used alone in a water-soluble methylcellulose base (Methocel).

The number of substances recommended for application to the ulcer site is proof that the ideal has not yet been found. Gentian violet, 3 percent solution, is used for its bacteriostatic effect. It is probable that the supporting bandage is the important factor in the success of any of these local treatments. Without relief of venous stasis, none of them succeeds.

STASIS DERMATITIS

Many patients with edema of the lower leg develop a scaling which often develops into a weeping, crusting dermatitis associated with marked itching. This group of symptoms often is called a stasis dermatitis, although varicose veins may not be a prominent feature when the patient is examined. This change seems to be the result of edema, and whatever measures are used to relieve the edema relieve also the stasis dermatitis.

If varicose veins are present, they should be treated, but the essential therapy is some form of dressing that supports the lower leg. A gelatin boot is probably the most effective form of support, but in many cases, because of the marked itching and the secretion, a boot cannot be used as the primary dressing.

The itching and redness often respond very rapidly to applications of corticosteroids. These are available in forms of ointments or creams. The author prefers that the creams be applied generously, covered with Saran Wrap, and held in place with elastic bandage. This may be changed daily or every other day. When the weeping stops, the Saran Wrap may not be necessary, but the cream may be applied morning and night if the itching persists.

Stasis dermatitis usually clears up rather slowly, even with adequate supportive dressings, and these should be maintained for from 4 to 6 weeks after all the scaling has cleared up to permit the skin to return to its normal texture.

AMBULATORY TREATMENT OF THROMBOPHLEBITIS OF THE SUPERFICIAL VEINS

Thrombophlebitis of superficial veins may occur as the result of trauma, or it may develop spontaneously as the result of a latent infection. The portion of the vein involved is a firm, hard, painful cord, often surrounded by a considerable area of tender edematous fat. The skin overlying the vein may also be tender and red. In some patients, there is no systemic reaction, but in others there is a temperature elevation of considerable degree. Most patients are treated by bed rest, elevation, and the use of hot packs, and the process subsides gradually in from 2 to 3 weeks.

A much more satisfactory and immediate therapy is available. If a firm elastic adhesive bandage is applied to the leg, the entire painful process will subside within 24 to 48 hours. The elastic adhesive is applied snugly, and, as a rule, it is begun at the foot and carried up the leg in spiral fashion to the groin, two 3-inch bandages being used. It is wise to insert a 4 x 8 inch gauze compress at the back of the knee under the bandage; otherwise, pinching of the skin in this area may cause discomfort.

By this method of therapy, the patient's fever subsides within 24 hours, and the pain and the discomfort associated with thrombophlebitis are relieved almost immediately. The patient may be ambulatory throughout the entire period of treatment. From wide experience in treating thrombophlebitis of superficial veins in this manner, the author has never seen a case in which there was even a suggestion of embolism.

The bandage is worn for from 2 to 3 weeks and then removed, and if the area is still tender on palpation, a new one is applied. In a few cases in which the patient's skin does not tolerate the elastic adhesive bandage, a gelatin boot may be substituted.

A second method of treatment is by ligation and division of the vein above the area of phlebitis. This is performed best at the saphenofemoral junction, but ligation immediately above the area of thrombosis produces equally good results so far as relief of pain and prevention of embolism are concerned. Probably the best treatment is a combination of the two methods, that is, ligation followed by the application of a snug elastic or elastic adhesive bandage. The patient must be up and about throughout his period of treatment; the worst thing he can do is to stay in bed with the foot elevated. This slows the blood flow and favors thrombus propagation and embolism.

With the almost complete relief of symptoms obtained by these methods of treatment, other methods, such as lumbar sympathetic block, have not been found necessary.

Phlebitis and thrombosis of the deep veins of the leg in the acute stage is a disease entity not frequently encountered in ambulatory patients, and the treatment must be carried out in the hospital.

REFERENCES

Varicose Veins

Adams, J. C.: Etiological factors in varicose veins of the lower extremities. Surg., Gynec. Obstet., *69*:717, 1939.

Beesley, W. H., and Fegan, W. G.: An investigation into the localization of incompetent perforating veins. Brit. J. Surg., *57*:30, 1970.

Biegeleisen, H. I.: End results of surgery for varicose veins. New York J. Med., *60*:2387, 1960.

Carter, B. N., II, and Johns, T. N. P.: Recurrent varicose veins: anatomical and physiological observations. Ann. Surg., *159*:1017, 1964.

Cotton, L. T.: The treatment of varicose veins. Practitioner, *206*:352, 1971.

Dodd, H.: The Pathology and Surgery of the Veins of the Lower Limb. London, E. & S. Livingston, 1956.

Edwards, E. A.: Thrombophlebitis of varicose veins. Surg., Gynec. Obstet., *66*:226, 1938.

Edwards, J. E., and Edwards, E. A.: The saphenous valves in varicose veins. Am. Heart J., *19*:338, 1940.

Fegan, W. G.: The complications of compression sclerotherapy. Practitioner, *207*:797, 1971.

Haeger, K.: Venous and Lymphatic Disorders of the leg. Philadelphia, J. B. Lippincott, 1966.

Halliday, P.: The place of subfacial ligation of perforating veins in the treatment of post-phlebitic syndrome. Brit. J. Surg., *58*:104, 1971.

Heller, R. E.: The pathological physiology of varicose veins. Surg., Gynec. Obstet., *71*:566, 1940.

Len, J. J.: The modern conception of therapy of varicose veins. Angiology, *15*:371, 1964.

Linn, B. S.: Subfascial ligation of incompetent perforating veins: a rational therapy to prevent recurrence of venous stasis ulcers. Southern Med. J., *65*:1063, 1972.

Ludbrook, J.: Obesity and varicose veins. Surg., Gynec. Obstet., *118*:834, 1964.

Mahorner, H. R., and Ochsner, A.: The modern treatment of varicose veins as indicated by the comparative tourniquet test. Ann. Surg., *107*:927, 1938.

Moosman, D. A., and Hartwell, S. W.: The surgical significance of the subfascial course of the lesser saphenous vein. Surg., Gynec. Obstet., *118*:761, 1964.

Nabatoff, R. A.: The current status of therapy for varicose veins. Curr. Med. Dig., Oct., 1961.

Nabatoff, R. A., and Pincus, J. A.: Management of varicose veins during pregnancy. Obstet. Gynec., *36*:928, 1970.

Pattisson, P. H., and Tretbar, L. L.: The injection treatment of varicose veins: a follow-up study of 264 patients. Vasc. Surg., *5*:1, 1971.

Pratt, G. H.: Test for incompetent communicating branches in surgical treatment of varicose veins. JAMA, *117*:100, 1941.

————: Results of surgical treatment of varicose veins. JAMA, *112*:797, 1943.

Rhodes, D. J., and Hadfield, G. J.: Treatment of varicose veins by injection and compression. Practitioner, *208*:809, 1972.

Stalker, L. K.: The management of varicose veins and their related problems during pregnancy. New York J. Med., *52*:729, 1952.

Veal, J. R., and Van Werden, B. deK.: The physiologic basis for ligation of the great saphenous vein in the treatment of varicose veins. Am. J. Surg., *40*:426, 1938.

Weddell, J. M.: A comparison of two methods in the treatment of varicose veins. Brit. J. Prev. Soc. Med., *24*:65, 1970.

Wood, J. E.: The Veins: Normal and Abnormal functions. Boston, Little, Brown & Co., 1965.

Phlebitis

Cockett, F. B.: The post-phlebitic syndrome. Proc. Roy. Soc. Med., *63*:131, 1970.

Linton, R. R.: The post-thrombotic ulceration of the lower extremity; its etiology and surgical treatment. Ann. Surg., *138*:415, 1953.

Williams, R. D., and Zollinger, R. W.: Surgical treatment of superficial thrombophlebitis. Surg., Gynec. Obstet., *118*:745, 1964.

Leg Ulcers

Besznyak, I., Nemes, A., and Sebesteny, M.: The use of hyperbaric oxygen in the treatment of experimental hypoxaemic skin ulcers of the limb. Acta Chir. Acad. Sci. Hung., *11*:15, 1970.

Chilvers, A. S., and Freeman, G. K.: Outpatient skin grafting of venous ulcers. Lancet, *2*:1087, 1969.

Dale, W. A., and Foster, J. H.: Leg ulcers—comprehensive plan of diagnosis and management. Med. Sci., 56, July, 1964.

Fegan, W. G.: Treatment of varicose ulceration. Lancet, *1*:780, 1970.

Henry, M. E., Fegan, W. G., and Pegum, J. M.: Five-year survey of the treatment of varicose ulcers. Brit. Med. J., *2*:493, 1971.

Hines, E. A.: How to treat chornic leg ulcer. Consultant, 11, Sept., 1964.

Husni, E. A., and Goyette, E. M.: Elastic compression of the lower limbs: merits and hazards. Am. Heart J., *82*:132, 1971.

Lofgren, K. A., and Lofgren, E. P.: Extensive ulcerations in the postphlebitic leg. Surg. Clin. N. Am., *49*:1033, 1969.

Milberg, I. L., and Tolmach, J. A.: Treatment of chronic leg ulcers with absorbable gelatin sponge (Gelfoam) powder. JAMA, *155*:1219, 1954.

Myers, H. L.: Further observations of a modified elastic support for stasis and stasis ulcers of the legs. Angiology, *21*:700, 1970.

Recek, C.: A critical appraisal of the role of ankle perforators for the genesis of venous ulcers in the lower leg. J. Cardiovasc. Surg. (Torino) *12*:45, 1971.

Robinson, H. M., Sr.: A medical treatment for stasis ulcers. JAMA, *157*:27, 1955.

Robnett, A. H.: Chronic ulcers of the leg of venous origin. Cleveland Clin. Quart., *22*:309, 1955.

Rutter, A. G.: Chronic ulcer of the leg in young subjects. Surg., Gynec. Obstet., *98*:291, 1954.

Silver, D., Gleysteen, J. J., Rhodes, G. R., Georgiade, N. G., and Anlyan, W. G.: Surgical treatment of the refractory postphlebitic ulcer. Arch. Surg., *103*:554, 1971.

Spier, I. R., antl Cliffton, E. E.: Local ambulatory treatment of chronic leg ulcers with hyaluronidase, plasminogen, and antibiotics. Surg., Gynec. Obstet., *98*:667, 1954.

Zimmerman, L. M., and Faller, A.: Etiology and treatment of ulcers of the leg. Surg., Gynec. Obstet., *70*:792, 1940.

Sprains and Ligament and Muscle Injuries

Arner, O., and Lindholm, A.: What is tennis leg? Acta Chir. Scand., *116*:73, 1958.

Böhler, L.: The Treatment of Fractures. ed. 4. Baltimore, Wm. Wood, 1935.

Crenshaw, A. H.: Campbell's Operative Orthopaedics. St. Louis, C. V. Mosby, 1963.

Cole, J. P.: A study of Osgood-Schlatter disease. Surg., Gynec. Obstet., *65*:55, 1937.

Fahrni, W. H.: Treatment of tennis leg. Canad. J. Surg., 7:157, 1964.

Ferguson, L. K., and Thompson, W. D.: Internal derangements of the knee joint. Ann. Surg., *112*:454, 1940.

Leriche, R.: De l'entorse et de la luxation du genou. J. Chir., *54*:593, 1939.

Lewin, P.: Manipulative maneuvers of the knee for replacing displaced meniscuses. JAMA, *156*:1105, 1954.

Mennell, J. McM.: Joint Pain. Boston, Little, Brown & Co., 1964.

O'Donoghue, D. H.: Treatment of Injuries to Athletes. Philadelphia, W. B. Saunders, 1962.

Rix, R. R.: Accuracy in the diagnosis of torn meniscus in the knee. JAMA, *180*:140, 1962.

Salter, R. B.: Textbook of Disorders and Injuries of the Musculoskeletal System. Baltimore, Williams & Wilkins, 1970.

Schmier, A. A.: Fascial herniae of both lower extremities; injection with sodium morrhuate. JAMA, *109*:28, 1937.

Schutz, N., Dohrmann, R., and Flemming, G.: Die myositis ossificans traumatica: an beitrag zur differential diagnose gegenüber dem osteo-genen sarkom. Chirurg, *32*:97, 1961.

Truslow, W.: Simplified support for knee injuries. JAMA, *110*:285, 1938.

25

Lower Limb

Part II—Fractures

Andrew C. Ruoff, M.D.

FRACTURES OF THE PATELLA

ANATOMY

The patella is an ovoid sesamoid bone which is an integral part of the quadriceps tendon. Anteriorly, it is covered by the fibers of the tendon; posteriorly, its upper portion is covered by articular cartilage. Strong expansions of the quadricep-stendon lie to each side. The portion of the tendon that extends from the patella to the tibial tubercle is called the patellar ligament.

ETIOLOGY

The bone may be fractured by direct violence, such as a fall or a blow on the knee, or indirectly by violent abrupt contraction of the extensor muscles, as in stumbling or in falling on the feet with the knees semi-flexed. The fracture line is likely to be stellate when due to direct violence and transverse when due to muscular action. The amount of separation of the fragments depends on the extent to which the lateral expansions of the quadriceps tendon are torn. The fracture line may be a simple fissure 1 or 2 mm. wide (Fig. 25-28, *left*), or there may be separation of 1 cm. or more, accompanied by extensive lacerations of the lateral expansions of the quadriceps tendon and a wide opening of the knee joint (Fig. 25-28, *right*). The proximal fragment is drawn

upward by the extensor muscles. There may be an infolding of torn portions of the tendon, or, after comminuted fractures, loose fragments may fall into the joint. There is always hemorrhage into the joint.

DIAGNOSIS

Following a fall or a blow, there is severe pain at the knee, rapid swelling, and inability to extend the knee and to stand. Acute localized tenderness is present over the fracture line, and there may be palpable separation of the fragments. The knee joint usually is distended by blood.

Acute traumatic prepatellar bursitis may simulate fracture, but the swelling is localized anterior to the patella. A traumatized villus in the floor of the bursa may be acutely tender.

TREATMENT

The knee should be protected with a posterior splint, applied with the knee in extension, and ice should be applied to the area of tenderness. Roentgenograms should be obtained.

Treatment of Simple Fissure Fractures. When the fracture is a simple or stellate fissure in the bone, the splint, a pressure dressing, rest, and elevation may be continued until the swelling has subsided. Aspiration may be repeated as nec-

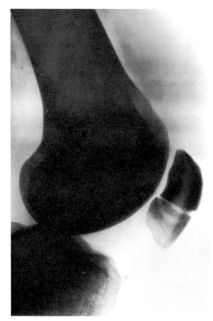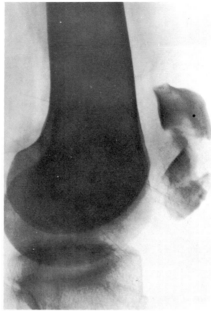

Fig. 25–28. (*Left*) Fracture of the patella with slight separation of the fragments. (*Right*) Fracture of the patella with comminution and wide separation of the fragments.

essary, and the patient is ambulatory on crutches.

After 5 to 7 days, a cylinder cast (Fig. 25-29) or a long leg cast may be applied to maintain the knee in full extension. A cylinder cast can be a problem unless it is well padded just above the malleoli and the portion of the padding next to the skin is made of some adherent material. An excellent mechanism for obtaining this is to apply two long strips of Foamtrac (1/8-inch foam rubber on an elastic backing) along the medial and lateral aspects of the leg from the thigh to the ankle; the leg is then covered with stockinet, appropriate padding being placed over the patella and the head of the fibula, and about the proximal and distal ends of the cast. A plaster of Paris cast is applied, and the ends of the Foamtrac are turned down and incorporated in the plaster. This gives excellent protection and does not allow the cast to slide distally. The use of elastifoam (a similar bandage made with an elastic backing) is very satisfactory as shown in Fig. 25-29.

After 5 to 6 weeks, the cylinder cast may be removed; a supportive elastic compression dressing is applied from the toes to above the knee, and quadriceps exercises are initiated. The patient may be able to do moderate work after the cast is applied, and he may be able to do more strenuous work after 8 to 12 weeks.

Treatment of Fractures with Separation of the Fragments. When the separation of the fragments is more than 2 mm., operation is indicated. The fragments may be sutured if the fracture is transverse and near the middle. Fracture through the upper or lower pole may be best treated by excision of the smaller fragment and repair of the torn tendon.

Total patellectomy gives good results in severely comminuted or neglected fractures. Hospitalization is necessary.

DISLOCATIONS OF THE PATELLA

Dislocation of the patella is usually due to direct violence. Most often the dislocation is to the lateral side; in some instances, the medial edge of the patella is

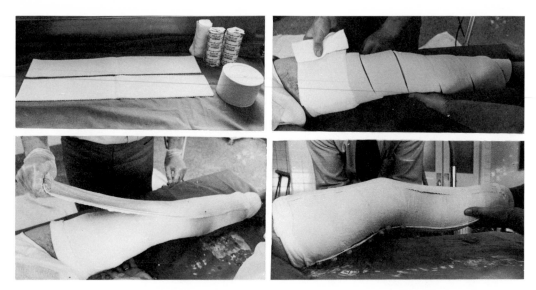

Fig. 25–29. Application of a cylinder cast. (*Top, left*) Plaster splint, sheet wadding. (*Top, right*) Application of sheet wadding; 5-inch plaster rolls. (*Bottom, left*) Application of plaster splint anteriorly after one layer of circular plaster. (*Bottom, right*) Application of plaster splint, posterior. Another layer of circular plaster completes the cast.

depressed and caught in the intercondylar notch of the femur, making the lateral edge unusually prominent. Rarely is displacement to the lateral side so complete that the medial edge of the patella lies against the lateral side of the lateral condyle of the femur. A dislocation implies some laceration of the quadriceps extensor tendon, which is manifested by hemorrhage or effusion into the knee joint. Dislocation of the patella to the medial side of the knee is rare.

Diagnosis. Pain and swelling at the knee, visible or palpable displacement of the patella, and severe pain on attempting to walk are characteristic. Attempts to move the knee are painful.

Treatment. The knee joint is aspirated if it is distended and painful. Usually, the dislocation may be reduced without anesthesia. An assistant flexes the thigh on the abdomen with the knee hyperextended. This relaxes the quadriceps extensor muscle completely and allows the surgeon to reduce the displacement by pressing the patella toward its normal position.

A padded posterior splint and a pressure dressing or a cylinder cast are applied, and the patient is allowed to walk immediately. Ice bags may be applied for from 24 to 48 hours if there has been much pain and swelling. Quadriceps sitting exercises must be started promptly. The splint should be worn for 4 weeks to secure good healing and so avoid recurrence of the dislocation.

If the dislocation becomes recurrent, operation is usually required.

FRACTURES OF THE SHAFT OF THE TIBIA ALONE

Many fractures of the shaft of the tibia, both in adults and in children, need only ambulatory treatment (Fig. 25-30). In this class belong transverse, oblique, and slightly comminuted fractures in good position. In the case of displaced fractures that can be reduced easily and that are stable after reduction, the patient can sometimes become ambulatory after two or three days in the hospital. Extensive

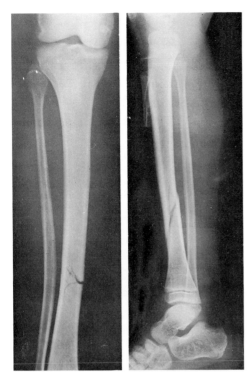

Fig. 25–30. (*Left*) Incomplete fracture of the tibia. (*Right*) Spiral fracture. These fractures can be treated well with a well-molded cast and immediate walking.

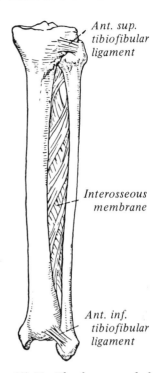

Ant. sup. tibiofibular ligament

Interosseous membrane

Ant. inf. tibiofibular ligament

Fig. 25–31. The bones and the ligaments of the leg. The fibula is bound securely to the tibia by the interosseous membrane and by ligaments at the proximal and the distal articulations.

crushing or laceration of soft parts, signs of impaired circulation, or signs of nerve injury make immediate hospitalization necessary. An open fracture, actual, threatened, or suspected, is a surgical emergency.

Anatomy and Etiology. Fractures of the shaft of the tibia follow direct and indirect violence, such as that due to blows, falls, and vehicular trauma. The bone has large proximal and distal ends and is narrowest at the junction of the middle and the lower thirds, at which point it is most often fractured. The fracture line may be oblique, transverse, or comminuted. The fibula is attached to the tibia by ligaments at the proximal and distal articulations and by a strong interosseous membrane (Fig. 25-31).

When the tibia alone is fractured, the fibula may act as a splint and prevent very great displacement or shortening. In more severe injuries, there is an associated fracture of the fibula.

Displacement. Displacement varies with the causative force. In oblique fractures, the line often runs from before upward and backward, the proximal fragment becomes prominent, and there may be slight angulation. Transverse fractures may exhibit little displacement.

Diagnosis. After an injury, there is pain and swelling over the tibia and pain on attempting to bear weight on the foot. There may be visible angulation. Children often have incomplete fractures, and they are able to walk with a limp.

For examination, the legs are placed parallel to each other on a table or a bed, and the visible signs of injury are noted. The crest of the tibia is subcutaneous, and it can be palpated for tenderness and irregularity and compared with the uninjured side. The tenderness due to fracture

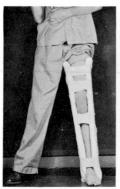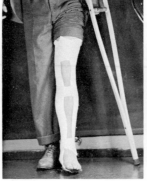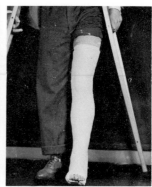

Fig. 25–32. (*Left*) Temporary splints for fractures of the shaft of the tibia or of both bones of the leg. (*Center*) Molded plaster splints for a fracture of the shaft of the tibia. (*Right*) The molded splints have been covered with plaster bandage to make a cast. This is a variation of the method described in the text.

is acute and well localized, except in spiral fractures, when it extends over the length of the fracture site. Percussion of the heel causes pain at the fracture site. It is inadvisable to attempt to elicit crepitus or preternatural mobility. In many instances, the diagnosis must depend on roentgen examination.

Treatment. The treatment aims at reducing any displacement and at immobilizing the fragments until union is solid. As a general rule, both the knee and the ankle must be immobilized. The limb is exercised from the beginning by walking; in this way, stiffness, muscle atrophy, and circulatory disturbances are avoided.

Immobilization for transportation is provided by applying well-padded wood or metal splints or an air splint from the heel to the upper thigh to prevent motion of the fragments (Fig. 25-32). The roentgen examination is made as soon as possible.

Reduction, if necessary, is performed by traction and local pressure; in young children, general anesthesia is often indicated; in older people, the fracture hematoma is infiltrated with local anesthetic solution. A well-padded long leg cast is applied until the acute swelling has subsided, and then a well-fitting long leg walking-cast or a patellar-tendon-bearing cast is utilized.

Residual angulation after application of the long leg cast may sometimes be corrected by wedging of the cast (Fig. 25-33). It is helpful prior to wedging to obtain an x-ray film, using a small metallic marker in order to locate the level of the wedge accurately.

From 6 to 8 weeks' immobilization for children, and from 8 to 10 weeks' immobilization for adults, is usually adequate.

After the cast is removed, an elastic compression dressing is applied from the toes to the knee; this is used until the tendency to swelling ceases. If roentgen examination shows that healing is satisfactory, the patient is permitted to bear weight after removal of the cast. If there is any indication of a delay in union, a new cast is applied for an additional 4 weeks and roentgen examination is repeated. Full mobility of the knee and the ankle usually returns in a few weeks. Badly displaced, severely comminuted, and otherwise unstable fractures should be treated in the hospital.

If the technique has been mastered and understood, a patellar tendon bearing cast (PTB) is applicable in 10 to 14 days after swelling has subsided.

FRACTURES OF THE SHAFT OF THE FIBULA ALONE

Common fibular fractures occur just above and below the distal tibiofibular articulation. Isolated fractures in the

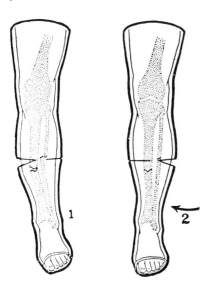

Fig. 25–33. Residual angulation of both bones of the leg may be corrected by removing a wedge of the cast on one side and incising the cast on the opposite side (1). The cast then is bent enough for correction (2) and is repaired with a few circular turns of plaster bandage.

proximal two thirds of the shaft of the fibula may follow direct violence (Fig. 25-34). A heavy layer of fibrous tissue and muscle surrounds the bone and prevents any considerable displacement, unless the violence has been great. Fractures at the neck of the fibula may be complicated by injuries to the peroneal nerve. When displacement is present, it is usually toward the tibia.

Diagnosis. A history of direct violence with local pain and tenderness suggests fracture. Roentgen examination is usually necessary to confirm the diagnosis.

Treatment. Reduction is seldom indicated, but it may be attempted for wide displacement. A local anesthetic may be infiltrated into the fracture site. Traction on, and forcible inversion of, the foot while the knee is flexed may improve the position of the fragments.

A cast is rarely needed for these cases. An elastic compression bandage from the toes to the knee may be useful. Persistent discomfort often responds to repeated injection of local anesthetic solution. The prognosis is excellent, except in fractures

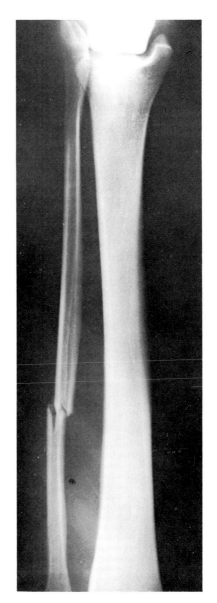

Fig. 25–34. Fracture of shaft of fibula with slight displacement.

of the neck of the bone; the possibility of late peroneal nerve involvement must be kept in mind in these cases.

AMBULATORY TREATMENT OF FRACTURES OF THE LEG AFTER DISCHARGE FROM THE HOSPITAL

Every effort should be made to apply a cast that will permit walking on the leg as soon as the fracture site is considered sufficiently stable. Usually, this is done while the patient is in the hospital, but, in some instances, it is applied after discharge. Active use of the leg is the best available form of physiotherapy and the best stimulus to union. The newly developed patellar-tendon-bearing cast and cast braces have been a marked step in improving early ambulation and more prompt union.

AMBULATORY TREATMENT OF DELAYED UNION OR NONUNION IN FRACTURES OF THE LOWER LEG

In many fractures of the lower limb involving one or both bones, especially when the fractures are open, there is a long delay in union. These patients may be treated very satisfactorily by ambulatory methods. Active use stimulates the circulation and appears to stimulate bony union. Edema must be prevented and adequate support given so that walking is possible.

Operation for nonunion should not be considered until this treatment has been tried for six to twelve months. Many fractures will respond with union after several months.

BIBLIOGRAPHY

Removal of Plaster Casts

Geyerhahn, G.: Removal of plaster casts used in walking. (Correspondence). JAMA, *169*:164, 1959.

Fractures of the Patella

Böhler, J.: Behandlung der kniescheibenbrüche (Treatment of patellar fractures). Deutsch. Med. Wschr., *86*:1209, 1961.
MacAusland, W. R.: Total patellectomy—a report of 28 cases. Am. J. Surg., *85*:221, 1954.
Nummi, J.: Fracture of the patella; a clinical study of 707 patellar fractures. Ann. Chir. Gynaec. Fenn. (179 Suppl.), *179*:1, 1971.
O'Donohghue, D. H.: Treatment of fractures of the patella. Northwest. Med., *57*:1592, 1958.
Reich, R. S., and Rosenberg, N. J.: Treatment of patellar fractures. Surg., Gynec. Obstet., *98*:553, 1954.•

Fractures of the Upper End of the Tibia

Bradford, C. H., Kilfoyle, R. M., Kelleher, J. J., and Magill, H. K.: Fractures of the lateral tibial condyle. J. Bone Joint Surg., *32A*:39, 1950.
Hohl, M., and Luck, J. V.: Fractures of the tibial condyle. J. Bone Joint Surg., *38A*:1001, 1956.
Turner, V. C.: Fractures of the tibial plateaus. JAMA, *169*:923, 1959.

Fractures of the Shaft of the Tibia

Boylston, B. F., and Knight, R. M.: Short oblique fracture of the tibia. JAMA, *167*:1477, 1958.
Hamilton, R. L., and Jahna, H.: A simple proven method for treatment of fractures of shaft of tibia (with or without fracture of fibula). Am. J. Surg., *88*:218, 1954.
Lithgow, W. C.: Fractures of the tibia and fibula. Surg. Clin. N. Am., *45*:69, 1965.
Travis, L. O.: Tibial shaft fractures—problems in management. JAMA, *164*:1175, 1957.
Urist, M. R.: End-result observations influencing treatment of fractures of the shaft of the tibia. JAMA, *159*:1088, 1955.
Winston, M. E.: The results of conservative treatment of fractures of the femur and tibia in the same limb. Surg., Gynec. Obstet., *134*:985, 1972.

26

Foot and Ankle

Part I—Soft Tissues

Mark W. Wolcott, M.D.

INFECTIONS

Infections of the foot correspond roughly to those of the hand, except that tenosynovitis is not a frequent lesion in the lower extermity.

CELLULITIS AND LYMPHANGITIS

Etiology and Symptoms. A common infection in the foot is cellulitis with an associated lymphangitis, which arises from an infection of the toes or from a dermatophytosis between them. This is either primarily or secondarily streptococcal in origin, and the usual history is of some small, often insignificant, abrasion or crack in the skin followed by the development of edema and cellulitis of the dorsum of the foot and of the typical red streaks due to lymphangitis up the leg. The subinguinal nodes overlying the saphenous opening are the ones involved most frequently, and these become enlarged and painful, often without any apparent intervening lymphangitis. The same type of infection may arise from an infected blister over the heel or over the metatarsophalangeal joint of the great toe.

Treatment. The treatment of streptococcal infection of the foot consists of elevation, hot wet dressings over the foot, the leg, and the involved lymph nodes, and administration of antibiotics, usually penicillin. This therapy necessitates rest in bed, but usually it can be carried out safely at home and results in a rapid subsidence of the infection in 2 or 3 days. However, the possibility of the later development of a suppurative adenitis in the lymph nodes involved should be remembered, and the patient should be seen frequently, since this may demand incision.

INFECTED CALLUS

A second type of infection that is seen occasionally in the foot is a local one about a callus on the plantar surface. This lesion is similar to the collar-button abscess seen in the hand, and it is treated in the same manner.

Treatment. The overlying thickened skin is incised, and the subcutaneous abscess is drained by spreading the small opening through the true skin with a hemostat. Treatment with a small drain and hot wet dressings usually results in a rapid subsidence of the infection. Antibiotics are useful adjuncts. During the course of this treatment, the patient should be off his feet, with the part elevated.

CHRONIC ULCERS OF THE PLANTAR SURFACE OF THE FOOT

Diagnosis. Chronic ulcers in the center of callosities on the plantar surface of the foot occur especially in older individuals, and most often in diabetics. They may develop in any foot in which there is a neurological deficit, whether this be due to the diabetic neuropathy or to other causes. These ulcers are characterized by a heaping up of thickened epithelium, in the center of which is a punched-out ulceration (Fig. 26-1). When they occur over the ball of the foot, they extend sometimes to the heads of the metatarsal bones. In addition, there often are roentgen changes in the bone, and these frequently are misdiagnosed as osteomyelitis. In reality, they are the changes of osteoporosis, although a secondary infection may lead to a true inflammation of the bony tissue.

Treatment. These ulcers are very resistant to all forms of treatment, and often they become infected secondarily. In diabetic patients, they may have serious consequences, leading to amputation.

The ulcer is probably the result of a reduced blood supply in the area, with a consequent decrease in healing power, even though pulsations may be palpable in the arteries in many cases.

Treatment by rest in bed is advised by some. The ulcer may heal, but tends to recur with weight bearing. We have suggested the use of felt or sponge-rubber arch supports, with a high pad under the scaphoid bone to shift the excessive pressure from the prominent metatarsal head to the soft tissues of the instep. Operation has been found useful by Classen: excision of the metatarsal head and the base of the phalanx through a dorsal incision, packing and drainage through the plantar ulcer. "A distressing aspect of the problem is the rapidity with which calluses develop under other metatarsal heads. Some go on to frank ulcerations." Aftercare and the need for foot supports to redistribute weight bearing are emphasized. The possibility of improving

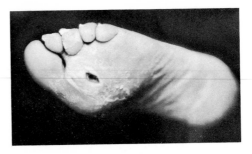

Fig. 26–1. Chronic ulcer and callosity of the plantar surface of the foot in a diabetic. Note the punched-out appearance of the ulcer, which extends deeply, even into the bone of the foot. This patient was treated with gelatin boots, and for more than a year and a half was able to get about on the foot. Eventually, infection necessitated amputation.

the vascular supply by means of the various revascularization procedures should be investigated. Femoral popliteal arterial bypass or endarterectomy may frequently improve the blood supply enough to permit healing of these ulcers.

TRAUMATIC LESIONS

INCISED WOUNDS

Incised wounds of the feet occur most commonly from stepping with the bare foot on some sharp object, such as glass or a razor blade.

Treatment. The care of such injuries does not differ from that for incised wounds elsewhere in the body. As a rule, the preparation of the surrounding area, followed by cleaning of the wound itself, permits primary suture. A pressure bandage is applied, and the patient usually is provided with crutches for a time to limit weight bearing.

PUNCTURE WOUNDS

Etiology. Puncture wounds probably are more common in the foot than elsewhere in the body. Pointed objects may enter the foot through the shoe, as when one steps on a nail in a board, or needles or other sharp-pointed objects left lying on the floor may enter the foot directly when one walks barefoot about a room. Often the patient does not seek treatment for several hours, or even days.

Treatment. As a rule, it is safer to administer a prophylactic dose of tetanus immune globulin (human) or to give a booster dose of toxoid. The treatment of the wound itself depends somewhat upon its condition. At the time of the primary dressing, it is usually unwise to probe the wound, and in a large majority of cases in which a simple protective dressing is applied, healing occurs without infection. If there is reason to believe that considerable contamination has been introduced with the puncturing object, it is wise to incise the wound under local anesthesia and to perform a radical wound cleansing. Prophylactic use of antibiotics is the rule in such cases.

Many puncture wounds are complicated by the presence of foreign bodies (see Chapter 10). Needles and splinters are the most common offenders.

CONTUSIONS

Contusions of the foot and the toes are common industrial accidents, the foot being caught under heavy machines, rolling barrels, or trucks. Often there is fracture of the distal phalanx of the great toe and of other bones of the toes. Therefore, such injuries should always be examined by roentgenography. The swelling is usually quite marked on the dorsum of the toes and on the dorsum of the foot. Frequently there is a subungual hematoma, or the base of the nail may be torn free and lie on top of the eponychium.

Treatment. Following roentgenography, the lesion is cleaned if there are open wounds, and any part of the nail base that lies on the eponychium is excised. The wounds are then protected with petrolatum gauze, and the whole foot and ankle are enclosed in a compression dressing.

The advantage of this dressing is that it supplies comparative immobilization, as well as pressure, and, with this therapy, the swelling and the pain subside rapidly and the patient, even in the case of severe contusion and fracture, may be able to walk without too much discomfort in 2 or 3 days to a week. The dressing is allowed to remain in place as long as it is in good condition. During this time, the patient can be ambulant without much disability with a shoe cut out at the toe.

CORNS

Description. Corns are a variety of callosity in which there is a central piling up of epithelial cells forming what frequently is called a core. They are the result of pressure and friction, and they are seen most commonly over the lateral and the dorsal surfaces of the fifth toe, though they may occur also over any bony prominence. Corns are described as being either hard or soft; this differentiation is due only to the amount of moisture in the area. Those occurring between the toes become macerated and are called soft corns, whereas those on the dorsum of the foot and the toes have a hard, horny epithelial covering. Soft corns are often associated with dermatophytosis.

Treatment. In the treatment of corns, the most important factor is the removal of the cause. Frequently, the correction of ill-fitting shoes or improper weight bearing of the feet permits the corn to disappear. However, if corns are to be removed, a scalpel or electrocoagulation may be used. A most conservative method, that of shaving away the hardened epithelium followed by an application of trichloracetic acid, is sometimes effective. Any local therapy without removal of the cause of the pressure is almost sure to be followed by a reappearance of the corn.

SPRAINS AND RUPTURES OF LIGAMENTS ABOUT THE ANKLE JOINT

Etiology and Symptoms. Sprains at the ankle occur most commonly at the lateral side (Fig. 26-2). Sudden inversion of the foot causes an injury to the lateral liga-

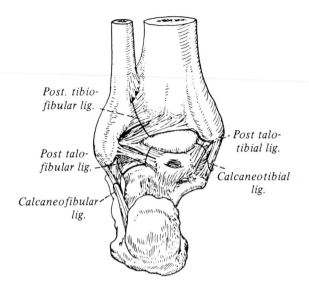

Post. tibio-fibular lig.

Post talo-fibular lig.

Calcaneofibular lig.

Post talo-tibial lig.

Calcaneotibial lig.

Fig. 26–2. Semidiagrammatic posterior view of the ligaments at the ankle (after Spalteholz). The lateral malleolus is bound strongly to the posterior aspect of the astragalus and to the os calcis, and it is often displaced with them after fractures.

ment, manifested by limping and pain and by swelling, ecchymosis, and tenderness at the lateral side of the ankle. Ecchymosis may not appear for a day or two after injury. A similar condition may occur at the medial side of the ankle. Sprains can usually be differentiated from fractures by the location of the most acute tenderness. In sprains, this is the area in front of and below the lateral malleolus; in fractures, it is definitely over the bone.

Very often, the anterior tibiofibular ligament is found to be tender, and there may be tenderness over the dorsum of the foot in front of the ankle. Tenderness at these sites indicates sprains of the tibiofibular ligament and the ligaments of the dorsum of the foot. Occasionally, the lateral ligament tears away from the malleolus and takes with it a small portion of the tip of the bone. This condition is called a sprain fracture.

When the signs of sprain at the lateral or the medial side of the joint are severe, a very extensive laceration of the ligament involved may be present. Similarly, great tenderness at the tibiofibular ligament indicates possible rupture. These lacerations are suspected more strongly when the foot can be inverted or everted forcibly beyond its normal limit and when the astragalus is felt to rotate excessively between the malleoli, indicating that the

injury is a reduced dislocation. Normally, the astragalus does not move mediolaterally.

The test is performed best after the tender areas have been infiltrated with 10 ml. of 1 percent procaine solution. When excessive mediolateral mobility is found or is suspected, it should be verified by making an anteroposterior roentgenogram of the ankle with the foot inverted or everted forcibly, as the case may require, so as to put the ligament affected on tension.

Prevention of Ankle Injuries in Sports. Many players believe that "ankle wraps" afford some protection against injury. A nonelastic bandage is applied by the player or the trainer over the inner of two pairs of socks, with a turn around the heel (Fig. 26-3). Its purpose is to limit mediolateral mobility without restricting flexion-extension. Quigley believes that the incidence of ankle injuries can be reduced by 50 percent by the use of such a bandage.

Treatment. Sprains and sprain fractures without abnormal mobility of the astragalus require support of the ankle joint and measures to control swelling. A strapping (Figs. 26-4 and 26-5), provides a firm supportive dressing; this is renewed when it becomes loose. Elevation and application of ice bags for from 24 to

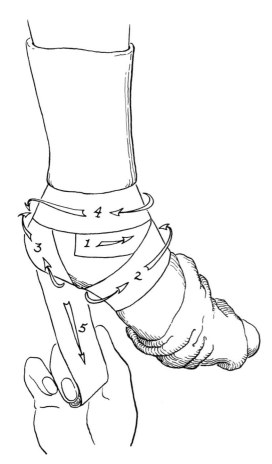

Fig. 26–3. Technique of the ankle wrap.

48 hours will control swelling. The patient continues his usual activities so far as possible. Recovery takes place in 3 to 14 days as a rule. Another method of treatment is to have the patient begin vigorous active use after the strapping has been applied. Often, there is striking subsidence of symptoms after a few hours.

Procaine injections may be used in treating these injuries, 10 ml. of 1 percent solution being injected at the site of the most acute tenderness. The joint is then moved to find any other painful areas and is palpated for additional tender spots. Any such areas should be injected also with from 5 to 10 ml. of the local anesthetic solution. Immediate relief of pain and the ability to walk freely result. The pain may return after some hours; it may or may not be severe. Additional injec-

tions may be given at intervals of 24 hours or more. Recovery is expedited by strapping the ankle as described.

There is some question as to whether injection of procaine should be used in the treatment of ankle sprains in sports. Quigley, after a large experience with such injuries at the Harvard Athletic Association, feels that anesthetization with procaine produces a loss of a sense of timing and coordination which predisposes to other injuries if the player goes back into the game immediately.

Lettin uses hyaluronidase instead of procaine injected at the most tender spot. He uses 1500 I.U. of hyaluronidase in 5 ml. of normal saline. This gives relief of pain and permits return to normal function faster than does strapping. In a 2-year follow-up of 85 cases, no ankle instability resulted from this treatment.

Some advise plaster-cast immobilization for ankle sprains. However, Nevin, in a large experience with paratroopers, had much better results with immediate ambulation than with casting.

Caro, Craft, Howells, and Shaw made a study of 172 patients with inversion injuries of the ankle. Fourteen of these were severe tears of the lateral ligament diagnosed roentgenologically after injection of the area with local anesthesia and 1500 I.U. of hyaluronidase. There were 28 fractures. In these cases, three types of treatment were used:

1. Hydrocortisone, 50 mg., injected into the site of maximum tenderness and spread into the injured ligament. An elastic bandage was applied, and weight bearing and gentle exercise advised.

2. Strapping and elastic adhesive bandage to produce strong eversion of the ankle. Weight bearing and gentle exercise were encouraged.

3. Plaster of Paris cast with walking rocker. Full weight bearing was permitted after 48 hours. The cast was worn for 2 weeks.

They found that the treatment by hydrocortisone injection gave the best results.

When signs of sprain are associated with abnormal mobility of the astragalus,

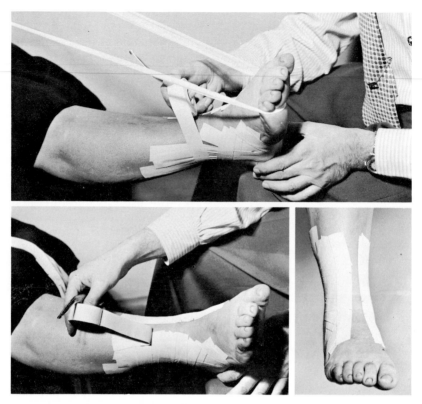

Fig. 26–4. Ankle strapping (Gibney boot). (*Top*) The heel is supported on the surgeon's knee, and the foot is held in a bandage loop at right angles to the leg by the patient. Alternate longitudinal and transverse strips of 1-inch-wide adhesive are applied from a roll. Each strip should lie flat on the part. Except for the dorsum of the foot, the entire area is covered by varying the direction of the adhesive strips. (*Bottom, left*) Rolling of the adhesive edges is prevented by longitudinal binding strips; these are nicked with scissors to permit them to conform to the part. (*Bottom, right*) Completed strapping.

rupture of the lateral ligament, the deltoid (medial) ligament, or of the tibiofibular ligaments must be suspected and verified by means of roentgenograms. Prolonged immobilization is necessary to secure firm healing of the rupture. When the swelling subsides, an unpadded case is applied from the toes to the knee, the malleoli being compressed firmly together with the flats of the hands and the plaster being molded well. A total of 6 weeks of immobilization is required. The patient begins to bear weight immediately after the cast is hard and the walking heel has been applied. The aftercare is

similar to that for ankle fractures without displacement. If prolonged immobilization and the walking prescribed are carried out, the prognosis is usually good.

SPRAINS OF THE
METATARSOPHALANGEAL JOINT

Treatment. Stubbing the toes, especially when walking barefoot or in soft slippers, often results in a sprain of the metatarsophalangeal joint, especially that of the great toe. This causes swelling and pain on motion. The pain may often be relieved by the injection of a local anes-

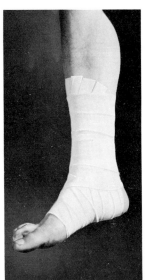
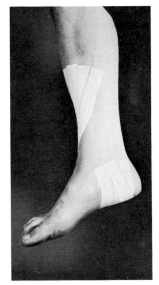

Fig. 26–5. Simple strapping and elastic adhesive bandage dressing for sprains of the lateral ligament or sprain fractures of the tip of the lateral malleolus. Both injuries are caused by inversion, which the strapping prevents.

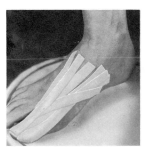
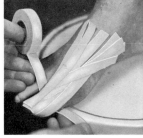
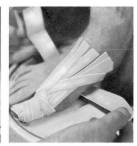

Fig. 26–6. Adhesive strapping for sprains of the metatarsophalangeal joint and of the joints of the toes. This strapping also is used frequently for fractures of the phalanges of the toes. It is a most effective dressing and much better than any form of splint. It should be applied with the patient standing on a stool and bearing his weight on the affected foot. (*Left*) Cross strappings extending from the dorsum of the foot to the end of the toe are applied. (*Center*) The longitudinal strips are anchored with circular turns of adhesive, applied with the patient extending his toes beyond the stool on which he is standing. A loop of adhesive is placed under the toe. The patient again places the entire foot on the stool and bears his weight on the foot, and the circular turn is completed. If these circular turns are put on while the patient's weight is borne on the foot, the strapping will be comfortable; otherwise, the tendency is for the toe to be held in extension and make the patient uncomfortable. (*Right*) The circular turns of the upper portion of the strapping are placed round the foot while it is lifted off the stool. With the patient's weight on his foot, the turns are completed.

thetic, usually procaine, 1 or 2 percent. A strapping applied along the dorsum of the foot and the toe provides relative immobilization, gives comfort, and results in rapid subsidence of the painful symptoms. It is essential that the patient bear his weight on the foot while the strapping is being applied; otherwise, the toe often is strapped in the hyperextended position, which gives more discomfort than the original lesion (Fig. 26-6). Local infiltration of 1 percent Xylocaine may be all that

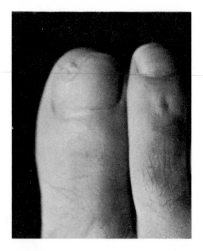

Fig. 26–7. Subungual wart of the great toe. This wart was cured by electrocoagulation under local anesthesia.

is necessary. This may be repeated on several occasions.

LESIONS OF THE TOENAIL

SUBUNGUAL WARTS

Warts under the toenails are troublesome lesions (Fig. 26-7). By pressing on the undersurface of the nail, they frequently cause pain and disability. Patients usually attempt to relieve their discomfort by cutting away the nail round the wart, but as the nail grows out, it tends to cut into the wart, causing pain and, sometimes, infection.

Treatment. The warts may be removed either by cauterization with an electrocoagulating needle under local anesthesia or by the injection into the base of the wart of a drop or two of a sclerosing solution, such as sodium morrhuate. The nail should be cut back from the area until the wart separates and comes away.

INGROWN TOENAIL

Etiology. Ingrown toenail is a painful lesion caused by the pressure of tight shoes on the soft tissues at the edge of the nail of the great toe. The secondary, or exciting, cause of the difficulty is the frequent mistake of cutting the nail too short, so that its corner may be overlain easily by the soft tissues at the edge of the nail. In teen-aged boys, when wear and tear on the feet is high and foot care is poor, and when canvas shoes are frequently worn, ingrown toenails are especially common. As the nail grows out, the uncut corner is pushed into the soft tissues (Fig. 26-8), and the pressure of the shoe on the tissues produces marked pain. Frequently, the sharp projecting tip of the nail produces an ulceration in the skin overlying the nail edge, and this causes a chronic infection (Fig. 26-9, *left*). Granulations form over the nail edge, and there is a constant discharge of a small amount of purulent secretion (Fig. 26-9, *right*). In this type of lesion, the discomfort is more or less constant, but it is made much worse by the pressure of shoes.

Treatment. The treatment of ingrown toenail may be divided into the conservative and the operative.

In most minor cases of ingrown toenail, the soft tissues may be pushed away from the projecting tip of the nail with the tip of a scalpel. When the offending corner of the nail has been demonstrated, a wisp of cotton may be introduced between the soft tissues and the nail to hold the soft tissues away from the nail; it should be packed under the projecting corner of the nail. The author has used a small piece of cotton pulled from an alcohol sponge for this purpose. This elevation of the nail permits it to grow out beyond the soft tissues, and if the nail is permitted to grow so that its entire end appears, and if this is then cut at right angles to the axis of the toe, the symptoms are relieved and there is no recurrence. In some people, the discomfort may be relieved without anesthesia by excising the side of the nail with the tip of a scalpel, thus removing the factor that causes the pain. It is important to remove the corner of the nail that projects into the soft tissues, which is often found as a sharp point. The overhanging granulations may be cauterized with a silver nitrate stick, and if precautions are taken to prevent pressure by

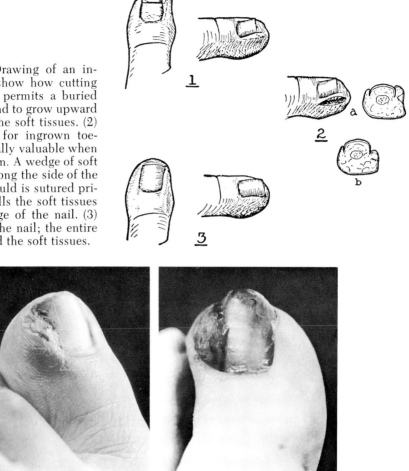

Fig. 26–8. (1) Drawing of an ingrown toenail to show how cutting the nail too short permits a buried corner to remain and to grow upward as a point under the soft tissues. (2) Bartlett operation for ingrown toenail; this is especially valuable when there is no infection. A wedge of soft tissue is excised along the side of the toe (a), and the would is sutured primarily (b). The pulls the soft tissues away from the edge of the nail. (3) Proper cutting of the nail; the entire nail edge is beyond the soft tissues.

Fig. 26–9. (*Left*) Infection along the edge of the nail in a typical ingrown toenail. (*Right*) Neglected ingrown toenail, with growth of hypertrophic infected granulation tissue along the edge of the nail.

wearing shoes that fit properly, the patient's symptoms may be relieved completely and often permanently.

In many cases, it may be wise not to attempt conservative therapy, but, rather, some form of operative treatment. Two methods of operation have been employed, and we have found specific indications for each type. The operation described by Bartlett has been found to be of particular value in those patients in whom the pain from the ingrown toenail is not associated with an infection along the edge of the nail (Fig. 26-8). In this operation, using local anesthesia, an ellipse of skin and subcutaneous tissue is excised along the side of the toe. The wound is sutured primarily, and a simple pressure dressing is applied with adhesive. The sutures are permitted to remain in place for 7 days at least, and often the dressing is not changed until this time. The advantages of this operation are the rapid, usually primary, healing and the relatively short period of disability, not more than a day or two. Excellent per-

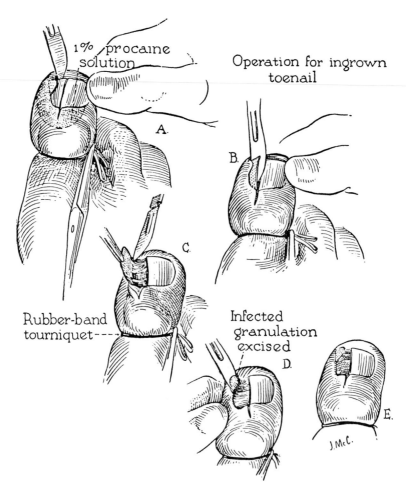

Fig. 26–10. Operation for ingrown toenail. (*A*) The eponychium at the base and the sides of the nail is infiltrated with 1 percent procaine solution. The anesthesia should extend upward to the soft tissues at the tip of the toe. An incision is made through the nail and the eponychium with a knife or scissors. (*B*) The nail is reflected from the phalanx throughout its entire length, including the matrix. (*C*) The nail is dissected away, tension being kept upon it with forceps or a hemostat. (*D*) After the entire nail and its matrix have been removed, the infected granulation tissue is excised. (*E*) Petrolatum gauze or a small piece of Gelfoam is applied.

manent results are obtained by means of this treatment, which is designed to pull the soft tissues away from the edge of the nail.

For ingrown toenails in which there is a definite infection along the edge of the nail, with a heaping up of chronic granulation tissue, a much better operation is excision of the side of the toenail and of the overhanging soft tissues (Figs. 26-10 and 26-11). The operation is performed under a block anesthesia at the base of the nail and round the edges of the toe. A tourniquet at the base of the toe provides hemostasis. With a knife or scissors, the toenail is divided down to and through the matrix. This includes also an incision through the eponychium, which is turned

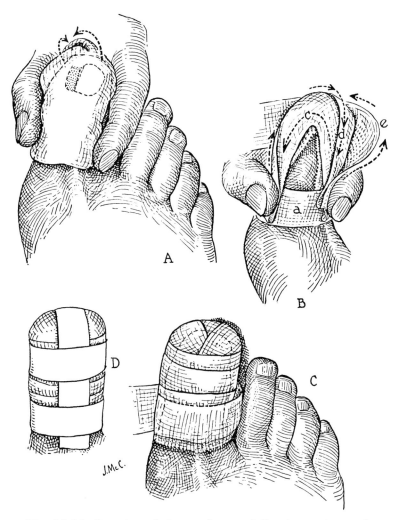

Fig. 26–11. Dressing of the toe for use following excision of an ingrown toenail. (*A*) A gauze dressing, 2 × 3 inches, is cut at the top and folded over the end of the toe. (*B*) A circular anchor-turn of bandage is applied, followed by a reverse turn of the bandage over the toe. (*C*) The bandage is finished by making circular turns. (*D*) Adhesive strips are applied: 1 longitudinaly strip, which extends beyond the bandage front and back; and 2 circular strips, which anchor the bandage and the longitudinal adhesive strip in place.

back with an Allis forceps. The scalpel is then inserted under the uplifted cut edge of the nail, and the offending portion of the nail is removed together with its matrix. The hypertrophic granulation tissue and the soft tissues that overhang the nail are excised, and a small piece of Gelfoam is laid over the resulting wound. A pressure dressing is applied. The gauze is changed in about 3 days; after that, small protective dressings are continued until the wound has healed; this occurs in about 2 to 3 weeks.

In the ambulatory care of patients with ingrown toenail, the toe of an old shoe can be cut out to permit the application of a bandage without pressure on the toe. Obtaining an old shoe often makes it necessary to delay operation for 24 hours. During this time, hot soaks are suggested to relieve the infection and the local cellulitis that may surround the nail edge.

After operation, the patient should be warned that the wearing of tight shoes that cause pressure on the edge of the nail may cause recurrence of an ingrown nail. Instructions should also be given about permitting the nail to grow so that the edge extends beyond the soft tissues.

HYPERTROPHIED TOENAIL

(Onychogryphosis)

Etiology and Symptoms. Hypertrophy of the toenail occurs most frequently in the nail of the great toe. As a rule, the cause of the overgrowth is some trauma to the nail bed, with subsequent marked thickening of the nail. Often, an almost hornlike nail develops, especially in older people who have a tendency to neglect themselves. The hypertrophy may cause pain by causing pressure upon the toe by the shoe, and it is for this reason that many patients seek treatment.

Treatment. If it is recognized that the symptoms may be relieved by relief of pressure, then conservative therapy, consisting of the simple cutting away of the hypertrophied nail, may be tried. Bone-cutting forceps are used to cut off the excessive nail, and the patient is taught to file away the overgrowth as necessary. This will not produce a cure, but it will relieve the symptoms.

Removal of the nail often is a disappointing procedure because the deformity sometimes recurs. For this reason, careful excision of the nail matrix must be performed, in addition to removing the nail, as a further precaution against regrowth. Some authors advise cauterization of the nail base. This operation can be done under local anesthesia.

SUPERNUMERARY TOES

Supernumerary toes are not at all uncommon, and, because of the difficulty they may cause in wearing shoes, it is frequently necessary to remove the extra digit. This can be done best in childhood because the growing child is able to adjust to the joint deformity that may follow the removal of the extra toe and its articulation.

Treatment. The operation is performed easily under local anesthesia. A roentgenogram is an aid in deciding which portion of the several toes should be removed. The toe is given a block anesthesia at its base for excision. It is wise to carry the skin incision fairly high along the toe to be removed. This flap of skin is reflected back sufficiently from the toe articulation to ensure that there will be sufficient skin and subcutaneous tissue to close over the defect resulting from removal of the extra toe. Skin sutures that pass through the entire thickness of the underlying soft tissues and to the bone are necessary. Fine steel wire is an excellent suture material. A pressure dressing is applied without a splint. The patient may be ambulatory throughout the period of treatment.

PLANTAR WARTS

Etiology and Diagnosis. Warts occurring on the plantar surface of the foot are among the frequent and painful lesions of this area (Fig. 26-12). Dermatologists believe that they are due to a type of virus; however, their appearance at sites of irritation is not infrequent. Often they are found to be associated with fallen arches. When they are associated with problems of faulty weight bearing, measures that improve the weight bearing often relieve the discomfort, and the wart disappears and exercise may prevent recurrence.

They occur more often in younger people, and they are important because of the pain produced by pressure upon them. Plantar warts may be small, or they may reach considerable size. Usually they are surrounded by an area of thickened epithelium, and in their center is a papillary growth that bleeds easily when it is pared with the scalpel. Pressure over this central core causes definite pain.

Treatment. There are several methods of treatment. The discomfort of a plantar wart is due to the pressure on its central

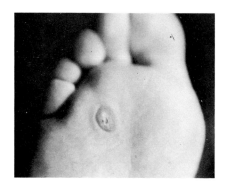

Fig. 26–12. Plantar wart of the foot.

core. This can often be relieved by shaving the wart. The author has used a double-edged safety razor blade for this purpose, bending it in the fingers so that the shaving may be done with the curved blade. After very thin slices of the epidermis have been shaved from the wart and the surrounding skin, the core of the wart can be plainly seen. There often may be a very slight capillary ooze from the core. After the surrounding skin has been protected with Vaseline, the core of the wart is treated with bichloroacetic acid. This is applied with a toothpick, which is dipped in the solution, and is worked into the soft tissues of the core carefully and deeply. This may cause slight discomfort. After the bichloroacetic acid has had a chance to be absorbed into the tissues, the area is covered with a Band-Aid. There may be slight soreness in the area for a day, but when the patient returns in 6 or 7 days, the core of the wart is black and can be removed with the tip of a knife or a small curette. This treatment may have to be repeated if the entire wart cannot be removed after one treatment.

An ointment of 20 percent linseed oil and 20 percent podophyllin in lanolin has been used with success by British authors. They claim that the linseed oil disrupts the keratin layer of the skin and allows podophyllin to destroy the wart. The ointment is applied to a piece of gauze a little larger than the wart, placed on the wart, and retained in place by waterproof adhesive. This dressing is not changed for a week. Thereafter, the foot is washed daily with soap and water.

Branson and Rhea inject 2 to 3 ml. of 1 percent procaine, under pressure, with a 26-gauge needle at the base of the wart. If the needle tip is properly placed at the stratum germinativum, there is marked blanching of the skin and elevation of the wart. The curative effect probably results from interruption of the blood supply of the wart.

The slight soreness produced by the injection disappears in 24 hours, and, if the injection has been properly placed, the wart may be lifted out of its site in about a week. The author has used this method of treatment with success in several cases.

Other methods of therapy are removal of the wart by electrodesiccation after anesthetization with procaine solution, or by the application of carbon dioxide snow. In many cases, the wart disappears with a minimum of discomfort by the injection into its base of a drop or two of quinine and urethane solution. The wart becomes dark or black in a few days and peels out of its crater without difficulty. Suitable arch supports should be prescribed when necessary. Often this alone will effect a cure.

CALLOSITIES (CALLUSES)

Callosities are masses of hypertrophied epithelial tissue, hard and yellowish in appearance, that occur over areas subjected to long-continued pressure or friction. They are seen most commonly over the ball of the foot, and they arise in this area due to imperfect weight bearing. Frequently they become tender and painful due to long-continued trauma.

Treatment. The treatment of callosities is removal of the cause. Since there usually is defective weight bearing, suitable arch supports must be prescribed. Painful areas subjected to pressure may be shaved with a razor blade or reduced by filing with an emery board.

BUNIONS

Etiology. This is the name given to hypertrophy of the metatarsophalangeal joint of the great toe. This joint becomes

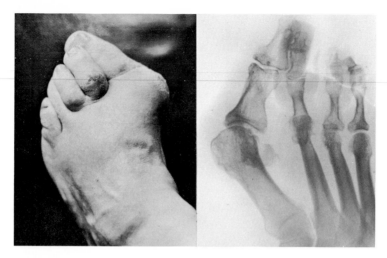

Fig. 26–13. Typical deformity of a bunion. The photograph shows the infected callus over the prominence of the metatarsal head. The roentgenogram shows the marked bony deformity.

deformed as a result of the wearing of shoes that do not fit properly and that cause a lateral deviation of the great toe. As the joint becomes more and more prominent, pressure over the hypertrophied bone produces either a callus or a subcutaneous bursa. As the condition continues, the joint becomes painful, and frequently the bursa becomes the site of an infection (Fig. 26–13).

Treatment. In the conservative treatment of bunions, attempts are made to reduce the deformity by placing a pad of lamb's wool between the great and the second toes and by preventing pressure over the metatarsophalangeal joint with felt pads. The wearing of shoes with toes that are wide enough may relieve the symptoms, but it rarely relieves the entire pathologic process.

Operation is usually necessary to produce a cure, and this necessitates hospitalization.

PAINFUL HEEL

A heel that is painful in walking is a troublesome clinical entity for both patient and surgeon. This condition occurs in two groups of patients.

PAINFUL HEEL IN CHILDREN

Symptoms and Diagnosis. In the first group are the young children between 8 and 12 years of age, most of them boys. In this group there rarely is any history of injury, but the patient usually is active and vigorous. The pain is at the back of the heel; the patient walks with a slight limp and often notes that he is more comfortable when walking on his toes. On examination, the heel is found to be tender posteriorly, and there is a slight thickening at the insertion of the Achilles tendon.

This symptom complex in children has been found to be due to an epiphysitis of the heel. A lateral roentgen film shows definite changes in the region of the calcaneal epiphysis and in the epiphyseal line.

Treatment. In milder cases, elevation of the heel with pads relieves the pressure on the Achilles tendon, and if strenuous exercise is avoided, usually the symptoms disappear rapidly. Local heat in the form of footbaths may be of value. As a rule, the pain disappears spontaneously, but the patient should be warned that shoes with heels should be worn to avoid recurrence.

PAINFUL HEEL IN ADULTS

Etiology and Pathology. In adults, this lesion has been regarded as resulting from the development of a calcaneal spur. However, this finding in the roentgen film probably is of no great clinical significance, and its presence appears to be incidental. Current belief is that the pain is due either to the development of a bursitis in the region of the spur or to a painful fasciitis of the plantar fascia and of the flexor digitorum brevis, which have their points of attachment near the site of the calcaneal spur. The pathologic process in this type of change may be similar to that which occurs at the lateral epicondyle in tennis elbow. It is often seen following prolonged and unusual periods of time on the feet. It is worse on first arising in the morning and improves as the day progresses.

Treatment. Various types of pads, springs, and other devices to relieve pressure have been used, but usually without much success. Two methods of therapy are of value—injection and needling, or actual division of the fascia and the muscles attached to the os calcis.

In injection and needling, the painful area is infiltrated with 0.5 or 1 percent procaine solution, and a large 14- or 16-gauge needle is introduced into the painful area. The needle is inserted from either side and is passed a sufficient distance into the painful area to puncture and drain the bursa that may be present. In a fair percentage of cases, this results in a cure of the painful heel.

In some cases, hydrocortisone is added to the procaine for injection into the painful area. A convenient preparation for this type of injection is a combination of dexamethasone 21-phosphate and lidocaine hydrochloride (Decadron phosphate injection with Xylocaine). This combination of an anti-inflammatory steroid and local anesthetic is injected in amounts of 1 to 2 ml. and gives excellent results in some cases.

Lapidus and Guidotti recommend phenylbutazone, 0.1 g. three times daily for a maximum of 20 doses.

Conservative treatment, including rest and avoidance of excessive standing, especially on hard surfaces, plus foot exercises, is usually successful.

BIBLIOGRAPHY

Plantar Ulcers

Classen, J. N.: Neurotrophic arthropathy with ulceration. Ann. Surg., *159*:891, 1964.
Radow, R. B., and Friedman, S. A.: Methods to avoid pressure on chronic foot ulcers. Arch. Phys. Med., *51*:304, 1970.

Ankle Sprains and Injuries

Blain, A., III, Razi, M., and Teves, M.: Use of walking casts for ankle sprains. J. Michigan Med. Soc., *61*:321, 1962.
Caro, D., Craft, I. L., Howells, J. B., and Shaw, P. C.: Diagnosis and treatment of injury of the lateral ligament of the ankle joint. Lancet, *2*:720, 1964.
Cave, E. F.: Treatment of ankle injuries. GP, *25*:85, 1957.
Hilsinger, E. A.: Partial plaster splint for the sprained ankle. JAMA, *214*:1326, 1970.
Kendall, P. H.: Hyaluronidase in the treatment of acute sprained ankle: a preliminary report. Ann. Phys. Med., *2*:95, 1954.
Lettin, A. W. F.: Diagnosis and treatment of sprained ankle. Brit. Med. J., *1*:1056, 1963.
Litton, L. O.: How to treat the sprained ankle. Consultant, p. 10, June, 1965.
Nevin, J. E.: Immediate ambulation of ankle sprains. Surg., Gynec. Obstet., *117*:368, 1963.
Quigley, R. B.: Management of athletic ankle injuries. JAMA, *169*:1431, 1959.
Staples, O. S.: Result study of ruptures of lateral ligaments of the ankle. Clin. Orthop., *85*:50, 1972.

Plantar Warts

Branson, E. C., and Rhea, R. L., Jr.: Plantar warts; cure by injection. New Eng. J. Med., *248*:631, 1953.
Carslaw, R. W., Neill, J., and Thom, J. A.: Linseed oil treatment of plantar warts. Brit. J. Derm., *75*:380, 1963.
Kerr, P. R.: Care of the feet. Practitioner, *206*:626, 1971.
LoCricchio, J., and Haserick, J. R.: Hot water treatment for warts. Cleveland Clin. Quart., *29*:156, 1962.

Ingrown Toenail

Bartlett, R. W.: A conservative operation for the cure of so-called ingrown toenail. JAMA, *108*:1257, 1937.

Lloyd-Davies, R. W., and Brill, G. C.: Management of ingrown toenail. Brit. J. Surg., *50*:592, 1963.

Vandenbos, K. Q., and Bowers, W. F.: Ingrown toenail: a result of weight bearing on soft tissue. U. S. Armed Forces Med. J., *10*:1168, 1959.

Wright, W.: Verruca plantaris. Calif. Med., *86*:450, 1955.

Painful Heel

Lapidus, P. W., and Guidotti, F. P.: Painful heel: report of 323 patients with 364 painful heels. Clin. Orthop., *39*:178, 1965.

26

Foot and Ankle

Part II—Fractures

Andrew C. Ruoff, M.D.

FRACTURES ABOUT THE ANKLE JOINT

ANATOMY

The tibia and the fibula are bound together just above the ankle joint by the tibiofibular ligaments (Fig. 26-14). These ligaments are often stronger than the fibula and resist widening of the space between the malleoli, in which the astragalus fits snugly. The astragalus tapers slightly from before backward. This tight mortise and tenon joint, between the tibiofibular unit above and the astragalus below, permits free flexion and extension but practically no mediolateral or rotary movement of the astragalus. Strong medial and lateral ligaments reinforce the sides of the capsule of the ankle joint. A strong posterior portion of the lateral ligament inserts on the posterior aspect of the astragalus, making the attachments of this bone to the fibula much stronger than those to the tibia. When the lateral malleolus is displaced, the astragalus tends to move with it. The articular surface of the astragalus fits exactly into the articular surface of the distal end of the tibia. When the astragalus becomes displaced, the weight-bearing axis shifts, and, if this is not corrected, serious impairment of ankle function follows. When the space between the malleoli increases as the result of displacement, the astragalus wob-

bles with each step, and again serious impairment of function will be the result.

ETIOLOGY

Most fractures about the ankle joint are caused by indirect violence, the force usually being applied to the foot and transmitted to the astragalus. They are classified according to the violence causing them: (1) fractures due to eversion and external rotation; (2) fractures due to inversion and internal rotation; (3) fractures due to forward or backward thrust against the articular surface of the tibia; and (4) fractures due to upward thrust against the articular surface of the tibia.

Fractures due to Eversion (Abduction) and External Rotation

Forcible eversion of the foot, that is, elevation of the lateral border, rotates the astragalus about its long axis so as to wedge the malleoli apart. The strain is applied to the tibiofibular ligament, which becomes a fulcrum at which the lever action works. The lateral malleolus is pressed outward. When it breaks, there is tension on the deltoid (medial collateral) ligament (Fig. 26-14, *A*). The ligament may tear, or the medial malleolus may be fractured. External rotation of the foot, that is, forefoot outward, forces the astragalus to rotate about a vertical axis, and also it acts to wedge the malleoli apart.

Eversion and external rotation are usually combined to cause typical fractures. When the force is not great, there is a fracture of the fibula at or above the tibiofibular ligaments, the fracture line being irregularly transverse or, from in front upward and backward, oblique. When the force is greater, there is a fracture of the fibula complicated by disruption of the mortise because of (1) fracture of the medial malleolus below the level of the ankle joint, (2) rupture of the deltoid ligament, or (3) rupture of the tibiofibular ligaments causing disruption of the tibiofibular unit.

Fractures Due to Inversion and Internal Rotation

Forcible inversion of the foot, that is, elevation of the medial border, acts to press the malleoli apart (Fig. 26-14, *B*). The strain falls on the tibiofibular ligaments and the lateral ligament. Internal rotation may occur at the same time and add to the wedging action. When the force is not great, the medial malleolus alone may be fractured, the fracture line running almost vertically upward. When the force is greater, the fracture of the medial malleolus is complicated by (1) fracture of the fibula below the tibiofibular ligaments, (2) rupture of the lateral ligament, or (3) rupture of the tibiofibular ligaments.

Fractures Due to Forward or Backward Thrust Against the Articular Surface of the Tibia

When the foot is plantar flexed and is thrust backward, (Fig. 26-14, *C*), the posterior margin of the articular surface of the tibia may be broken off, and the foot may be dislocated posteriorly. When the foot is dorsiflexed and thrust forward, the anterior margin of the articular surface of the tibia may be broken off, and the foot may be dislocated anteriorly. Fractures of an articular margin occur less frequently

alone than in combination with fractures of the malleoli.

Fractures Due to Upward Thrust Against the Articular Surface of the Tibia (Explosion Fracture)

These fractures are very rare and they follow falls on the feet. The inferior tibiofibular ligaments may be ruptured and the astragalus driven up between the two bones. The articular surface of the tibia may be crushed or split, and the astragalus displaced upward between the fragments that lie in front of it and behind it.

DIAGNOSIS OF FRACTURES ABOUT THE ANKLE

The history of an injury causing violent torsion of the foot, followed by severe pain and swelling of the ankle and an inability to walk, suggests a fracture. The ankle must be examined with definite points in mind. Characteristic deformity indicating displacement of the foot may be visible before swelling becomes great. Lateral, medial, anterior, or posterior displacement indicates disruption of the mortise. The condition of the soft tissues, that is, swelling, ecchymosis, and bleb formation, should be noted.

Points of acute tenderness indicate points of injury. Acute tenderness over the deltoid, lateral, or tibiofibular ligaments indicates sprain or rupture of these ligaments (Fig. 26-15); over the malleoli, below or above the level of the joint, it indicates fracture. The entire fibula should be examined, as it may be fractured high in its shaft. Acute tenderness in the space anterior to the insertion of the Achilles tendon suggests posterior marginal fracture of the tibia or fracture of the posterior lip of the astragalus. Similarly, the anterior margin of the tibia is tender when fractured.

Increased mediolateral mobility should be sought by grasping the heel, not the foot, and pressing it firmly to the lateral side, to the medial side, toward eversion, and toward inversion. Increased mobility

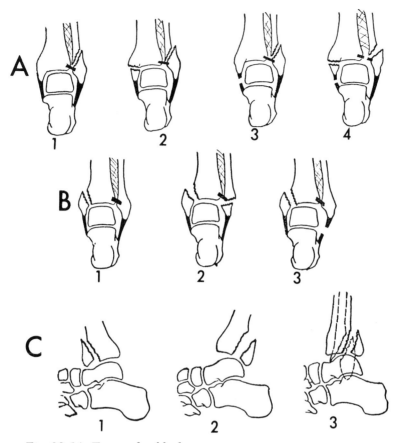

Fig. 26–14. Types of ankle fractures.

(*A*) Fractures due to eversion-external rotation: (1) simple fracture of the fibula above the ankle joint; (2) fracture of the fibula with fracture of the medial malleolus at or below the level of the ankle joint; (3) fracture similar to 2—the medial malleolus has not been fractured, but the deltoid ligament has been torn instead; (4) the most severe type of injury, fractures of both malleoli with rupture of the tibiofibular ligament and, sometimes, rupture of the deltoid ligament. (2, 3, and 4), These often are complicated by a posterior marginal fracture of the tibia as shown in *C*, 2 and 3.

(*B*) Fractures due to inversion-internal rotation: (1) simple fracture of the medial malleolus running upward from the joint; (2) similar fracture of the medial malleolus with fracture of the lateral malleolus below the level of the ankle joint; (3) fracture similar to (2)—the lateral malleolus has not been fractured, but the lateral ligament has been torn instead.

(*C*) (1) Fracture of the anterior margin of the tibial articular surface—this is caused by a forward thrust on the foot, excessive dorsiflexion, or a fall on the foot. (2 and 3) Fracture of the posterior margin of the tibial articular surface with posterior dislocation of the foot—this is caused by a backward thrust on the foot or excessive external rotation of the foot, and very often it is associated with *A*, 1 through 4.

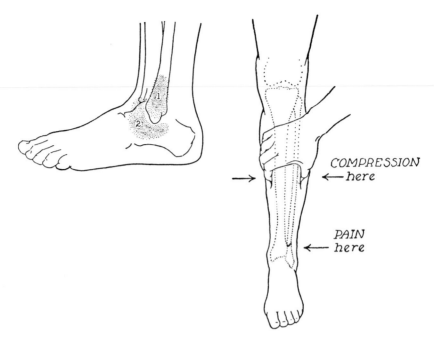

Fig. 26–15. (*Above*) The tender areas in ankle sprains and fractures. (1) The site of tenderness in fractures of the lateral malleolus; (2) the site of tenderness in sprains of the lateral ligament. (*Right*) Compression of the bones at the middle of the leg causes pain at the ankle when the lower end of the fibula is fractured.

points to disruption of the mortise. This may be checked in roentgenograms by having additional anteroposterior views made with the foot in forced eversion and forced inversion after the tender points have been anesthetized with local anesthetic solution.

The bowlike relation of the fibula to the tibia may be used to demonstrate the pain produced by movement at the fracture site. The test is performed by pressing the bones together in the middle of the leg. This causes no particular discomfort in the ankle in cases of sprain, but when the fibula is fractured, there is definite pain at the fracture site (Fig. 26-15).

The roentgen examination is extremely important. Exact anterioposterior and lateral views from the lower third of the leg to the os calcis are the minimum requirement. These may be supplemented by views made with the foot in forced eversion and inversion. The films should be examined for fracture of the malleoli and

of the articular margins of the tibia, for separation of the tibia from the fibula, and for mediolateral and anteroposterior displacement of the astragalus. Normally, the articular surface of the astragalus lies exactly beneath the articular surface of the tibia, and it is fitted accurately between the malleoli. Widening of the space between a malleolus and the astragalus indicates disruption of the mortise. When there is any doubt, the uninjured side should be examined for comparison.

TREATMENT

Preliminary Treatment of Fractures About the Ankle

When the examination has been completed, the ankle must be adequately splinted for transportation (Fig. 26-16). The foot, the ankle, and the lower third of the leg should be wrapped firmly in an elastic compression dressing to control

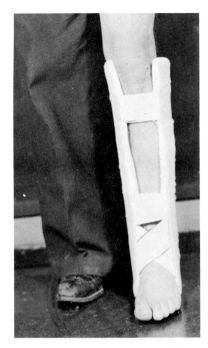

Fig. 26–16. Application of splints for preliminary treatment of ankle fracture. The pressure dressing has been omitted for clarity.

swelling. Two well-padded board splints, long enough to reach from the heel to the knee, are secured to the medial and lateral aspects of the leg with wide adhesive straps. The foot should be secured to the splints with a figure-of-eight strap, and, as a general rule, it is best to splint the injured ankle with the shoe in place. While waiting for further treatment, the leg should be elevated, and ice bags applied. An inflatable plastic splint may be used if available. Air splints should never be inflated by mechanical means, but always by lung pressure.

For further treatment, the fractures about the ankle are classified according to the severity of the injury as follows:

1. Fractures without displacement of the malleoli and without displacement of the astragalus. These include fractures of the lateral malleolus, the fibula above the tibiofibular ligaments, the medial malleolus, both malleoli, and the anterior or the posterior margin of the tibia.

2. Fractures with displacement of the malleoli and the astragalus. These include fractures due to eversion-external rotation, the astragalus being displaced laterally; fractures due to inversion, the astragalus being displaced medially; marginal fractures of the tibia, with anterior or posterior displacement of the astragalus; and fractures of the tibial articular surface, or tibiofibular separation, with upward displacement of the astragalus.

Treatment of Fractures of the Medial or Lateral Malleolus Alone (Fig. 26-17)

When in good position, and without torn ligaments, these require only support and a pressure dressing to maintain a useful extremity and to enable the patient to walk without crutches during treatment. When the fracture is slight, such as a fissure in the bone, a local anesthetic may be injected into the site of most acute tenderness. A firm adhesive strapping may be applied. An elastic adhesive bandage or a gelatin boot may be all that is required to make the patient comfortable. Additional local anesthetic injections may be necessary at intervals of 1 or 2 days. After a few days, the patient should be able to walk with little discomfort. The dressing is reapplied when it becomes loose, and, after 3 or 4 weeks, it may be replaced by an elastic ankle support.

If the fracture is comminuted, or if displacement seems likely with active function, the strapping and the pressure dressing are replaced with a boot cast as soon as the swelling subsides.

Application of the Boot Cast. As a general rule, the patient is allowed to sit with the injured leg flexed over the side of the table, and the surgeon sits on a low stool facing the patient. He may support the toes of the affected foot with his knee. Stockinet is placed over the leg from above the knee to beyond the toes. A strip of felt is placed about the proximal tibia and fibula to protect the fibular head. A thin layer of sheet wadding is wrapped about the malleoli and around the fore-

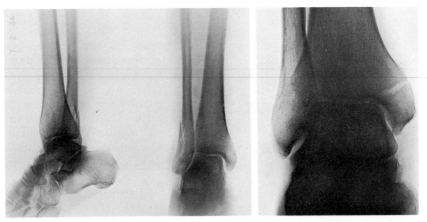

Fig. 26–17. (*Left*) Comminuted fracture of lateral malleolus caused by eversion-external rotation. (*Right*) Fracture of medial malleolus in good position.

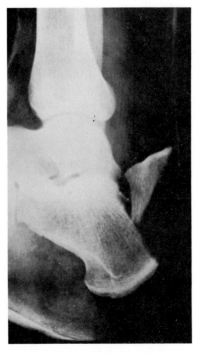

Fig. 26–18. Posterior marginal fracture of the tibia at the ankle in good position.

foot. With the knee flexed at 90° and the ankle maintained at approximately neutral position between flexion and extension, a circular plaster cast is applied and is molded well behind and below the malleoli. The cast is allowed to extend beyond the toes and, while still wet, is cut back on the dorsum to allow toe extension. The stockinet is folded back over the cast proximally and distally and is held firmly with a small additional circular plastic bandage. The cast should be molded well to maintain a satisfactory plantar arch and, for additional comfort, should also be molded slightly behind the second, third, and fourth metatarsal heads. A walking heel may be attached to the cast, and the patient may be allowed to begin to walk after the plaster is thoroughly set.

After 4 to 6 weeks the cast may be removed. Following removal of the cast, elastic support from the toes to the knees should be used until the circulation readjusts to its unprotected condition. These injuries rarely require any physiotherapy, but when they do, the patient is instructed to immerse the foot in hot water for 15 minutes and to massage it for 5 minutes twice daily at home.

Treatment of Fractures of Both Malleoli in Good Position and of Fractures of the Anterior or the Posterior Articular Margin of the Tibia in Good Position (Fig. 26-18)

These may also be treated with a boot cast applied with the foot and ankle in

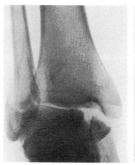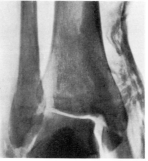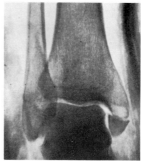

Fig. 26–19. Fractures following eversion-external rotation. (*Left*) An oblique fracture of the fibula and a fracture of the medial melleolus are seen. The astragalus has moved laterally, and the intermalleolar space has widened greatly. (*Center*) The position of the fragments has been improved, but residual displacement still can be seen in the wide space between the medial margin of the astragalus and the unbroken portion of the medial malleolus. (*Right*) Almost full correction by pressure 1 week after injury, when the swelling had subsided. An unpadded cast was applied. If the medial malleolus shows any considerable residual displacement, it may be advisable to operate for reduction and fixation.

neutral position. The cast should be left in place for 6 to 8 weeks, and follow-up care is similar to that described above.

Treatment of Fractures with Displacement of the Malleoli and/or the Astragalus

These fractures are serious injuries, since the mortise of the ankle is disrupted and/or the astragalus is moved from the weight-bearing axis. The soft tissues usually exhibit evidence of severe injury. Without extremely accurate reduction and careful after-treatment, there may be great disability. When there is any doubt concerning the ability to manage these patients on am ambulatory basis, they should be given hospital care. Closed reduction methods can fail, due to infolding of soft tissue between the fragments or due to bony irregularities. If necessary to obtain a good ankle mortise, open reduction is indicated.

The basic requirements for a good result are (1) adequate roentgen study, (2) accurate reduction, (3) adequate measures for reducing the swelling, (4) prolonged uninterrupted immobilization of the fragments until union occurs, and (5) active use of the limb during the period of immobilization whenever possible.

Treatment of Eversion-External Rotation Fractures with Displacement (Fig. 26-19) (Pott's Fracture)

The most common of these is the so-called Pott's fracture. The fibula is broken at or above the tibiofibular ligament, the medial malleolus is fractured below the level of the joint, and the astragalus is shifted laterally. Reduction is performed without delay, each fracture site being infiltrated with local anesthetic solution, and from 10 to 15 minutes being allowed to elapse before proceeding; or general anesthesia may be used if preferred. With the knee flexed and the leg hanging over the edge of the table, the surgeon grasps the medial side of the leg above the ankle with one hand, and presses strongly medially on the heel and on the lateral malleolus with the other. Internal rotation of the foot is usually also necessary. A strip of felt is fastened around the leg just below the knee to protect the peroneal nerve as it passes around the neck of the fibula. A lightly padded boot cast is applied with the ankle at 90° and firm pressure holding the foot medially. After the cast is firm, it should be extended to the upper thigh with the knee in 30° of flexion. Roentgen evaluation is then made, and if the posi-

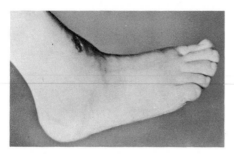

Fig. 26–20. Typical deformity after a posterior marginal fracture of the tibia with posterior dislocation of the foot. An ulceration is present over the prominent lower end of the tibia; this was due to excessive pressure from a dressing that had been applied incorrectly.

tion is not satisfactory, manipulation should be repeated. This cast should be replaced with a short leg walking-cast in 4 to 6 weeks. At any sign of circulatory difficulty, the cast should be bivalved to the skin and it should be replaced with a snug long leg cast when the initial swelling has subsided. Care must be taken to instruct the patient as to proper elevation of the foot and avoiding pressure on the heel.

The leg is kept elevated, and ice bags are applied for from 24 to 48 hours after injury. No weight bearing should be permitted early.

When the cast is removed, an elastic support should be used until the circulation adapts to the changed situation, and alternate elevation and dependency should be allowed.

Treatment of Inversion-Internal Rotation Fractures with Displacement

The medial malleolus is fractured along a line running upward from the articular surface, and the fibula is broken below the level of the ankle joint. The malleoli and the astragalus are displaced toward the medial side. When the lateral malleolus shows no fracture and the intermalleolar space is widened, rupture of the lateral and the tibiofibular ligaments must be suspected. This may be confirmed by

taking an anteroposterior roentgenogram with the foot forcibly inverted, again using a local anesthetic.

The treatment of these fractures is similar in all respects to that for the eversion-external rotation fractures, except that the reduction maneuvers are reversed. The surgeon forces the heel and the medial malleolus laterally strongly, and repeats this pressure when the plaster is applied. Persistent displacement of the medial malleolus may be due to soft-part interposition, and requires open reduction and internal fixation.

Treatment of Marginal Fractures with Anteroposterior Displacement of the Foot (Figs. 26-20 and 26-21)

Although fractures of the posterior margin of the articular surface of the tibia with posterior displacement of the foot are usually associated with fractures of the malleoli, they may occur without them. If the posterior fragment of the tibia includes less than 20 percent of the joint surface, the fracture may be treated by closed reduction; but if more of the articular surface is involved, accurate reduction is required, and open reduction is usually necessary.

Reduction is obtained with the knee flexed, by making backward pressure on the leg above the ankle and a strong forward pull on the foot, accompanied by dorsiflexion. The displacement will tend to recur very easily. Immediate roentgenograms must show complete reduction of the posterior dislocation and complete or almost complete replacement of the posterior fragment. In rare instances, there may be a fixed displacement of the fibula behind the tibia that blocks reduction and may require open reduction. Failure to maintain reduction indicates the need for hospitalization. Roentgenograms should be repeated in from 7 to 10 days so that recurrent displacement may be identified and corrected. The aftercare is similar to that for displaced malleolar fractures except that the cast remains in place for 8 weeks.

Fracture of the posterior margin of the

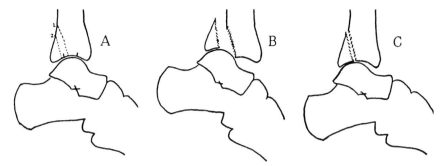

Fig. 26–21. *A*: (1) The "classical" type of posterior marginal fracture (after Nelson and Jensen); (2) the "minimal" type of fracture. *B*: Typical displacement. *C*: Incomplete reduction. The articular surface of the astragalus is not concentric with the main articular surface. Unless the foot is brought forward to its correct position, the result will be very unsatisfactory.

Fig. 26–22. The tuberosity-joint angle. (*a*) The dotted line drawn from the tuberosity to the posterior margin of the articular surface intersects the broken line from the anterior margin of the articular surface to the posterior margin. These lines make an angle of about 30°. When the os calcis is crushed, the angle is decreased or reversed, as shown in (*b*).

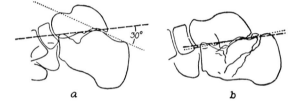

articular surface of the tibia occurs frequently in parachute jumpers. It may occur alone or associated with malleolar fractures, as described above. When it occurs alone, displacement is apt to be slight, and from 4 to 6 weeks' immobilization in a walking cast seems to be sufficient.

Fractures of the anterior margin of the articular surface of the tibia with anterior displacement of the foot require that the foot be pushed posteriorly and plantar flexed while the leg above the ankle is pulled forward. Displacement recurs readily, and this makes it necessary to use the same precautions and roentgen criteria as are used in the treatment of posterior marginal fractures. When displacement of the astragalus tends to recur, a Kirschner wire may be inserted through the heel, and traction distally and posteriorly may maintain reduction. The wire may be incorporated in a cast, and traction posteriorly and distally maintained for 10 to 14

days. The after-treatment is similar to that described above.

FRACTURES OF THE OS CALCIS

Etiology. The os calcis is fractured by falls on the feet from a height, rarely by other means. Bilateral fracture occurs frequently, and both heels must be examined when one is injured. Fractures of the lumbar spine are frequently caused by the same violence, and patients with fracture of the os calcis should always be examined for possible fracture of the spine and vice versa.

A properly functioning os calcis is ordinarily essential for painless weight bearing and walking. Violence may so compress (Fig. 26-22), widen, or shatter the bone that its articulations no longer fit, or they become roughened; its weight-bearing axis is also distorted. Many fracture patterns occur. The constant pull of

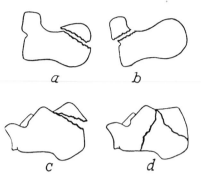

Fig. 26–23. Some varieties of fracture of the os calcis that can be treated by ambulatory methods (after Watson-Jones): (*a*) simple fracture of the posterior portion of the base; (*b*) fracture of the sustentaculum tali without displacement; (*c*) "Beak" fracture of the tuberosity; (*d*) fissure fractures without displacement.

the gastrocnemius muscle often maintains the displacement. To reduce these displacements and to maintain good position, skeletal traction and pin transfixion may be required.

Diagnosis. Pain in the heel after a fall or a jump from a height suggests fracture of the os calcis. Swelling occurs after a few hours, and ecchymosis appears later. Weight bearing on the heel causes severe pain. The bone is tender on mediolateral compression. Comparison with the uninjured side may disclose widening of the heel. Anteroposterior, as well as lateral, roentgenograms must be made.

Treatment. Only those cases of single or multiple fissure fractures without displacement (Fig. 26-23) and those of isolated fractures of a small portion of the bone are suitable for ambulatory treatment. Narrowing of the tuber-joint angle (Fig. 26-22), displacement, or depression of the joint surfaces and widening of the tuberosity require hospitalization and expert care.

The ambulatory patients receive a firm compression dressing immediately to control swelling. A thick flannel or elastic bandage is applied from the toes to the middle of the leg, or the part may be

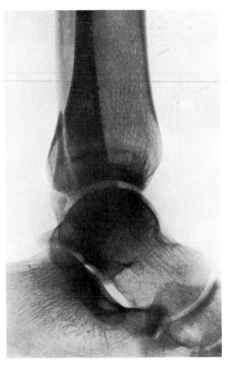

Fig. 26–24. "Beak" fracture of the os calcis.

wrapped in a heavy layer of cotton and bandaged tightly with gauze or muslin. The leg is kept elevated, and ice bags are applied for from 24 to 48 hours after injury. After from 5 to 7 days, when the swelling has subsided, a lightly padded cast from the toes to the knee and a walking heel are applied. No manipulation is required in the case of fissure fractures without displacement.

A "beak" fracture of the tuberosity (Fig. 26-24) is reduced by moderate plantar flexion of the foot and direct pressure of both thumbs above the fragment at the sides of the Achilles tendon. If the displacement cannot be corrected, operation may be required.

Medial displacement of a fragment of the sustentaculum tali or a fragment of the tuberosity may be reduced by strong pressure with the thumbs. The cast must be well molded about the heel and the ankle. The foot should be kept at a right angle to the leg, except after reduction of a "beak" fracture, in which case some plantar flexion is preferable. The cast

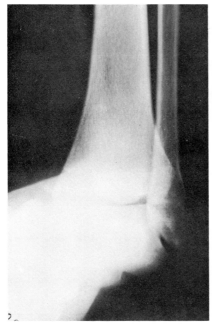 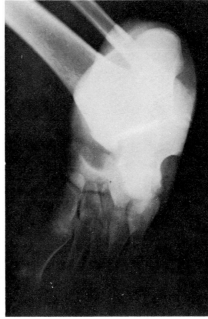

Fig. 26–25. Subastragaloid dislocation. (*Left*) Anteroposterior view of the ankle. The astragalus lies in its normal position between the malleoli, and the foot is dislocated to the medial side. (*Right*) View taken with the foot placed flat on the film. The head of the astragalus lies over the tarsal bones on the lateral side of the foot, and not in the concave facet of the scaphoid on the medial side.

should be maintained for from 6 to 8 weeks. The aftercare is similar to that for fractures about the ankle. If the plantar surface remains tender, a pad of felt or sponge rubber may be worn in the heel of the shoe.

The prognosis in the simple types of fracture is usually good. Full return of function is usually anticipated.

SUBASTRAGALOID DISLOCATIONS

Etiology. Inversion and eversion of the foot take place at the subastragaloid joint (Fig. 26-25). When the normal range of motion is exceeded suddenly, there may be a dislocation of the foot at this joint. The astragalus remains between the malleoli, while the os calcis and the scaphoid dislocate with the foot. The dislocation usually is to the medial or the lateral side, rarely forward. Fracture of the astragalus

or of the surrounding bones may also be present.

Diagnosis. There is severe pain at the ankle following a violent injury. The dislocation, lateral or forward, presents a striking deformity quite unlike that of ankle fractures. The malleoli are usually intact and painless. Roentgen study is required to exclude fractures.

Treatment. The dislocation must be reduced promptly. Under general or local anesthesia, the knee is flexed, the foot is plantar flexed, and strong traction is made on the foot, which then is pulled quickly and gently toward its normal position. A well-padded boot cast is applied and immediately bivalved. The leg is elevated, and the ankle is surrounded with ice bags for from 24 to 48 hours. When the swelling subsides, a lightly padded plaster cast and a walking heel are applied. The patient begins to walk as soon as the cast is hard and dry. The cast is removed after

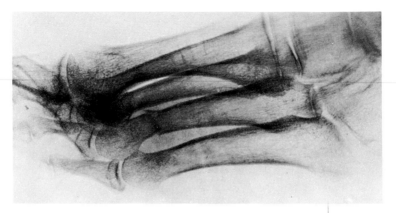

Fig. 26–26. Fracture of the neck of the fourth metatarsal without displacement.

six weeks, and the aftercare is similar to that for ankle fractures.

The prognosis is good if there are no complicating fractures of the astragalus. Failure to reduce the dislocation, associated fractures, or open wounds are indications for hospital care.

FRACTURES OF THE METATARSALS

Etiology (Fig. 26-26). These fractures often follow direct violence, such as the impact of a heavy object or being run over by a wheel. They may also be caused by indirect violence. Fracture of the base of the fifth metatarsal often follows sudden inversion of the foot. Most metatarsal fractures exhibit little or no displacement unless the violence has been very great.

Diagnosis. A history of violence followed by pain, swelling, ecchymosis, and inability to bear weight is suggestive of fracture. There is acute localized tender ess over the fracture line and increased pain when the toe is pressed proximally in the long axis of the metatarsal. Fractures with great displacement swell very rapidly. The deformity is readily palpable. The site of the fracture becomes acutely tender. In children of from 11 to 16 years of age, it is important to differentiate in the roentgenogram between a fracture and a normal epiphysis of the tuberosity at the base of the fifth metatarsal.

Treatment. When there is a fracture in good position, a felt pad is applied to the plantar surface to conform to the arch, and a firm flannel or elastic bandage or a gelatin boot is applied from the toes to the knee. Ice bags are then applied for from 24 to 48 hours, and the leg is elevated until the swelling subsides. When there are multiple fractures, a snug boot cast and a walking heel may be applied from the toes to below the knee. This should remain in place for from 4 to 8 weeks. The longitudinal arch must be molded well, and the foot must be at right angles to the leg. Walking begins when the cast is hard. An arch support is used in the aftercare, in addition to the other measures for fractures at the ankle. Many of these patients with metatarsal fractures may be treated well with nothing more than a gelatin boot or an elastic adhesive bandage. The gelatin is applied in a heavy layer from above the ankle to include the toes. Felt pads are cut to conform to the plantar arch, and they are applied over the first layer of gauze bandage. Usually, two layers of gelatin are sufficient. The patient may wear a cutout shoe, which will allow him to walk comfortably after from 7 to 10 days.

Fractures of the base of the fifth metatarsal (Fig. 26-27) may require only firm

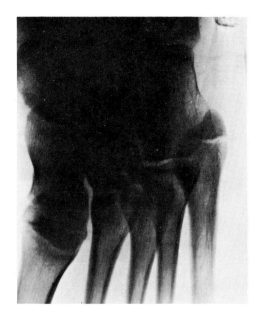

Fig. 26–27. Fracture of the tuberosity of the fifth metatarsal.

strapping with adhesive or with an elastic adhesive bandage, the foot being held in eversion while the bandage is applied. A procaine injection at the fracture site usually relieves pain and discomfort. Most of these patients walk without disability in from 6 to 8 days.

When there is considerable displacement complicating fracture of a metatarsal, it must be reduced as accurately as possible. With the patient under local or general anesthesia, assistants make traction on the toe and countertraction on the foot and leg above the ankle. The toe or the toes may be wrapped in adhesive to obtain a better grip. The surgeon presses on the fragments to restore normal position. In the presence of great swelling, reduction may be deferred for a few days while the part is elevated. Oblique and unstable fractures require continuous skeletal traction, as is required for similar fractures of the metacarpals.

Since the first metatarsal bears a large share of the weight of the body, it is particularly important to correct any angulation of its fragments. Some slight displacement of the other metatarsals is not of such importance.

Prognosis. When there is no displacement, the prognosis is excellent. When there is great displacement, the prognosis depends on accurate reduction and adequate aftercare. There may be prolonged discomfort in the foot when angulation remains, particularly when the angle is open toward the dorsum of the foot.

FRACTURES OF THE SESAMOID BONES OF THE FOOT

There usually are two sesamoid bones in the flexor tendons beneath the head of the first metatarsal. In rare instances, a congenitally divided, "bipartite," sesamoid bone may be found; this should not be mistaken for a fracture. After a fall on the feet, the fracture of a sesamoid bone may be identified by acute tenderness on the plantar surface just to the medial side or to the lateral margin of the head of the first metatarsal. Treatment is identical with that for fracture of a metatarsal.

MARCH FRACTURES OF THE METATARSALS

Fractures of the second, the third, and the fourth metatarsals may occur without a single acute trauma; but a history of unusual exertion or of a long walk may be elicited on pointed questioning. In soldiers, symptoms sometimes begin during a long march. The etiologic background appears to be a functional overload on a poorly conditioned foot.

Diagnosis. The first symptom is usually a crampy ache or a burning pain in the forepart of the foot. It may be felt only on weight bearing, or it may be constant. Swelling is present over the dorsum of the foot in mild cases, and also on the plantar aspect in the severe ones. There is acute tenderness at the site of the fracture. There may be a history of onset during or after a prolonged or a forced march. Roentgenograms may not show the crack in the bone in the first few days, or until some decalcification takes place. After 3 weeks, periosteal proliferation may be visible. This may be confused with syphilitic periostitis or bone tumor, but careful inspection of the films will show the fine fissure in the bone.

Treatment. An elastic bandage, rest, elevation of the foot, and avoidance of weight bearing are advisable until the acute symptoms subside. Following this, in very mild cases, a gelatin boot and an arch support may be used, with a pad beneath the head of the first metatarsal if it is shorter than the second, or if the medial side of the foot flattens excessively on standing. For the more severe cases, the application of a snug boot cast from the toes to the knee for from 4 to 6 weeks or longer is the method of choice. An elastic compression dressing should be used after removal of the cast. When necessary, a pad is used as described previously, or a well-fitted arch support may be worn.

FRACTURES OF THE TOES

Fractures of the toes result from the impact of a falling object or from stubbing the toe. The great toe is involved most often by crush injuries. Displacement is seldom great. When present, it is seen in fractures of the proximal phalanges, and is similar to the displacement seen in the phalanges of the fingers. There is a history of a characteristic injury followed by pain, swelling, and tenderness of the toe involved. The toe may be abnormally mobile, and crepitus may be felt.

Treatment. Unless there is considerable displacement which is likely to lead to deformity, no reduction is required. When the phalanges of the great toe are involved, a medial plaster splint may be molded about the toe, a small soft pad applied between the great toe and the second toe, and the forefoot bandaged with elastic adhesive. When the second to the fifth toes are involved, these may be best treated by placing a small soft padding between the injured toe and the adjacent toe and bandaging the two toes together, using small strips of elastic adhesive bandage. Care must be taken when using regular adhesive to avoid abnormal pressure, and the rest of the foot may be protected with an elastic bandage. The uninjured toe can be used very successfully as a mold or a splint. Local anesthetic injections sometimes relieve pain and disability. A shoe may be worn; a larger shoe, or a slit in the shoe may be necessary to avoid pain due to pressure. An excellent dressing is the type of sandal that has a strap between the great toe and the other toes.

Displacements of the distal or middle phalanges are reduced easily by traction and pressure or molding, and the position is maintained by a dressing similar to that mentioned above. Fractures of the proximal phalanges sometimes prove to be troublesome, but they rarely need dressings other than the simple ones described above.

Support should be continued until there is no tenderness or pain. A firm-soled shoe should always be prescribed, and if one is not available, an additional sole can easily be applied to a shoe that fits over the dressing. In the case of simple fractures, only the adhesive dressing may be needed for two weeks, and the patient may wear his regular shoe if there is sufficient room for his foot.

BIBLIOGRAPHY

Fractures of the Ankle

Ahstrom, J. P., Jr.: Epiphyseal injuries of the lower extremity. Surg. Clin. N. Am., *45*:119, 1965.

Bosworth, D. M.: Fracture dislocation of the ankle with fixed displacement of the fibula behind the tibia. J. Bone Joint Surg., *29*:130, 1947.

Cave, E. F.: Treatment of ankle injuries. GP, *15*:85, 1957.

Glick, B. W.: The ankle fracture with inferior tibiofibular joint disruption. Surg., Gynec. Obstet., *118*:549, 1964.

Lauge-Hansen, M.: Fractures of the ankle. Arch. Surg., *67*:813, 1953.

Nelson, M. C., and Jensen, N. K.: The treatment of trimalleolar fractures of the ankle. Surg., Gynec. Obstet., *71*:509, 1940.

Quigley, T. B.: Management of the ankle injuries sustained in sports. JAMA, 169: 1431, 1959.

————: A simple aid to the reduction of abduction-external rotation fractures of the ankle. Am. J. Surg., *97*:488, 1959.

Scuderi, C., and Schrey, E. L.: Posterior lipping fractures of the tibia involving the ankle mortice. Illinois Med. J., *97*:310, 1950.

Vahvanen, U., and Rokkanen, P.: Arthrodesis of the ankle; a follow-up study on 28 patients. Ann. Chir. Gynaec. Fenn., *61*:37, 1972.

March Fractures

Wang, C. C., Lowere, C. W., and Severance, R. L.: Fatigue fracture of the pelvis and the lower extremity. New Eng. J. Med., *260*:958, 1959.

Fractures of the Foot

Bennett, R. J.: Fractures of the metatarsals and tarsals. Indust. Med. Surg., *20*:423, 1951.

Carey, E. J., Lance, E. M., and Wade, P. A.: Extra-articular fractures of the os calcis. J. Trauma, *5*:362, 1965.

Eichenholtz, S. N.: Management of avulsion fractures at the base of the fifth metatarsal bone. JAMA, *184*:236, 1963.

Fahey, J. J., and Murphy, J. L.: Dislocations and fractures of the talus. Surg. Clin. N. Am., *45*:79, 1965.

Hawkins, L. G.: Fracture of the lateral process of the talus. J. Bone Joint Surg., *47A*:1170, 1965.

Lindsay, W. R. N., and Dewar, F. P.: Fractures of the os calcis. Am. J. Surg., *95*:555, 1958.

Rowe, C. R., Sakellarides, H. T., Freeman, P. A., and Sorbie, C.: Fractures of the os calcis—a long-term follow-up study of 146 patients. JAMA, *184*:920, 1963.

Sarrick, C. K., and Bremmer, A. E.: Fractures of the calcaneum. J. Bone Joint Surg., *35B*:33, 1953.

Index